AF413050

IMMUNOGENICITY

FRONTIERS OF BIOLOGY

VOLUME 25

Under the General Editorship of
A. NEUBERGER
London
and
E. L. TATUM
New York

Consultant for Immunology
E. J. HOLBOROW
Taplow

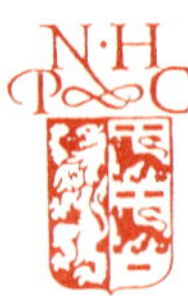

NORTH-HOLLAND PUBLISHING COMPANY – AMSTERDAM · LONDON

IMMUNOGENICITY

Edited by

FELIX BOREK

Albert Einstein College of Medicine, Yeshiva University, Bronx, N.Y.

1972

NORTH-HOLLAND PUBLISHING COMPANY – AMSTERDAM · LONDON
AMERICAN ELSEVIER PUBLISHING CO., INC. – NEW YORK

Library of Congress Catalog Card Number: 78–157040
ISBN North-Holland : 0 7204 7125 7
ISBN American Elsevier: 0 444 10104 7

25 illustrations and graphs, 30 tables

PUBLISHERS:

NORTH-HOLLAND PUBLISHING COMPANY – AMSTERDAM
NORTH-HOLLAND PUBLISHING COMPANY, LTD. – LONDON

SOLE DISTRIBUTORS FOR THE U.S.A. AND CANADA:
AMERICAN ELSEVIER PUBLISHING COMPANY, INC.
52 VANDERBILT AVENUE, NEW YORK, N.Y. 10017

PRINTED IN THE NETHERLANDS

There was a king reigned in the East:
There, when kings will sit to feast,
They get their fill before they think
With poisoned meat and poisoned drink.
He gathered all that springs to birth
From the many-venomed earth;
First a little, thence to more,
He sampled all her killing store;
and easy, smiling, seasoned sound,
Sate the king when healths went round.
They put arsenic in his meat
And stared aghast to watch him eat;
They poured strychnine in his cup
And shook to see him drink it up.
They shook, they stared as white's their shirt;
Them it was their poison hurt.
– I tell the tale that I heard told.
Mithridates, he died old.

From 'A Shropshire Lad' by A. E. Housman

General preface

The aim of the publication of this series of monographs, known under the collective title of '*Frontiers of Biology*', is to present coherent and up-to-date views of the fundamental concepts which dominate modern biology.

Biology in its widest sense has made very great advances during the past decade, and the rate of progress has been steadily accelerating. Undoubtedly important factors in this acceleration have been the effective use by biologists of new techniques, including electron microscopy, isotopic labels, and a great variety of physical and chemical techniques, especially those with varying degrees of automation. In addition, scientists with partly physical or chemical backgrounds have become interested in the great variety of problems presented by living organisms. Most significant, however, increasing interest in and understanding of the biology of the cell, especially in regard to the molecular events involved in genetic phenomena and in metabolism and its control, have led to the recognition of patterns common to all forms of life from bacteria to man. These factors and unifying concepts have led to a situation in which the sharp boundaries between the various classical biological disciplines are rapidly disappearing.

Thus, while scientists are becoming increasingly specialized in their techniques, to an increasing extent they need an intellectual and conceptual approach on a wide and non-specialized basis. It is with these considerations and needs in mind that this series of monographs, '*Frontiers of Biology*' has been conceived.

The advances in various areas of biology, including microbiology, biochemistry, genetics, cytology, and cell structure and function in general will be presented by authors who have themselves contributed significantly to these developments. They will have, in this series, the opportunity of bringing together, from diverse sources, theories and experimental data, and of integrating these into a more general conceptual framework. It is unavoidable, and probably even desirable, that the special bias of the individual authors will become evident in their contributions. Scope will also be given for presentation of new and challenging ideas and hypotheses for which complete evidence is at present lacking. However, the main emphasis will be on fairly complete and objective presentation of the more important and more rapidly advancing aspects of biology. The level will be advanced, directed primarily to the needs of the graduate student and research worker.

Most monographs in this series will be in the range of 200–300 pages, but on occasion a collective work of major importance may be included exceeding this figure. The intent of the publishers is to bring out these books promptly and in fairly quick succession.

It is on the basis of all these various considerations that we welcome the opportunity of supporting the publication of the series '*Frontiers of Biology*' by North-Holland Publishing Company.

E. L. TATUM
A. NEUBERGER, *General Editors*

Editor's preface

The objective of this book is to present a comprehensive and up-to-date review of various aspects of the question why a particular host responds immunologically to a certain antigen and what are the factors influencing the type, intensity and duration of the response. Each of these aspects is discussed in separate chapters contributed by a number of investigators reputed for their knowledge of different facets of immunology and of related disciplines. Thus the problems of immunogenicity are elucidated from various viewpoints. The contributors have been provided with an opportunity to express their opinions on the subject matter, in the hope of achieving a stimulating and occasionally controversial presentation, especially of the topics still under investigation.

The book is divided into two major parts, one devoted to the function of antigen and the other to the function of the host. This has been done in view of the increasing importance ascribed nowadays to the role of host in immune response. The heterogeneity of the immune response and the cellular aspect of the latter have been accorded their due recognition, consistent with the contemporary trends in the field. Immunological tolerance in considered throughout the book as an important phenomenon, side by side with immunity.

Attempts have been made during the planning and editing of the book to make it accessible to a fairly wide circle of interested readers. At the same time, thanks to the contributing authors, a high standard of presentation of the subject matter has been maintained with the aim of providing researchers in the field with new and useful information and with concepts likely to assist them in their work. Nevertheless this book makes no claim to being a complete encyclopaedia of modern immunology. Indeed there may be a need for such a book, but it still remains to be written.

A collective volume of this kind is always a product of the efforts of numerous individuals. I would like to thank all the contributing authors for their excellent work and co-operation in making the realization of the book possible by providing it with most valuable contents. I wish to express my gratitude to Dr. E. J. Holborow for having suggested the original idea of preparing this book; his helpful advice offered later is also greatly appreciated. Thanks are due Sir Macfarlane Burnet, Prof. P. G. H. Gell and Dr. David A. Long, for their generous help in various stages of the work on the book. I must also thank my wife, Dr. Carmia Borek, for her useful suggestions during editing the book. Messrs. H. L. Woudhuysen and A. T. G. van der Leij of the North-Holland Publishing Company have been most helpful in dealing with the technical matters connected with planning and editing this volume.

On completing my task as the editor, I express the hope that the prospective readers will derive enjoyment from this book and will profit from the information contained therein.

F ELIX B OREK

List of contributors

ALLISON, ANTHONY C., Clinical Research Centre Laboratories, National Institute for Medical Research, Mill Hill, London, England.

BALIS, M. EARL, Sloan-Kettering Institute for Cancer Research, Walker Laboratory, Rye, New York, N.Y., U.S.A.

BATCHELOR, J. R., McIndoe Memorial Research Unit, Queen Victoria Hospital, East Grinstead, Sussex, England.

BATTISTO, JACK R., Department of Microbiology and Immunology, Albert Einstein College of Medicine, Bronx, N.Y., U.S.A.

BOREK, FELIX, Department of Microbiology and Immunology, Albert Einstein College of Medicine, Bronx, N.Y., U.S.A.

BRENT, LESLIE, Department of Immunology, St. Mary's Hospital Medical School, London, England.

BURNET, SIR MACFARLANE, School of Microbiology, University of Melbourne, Parkville, Victoria, Australia.

BURNS, W. H., Department of Medicine, Stanford University Medical School, Stanford, Calif., U.S.A.

FELDMAN, MICHAEL, Department of Cell Biology, The Weizmann Institute of Science, Rehovoth, Israel.

FRANKS, DAVID, Department of Pathology, University of Cambridge, Cambridge, England.

GELL, PHILIP, G. H., Department of Experimental Pathology, The Medical School, University of Birmingham, Birmingham, England.

GILL, THOMAS J., III, Department of Pathology, University of Pittsburgh, School of Medicine, Pittsburgh, Pa., U.S.A.

GLOBERSON, AMIELA, Department of Cell Biology, The Weizmann Institute of Science, Rehovoth, Israel.

GOLDSTEIN, ALLEN, L., Department of Biochemistry, Albert Einstein Einstein College of Medicine, Bronx, N.Y., U.S.A.

LESKOWITZ, SIDNEY, Department of Pathology, Tufts Medical School, Boston, Mass., U.S.A.

LILLY, FRANK, Department of Genetics, Albert Einstein College of Medicine, Bronx, N.Y., U.S.A.

MITCHISON, N. AVRION, National Institute for Medical Research, Mill Hill, London, England.

SALVIN, SAMUEL, B., Department of Microbiology, School of Medicine, University of Pittsburgh, Pittsburgh, Pa., U.S.A.

STARK, J. MARSHALL, Department of Bacteriology and Immunology, University of Glasgow, Glasgow, Scotland.

WARNER, NOEL, L., Laboratory of Immunogenetics, The Walter and Eliza Hall Institute of Medical Research, Melbourne, Australia.

WEIR, DONALD, M., Department of Bacteriology, University of Edinburgh, Medical School, Edinburgh, Scotland.

WHITE, ABRAHAM, Department of Biochemistry, Albert Einstein College of Medicine, Bronx, N.Y., U S.A.

WHITE, ROBERT, G., Department of Bacteriology and Immunology, University of Glasgow, Glasgow, Scotland.

Introductory remarks

F. M. BURNET

School of Microbiology, Parkville, Victoria, Australia

One of the virtues of the modern approach to immunity is that it allows one to give a rather more precise meaning to the work 'immunogenicity' and to ask more meaningful questions about that quality. In the first place 'immunogenicity' must always be considered in relation to the individual host animal being immunized as well as in relation to the substance being used as antigen. A substance is immunogenic in relation to an individual host when its appropriate administration provokes a demonstrable and specific immunological effect, either production of antibody or changed cellular reactivity. At the cellular level this can be restated as follows. An immunogenic substance is one bearing antigenic determinants which are capable of reacting with 'antibody-like' receptors on certain immunocytes or antigen-reactive cells (ARC) and inducing them to proliferate to clones large enough to allow demonstrable effects – an increase in antibody, development of skin sensitivity or capacity for accelerated rejection of homograft tissue. Based largely on the work of Gowans, it is clear that most immunocytes present the morphological character of small lymphocytes. The indications are that specific stimulation can under certain conditions convert a small lympho-cyte to a blast form and that some blasts can give rise to a descendant clone of plasmacytes, some to a standard lymphocytic progeny. There is also evidence that many blast cells proliferating in relation to antigenic stimulation die with morphological necrosis in the immediate post-mitotic phase.

In dealing with immunogenicity we are concerned at one remove with most of the basic problems of immunology: the nature of immune receptors on ARC and their structural relation to the immunoglobulins: the processes by which diversity of immune pattern is generated at the genetic level and the significance of the genetic differences recogniz-able when synthetic antigens are tested for immunogenicity in pure line strains: the nature of tolerance and other forms of immunological nonresponsiveness. Limiting ourselves more specifically to immuno-genicity as a definable area of study it may be useful to mention the main fields of current study from which definitive answers are still to be obtained:

(1) Accepting as a fact that all antigen-reactive cells (immunocytes) carry specific (antibody-like) receptors and that all in the unstimulated condition have small lymphocyte morphology,

(a) Is each immunocyte before stimulation pre-programmed to produce only one Ig type of antibody (or to proliferate to T*-immunocytes concerned with cellular immunity)?

(b) What determines whether specific contact results in activation and proliferation or damage and death?

(2) Accepting that the phenomena of tolerance, paralysis and immunological unresponsiveness depend essentially on the absence of adequate numbers of immunocytes of the appropriate specificity, what are the circumstances giving rise to various degrees of partial tolerance?

(3) There are many instances where it is known that a chemical configuration capable of acting as an antigenic determinant when related to an appropriate 'carrier', is not immunogenic when in small molecular form or with an inappropriate carrier. This is closely related to the question of co-operation between B-** and T-immunocytes in antibody production. One senses that valid generalization here may require more extensive study in animals other than in the mouse.

(4) Where the antigen or antigenic determinant forms part of the surface of a living vertebrate cell, as in relation to homograft and tumour immunity, conditions become extremely complex. Since there is evidence that on the surface of dendritic phagocytic cells of lymph follicles a variety of antigens are held available to act as selectors of appropriate immunocytes, and that delayed hypersensitivity is also induced by antigenic determinants on the surface of mobile cells, questions of interaction between different cells of the host become important in most aspects of immunogenicity.

(5) Finally there is an almost untouched field in the study of the antigen-immunocyte interaction as a pharmacological phenomenon. The new approach to regarding cyclic-AMP as the 'second messenger' in many types of cell simtulations by hormones and drugs must have important immunological implications.

Most of these points are elaborated or at least touched on at various places in this volume but all remain open for further work. It is challenging, and in a sense cheering, that in cellular immunology we are confronted with a highly complex tangle to unravel. Most of the necessary experimental approaches are available but obviously long continued and detailed work on a wide range of species and antigens is still needed.

---

* Thymus-dependent.

** *Directly* derived from bone-marrow precursors.

Contents

Part I. Function of antigen

A. Soluble antigens

B. Particulate antigens

Part II. Function of host

Chapter 10.   *The inductive phase of antibody production, by M. Feldman and A. Globerson* *273*

Chapter 11.   *Hereditary aspects of the capacity to respond immunologically, by J. R. Battisto and F. Lilly* *302*

Chapter 12. *Hormonal regulation of host immunity, by A. White and A. L. Goldstein* *334*

Chapter 13. *Effects of antimetabolites and other pharmacological agents, by M. E. Balis* *365*

PART I

Functions of antigen

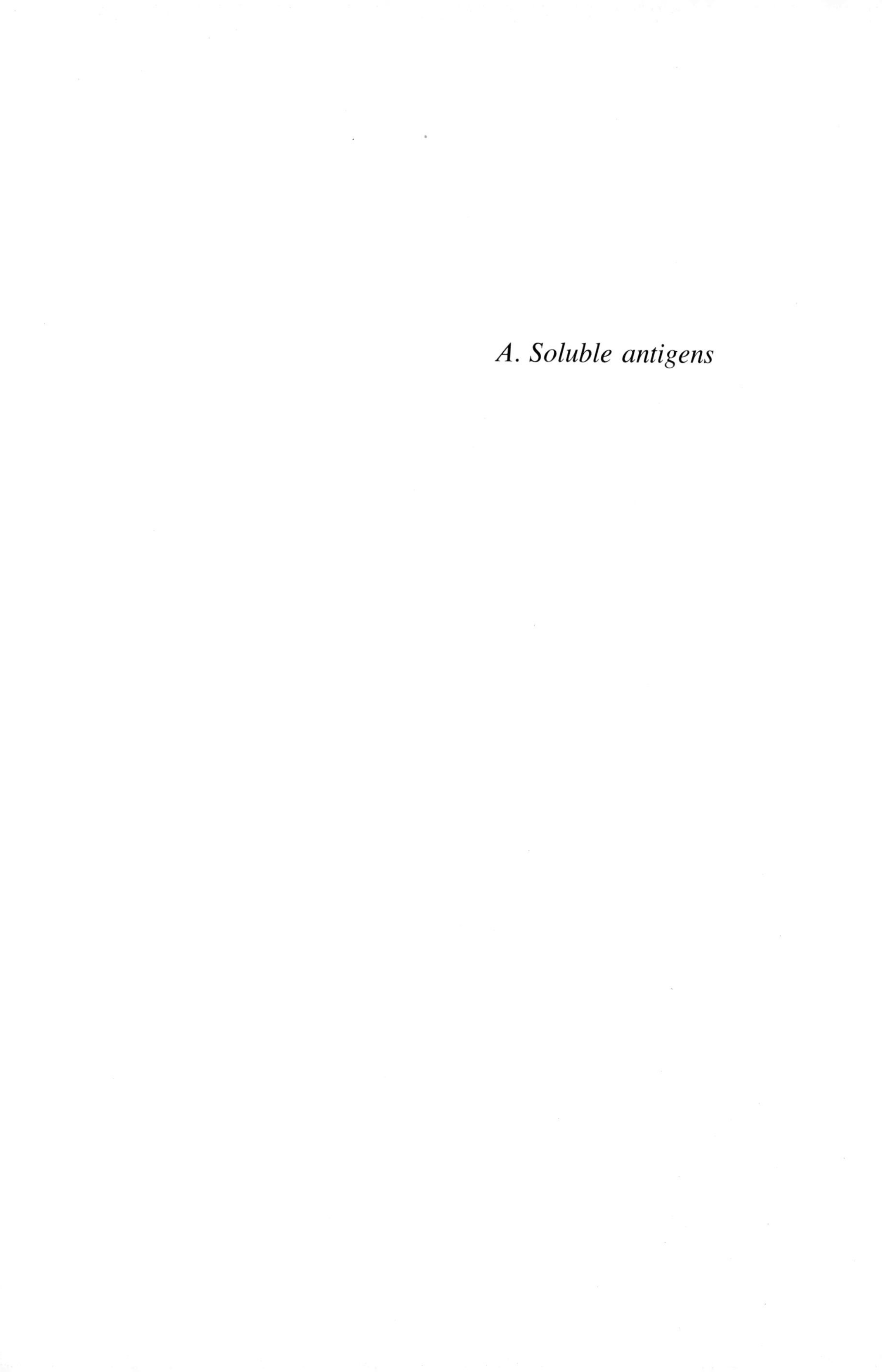

A. Soluble antigens

CHAPTER 1

The chemistry of antigens and its influence on immunogenicity

THOMAS J. GILL, III

Department of Pathology, University of Pittsburgh, School of Medicine, Pittsburgh, Pa.

1.1. Introduction

The ability of an animal to mount an immune response depends upon the interplay between the chemistry of the antigen and the physiological state of the host. The way in which the antigen is presented and the use of adjuvants greatly affect its action. The host's ability to respond can be altered by nutritional imbalances, disruption of the normal hormonal balances, administration of drugs or exposure to radiation. This chapter will focus on the role that the chemistry of the antigen plays in the induction of the immune response in the normal host. The major thesis proposes that there is a quantitative balance between the stimulation of an immune response and the induction of tolerance following the introduction of the antigen. This balance varies for each antigen, and the chemistry of the antigen is the crucial factor in determining its immunological activity. The effective amount of antigen depends upon the dose and method of administration and upon the degradation of the antigen *in vivo*. The major role of antigen metabolism is postulated to lie in the regulation of the amount of antigen left intact and capable of stimulating an immune response.

In discussing immunological phenomena, the term antigenicity will be used to encompass all of the immune capabilities of a molecule. The various manifestations of immunity can be classified as: (a) immunogenicity, which is the ability to elicit an antibody response; (b) reactivity with antibody, which is a function of the antigenic determinants on the macromolecule; (c) the induction of tolerance (paralysis); and (d) the induction of delayed hypersensitivity. These four properties can be operationally separated in some cases, and there is a growing body of evidence that each may be a function of a different portion of the antigen molecule. In studies of immunogenicity and the induction of tolerance, the major assay methods are those for detecting antibody, whereas for delayed hypersensitivity various manifestations of cellular immunity, such as skin reactivity or stimulation of cells *in vitro*, are used. A variety of techniques for detecting the antibody-antigen reaction have been summarized by Borek (1968a) and by Gill (1970). The maintenance of the antibody-antigen union depends upon the interplay of steric specificity and relatively weak binding forces which generate free energies in the range of -5 to -15 kcal/mole. The major contributions to the binding energy come from van der Waal's (dispersion) forces (-1 kcal/mole), hydrogen bonds (-1 kcal/mole), hydrophobic interactions (-3 to -4 kcal/mole) and electrostatic interactions (-1 to -4 kcal/mole).

1.2. Proteins

The chemical basis for the immunogenicity of proteins was amongst the earliest problems to be studied in immunology, and the results have been summarized in reviews by Marrack (1938) and by Landsteiner (1945). Some of the general chemical features which influenced the antibody response were delineated, but the chemical complexity of proteins made detailed studies impossible. One of the chemical requirements for immunogenicity was thought to be the presence of tyrosine; for example, the studies of Obermeyer and Pick indicated that gelatin was not immunogenic, but adding tyrosine made it so. There were, however, contradictory results: combination with phenylisocyanate did not convert gelatin into an immunogen, and insulin, which contains 12% tyrosine, and tyrosine-containing proteins which were degraded by alkali were poorly immunogenic or not immunogenic under the conditions used. In addition, chemical destruction of tyrosine residues decreased the immunogenicity of proteins in some cases, but not in others. Studies with many proteins differing in charge, shape, size and other chemical properties outlined some of the general molecular characteristics which affected immunogenicity, and a summary of these properties is given in Table 1.1. Because of the difficulties in manipulating discrete aspects of protein structure, most immunological studies were focused on determining the antigenic specificities of native and chemically modified macromolecules and of various haptenic groups on these molecules. In the few instances in which the effects of chemical modification on immunogenicity were explored, for example, deamination of ovalbumin (Maurer and Heidelberger 1951) and oxidation of the disulphide groups in ribonuclease (Brown et al. 1967), the chemically induced changes were so great that the overall structure of the molecule was drastically changed.

One of the major approaches to investigating the immunogenicity of

TABLE 1.1

General molecular characteristics affecting the immunogenicity of proteins*[a]

Property	Effect on immunogenicity	Experimental basis
(1) Presence of tyrosine	variable	chemical modifications of proteins and responses to different proteins.
(2) High charge	−	protamines, histones.
(3) Shape	0	globular and fibrous proteins are immunogenic.
(4) Size		
(a) small	−	insulin, ribonuclease
(b) large	+	haemocyanin
(5) Racemization	−	ovalbumin
(6) Easily degradable	−	gelatin
(7) Denaturation	−	albumin, ribonuclease[b]
(8) Chemical or enzymatic cleavage	−	albumin
(9) Species specificity	variable	ovalbumins

* The symbols are: −, decreased immunogenicity; +, increased immunogenicity; and 0, no effect.

[a] Marrack (1938) and Landsteiner (1945).   [b] Brown et al. (1967).

proteins involved the attachment of various chemical groups to poorly immunogenic molecules in an attempt to improve their ability to elicit antibody formation. The results of such studies using gelatin are summarized in Table 1.2. The attachment of various sugar residues by themselves did not alter the immunogenicity of gelatin, but when tyrosine was included, the ability of gelatin to elicit an antibody response was enhanced. Aromatic compounds generally enhanced immunogenicity with the exception of phenylisocyanate and benzoic acid. In addition, some non-aromatic peptides, such as leucine-glutamic acid and lysine-glutamic acid, were also effective. When only a small number of tyrosine residues was attached to gelatin, the antibody was directed toward the gelatin and not the tyrosine (Arnon and Sela 1960). However, if more than 2% of tyrosine residues was attached, the specificity of the antibody was progressively directed at the tyrosine; the attachment of tyrosine-glutamic acid greatly enhanced the immunogenicity of gelatin and provided a very strong determinant group. Since the attachment of leucine-glutamic acid, lysine-glutamic acid or cysteine also enhanced the immunogenicity of gelatin, the role of tyrosine in this regard was not exclusive. Thus, the study of poly-α-amino acids as immunogens was undertaken to provide a completely synthetic approach to exploring the

TABLE 1.2

The changes in the immunogenicity of gelatin caused by coupling with various haptens and peptides.*

Attached group	Effect on immunogenicity	Reference
0-β-glucosido-tyrosine	+	Clutton et al. (1938); Humphrey and Yuill (1939)
arabinose	0	Micheel and Schallenberg (1952)
arabinose-tyrosine	+	ibid.
cellulose-glycol	0	ibid.
cellulose-glycol-tyrosine	+	ibid.
pectin	0	ibid.
pectin-tyrosine	+	ibid.
aromatic diazonium compounds	+	Osborne et al. (1905)
azo-atoxyl	+	Adant (1930); Hooker and Boyd (1933)
phenylisocyanate	0	Hopkins and Wormall (1933)
benzoylation	0	Medveczky and Uhrovitz (1931)
tryptophan	+	Sela and Arnon (1960a)
L-tyrosine or D-tyrosine	+	Sela and Katchalski (1956); Sela and Haurowitz (1958); Sela and Arnon (1960a); Sela and Fuchs (1964)
tyrosine-glutamic acid	+	Arnon and Sela (1960b)
phenylalanine	+	Sela and Arnon (1960a)
cyclohexylalanine	+	Sela and Arnon (1960b)
methionine	+	Fuchs and Sela (1964)
leucine-glutamic acid	+	ibid.
lysine-glutamic acid	+	ibid.
cysteine	±	Sela and Arnon (1960a)
lysine	0	ibid.

TABLE 1.2 (continued)

Attached group	Effect on immunogenicity	Reference
glutamic acid	0	Sela and Arnon (1960a)
alanine	0	ibid.
serine	0	Sela and Arnon (1960b)

* The symbols are: +, increased immunogenicity; ±, slightly increased; and 0, no effect.

role that the chemistry of a macromolecule played in its ability to elicit an immune response.

1.3. Synthetic polypeptide antigens

1.3.1. Initial studies

The use of completely synthetic molecules for studying the chemical basis of immunogenicity and serological reactivity goes back to the work of Ivanovics, Bruckner and their collaborators (Ivanovics and Bruckner 1937; Bruckner and Kovacs 1957; Bruckner et al. 1958) who studied the anthrax bacillus and the poly-γ-D-glutamic acid which made up its capsule. They showed that immunization of rabbits with the intact anthrax bacillus elicited antibodies which were specific for poly-γ-D-glutamic acid, but that poly-γ-D-glutamic acid itself was not capable of eliciting an antibody response. The antibody was highly specific for the γ-D isomer of polyglutamic acid, since it showed only slight reactivity with the meso-form and no reactivity with the L-form. More recently, the immunochemistry of poly-γ-D-glutamic acid has been studied by Goodman and Nitecki (1966) and by Goodman (1969). They prepared antisera by immunizing rabbits with the intact organism but could not elicit an immune response with the polypeptide itself. The antibody was specific for the poly-γ-D-glutamic acid, and they explored its serological specificity in detail.

Several early attempts to detect immunogenic behaviour following the injection of synthetic polypeptides either failed or produced a low and erratic antibody response (Stahmann et al. 1955; Maurer 1957a). Following these attempts with polypeptides alone, Stahmann and his collaborators (Stahmann et al. 1959; Buchanan-Davidson et al. 1959a, b, c) turned to the use of polypeptidyl proteins to study the antigenic function of synthetic polypeptides. They found that the antibody response was directed in large measure toward the polypeptide sidechains, as Landsteiner (1945) had found earlier when he attached short peptides to protein carriers. They also found that the antisera to synthetic polypeptides alone would occasionally yield small precipitates with the polypeptidyl proteins. Sela and Katchalski (1956) and Sela and Haurowitz (1958) found that polytyrosine coupled to gelatin would induce the formation of antibodies detectable by anaphylactic shock in sensitized guinea pigs. Further studies showed that polypeptidyl gelatins induced the formation of precipitating antibodies with a fairly sharp antigenic specificity in rabbits (Table 1.2). At the same time, reinvestigation of the immunogenicity of polypeptides by Maurer et al. (1959) did reveal an occasional antibody response to a copolymer of glutamic acid and lysine; however, it could only be detected by the extremely sensitive passive cutaneous anaphylaxis test. Following these earlier studies, an unequivocal antibody response to synthetic polypeptide antigens in rabbits was shown by several groups: (a) Gill and Doty (1960) who used a linear polypeptide containing glutamic acid, lysine and tyrosine; (b) Sela and Arnon (1960c) who used a branched (multichain) polymer with tyrosine-glutamic acid sidechains; and (c) Maurer (1962) who used a linear polypeptide containing glutamic acid and lysine. Thus, a completely synthetic molecule could elicit an antibody response, and the systematic exploration of the various chemical features that affected immunogenicity would be possible (reviewed by Maurer 1964; Sela 1966, 1969).

1.3.2. Composition

The presence of tyrosine was not needed in order for a polypeptide to induce an antibody response (Gill and Doty 1961; Maurer 1962). For example, a polypeptide composed of glutamic acid and lysine, which was highly flexible (Omenn and Gill 1967), could elicit a moderately good antibody response. In general, however, aromatic amino acids consistently enhanced the amount of antibody formed (Gill and Doty 1961; Sela et al. 1962; Fuchs and Sela 1963; Gill et al. 1967). Tyrosine and phenylalanine were equally effective in enhancing immunogenicity, and there was no clear correlation between the amount of tyrosine or phenylalanine in the polypeptide and the amount of antibody formed. This ability to enhance antibody formation was consistent, but not exclusive, since copolymers of glutamic acid, lysine and alanine could elicit amounts of antibody comparable to those elicited by the tyrosine-containing polypeptides (Maurer et al. 1963a; Gill et al. 1967). In addition, poly $Glu^{63}Ala^{28}Tyr^9$ elicited more antibody than any of the (glutamic acid, lysine, tyrosine) or (glutamic acid, lysine, alanine) polymers (Gill et al. 1967).

1.3.3. Charge

The effects of charge on immunogenicity were examined with a series of (glutamic acid, lysine) and (glutamic acid, lysine, tyrosine) polymers in which the amounts of glutamic acid and lysine were systematically varied; the same schedule of immunization and bleeding was used for each polymer (Gill et al. 1967). The polypeptides containing tyrosine elicited more antibody than their counterparts containing only glutamic acid and lysine. The best immunogens fell in the range $+75\%$ to -75% net charge density, and within this range there was no effect of charge on the amount of antibody formed. This finding was the same in both classes of polypeptides, although the level of antibody formation was uniformly higher with the tyrosine-containing polypeptides. Using this immunization schedule, completely charged homopolymers (poly Lys and poly Glu) and a succinylated copolymer (poly $Glu^{59}LysS^{41}$) did not evoke an antibody response; using a different schedule, as discussed below, they did induce a weak antibody response. Highly charged polymers (e.g., poly $Lys^{96}Tyr^4$) elicited only small amounts of antibody whether or not they contained tyrosine. Polypeptides in which the net charge was zero elicited amounts of antibody comparable to those induced by polypeptides with a net charge between -75% and $+75\%$, and polypeptides which were completely uncharged (Sela and Fuchs 1963; Maurer et al. 1966) also evoked a good antibody response. Even various polyproline preparations were weakly immunogenic (Jasin and Glynn 1965; Brown and Glynn 1968). Therefore, charge is not a requirement for immunogenicity, and, over a wide range, charge does not influence the amount of antibody elicited; however, excessively high charge depresses the antibody response. Finally, there is an inverse relationship between the net charge of the antigen and that of the antibody without any apparent change in the specificity of the antibody (Sela and Mozes 1966; Rüde et al. 1968; Benacerraf et al. 1969).

1.3.4. Shape

The shape of a polypeptide does not affect its ability to elicit an antibody response, although it can alter the amount of antibody formed, and it greatly changes the specificity of the antibodies. Linear polypeptides, which have no organized conformational structure, can be potent immunogens (Gill et al. 1967). Ordered sequence polypeptides which have the α-helical conformation (poly Tyr-Ala-Glu) or which have the collagen triple helix (poly Pro-Gly-Pro) were immunogenic (Sela et al. 1968; Borek et al. 1969); the latter was rather weakly immunogenic. An α-helical, ordered sequence polymer of tyrosine, alanine and glutamic acid conjugated with the p-azobenzenearsonate hapten was considerably less immunogenic than the smaller, random polymer containing the same amino acids and the same hapten (Conway-Jacobs et al. 1970). Intramolecularly cross-linked synthetic polypeptides (Gill et al. 1968a), which have an ordered spatial structure, were potent immunogens. Finally, multichain polymers (Sela et al. 1963), which are compact, globular molecules, were highly immunogenic. Thus, all the levels of structure and surface topography can be present in immunogenic polypeptides. Presumably, the same conclusion holds true for proteins, and the loss in immunogenic potency with denaturation may be explained in part on grounds other than conformational change, e.g., rapid degradation *in vivo*.

1.3.5. Size

Small molecules can be immunogenic, and even a hapten-amino acid complex may elicit a weak response. However, studies of the immunogenicity of hapten-amino acid complexes must be approached with caution. Transconjugation occurred with many DNP-amino acids, such that the true immunogen was a hapten-protein conjugate, and many DNP-amino acid preparations contained higher molecular weight, immunogenic impurities (Frey et al. 1966, 1969). The immunological capabilities of a variety of small molecules are summarized in Table 1.3.

Molecular weight plays an important role in the relative immunogenicity of small molecules, but above a certain threshold, it does not appear to be a determining factor. This limit is a function both of size and of amino acid composition: for (glutamic acid, lysine) polymers, the threshold is around 30,000 or 40,000 and for (glutamic acid, lysine, tyrosine) polymers, between 10,000 and 20,000. Both types of polypeptides elicited the same antibody response over a three-fold variation in molecular weight once the molecular weight threshold was exceeded (Gill et al. 1967). Since a poly $Glu^{50}Ala^{40}Tyr^{10}$ of molecular weight 4,000 was a good immunogen (Sela et al. 1962), the presence of both tyrosine and alanine appears to lower the molecular weight threshold even more. In the cases where a very high molecular weight contributed to a greater antibody response, for example, with haemocyanin or tobacco mosaic virus (Landsteiner 1945), the effects might be due in some measure to aggregation.

1.3.6. Optical isomerism

In several of the earlier studies of D-amino acid polymers (Gill et al. 1963a; Maurer 1963c, 1965) in which rabbits were immunized with moderate amounts of antigen, the animals did not make any antibody. The one exception to these findings was the antibody response to poly

TABLE 1.3
Effect of size on immunogenicity.

Immunogen	Molecular weight	Species	Test*	Reference
Native peptides				
angiotensin II	1031	guinea-pig	DH, Arthus	Dietrich (1966)
fibrinopeptide B (on acrylic particles)	1400	rabbits	Gel	Berglund (1965)
DNP_3-bacitracin	1928	guinea-pig	PCA, Gel	Abuelo and Ovary (1965)
ACTH peptides				
(a) 11-24	1670	guinea-pig	DH	Salvin and Liauw
(b) 1-24	2800			(1967)
(c) P-16	2070	guinea-pig	PCA, DH, HA	Axelrod et al.
(d) P-20	2580			(1963)
(e) P-23	3000			
Synthetic polypeptides and amino acids				
$Rp-N-Ac-Tyr-NH_2$	450	guinea-pig	PCA, DH, SA	Borek et al. (1965b); Leskowitz et al. (1966, 1970)
$Rp-N-Ac-DTyr-NH_2$	450	guinea-pig	PCA, DH, SA	Leskowitz et al. (1966); Borek et al. (1967b)
$(Rp)_1-Tyr_2$	610	guinea-pig	DH, SA	Leskowitz et al. (1966)
$(Rp)_1-Tyr_3$	900	guinea-pig	PCA, DH	Borek et al. (1965b)
$(Rp)_1-Tyr_6$	1200	guinea-pig rabbit	PCA, DH Ppt	Borek et al. (1965b, 1967b)
$\alpha-DNP-Lys_7$	1136	guinea-pig	PCA, DH Arthus	Schlossman et al. (1965)
poly $Glu^{50}Ala^{40}Tyr^{10}$	4000	rabbit	Ppt	Sela et al. (1962)
poly $Glu^{60}Lys^{40}$	5000	rabbit	Ppt	Maurer (1963a)
Other compounds				
catechols	120 – 320	guinea-pig	DH	Baer et al. (1966)
arsphenamine	367	guinea-pig	SA, DH	Landsteiner and Jacobs (1935, 1936)
neoarsphenamine	466	guinea-pig humans	SA, DH DH	Frei (1928); Frey et al. (1966)
tetracyclines	440 – 500	rabbits	HA, SD	Queng et al. (1965)

* Abbreviations: DNP: 2,4-dinitrophenyl; Rp: *p*-azobenzenearsonate; ACTH: adreno-corticotropic hormone; Ac: acetyl; NH_2: amide; Arthus: Arthus skin reaction; DH: delayed hypersensitivity; PCA: passive cutaneous anaphylaxis; HA: haemagglutination; SA: systemic anaphylaxis; Ppt: precipitin reaction; Gel: diffusion in agar gel or immuno-electrophoresis; SD: Schultz-Dale test on guinea-pig ileum.

DGlu^{55}DLys^{39}DTyr^6, which elicited about one quarter as much antibody as the L-enantiomorph (Gill et al. 1964b). In an effort to understand the immunogenic differences of the D- and L-polymers, studies of their metabolism were undertaken in the rabbit (Gill et al. 1964c, 1965; Papermaster et al. 1965; Carpenter et al. 1967) and in the mouse (Janeway and Sela 1967; Janeway and Humphrey 1968; Janeway 1969). In the rabbit, the metabolic fate of intravenously injected, ^{131}I-labeled poly DGlu^{55}DLys^{39}DTyr^6 differed markedly from that of its enantiomorph poly Glu^{56}Lys^{33}Tyr^6. Although both polymers were rapidly cleared from the circulation, only 32% of the D-polymer was degraded in three weeks, whereas over 85% of the L-polymer was degraded by the seventh day. Previous injection of one isomer did not affect the metabolism of the other isomer. Large amounts of the D-polymer were retained in the liver and in the kidneys. The amount of D-polymer in the liver slowly declined from a maximum of 16% at five days, but the amount in the kidney continued to increase for two to three weeks and ultimately reached 30% to 35% of the injected dose. Chromatographic analyses of the dialysable radioactivity in the urine and in the homogenates of liver and kidney showed the presence of labeled peptides of molecular weight approximately 1,000; they were derived from the degradation of the D-polymer or of the L-polymer. Studies with a second external label, ^{59}Fe-ferrocene, confirmed the serum elimination, urine excretion and organ retention patterns obtained with the iodine label. There was no evidence for specific binding between the polypeptides and serum proteins, although there was some non-specific binding *in vivo* and *in vitro*; hence, the polypeptides alone acted as immunogens. Finally, radioautographic studies showed that both polymers entered the proximal tubules of the kidney: the D-polymer persisted, whereas the L-polymer was quickly eliminated. Ureteral ligation to stop glomerular filtration demonstrated that the polymers were filtered through the glomerulus and then reabsorbed by the tubules. In rabbits whose kidneys had been removed, there was a slower serum elimination of the D-polymer than in normal animals.

These metabolic studies suggested that the apparent lack of immunogenicity of D-amino acid polymers was due to their prolonged retention in the organs and gradual release over a long period of time: this caused immunological paralysis. In order to verify this hypothesis, small doses of a variety of D-polypeptides were injected over a long period of time, and all of the polymers consistently elicited an antibody response; continued administration of antigen depressed and finally abolished the antibody response (Gill et al. 1967; Stupp and Sela 1967; Jaton and Sela 1968). An inbred strain of rabbits (strain C) which gave the highest antibody response to poly Glu^{56}Lys^{38}Tyr^6 (Gill 1965) did not form antibody when immunized with poly DGlu^{55}DLys^{39}DTyr^{6} (Gill et al. 1967). Studies in monkeys (Gill et al. 1967), mice (Janeway and Sela 1967), guinea-pigs (Stupp and Sela 1967) and rats (Simonian et al. 1968) showed that all of these species responded to the D-amino acid polymers. The studies on the immunogenicity and metabolic fate of the D-amino acid polymers in mice yielded results consistent with those obtained in rabbits. In addition, Janeway (1969) found that if mice were left for a long time prior to receiving a booster injection, they displayed an anamnestic response; this behavior is similar to that seen with pneumococcal polysaccharides (Paul et al. 1967, 1969). A similar finding was noted when poly DGlu^{48}DLys^{38}DTyr^{14} was administered to rabbits as an aggregate with methylated bovine serum albumin (MeBSA) and emulsified with Freund's complete adjuvant (Gill et al. 1967). There was a booster response early in the course of immunization, as shown by a higher antibody concentration and a more intense Arthus skin reaction; however, there was no such booster response in rabbits immunized with the unaggregated D-polypeptide antigen.

Using low doses of antigen over a relatively long period of time, polyglutamic acid and polylysine of both the L- and D-configurations elicited an antibody response (Gill et al. 1967). Racemic polymers also elicited an antibody response (Borek et al. 1965a; Stupp and Sela 1967), including a branched polymer of DL-alanine and lysine which was used as the backbone of multichain polypeptides (Rimon et al. 1967).

Some interesting differences in the biological properties of rabbit antibodies to L- and D-polypeptides have been found (Gill and Kunz 1966; Gill et al. 1967). The antibodies elicited by poly Glu^{58}Lys^{36}Tyr^{6} and by poly DGlu^{55}DLys^{39}DTyr^{6}, both alone and when aggregated with MeBSA, are IgG immunoglobulins. The antibody to the L-polymer precipitates, gives a passive cutaneous anaphylaxis (PCA) reaction and fixes complement. The antibody to the D-polymer precipitates and fixes complement, but it does not usually give a PCA reaction. On the other hand, the antisera elicited by the D-polymer aggregated with MeBSA precipitate and give PCA and complement fixation reactions. The antisera to poly DGlu^{55}DLys^{39}DTyr^{6} alone did not elicit a PCA reaction at antibody concentrations that were the same as those giving a reaction with antisera to the D-polymer aggregated with the MeBSA or to the L-enantiomorph. In addition, the amounts of antibody in the sera were quite adequate for PCA reactions with a variety of other systems (Ovary 1958). Antibody to poly DGlu^{55}DLys^{39}DTyr^{6} gave Arthus reactions which were somewhat less intense and more erratic than those seen in rabbits immunized with poly Glu^{56}Lys^{38}Tyr^{6} or with the D-polymer aggregated with methylated bovine serum albumin and having

a comparable amount of circulating antibody. Thus, there is probably
a difference in the biological properties of the antibody elicited by poly
$DGlu^{55}DLys^{39}DTyr^6$ alone from that elicited by the D-polymer aggregated
with MeBSA or by the L-polymer.

1.3.7. Delayed hypersensitivity

Essentially all of the investigations on the mechanism of delayed
hypersensitivity have been carried out in guinea-pigs immunized with
antigen in Freund's complete adjuvant. The investigations of delayed
hypersensitivity and of the molecular requirements for its elicitation
have utilized three systems: hapten-amino acid complexes, hapten-
protein or hapten-synthetic polypeptide conjugates (Kantor et al. 1963;
Levine et al. 1963a; Leskowitz 1963c; Schlossman et al. 1965) and
synthetic polypeptides (Gill and Doty 1961; Ben-Efraim et al. 1963;
Maurer 1963a; Borek and Stupp 1965; Brown and Glynn 1968). These
studies have been reviewed in detail by Borek (1968b), and they are
summarized in Table 1.3. The results in each of these areas lead to
somewhat different conclusions. It seems, however, that the requirements for eliciting a delayed response are more complex than those for
eliciting an antibody response.

A variety of small molecules, for example, hapten-amino acid complexes, can elicit delayed hypersensitivity. There is some evidence that
these materials may act by themselves and not by becoming attached to
macromolecules in the host (Borek 1968b).

The case with hapten-protein conjugates is more complex, and the
specificity of the delayed hypersensitivity reaction is apparently directed
at a larger area than just the haptenic group (the carrier effect). The same
protein carrier was needed to elicit a delayed response to a hapten-protein
conjugate, and there was no cross-reaction between conjugates containing identical haptens on unrelated protein carriers (Salvin and Smith
1960; Gell and Benacerraf 1961; Benacerraf and Levine 1962; Gell and
Silverstein 1967). There were, however, cross-reactions between
chemically related haptens on the same protein carrier (Silverstein and
Gell 1962). The strongest delayed reactions were elicited when the test
antigen contained the same relative amount of hapten as the sensitizing
antigen (Benacerraf and Levine 1962). There is evidence, however,
that this carrier effect is not present in some complexes of the *p*-azo-
benzenearsonate (Rp) hapten (Leskowitz 1963a). For example, guinea-
pigs sensitized with Rp-guinea-pig albumin gave cross-reactions with
several antigens containing the Rp-hapten attached to unrelated protein
carriers; no such cross-reactions were observed in guinea-pigs sensitized
with azobenzoate-guinea-pig albumin.

Studies of delayed hypersensitivity using the α-DNP-oligolysine system showed that Hartley or strain 2 guinea-pigs could not be sensitized with any α-DNP-oligolysine derivatives containing less than seven lysine residues (Schlossman et al. 1966; Schlossman and Levine 1967; Yaron and Schlossman 1968). Animals sensitized with α-DNP-Lys$_7$ gave delayed hypersensitivity and Arthus reactions when skin tested with the immunizing compound. If skin tested with α-DNP-lysine derivatives containing three to six lysine residues, only the Arthus reaction was elicited. Thus, the chemical basis for immunogenicity was the same for antibody formation and delayed hypersensitivity, but the chemical specificity for eliciting the response was different in the two cases. Furthermore, immunization with α-DNP-Lys$_4$-DLys-Lys$_4$ did not sensitize guinea-pigs, whereas immunization with α-DNP-Lys$_9$ sensitized them very strongly (80 to 120 μg Ab/ml). The racemic polypeptide could elicit an Arthus reaction but not a delayed reaction in a sensitized animal. Finally, guinea-pigs immunized with α-DNP-oligolysines did not give a delayed hypersensitivity response when skin tested with α-DNP-oligo-D-lysine (Schlossman et al. 1966). Thus, this hapten-polypeptide system showed a high degree of specificity for optical configuration in the induction and in the elicitation of delayed hyper-sensitivity.

From a variety of studies using hapten conjugates of proteins or synthetic polypeptides there is evidence for hapten-specific delayed hypersensitivity when the p-azobenzenearsonate hapten is used; there is also a report (Leskowitz and Zak 1966) that two other haptens, p-azobenzenephosphonate and p-azobenzene-mercuri-thioglycolate, can elicit hapten-specific delayed hypersensitivity. The delayed response produced by sensitization with Rp-polytyrosine could be elicited by skin testing with the hapten attached to various proteins (Leskowitz 1963b). With animals sensitized to a variety of synthetic polypeptides containing the Rp-hapten, a delayed response could be elicited by Rp-bovine serum albumin, but not by other haptens attached to bovine serum albumin (Borek and Stupp 1965). Guinea-pigs sensitized by an Rp-synthetic polypeptide showed a delayed response when skin tested with the conjugate of the optical enantiomorph: (a) animals sensitized with Rp-poly-D-tyrosine responded to Rp-poly Glu^{60}Ala^{30}Tyr^{10} (Leskowitz et al. 1966); (b) animals sensitized with Rp-poly-L-tyrosine showed a reaction when skin tested with Rp-poly-D-tyrosine (Borek et al. 1967a); and (c) animals sensitized with Rp-poly Glu^{60}Ala^{30}Tyr^{10} responded to skin testing by Rp-poly DGlu^{60}DAla^{30}DTyr^{10} (Benacerraf et al. 1963).

The more fastidious structural requirements for delayed hypersensitivity are further illustrated in guinea-pigs sensitized to polypeptides related to collagen – poly Pro, poly (Pro, Gly) and poly (Pro, Gly, HypAc) (Brown and Glynn 1968). Poly Pro less than 14,000 in molecular weight did not induce delayed hypersensitivity nor did it elicit a skin reaction in animals sensitized with higher molecular weight poly Pro (M = 40,000). The skin reactivity in all cases was quite specific, since only the sensitizing antigen elicited a response; the one exception was the cross-reactivity to poly Pro in animals sensitized to poly (Pro, Gly). In contrast, immediate skin reactivity was far more catholic: animals sensitized with each of the three polypeptides showed a high degree of cross-reactivity with all of the polypeptides and with polyhydroxyproline.

The conformation of the sensitizing and skin testing antigen is important. There was no cross-reactivity in strain 2 guinea-pigs between linear and multichain copolymers containing glutamic acid, lysine and tyrosine (Ben-Efraim et al. 1967). There was also no cross-reactivity in guinea-pigs immunized with an ordered sequence copolymer of proline and glycine (poly Pro-Gly-Pro) when skin tested with a random copolymer of proline and glycine (Borek 1968b).

In summary, then, delayed hypersensitivity can be induced against relatively small groups, for example, hapten-amino acids or haptens on synthetic polypeptides. However, this appears to be a function of the particular hapten involved and the chemical simplicity of the carrier molecule. When haptens are attached to structurally complex proteins, it appears as if the requirements for inducing delayed hypersensitivity involve a larger part of the molecule – the hapten and the area adjacent to it. The requirements for the induction of delayed hypersensitivity may involve a complex group of factors related to the interplay of the hapten and the particular carrier: with a potent hapten and a simple carrier, the specificity is directed mainly at the hapten, but with a structurally complex carrier, part of the carrier may be involved both in inducing the delayed reaction and in eliciting the skin test.

1.3.8. Tolerance

Synthetic polypeptides have been used in attempts to probe the structural basis underlying the induction of tolerance (see review by Dresser and Mitchison 1968). Most of the experiments were carried out in newborn rabbits using approximately 100–200 mg. of polymer administered intraperitoneally or intravenously to induce tolerance; the antibody forming capability of these animals was then assayed by immunization with the antigen in complete Freund's adjuvant. A variety of linear (Maurer et al. 1963b; Brown and Glynn 1968) and multichain (Sela et al. 1963; Janeway and Humphrey 1969) synthetic polypeptides and polypeptidyl proteins (Bauminger et al. 1967) induced tolerance; however, it was not possible to induce tolerance with a tetrapeptide of alanine (Bauminger and Sela 1969). In addition, adult rabbits treated with 6-mercaptopurine could be made tolerant to branched chain polypeptides (Sela et al. 1963). None of these studies showed any clear correlation between antigenic specificity and specificity for the induction of tolerance (Bauminger and Sela 1969). There is some evidence that the specificity for tolerance with respect to antibody formation and to delayed hypersensitivity may be different (Brown and Glynn 1968, 1969). Guinea-pigs sensitized with poly Pro, poly (Pro, Gly) or poly (Pro, Gly, HypAc) in complete Freund's adjuvant developed both delayed hypersensitivity and Arthus reactions. Tolerance induced by poly Pro (M = 14,000, but not with M = 1600) in incomplete Freund's adjuvant provided effective blocking of both immediate and delayed reactions following immunization with poly Pro (M = 14,000 or higher). Immunization with poly (Pro, Gly, HypAc) broke tolerance with respect to both. The administration of poly (Pro, Gly) in saline induced partial tolerance to poly Pro and to poly (Pro, Gly), but none to poly (Pro, Gly, HypAc). Finally, poly (Pro, Gly, HypAc) in saline did not induce tolerance to poly Pro or to poly (Pro, Gly, HypAc), and it induced only partial tolerance to poly (Pro, Gly). During the recovery from tolerance, the antibodies formed by the partially tolerant guinea-pigs differed from those of the normally immune animals by having a lower avidity (Brown and Glynn 1969).

Cross-tolerance could be induced using a variety of different polypeptide combinations (Maurer et al. 1965). Tolerance to poly glutamic acid gave cross-tolerance to poly $Glu^{60}Ala^{40}$, but not to poly $Glu^{42}Lys^{28}$-Ala^{30}. Tolerance to the latter polymer produced cross-tolerance to poly $Glu^{60}Ala^{40}$. The induction of tolerance to polypeptidyl proteins gave a variable pattern of tolerance to the protein carrier and to the polypeptide sidechain (Bauminger et al. 1967). Tolerance to (poly DLAla) – ribonuclease was directed at the protein carrier and partially at the poly-DL-alanine sidechains. On the other hand, the induction of tolerance to (poly DLAla) – human serum albumin gave tolerance to human serum albumin but not to the poly-DL-alanine sidechains. The induction of tolerance to the graft polymer of DL-alanine and lysine used as a backbone for multichain polypeptides produced tolerance to the poly-DL-alanine sidechains of a variety of alanylated proteins. Finally, immunization of rabbits with polypeptidyl derivatives of their own serum proteins elicited antibody against the polypeptide sidechains only: immunization with (poly Tyr)-rabbit serum albumin elicited antibody to polytyrosine (Schechter et al. 1964).

Tolerance to human serum albumin can be terminated by immunization with the polytyrosine derivative of human serum albumin but not with the polyalanine derivative (Schechter et al. 1964). The amount of tyrosine added was crucial in determining the ability of the polypeptidyl protein to break tolerance: the attachment of 3% or 13% tyrosine residues was only modestly effective, whereas a derivative containing 7% tyrosine was very effective.

1.3.9. Conjugates of synthetic polypeptides and small molecules

A variety of small molecules attached to a poorly immunogenic synthetic polypeptide can enhance the immunogenicity of the polypeptide in the rabbit, and the complex can elicit antibody specific for the small molecule (Sela 1969). In general, aromatic haptens, coenzymes, drugs, nucleosides and cytolipin H enhanced immunogenicity. On the other hand, the attachment of peptide hormones or of monosaccharides only slightly affected immunogenicity. Ferrocene (biscyclopentadienyl iron), which is one of the metallocenes, displayed unique behaviour in that it enhanced the immunogenicity of the potent immunogen poly $Glu^{58}Lys^{36}$ Tyr^6 (Gill and Mann 1966). As in the case with the attachment of tyrosine to gelatin (Arnon and Sela 1960), small amounts of ferrocene (2 residues/molecule of polypeptide) enhanced the amount of antibody only slightly, and most of the antibody was directed at the polypeptide carrier. The attachment of 10 to 16 ferrocene residues per polypeptide molecule markedly increased the amount of antibody elicited, and 60% to 70% of the antibody was directed against ferrocene. The attachment of the dinitrophenyl hapten to polylysine or to a copolymer of glutamic acid and lysine enhanced the immunogenicity of these polypeptides in guinea-pigs (Kantor et al. 1963). However, if more than 10% of the lysine residues in polylysine were dinitrophenylated, the immunogenicity of the complex decreased. The attachment of DNP-residues to poly $Glu^{60}Lys^{40}$ or to poly $Glu^{52}Lys^{33}Tyr^{15}$ did not enhance the immunogenicity of these polypeptides in rabbits, and if more than 40% of the lysine residues in poly $Glu^{60}Lys^{40}$ were dinitrophenylated, the immunogenicity of the complex decreased (Gill et al. 1967).

1.3.10. Summary

The studies on synthetic polypeptide antigens have delineated some of the molecular characteristics which influence the induction and magnitude of the antibody response. A summary of these properties is given in Table 1.4.

TABLE 1.4

Summary of the chemical properties affecting the immunogenicity of synthetic antigens.*

Property	Effect on immunogenicity	Comment
(1) Composition		
(a) three or more different types of amino acids	+	poly $Glu^{56}Lys^{38}Tyr^6$ = poly $Glu^{42}Lys^{28}Ala^{30}$ > poly $Glu^{60}Lys^{40}$ > poly Glu = poly Lys
(b) presence of tyrosine or phenylalanine	+	not necessary, but enhances amount of antibody in most cases
(c) presence of alanine + tyrosine	+	poly $Glu^{63}Ala^{28}Tyr^9$ > poly $Glu^{56}Lys^{38}Tyr^6$ = poly $Glu^{42}Lys^{28}Ala^{30}$
(2) Charge		
(a) high	−	completely charged polymers are weakly immunogenic
(b) none	0	uncharged polymers are immunogenic
(3) Shape	0	polypeptides of all conformations are immunogenic
(4) Size		
(a) small	−	hapten-peptide can elicit a weak immune response
(b) large	±	molecular size over 5,000–20,000, depending upon the composition, is not critical
(5) D-amino acids	−	less immunogenic than L-counterpart
(6) Metabolism	variable	role in regulating the amount of antigen available
(7) Non-biological components	−	vinyl polymers are weakly immunogenic

* The symbols are: +, increased immunogenicity; ±, slightly increased; 0, no effect; and −, decreased.

1.4. Other macromolecules

1.4.1. Vinyl polymers

The hypothesis developed from the study of D-amino acid polymers –
that low doses of antigen over long periods of time can elicit an immune
response to poorly immunogenic macromolecules – was tested further
with four vinyl polymers, each of which possessed particular properties

of interest (Gill and Kunz 1968). Polyvinylpyrrolidone (M = 180,000) is the most peptide-like of the vinyl polymers because it contains a substituted amide group and a heterocyclic ring, which is a model for aromatic amino acids. Poly (methacrylic acid-2-dimethylaminoethyl methacrylate) (M = 360,000) is a polyampholite which resembles proteins in respect to charge distribution; it is the vinyl analogue of a synthetic polypeptide containing glutamic acid and lysine. Lastly, polymethacrylic acid (M = 15,000) and polyvinylamine (M = 43,000) are completely charged vinyl homopolymers – a combination of characteristics that should produce the most unfavourable type of immunogen – and they are the vinyl analogues of polyglutamic acid and polylysine, respectively. Polyvinylpyrrolidone and poly (methacrylic acid-2-dimethylaminoethyl methacrylate) consistently elicited a moderate amount of antibody (100–200 μg Ab/ml), and polymethacrylic acid and polyvinylamine elicited a low and variable antibody response (5–20 μg Ab/ml). The amounts of antibody elicited by these vinyl polymers were in the same relative proportions as the amounts elicited by their polypeptide analogues. The antibody responses decreased and were eventually abolished as more antigen was administered. The passive cutaneous anaphylaxis test in guinea-pigs showed weak reactions with antisera to polyvinylpyrrolidone and equivocal reactions with antisera to poly (methacrylic acid-2-dimethylaminoethyl methacrylate). The amounts of antibody used would ordinarily give very strong reactions with protein or polypeptide antigens. This deficiency in the biological capability of the antibody is the same as that noted with antibody elicited by D-amino acid polymers (Gill and Kunz 1966; Gill et al. 1967).

An immune reaction against polyvinylpyrrolidone was demonstrated in four strains of mice by serological methods and by the immune elimination technique; each strain had a somewhat different dose range for maximal immunogenicity (Andersson 1969). Preparations with molecular weights of 24,000 to 360,000 were immunogenic, and immunological paralysis could be induced in adult mice with 100 μg of antigen in saline given intravenously. The haemagglutination reactions could be inhibited by polyvinylpyrrolidone preparations with molecular weights less than 10,000.

Three implications can be drawn from the demonstration that vinyl polymers are immunogenic. First, the antigen does not have to be fragmented in order to induce antibody formation, since there is no evidence that vinyl polymers can be enzymatically or in any other way physiologically attacked. Secondly, the surface topography of the molecule is probably the crucial structural parameter for interaction with the immunocompetent cell, regardless of how the surface is constructed.

Thirdly, immunogenicity is probably a general property of most, if not all, macromolecules, since the vinyl polymers which elicited an antibody response are biologically quite alien substances.

A number of previous studies on the immunogenicity of vinyl polymers (reviewed in Maurer 1964; Gill and Kunz 1968) – for example, on polyvinylpyrrolidone, polyvinylpyrrolidone coupled with amino acid or sugar determinants, or polystyrene – failed to demonstrate antibody formation in the rabbit or in any other species, with one exception. High molecular weight polyvinylpyrrolidone ($M = 1,000,000$) elicited antibody formation in 25 of 66 humans, but a lower molecular weight preparation ($M = 250,000$) did not (Maurer 1956, 1957b). The apparent lack of immunogenicity of the polymer in rabbits and of the lower molecular weight preparation in humans was probably due to the administration of too much antigen; hence, it induced immunological paralysis (Gill and Kunz 1968). In those humans who responded to a first course of immunization with polyvinylpyrrolidone, a second course a year later failed to elicit any antibody at all. Thus, the data on both humans and rabbits are quite compatible with the postulate concerning the relationship between the chemistry of the antigen and the dose required for immunization.

1.4.2. Carbohydrates

A variety of purified carbohydrates are immunogenic in several different species. The pneumococcal polysaccharides which have high molecular weights (Heidelberger et al. 1936, 1946) can induce an immune response in humans, rabbits, and mice when given in small amounts (Kabat 1961, 1968; MacLeod 1965). The dose of antigen was most critical in the rabbit and the mouse, since these species are quite susceptible to the induction of immunological paralysis. In rabbits immunized with small amounts of material, an anamnestic response can be demonstrated several months after the primary course of immunization by giving a small amount of antigen (Paul et al. 1967, 1969). Highly purified type II pneumococcal polysaccharide and penicilloylated dextran can induce delayed hypersensitivity very efficiently in random-bred guinea-pigs (Gerety et al. 1970, Schneider and de Weck 1967). A complex of pneumococcal polysaccharide with methylated bovine serum albumin can elicit in the rabbit a potent antibody response against the pneumococcal polysaccharide (Plescia et al. 1964). Thus, the immunogenic properties of pneumococcal polysaccharides are like those of the D-amino acid and vinyl polymers. Purified blood group substances are immunogenic both in animals and in man (Kabat 1956). Finally, several other purified carbohydrates are immunogenic in man: dextrans and levans (Kabat and Bezer 1958; Kabat 1968), teichoic acids (Torii et al.

1964), and high molecular weight (M = 100,000) meningococcal group A and group C polysaccharides (Gotschlich et al. 1969).

In most cases where a purified polysaccharide was immunogenic in man, its molecular weight was in excess of 75,000 to 100,000. In a systematic study of the effect of molecular weight on the immunogenicity of dextran, Kabat and Bezer (1958) found that dextrans larger than 90,000 were consistently immunogenic in man, whereas if the molecular weight was less than 51,000, the antibody response was erratic and very low. A similar study in mice using type III pneumococcal polysaccharide as the antigen showed that the molecular weight had to exceed 18,000 in order for the polysaccharide to elicit antibody formation or to induce immunological paralysis (McMaster et al. 1970). Thus, it appears that molecular weight is a much more important factor in the immunogenicity of carbohydrates than in the immunogenicity of proteins or synthetic polypeptides.

1.4.3. Nucleic acids and polynucleotides

Purified nucleic acids or polynucleotides have not been reported to elicit antibody formation by themselves (reviewed in Plescia and Braun 1967, 1968; Levine and Stollar 1968). The one exception is a report that a trinitrophenyl-DNA complex elicited anti-TNP antibodies in rabbits (Voss et al. 1969). In the serum of patients with systemic lupus erythematosus, there are naturally occurring antibodies against DNA and RNA, and specificities vary in different patients. The anti-DNA antibody can react with denatured or with native DNA, and the anti-RNA antibody can react with RNA, double-stranded viral RNA, ribosomes and the single-stranded polynucleotides polyinosine, polyadenosine, and polyguanosine (Schur et al. 1967; Koffler et al. 1969; Steinberg et al. 1969). The same types of anti-RNA antibodies have been found also in NZB/NZW mice (Steinberg et al. 1969).

Antibodies against denatured DNA have been elicited by denatured DNA or by oligonucleotides complexed with methylated bovine serum albumin (Plescia et al. 1964; Plescia and Braun 1968) or by sonicated bacteriophage (Levine et al. 1960). Antibodies have been elicited by double-stranded polynucleotides complexed with MeBSA which reacted with double-stranded polynucleotides or nucleic acids (Seaman et al. 1965; Lacour et al. 1968; Schwartz and Stollar 1969; Steinberg et al. 1969); reactions with single-stranded polynucleotides or nucleic acids have also been reported (Lacour et al. 1968). Anti-RNA antibodies have been elicited by immunization with ribosomes (Barbu and Panijel 1960; Plescia and Braun 1967). Antibodies specific to the nucleotide bases or to small oligonucleotides can be produced by immunizing with the bases or oligonucleotides coupled to proteins (Plescia et al. 1965; Plescia and Braun 1967, 1968; Levine and Stollar 1968; Garro et al. 1971; Wallace et al. 1971) or to a multichain polymer of DL-alanine and lysine (Ungar-Waron et al. 1967). These anti-nucleotide antibodies will react with single-stranded polynucleotides and with thermally denatured nucleic acids. Finally, the double-stranded polyinosinic poly-cytidylic acid can elicit immunological tolerance in NZB/NZW mice treated with cyclophosphamide (Steinberg et al. 1970).

The immunogenic properties of nucleic acids *per se* have still not been defined, since the antigen in lupus is not known and, in the other cases, nucleic acids or polynucleotides complexed with proteins had to be used as the immunogen. One possibility for the difficulty in clearly demonstrating immunogenicity to nucleic acids may be their rapid degradation by serum and tissue nucleases.

1.4.4. Lipids

No purified lipid has yet been shown to be immunogenic (Rapport and Graf 1969, Landsteiner 1945), although the apparent, very weak immune response to purified glycolipid from *M. pneumoniae* may be an exception (Razin et al. 1970). To obtain an antibody directed against a lipid, the latter must be complexed with serum (Landsteiner 1945), proteins (Graf et al. 1965; Koscielak et al. 1968; Kataoka and Nojima 1970), synthetic polypeptides (Arnon et al. 1969) or red blood cells (Landsteiner 1945; Yokoyama et al. 1963). In addition, antibodies to gangliosides have been reported in patients with central nervous lesions (Yokoyama et al. 1962). The best studied lipid haptens are the glycolipids cytolipin H from human epidermoid carcinoma (Graf et al. 1965; Arnon et al. 1969) and globoside from human red blood cells (Koscielak et al. 1968). Antibody was elicited by a cytolipin H-synthetic polypeptide conjugate (Arnon et al. 1969) or by a mixture of globoside with bovine serum albumin (Koscielak et al. 1968). The specificity of the antibody directed at cytolipin H was mainly to the lactose moiety, but with some toward the lipid part. In like manner, the specificity of the antibody to globoside was directed mainly at the sugar moiety, although a part of the lipid was also involved. The immunological reactivity of the anti-globoside antibody was best when the globoside was aggregated with a 'carrier' lipid, e.g., ganglioside, to form a micellar structure (Koscielak et al. 1968). Thus, the immunogenicity of lipids requires that the lipid be aggregated with some other macromolecule, and the immunochemical reactivity of lipids is best when the lipid is aggregated into a larger micellar structure. The low molecular weight and high degree of flexibility, which are two characteristics of poor immunogens, contribute to the difficulty in eliciting an antibody response to a purified lipid. In addition, lipids are readily adsorbed to a wide variety of molecules, and they may not be able to act independently to stimulate the antibody-producing mechanism.

1.4.5. *Cells and tissues*

The antigens characteristic of cells and tissues are quite complex, and they contain mainly carbohydrate and lipid with variable amounts of proteins. The best studied ones are the blood group antigens (reviewed in Marcus 1969), the histocompatibility antigens (Batchelor and Sanderson 1969; Boyle 1969; Kahan and Reisfeld 1969; Lange and Markowitz 1969; Mann et al. 1969; Manson and Simmons 1969; Summerell and Davis 1969; Hämmerling et al. 1971; Davies et al. 1971; McPherson et al. 1971; reviewed in Amos 1970 and in Ivanyi 1970), and the Forsmann and Wassermann antigens (Cushing and Campbell 1957; Landsteiner 1945). Their physiological functions are not well understood, but they play a role in a variety of clinically important immunological reactions.

1.5. *Antigenic competition*

When the immune mechanism is simultaneously presented with two strong antigenic determinants, there is a competitive effect which results in an alteration of the ability to make an immune response against one of the determinants. The physiological state of the animal and the method of immunization are important factors in determining the presence and the magnitude of such effects.

Antigenic competition exists between proteins and between synthetic polypeptides. In studies on mice injected intravenously with the antigen in incomplete Freund's adjuvant, there was competition between bovine γ-globulin and ferritin (Adler 1964). The injection of a variable dose of bovine γ-globulin decreased the antibody response to a standard dose of ferritin and vice versa. The strongest competition occurred when one antigen was injected before the other, although there was competition when both were injected together. The same conclusions were reached using bovine serum albumin and haemocyanin in a comparable type of experiment (Cremer 1963). Similar experiments were carried out in guinea-pigs using synthetic polypeptide antigens in Freund's complete adjuvant and using skin tests as the assay method (Ben-Efraim and Liacopoulos 1967, 1969a, 1969b). Competition was demonstrated between chemically related synthetic polypeptides and between D-amino acid polymers and their L-isomers.

Competition studies employing hapten-protein complexes or polypeptidyl proteins demonstrated discrete competition for the antibody response to the hapten. In mice, the injection of azobenzenearsonate (Rp)-mouse serum albumin and Rp-ferritin caused a decrease in the antibody response to ferritin (Adler 1964). When Rp-mouse serum albumin was injected before, or simultaneously with, ferritin, there was no effect on the amount of antibody elicited by ferritin. Finally, administration of Rp-mouse serum albumin, then ferritin plus Rp-mouse serum albumin, caused a decreased antibody response to the ferritin.

There is competition between the Rp- and the DNP-hapten when both of them are on the same protein carrier (Amkraut et al. 1966). In rabbits immunized with the antigens in complete Freund's adjuvant, the antibody response elicited in animals immunized with both haptens on the same carrier was compared to the response to the mixture of Rp-protein and DNP-protein. When comparable amounts of Rp- and DNP-haptens were attached to keyhole limpet haemocyanin, to bovine serum albumin or to sheep red cell stroma, the antibody response to the Rp-determinant was depressed, whereas the response to the DNP-determinant was unaltered. However, if the number of Rp-groups greatly exceeded that of the DNP-groups, the antibody response to the Rp-determinant was increased, and the response to DNP was either decreased or increased. Thus, the DNP-hapten is the more potent determinant.

A third type of study employed polypeptidyl proteins injected into rabbits in complete Freund's adjuvant. When the poly-DL-alanine derivative of ribonuclease, human serum albumin (HSA), or rabbit serum albumin (RSA) was injected simultaneously with the respective poly-DL-phenylalanine-containing protein, the antibody response to alanine was depressed and the response to phenylalanine was normal if the carriers were the same or related; if they were very different, no competition occurred (Schechter 1965, 1968). Tolerance to (poly DLPhe) –RSA did not affect the antibody response to the poly-DL-alanine sidechains following the injection of (poly DLAla) – RSA or (poly DLAla) – HSA. However, if both (poly DLAla) – RSA and (poly DLPhe) – RSA were injected into the tolerant animal at the same time, there was no antibody formed against the poly-DL-alanine sidechains. These experiments imply that the determinant and the carrier are both important in antigenic competition with these molecules. When poly-peptidyl conjugates of ribonuclease, human serum albumin or rabbit serum albumin with (poly DLTyr), (poly DLAla), or (poly DLPhe) sidechains were injected into rabbits in complete Freund's adjuvant, the antibody was directed mainly at the D-amino acid moiety; therefore, there is competition between the stereoisomers, and the D-form is the more potent immunogen (Schechter and Sela 1967).

Finally, studies in mice using intravenously injected antigens or cells demonstrated competition between haemocyanin and goose or rat red blood cells, between rat and goose red blood cells and between various red cells or haemocyanin and cellular immunity as measured by prolonged survival of skin grafts (Eidinger et al. 1968). Prior injection of sheep red blood cells decreased the response of mice to rat red cells (Albright and Makinodan 1965), and prior injection of horse red blood cells decreased the response to sheep red blood cells (Radovich and Talmage 1967).

Thus, antigenic competition can occur between haptens, proteins, polypeptides, or cells. The mechanism underlying this competition is not well understood, and it presents the same types of complexity that delayed hypersensitivity does. There is evidence, however, that antigenic competition is not due to competition for metabolites (Cremer 1963; Adler 1964) nor to competition for immunologically competent cells (Albright et al. 1970; Waterston 1970). There is some evidence that antigenic competition occurs locally at the site of antigenic stimulation, is dose dependent, is relatively independent of the carrier molecule in a hapten-carrier complex and does not alter the affinity of the antibody elicited compared to that formed in response to one antigen alone (Brody and Siskind 1969).

1.6. Aggregation

The physical form in which an antigen is used is an important factor in determining its immunogenic activity. Differences in the immunogenic capabilities of aggregated and unaggregated molecules have been demonstrated for proteins, nucleic acids and synthetic polypeptides. Dresser (1962) showed that in mice soluble bovine γ-globulin given intraperitoneally in saline induced tolerance, whereas the aggregated form induced an immune response. The same phenomenon was demonstrated with human γ-globulin in primates (Howard et al. 1969). Poorly immunogenic proteins, such as ribonuclease and human gonadotropin, could be made more immunogenically potent in the rabbit by intermolecularly cross-linking before giving them intravenously in saline (Anderer and Schlumberger 1969). The antibody elicited by these cross-linked proteins reacted completely with the native proteins.

The aggregation of a poor immunogen with a macromolecule of opposite charge greatly increased its immunogenicity (Gill and Doty 1962; Plescia et al. 1964; Gill and Kunz 1966; Green et al. 1967a). The most common molecules used for aggregation were methylated bovine serum albumin (Plescia et al. 1964), phosphorylated bovine serum albumin (Van Vunakis et al. 1966) and synthetic polypeptides (Gill and Kunz 1966). Most of the antibody was directed against the antigen (Gill and Kunz 1966), but when antibody was made against the carrier, it was produced by different cells (Green et al. 1967b). The induction of tolerance to the aggregating agent decreased or abolished the antibody response to the antigen (Green et al. 1968).

In guinea-pigs immunized with an aggregate of DNP-polylysine and ovalbumin, the responder strain developed delayed hypersensitivity to both the immunogen and the aggregating agent, whereas the non-responder strain developed a delayed reaction to the aggregating agent only (Green et al. 1967a). The same genetic difference in the pattern of response to skin testing was found in rats immunized with DNP-poly $Glu^{52}Lys^{33}Tyr^{15}$ aggregated with methylated bovine serum albumin or with polylysine, except that the poorly responding strain occasionally gave a weak delayed response when skin tested with the immunogen alone (B. P. Sloan and T. J. Gill, III, unpublished data). In rabbits immunized with poly-γ-D-glutamic acid aggregated with methylated bovine serum albumin, delayed reactions were elicited only by the aggregate or by the aggregating agent (Roelants et al. 1969).

The genetic differences in the primary and secondary responses to synthetic polypeptides in C57 and CBA mice were obliterated by complexing the antigens with MeBSA (McDevitt 1968). In inbred rats (Simonian et al. 1968), the aggregation of synthetic polypeptide antigens with MeBSA elicited an increased antibody response in those strains which produced a low titer of antibody to the polypeptide alone and reduced interstrain differences. Non-responding guinea-pigs formed antibodies when immunized with aggregates (Green et al. 1967a). In contrast to these findings, observations in rabbits (Gill et al. 1967) and in rats (Gill et al. 1970) indicated that the aggregate of a potent immunogen decreased the ability of the immunogen to elicit antibody formation.

Further studies on the effects of aggregation in genetically inbred rats showed that aggregating poly $Glu^{52}Lys^{33}Tyr^{15}$ with MeBSA had profound effects on the antibody responses in both the highly responding ACI strain and the poorly responding F344 strain (Gill et al. 1970). The major differences in the responses to the aggregated antigen compared with those to the unaggregated antigen were: (a) every rat in each strain and strain combination made antibody; (b) the heterogeneity of the antibody response was greatly restricted; (c) the antibody response in females, but not in males, of the poorly responding F344 strain was enhanced; (d) in contrast, there was either a decrease or there was no change in the amount of antibody formed by the highly responding ACI strain and by the various hybrids of the ACI and F344 strains;

and (e) the sex difference in the antibody response (female > male) was unaltered or enhanced. The effect of aggregation on the distribution of the antibody response among the different immunoglobulin classes was also quite striking. The F344 parental strain immunized with the antigen alone either did not respond or responded at a level too low to detect by radio-immunoelectrophoresis. When immunized with the aggregated antigen, this strain formed antibody almost exclusively in the IgG class. The highly responding ACI parental strain formed antibody in all immunoglobulin classes, as in the case of immunization with the unaggregated antigen. The various hybrids of the parental strains responded predominantly in the IgG class, in contrast to the findings following immunization with the unaggregated antigen, in which case the antibody response was distributed among all of the immunoglobulin classes. There were no significant sex differences in the amounts of antibody in the various immunoglobulin classes. An increase in the magnitude of the antibody response in the F344 strain and a decrease in the ACI strain following immunization with an aggregate of poly $Glu^{52}Lys^{33}Tyr^{15}$ also occurred with a variety of aggregating agents other than methylated bovine serum albumin (B. P. Sloan and T. J. Gill, III, unpublished data).

The changes in the antibody responses following immunization with the aggregated antigen are consistent with a dosage effect. Firstly, if aggregation protected the antigen from degradation, the amount of antigen available and the duration for which it was present could be greatly increased. The increased amount of antigen could then cause partial paralysis in the highly responding parental ACI strain and lead to a decrease in the amount of antibody formed. On the other hand, it could cause an enhanced antibody response in the parental F344 strain similar to that seen when this strain is immunized with high doses of antigen. In both of these cases, the antibody response was primarily in the IgG class. Secondly, this mechanism could also explain the restricted heterogeneity in the amount of antibody formed. When the antibody response became partially paralyzed (e.g., in the ACI strain) or a large amount of antigen was needed to force the formation of antibody (e.g., in the F344 strain), only a relatively restricted population of cells may be stimulated. Finally, if the effect of aggregation is one of increasing the effective antigen dosage, it would not alter the normal sex difference seen in the antibody response: such is the case.

The better antibody response of the poorly responding F344 strain with increasing dosage of poly $Glu^{53}Lys^{33}Tyr^{15}$ or with the aggregated antigen could be explained in one of two ways. The cells capable of interacting with the antigen may have receptors with a low binding affinity for the antigen. Therefore, large amounts of antigen would be needed to cause binding and the subsequent initiation of the antibody response, in accord with the principles of the mass action law. Alternatively, there may be only relatively few cells capable of interacting with poly $Glu^{52}Lys^{33}Tyr^{15}$, so that a large amount of antigen would increase the probability of an antigen-immunocompetent cell interaction. The probability of such an encounter is directly dependent upon the amount of antigen available, which is determined by the dosage and the rate of degradation of the antigen *in vivo*. Again, this mechanism is in accord with the principles of the mass action law.

1.7. Antigenic sites

All the various levels of organizations in proteins and polypeptides can provide the structural specificity for antigenic sites. Linear synthetic polypeptides have antigenic determinants which depend mainly upon the primary structure of the polypeptide (Gill et al. 1967; Sela 1969). More highly organized polypeptides provide antigenic sites based upon the secondary structure of the molecule: poly Tyr-Ala-Glu is α-helical (Sela et al. 1968), poly Pro-Gly-Pro has the triple helix of collagen (Borek et al. 1969) and polyproline can provide antigenic specificity in either the *cis* or the *trans* conformation (Jasin and Glynn 1965). Intramolecularly cross-linked synthetic polypeptides, which are models for the tertiary structure of proteins, have antigenic sites that depend upon the spatial organization of the polypeptide (Gill et al. 1968a).

The antigenic sites on polypeptides must be accessible to the antibody forming mechanism in order to be effective (Sela et al. 1962). All amino acids are not equally potent antigenically, and there is a hierarchy in which tyrosine is very potent, lysine moderately so and glutamic acid and alanine only modestly effective (Gill et al. 1963, 1968a). The amino acid composition of the antigenic combining site does not reflect the overall amino acid composition of the polypeptide (Gill et al. 1967). There appears to be an inverse relationship between the size of the antigenic site and the potency of the amino acid residues which constitute it (Gill et al. 1968b). Some of the antibody elicited by synthetic polypeptides is directed at the amino acid side-chains, especially that of tyrosine. This antibody accounts for the small amount of cross-reactivity between D- and L-polypeptides containing tyrosine (Gill et al. 1967) and between polyvinylpyrollidone and poly $Glu^{56}Lys^{38}Tyr^{6}$; the latter reaction is due to the structural similarities of the pyrolidone ring and the phenolic ring of tyrosine (Gill and Kunz 1968). Finally, there are cross-reactions between proteins and synthetic polypeptides due to side-chain cross-reactivity (Gill and Matthews 1963) or to conformational similarities (Borek et al. 1969).

Studies with native proteins also indicate that all levels of structural organization can provide antigenic determinants. Primary structure is the major factor in the antigenic sites of silk fibroin (Cebra 1961) and oxidized ribonuclease (Brown 1962). The completely helical paramyosin has antigenic sites whose residues are in the helical conformation (Kunz and Gill 1964). The spatial organization of globular proteins is a very important and subtle determinant in the structure of their antigenic determinants. The specificity of the oxygenated and deoxygenated forms of haemoglobin is different due to the conformational changes that occur when haemoglobin reacts with oxygen (Reichlin et al. 1964). The various mutations in the subunits of tryptophan synthetase either can or cannot change their antigenic specificity, depending upon where they occur (Yanofsky 1963; Suskind et al. 1963; Murphy and Mills 1965). If the tertiary structure of ribonuclease is disrupted by enzymatic digestion (Singer and Richards 1959) or by oxidation (Mills and Haber 1963; Brown 1963), its antigenic specificity is greatly altered. Finally, the quaternary structure of complex macromolecules provides unique antigenic determinants: immunochemical studies on the structure of the IgM macroglobulin showed that a certain fraction of the antibody elicited by the IgM molecule was directed at determinants which comprised parts of two subunits (Polmar and Steinberg 1964; Seligmann et al. 1966; Seligmann and Mihaesco 1967; Mihaesco and Seligmann 1968). The structure of all these antigenic sites depends upon the surface topography of the protein molecule, which acts as an immunogen in its native, intact form. The antigenic sites which are attributed to 'internal determinants' (Lapresle 1955; Lapresle and Webb 1960) are probably due to *in vivo* degradation of the protein and the subsequent action of the larger fragments as independent immunogens.

Two general approaches have been taken in investigating the more detailed aspects of the antigenic determinants on proteins. One technique is chemical modification. This method can give equivocal results, since there can be far-reaching effects on the entire structure of the molecule caused by modification of a given type of residue. In addition, it is difficult to obtain absolutely specific chemical reagents, and generally several amino acid residues can be affected by a particular reagent. Most modifications decrease the antigenic reactivity of proteins or polypeptides with antibody to the native molecule; some representative data are shown in Table 1.5. It is difficult to determine whether this loss of reactivity is due to modification of a specific type of residue or whether it is due to a change in the spatial organization of the molecule. The other

TABLE 1.5

Effects of chemical modification of proteins and polypeptides on the reactivity with antibody to the unmodiffied immunogen.*[a]

Antigen	*Acetylation* *(lysine)*	*Deamination* *(lysine)*	*Esterification* *(glutamic and aspartic acids)*	*Iodination* *(tyrosine)*
Bovine serum albumin	−	−	−	
Ovomucoid	−		−	−
Soy bean hemagglutinin	−			−
Ovalbumin	−	−		
Insulin	0		−	
Ribonuclease	−	−		
Poly Glu^{59}Lys^{41}		−	−	
Poly Glu^{49}Lys^{51}		+		
Poly Glu^{42}Lys^{58}		−		

* The symbols are: −, decreased reactivity; +, increased reactivity; and 0, no effect.
[a] Maurer (1963b) and Gill et al. (1964a).

approach is to use small peptides from the degradation of the native immunogen as the inhibitors of the antibody-antigen reaction. This procedure destroys the native conformation of the antigenic sites, especially in globular proteins. In order for the inhibiting fragment to approximate its structure in the native molecule, it probably has to be large enough to assume some ordered spatial structure. Therefore, the fragments causing significant amounts of inhibition probably over-estimate the size of the antigenic determinant. The proteins that have been most thoroughly studied by this approach are: albumin (Press and Porter 1962; Webb and Lapresle 1964; Kaminski 1965; Lapresle and Goldstein 1969); ribonuclease (Brown 1962); myoglobin (Crumpton and Wilkinson 1965; Crumpton and Small 1967; Givas et al. 1968; Atassi 1969); tobacco mosaic virus (Spitler et al. 1970); lysozyme (Fujio et al. 1968; Bonavida et al. 1969) and staphylococcal nuclease (Omenn et al. 1970). From a variety of different studies, the approximate size of the antigenic sites on macromolecules can be assessed. These estimates are summarized in Table 1.6.

1.8. Genetic aspects of immunogenicity

Studies on the genetic control of the antibody response using chemically defined, synthetic polypeptide antigens have been carried out mainly in

TABLE 1.6
Approximate size of the combining sites of various antigens.*

Antigen	Composition of the combining site	Approximate maximal size (Å)	References
Hapten	1 small organic molecule	5–15	Pressman and Grossberg (1968)
Protein	6–12 amino acid residues	25–45	Cebra (1961); Kabat (1966); Goodman (1969)
Synthetic polypeptide	4–9 amino acid residues	20–35	Gill et al. (1963b); Sage et al. (1964); Arnon et al. (1965); Schechter et al. (1966); Van Vunakis et al. (1966); Goodman (1969). Sela (1970), Sela et al. (1970)
Carbohydrate	6 sugar residues	35	Kabat (1966)
Nucleic acid	4–5 purine or pyrimidine residues	15–20	Stollar et al. (1962)
Lipid	not known		

* The induction of antibody formation and delayed hypersensitivity can both be achieved with a DNP-heptalysine (25–30 Å) complex. Smaller molecules have been reported to induce an immune response (Table 1.3), but the form in which they act is, as yet, unclear. No information is available on the minimal molecular size necessary for the induction of tolerance.

guinea-pigs, mice, rats and rabbits; many of these studies have been reviewed recently (Herzenberg et al. 1968; McDevitt and Benacerraf 1969).* The work of Benacerraf and his colleagues in random bred guinea-pigs (Levine et al. 1963b) indicated that the ability to respond to a given antigen was transmitted as a dominant Mendelian (unigenic) trait. The same conclusion was reached by Maurer and his collaborators (Ben-Efraim and Maurer 1966) using strain 2 and strain 13 guinea-pigs and by McDevitt and his colleagues using mice (McDevitt and Sela 1965, 1967; Mozes et al. 1969). However, studies of the antibody response to insulin in the guinea-pig (Arquilla and Finn 1965), to red cells in inbred mice (Playfair 1968) and to synthetic polypeptide antigens in inbred rats (Simonian et al. 1968; Gill and Kunz 1971; Gill et al. 1970, 1971a) indicated that the genetic control was complex and probably polygenic. One way to reconcile all of the findings is to postulate

* See also Chapter 11 of this volume.

that the control mechanism behaves as a dominant unigenic trait, but that it is governed by several genes which act essentially as one unit. Different strains of rabbits make significantly different amounts of antibody following immunization with a synthetic polypeptide antigen (Gill 1965) or with streptococcal polysaccharide (Braun et al. 1969). Finally, studies of the delayed hypersensitivity reaction to synthetic polypeptides in guinea-pigs suggested that the genetic control of the antibody response and of delayed hypersensitivity may be somewhat different (Gill and Doty 1961; Schlossman et al. 1965; Ben-Efraim and Maurer 1966; Ben-Efraim et al. 1967).

The amount of antibody formed by a genetically poorly responding strain of animals can be enhanced under certain circumstances. Immunization of female rats of the poorly responding, inbred F344 strain with poly $Glu^{52}Lys^{33}Tyr^{15}$ aggregated with methylated bovine serum albumin prior to mating led to an enhanced immune response by the first and second litters in the F1 generation and in the F2 generation (Gill et al. 1971b). When poly Lys was used as the aggregating agent, increased antibody formation occurred in only the first litter of the F1 generation and in the F2 generation. In both cases, antigen was transmitted from the immunized female to her offspring, where it localized in the bone marrow and, in a few cases, in the thymus and spleen also. The transplacental passage of antigen is probably the basis for the enhanced antibody response, which is a manifestation of immunological memory.

1.9. Generalizations

When an animal is injected with an antigen, there is a balance between immunological stimulation and paralysis which depends upon the chemistry of the antigen and the genetic background of the host. The chemical properties of the antigen set the level and range of dosage that can be used in stimulating an antibody response. The antigen acts intact, and the role of antigen catabolism is to function in concert with the original dose to regulate the amount of antigen available to stimulate antibody formation. A poor immunogen is probably a molecule that induces tolerance easily, but this proposition is a difficult one to test, since the mechanism of tolerance is not understood.

The properties of a molecule minimally necessary to induce antibody formation are those quite general to macromolecules. Even biologically alien macromolecules such as vinyl polymers can elicit antibody formation; hence, all macromolecules can probably elicit antibody formation if given in the proper dosage and by the proper schedule. The quantitative control of antibody formation depends upon both the general properties and the detailed composition of the immunogen. The presence of aromatic amino acids enhances immunogenicity, and there is a particular amount necessary for optimal enhancement. Too many aromatic amino acids residues can shift the specificity of the antigen and finally decrease its ability to elicit antibody formation. Other properties, such as D-configuration or high charge, depress immunogenicity but do not abolish it. Immunogenicity is a property which may involve portions of a macromolecule different from those required for the interaction with antibody. Studies on lactic dehydrogenase isoenzymes (Rajewsky and Rottlander 1967; Rajewsky et al. 1969), tobacco mosaic virus protein (Spitler et al. 1970), flagellin (Byrt and Ada 1969; Parish and Ada 1969) and glucagon (Senyk et al. 1971) and studies on the hapten-carrier relationship (Green et al. 1968; Rajewsky et al. 1969) indicate that a portion of the macromolecule different from the antigenic determinant is involved in interaction with the immunocompetent cell. In addition, the antigenic determinant appears to involve a smaller area of the molecule than the portion required for interaction with the immunocompetent cell.

The topography of a macromolecule is crucial in its ability to provide sites reactive with the immunocompetent cell and with antibody. In theory, the topography of a given site could be made up from several different types of components and still display the same immunochemical behavior. Such a concept could explain cross-reactivity among ostensibly unrelated antigens and could provide the rationale for there being a restricted number of antibody specificities to deal with an extensive repetoire of antigens. This hypothesis finds some support in the demonstration of cross-reactivity between vinyl polymers and synthetic polypeptides, between synthetic polypeptides and proteins, and between synthetic polypeptides of different optical configuration. The surface interaction involves relatively large areas of the molecules, since the volume change occurring during the antibody-antigen reaction is quite large (Ohta et al. 1970). Finally, the immunogenicity of vinyl polymers is in the same relative order as that of their synthetic polypeptide analogues; therefore, the van der Waals contour of the molecules, whether they are vinyl polymers or synthetic polypeptides, probably affects significantly the ability of the macromolecules to interact with the immunocompetent cell and to elicit antibody formation.

One hypothesis to explain the action of antigen at the cellular level and the effects of the factors modulating the immune response is shown in Fig. 1.1.* The amount of antigen that is available to stimulate the

---

* This hypothesis is consistent with several aspects of other hypotheses about the role of antigen in the immune response (Campbell and Garvey 1963; Siskind and Benacerraf 1969).

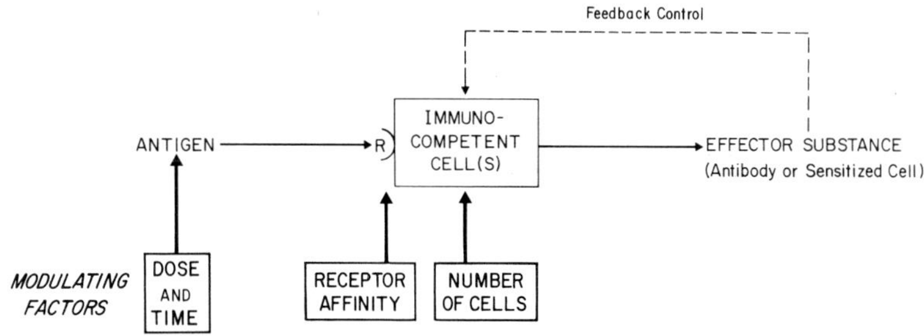

Fig. 1.1. Hypothetical scheme for the action of antigen and for the effects of the factors modulating the immune response. The hypothesis seeks to explain the various aspects of the immune response as quantitative, antigen-driven phenomena.

immunocompetent cell depends upon the dose, the time over which it is given, and the rate at which the antigen is degraded *in vivo* (Gill 1971). Aggregating the antigen would protect it from enzymatic degradation and provide for slow release over a long period of time; therefore, it would exert a dosage effect. Then, the ability of this effective concentration of antigen to stimulate an antibody response or to induce tolerance depends upon the genetically determined number of immunocompetent cells capable of reacting with the antigen and the binding affinity of the cellular receptors. The effector substances which are produced following stimulation exert a negative feed-back control. The population of immunocompetent cells capable of reacting with a given antigen and of producing antibody could be increased by periodic stimulation with the appropriate amount of antigen; in this way tolerance could be avoided. In like manner, immunological memory may be due to the continuous stimulation of the immunocompetent cell population by small amounts of antigen retained in the host. The retained antigen does not have to reside in the lymphoid tissue, but may just be released slowly from a variety of tissues. Thus, this scheme proposes to explain stimulation or tolerance on the basis of the same sequence of events which is governed by the mass action law and whose outcome depends upon multiple, interrelated equilibria.

Acknowledgment

The research carried out in the author's laboratory was supported by grants from the National Institutes of Health (HE 01771, AI 09520, K3-AM-5242 and K3-CA-5242) and from the National Science Foundation (GB-8379) and by a contract with the U.S. Army Research and Development Command (DADA 17-70-C-0046).

References

ABUELO, J. G. and Z. OVARY, 1965, J. Immunol. *95*, 113.

ADANT, M., 1930, Compt. Rend. Soc. Biol. *103*, 541.

ADLER, F. L., 1964, Progr. Allergy *8*, 41.

ALBRIGHT, J. F. and T. MAKINODAN, 1965, Dynamics of expression of competence of antibody-producing cells. *In*: J. Šterzl., ed.: Molecular and cellular basis of antibody formation. New York, Academic Press. pp. 427–446.

ALBRIGHT, J. F., T. F. OMER and J. W. DEITCHMAN, 1970, Science *167*, 196.

AMKRAUT, A. A., J. S. GARVEY and D. H. CAMPBELL, 1966, J. Exptl. Med. *124*, 293.

AMOS, D. B., ed., 1970: Human histocompatibility antigens, Federation Proc. *29*, 2010.

ANDERER, F. A. and H. D. SCHLUMBERGER, 1969, Immunochemistry *6*, 1.

ANDERSSON, B., 1969, J. Immunol. *102*, 1309.

ARNON, R. and M. SELA, 1960, Biochem. J. *75*, 103.

ARNON, R., M. SELA, E. S. RACHAMAN and D. SHAPIRO, 1969, European J. Biochem. *2*, 79.

ARNON, R., M. SELA, A. YARON and H. A. SOBER, 1965, Biochemistry *4*, 948.

ARQUILLA, E. R. and J. FINN, 1965, J. Exptl. Med. *122*, 771.

ATASSI, M. Z., 1969, Immunochemistry *6*, 801.

AXELROD, A. E., A. C. TRAKATELLIS and K. HOFMANN, 1963, Nature *197*, 146.

BAER, H., R. C. WATKINS and R. T. BOWSER, 1966, Immunochemistry *3*, 479.

BARBU, E. and J. PANIJEL, 1960, Compt. Rend. Acad. Sci. *250*, 1382.

BAUMINGER, S., I. SCHECHTER and M. SELA, 1967, Immunochemistry *4*, 169.

BAUMINGER, S. and M. SELA, 1969, Israel J. Med. Sci. *5*, 177.

BENACERRAF, B. and B. B. LEVINE, 1962, J. Exptl. Med. *115*, 1023.

BENACERRAF, B., V. NUSSENZWEIG, P. H. MAURER and W. STYLOS, 1969, Israel J. Med. Sci. *5*, 171.

BENACERRAF, B., A. OJEDA and P. H. MAURER, 1963, J. Exptl. Med. *118*, 945.

BEN-EFRAIM, S., S. FUCHS and M. SELA, 1963, Science *139*, 1222.

BEN-EFRAIM, S., S. FUCHS and M. SELA, 1967, Immunology *12*, 572.

BEN EFRAIM, S. and P. LIACOPOULOS, 1967, Immunology *12*, 517.

BEN EFRAIM, S. and P. LIACOPOULOS, 1969a, Immunology *16*, 573.

BEN-EFRAIM, S. and P. LIACOPOULOS, 1969b, Israel J. Med. Sci. *5*, 209.

BEN-EFRAIM, S. and P. LIACOPOULOS, 1969b, Israel J. Med. Sci. *5*, 209.

BEN-EFRAIM, S. and P. H. MAURER, 1966, J. Immunol. *97*, 577.

BERGLUND, G., 1965, Nature *206*, 523.

BONAVIDA, B., A. MILLER and E. E. SERCARZ, 1969, Biochemistry *8*, 968.

BOREK, F., 1968a, Methods for detection of antibody-producing cells and serum antibody. *In:* H. Sober, ed.: Handbook of biochemistry. Cleveland, Chemical Rubber Co. pp. K-19 to K-21.

BOREK, F., 1968b, Delayed-type hypersensitivity to synthetic antigens. *In*: Current Topics in Microbiology and Immunology, Vol. 43. New York, Springer-Verlag. pp. 126–161.

BOREK, F., J. KURTZ and M. SELA, 1969, Biochim. Biophys. Acta *188*, 314.

BOREK, F. and Y. STUPP, 1965, Immunochemistry *2*, 323.

BOREK, F., Y. STUPP, S. FUCHS and M. SELA, 1965a, Biochem. J. *96*, 577.

BOREK, F., Y. STUPP and M. SELA, 1965b, Science *150*, 1177.

BOREK, F., Y. STUPP and M. SELA, 1967a, Biochim. Biophys. Acta *140*, 360.

BOREK, F., Y. STUPP and M. SELA, 1967b, J. Immunol. *98*, 739.

BOYLE, W., 1969, Transplant. Proc. *1*, 491.

BRAUN, D. G., K. EICHMAN and R. M. KRAUSE, 1969, J. Exptl. Med. *129*, 809.

BRODY, N. I. and G. W. SISKIND, 1969, J. Exptl. Med. *130*, 821.

BROWN, P. C. and L. E. GLYNN, 1968, Immunology *15*, 589.

BROWN, P. C. and L. E. GLYNN, Immunology *17*, 943.

BROWN, R. K., 1962, J. Biol. Chem. *237*, 1162.

BROWN, R. K., 1963, Ann. N.Y. Acad. Sci. *103*, 754.

BROWN, R. K., M. MCEWAN, C. A. MIKORYAK and J. POLKOWSKI, 1967, J. Biol. Chem. *242*, 3007.

BRUCKNER, V., M. KATJAR, J. KOVACS, H. NAGY and J. WEIN, 1958, Tetrahedron *2*, 211.

BRUCKNER, V. and J. KOVACS, 1957, Acta Chim. Acad. Sci. Hung. *12*, 363.

BUCHANAN-DAVIDSON, D. J., E. E. DELLERT, S. E. KORNGUTH and M. A. STAHMANN, 1959a, J. Immunol. *83*, 543.

BUCHANAN-DAVIDSON, D. J., M. A. STAHMANN and E. E. DELLERT, 1959b, J. Immunol. *83*, 561.

BUCHANAN-DAVIDSON, D. J., M. A. STAHMANN, C. LAPRESLE and P. GRABAR, 1959c, J. Immunol. *83*, 552.

BYRT, P. and G. L. ADA, 1969, Immunology *17*, 503.

CAMPBELL, D. H. and J. S. GARVEY, 1963, Advan. Immunol. *3*, 261.

CARPENTER, C. B., T. J. GILL III and L. T. MANN, Jr., 1967, J. Immunol. *98*, 236.

CEBRA, J. J., 1961, J. Immunol. *86*, 190, 197, 205.

CLUTTON, R. F., C. R. HARINGTON and M. E. YUILL, 1938, Biochem. J. *32*, 1111.

CONWAY-JACOBS, A., B. SCHECHTER and M. SELA, 1970, Biochemistry *9*, 4870.

CREMER, N. E., 1963, J. Immunol. *90*, 685.

CRUMPTON, M. J. and P. A. SMALL, JR., 1967, J. Mol. Biol. *26*, 143.

CRUMPTON, M. J. and J. M. WILKINSON, 1965, Biochem. J. *94*, 545.

CUSHING, J. E. and D. H. CAMPBELL, 1957, Principles of immunology. New York, McGraw-Hill. pp. 91, 236–237.

DAVIES, D. A. L., U. HÄMMERLING and B. J. ALKINS, 1971, Immunochemistry *8*, 17.

DIETRICH, F. M., 1966, Int. Arch. Allergy *30*, 497.

DRESSER, D. W., 1962, Immunology *5*, 378.

DRESSER, D. W. and N. A. MITCHISON, 1968, Advan. Immunol. *8*, 129.

EIDINGER, D., S. A. KHAN and K. G. MILLAR, 1968, J. Exptl. Med. *128*, 1183.

FREI, W., 1928, Klin. Wschr. *7*, 539, 1026.

FREY, J. R., A. L. DE WECK and H. GELEICK, 1966, Int. Arch. Allergy *30*, 288, 385, 428, 521.

FREY, J. R., A. L. DE WECK, H. GELEICK and W. LERGIER, 1969, J. Exptl. Med. *130*, 1123.

FUCHS, S. and M. SELA, 1963, Biochem. J. *87*, 70.

FUCHS, S. and M. SELA, 1964, Biochem. J. *93*, 566.

FUJIO, H., M. IMANISHI, K. NISHIOKA and T. AMANO, 1968, Biken J. *10*, 89.

GARRO, A. J., B. F. ERLANGER and S. M. BEISER, 1971, J. Immunol. *106*, 442.

GELL, P. G. H. and B. BENACERRAF, 1961, Advan. Immunol. *1*, 319.

GELL, P. G. H. and A. M. SILVERSTEIN, 1967, J. Exptl. Med. *115*, 1037.

GERETY, R. J., R. W. FERRARESI and S. RAFFEL, 1970, J. Exptl. Med. *131*, 189.

GILL, T. J., III, 1965, J. Immunol. *95*, 542.

GILL, T. J. III, 1970, Immunochemistry *7*, 997.

GILL, T. J. III, 1971, Current Topics in Microbiology and Immunology *54*, 19.

GILL, T. J., III and P. DOTY, 1960, J. Mol. Biol. *2*, 65.

GILL, T. J., III and P. DOTY, 1961, J. Biol. Chem. *236*, 2677.

GILL, T. J., III and P. DOTY, 1962, Biochim. Biophys. Acta *60*, 450.

GILL, T. J. III, J. ENDERLE, R. N. GERMAIN and C. T. LADOULIS, 1971a, J. Immunol. *106*, 1117.

GILL, T. J., III, H. J. GOULD and P. DOTY, 1963a, Nature *197*, 746.

GILL, T. J., III. H. J. GOULD and H. W. KUNZ, 1964a, J. Biol. Chem. *239*, 3083.

GILL, T. J. III and H. W. KUNZ, 1966, Biochim. Biophys. Acta *124*, 374.

GILL, T. J., III and H. W. KUNZ, 1968, Proc. Natl. Acad. Sci. U.S. *61*, 490.

GILL, T. J. III and H. W. KUNZ, 1971, J. Immunol. *106*, 980.

GILL, T. J. III, H. W. KUNZ and C. F. BERNARD, 1971b, Science *172*, 1346.

GILL, T. J., III, H. W. KUNZ, E. FRIEDMAN and P. DOTY, 1963b, J. Biol. Chem. *238*, 108.

GILL, T. J., III, H. W. KUNZ, H. J. GOULD and P. DOTY, 1964b, J. Biol. Chem. *239*, 1107.

GILL, T. J., III, H. W. KUNZ and D. S. PAPERMASTER, 1967, J. Biol. Chem. *242*, 3308.

GILL, T. J., III, H. W. KUNZ, D. STECHSCHULTE and K. F. AUSTEN, 1970, J. Immunol. *105*, 14.

GILL, T. J., III and L. T. MANN, JR., 1966, J. Immunol. *96*, 906.

GILL, T. J., III and L. S. MATTHEWS, 1963, J. Biol. Chem. *238*, 1373.

GILL, T. J., III, D. S. PAPERMASTER, H. W. KUNZ and P. S. MARFEY, 1968a, J. Biol. Chem. *243*, 287.

GILL, T. J., III, D. S. PAPERMASTER, H. W. KUNZ and P. S. MARFEY, 1968b, The role of conformation in the structure of antigenic sites. *In*: O. J. Plescia and W. Braun, eds.: Nucleic acids in immunology. New York, Springer-Verlag. pp. 330–337.

GILL, T. J., III, D. S. PAPERMASTER and J. F. MOWBRAY, 1964c, Nature *203*, 644.

GILL, T. J., III, D. S. PAPERMASTER and J. F. MOWBRAY, 1965, J. Immunol. *95*, 794.

GIVAS, J., E. R. CENTENO, M. MANNING and A. H. SEHON, 1968, Immunochemistry *5*, 314.

GOODMAN, J. W., 1969, Immunochemistry *6*, 139.

GOODMAN, J. W. and D. E. NITECKI, 1966, Biochemistry *5*, 657.

GOTSCHLICH, E. M., I. GOLDSCHNEIDER and M. S. ARTENSTEIN, 1969, J. Exptl. Med. *129*, 1367.

GRAF, L., J. YARIV and M. M. RAPPORT, 1965, Immunochemistry *2*, 145.

GREEN, I., W. E. PAUL and B. BENACERRAF, 1967a, J. Exptl. Med. *126*, 959.

GREEN, I., W. E. PAUL and B. BENACERRAF, 1968, J. Exptl. Med. *127*, 43.

GREEN, I., P. VASSELLI and B. BENACERRAF, 1967b, J. Exptl. Med. *125*, 527.

HÄMMERLING, U., D. A. L. DAVIES and A. J. MANSTONE, 1971, Immunochemistry *8*, 7.

HEIDELBERGER, M., F. E. KENDALL and H. W. SCHERP, 1936, J. Exptl. Med. *64*, 559.

HEIDELBERGER, M., C. M. MACLEOD, S. J. KAISER and B. ROBINSON, 1946, J. Exptl. Med. *83*, 303.

HERZENBERG, L. A., H. O. MCDEVITT and L. A. HERZENBERG, 1968, Ann. Rev. Genetics *2*, 209.

HOOKER, S. B. and W. C. BOYD, 1933, J. Immunol. *24*, 141.

HOPKINS, S. J. and A. WORMALL, 1933, Biochem. J. *27*, 1706.

HOWARD, R. J., J. C. LANDON, S. F. DOUGHERTY, A. L. NOTKINS and S. E. MERGENHAGEN, 1969, J. Immunol. *102*, 266.

HUMPHREY, J. H. and M. E. YUILL, 1939, Biochem. J. *33*, 1826.

IVANOVICS, G. and V. BRUCKNER, 1937, Naturwissenschaften *25*, 250; Z. Immun.-Forsch. *90*, 304; *91*, 175.

IVANYI, P., 1970, Current Topics in Microbiology and Immunology *53*, 2.

JANEWAY, C. A., JR., 1969, Immunology *17*, 715.

JANEWAY, C. A., JR. and J. H. HUMPHREY, 1968, Immunology *14*, 225.

JANEWAY, C. A., JR. and J. H. HUMPHREY, 1969, Israel J. Med. Sci. *5*, 185.

JANEWAY, C. A., JR. and M. SELA, 1967, Immunology *13*, 29.

JASIN, H. E. and L. E. GLYNN, 1965, Immunology *8*, 95, 260.

JATON, J.-C. and M. SELA, 1968, J. Biol. Chem. *243*, 5616.

KABAT, E. A., 1956, Blood group substances. New York, Academic Press. pp. 67, 75.

KABAT, E. A., 1966, J. Immunol. *97*, 1.

KABAT, E. A., 1968, Structural concepts in immunology and immunochemistry. New York, Holt, Rinehart and Winston.

KABAT, E. A. and A. E. BEZER, 1958, Arch. Biochem. Biophys. *78*, 306.

KAHAN, B. D. and R. A. REISFELD, 1969, Transplant. Proc. *1*, 483.

KAMINSKI, M., 1965, Progr. Allergy *9*, 79.

KANTOR, F. S., A. OJEDA and B. BENACERRAF, 1963, J. Exptl. Med. *117*, 55.

KATAOKA, T. and S. NOJIMA, 1970, J. Immunol. 105, 502.

KOFFLER, D., R. I. CARR, V. AGNELLO, T. FIEZI and H. G. KUNKEL, 1969, Science *166*, 648.

KOSCIELAK, J., S. HAKOMORI and R. W. JEANLOZ, 1968, Immunochemistry *5*, 441.

KUNZ, H. W. and T. J. GILL, III, 1964, Biochim. Biophys. Acta *90*, 318.

LACOUR, F., A. M. MICHAELSON and E. NAHON, 1968, Specific antibodies to polynucleotide complexes and their reaction with nucleic acids. *In*: O. J. Plescia and W. Braun, eds.: Nucleic acids in immunology. New York, Springer-Verlag. pp. 32–46.

LANDSTEINER, K., 1945, The specificity of serological reactions, 2nd ed. Harvard Univ. Press. Reprinted in 1962 by Dover Publications, Inc., New York.

LANDSTEINER, K. and J. L. JACOBS, 1935, J. Exptl. Med. *61*, 643.

LANDSTEINER, K. and J. L. JACOBS, 1936, J. Exptl. Med. *64*, 717.

LANGE, C. F. and A. S. MARKOWITZ, 1969, Transplant. Proc. *1*, 502.

LAPRESLE, C., 1955, Ann. Inst. Pasteur *89*, 654.

LAPRESLE, C. and I. J. GOLDSTEIN, 1969, J. Immunol. *102*, 733.

LAPRESLE, C. and T. WEBB, 1960, Ann. Inst. Pasteur *99*, 523.

LESKOWITZ, S., 1963a, Nature *199*, 85.

LESKOWITZ, S., 1963b, J. Exptl. Med. *117*, 909.

LESKOWITZ, S., 1963c, Nature *199*, 291.

LESKOWITZ, S., V. E. JONES and S. J. ZAK, 1966, J. Exptl. Med. *123*, 229.

LESKOWITZ, S. and S. J. ZAK, 1966, Nature *211*, 246.

LESKOWITZ, S., H. B. RICHERSON and H. J. SCHWARTZ, 1970, Immunochemistry *7*, 949.

LEVINE, B. B., A. OJEDA and B. BENACERRAF, 1963a, Nature *200*, 544.

LEVINE, B. B., A. OJEDA and B. BENACERRAF, 1963b, J. Exptl. Med. *118*, 953.

LEVINE, L., W. T. MURAKAMI, H. VAN VUNAKIS and L. GROSSMAN, 1960, Proc. Natl. Acad. Sci. U.S. *46*, 1038.

LEVINE, L. and B. D. STROLLER, 1968, Progr. Allergy *12*, 161.

MACLEOD, C. M., 1965, The pneumococci. *In*: R. J. Dubos and J. G. Hirsch, eds.: Bacterial and mycotic infections of man, 4th ed. Philadelphia, Lippincott. p. 397.

MANN, D. L., G. N. ROGENTINE, J. L. FAHEY and S. G. NATHENSON, 1969, Transplant. Proc. *1*, 494.

MANSON, L. and T. SIMMONS, 1969, Transplant. Proc. *1*, 498.

MARCUS, D. M., 1969, New Eng. J. Med. *280*, 994.

MARRACK, J. R., 1938, The chemistry of antigens and antibodies. Medical Research Council Special Report No. 230. London, H. M. Stationary Office.

MAURER, P. H., 1956, J. Immunol. *77*, 105.

MAURER, P. H., 1957a, Proc. Soc. Exptl. Biol. Med. *96*, 394.

MAURER, P. H., 1957b, J. Immunol. *79*, 84.

MAURER, P. H., 1962, J. Immunol. *88*, 330.

MAURER, P. H., 1963a, J. Immunol. *90*, 493.

MAURER, P. H., 1963b, Ann. N.Y. Acad. Sci. *103*, 549.

MAURER, P. H., 1963c, Proc. Soc. Exptl. Biol. Med. *113*, 553.

MAURER, P. H., 1964, Progr. Allergy *8*, 1.

MAURER, P. H., 1965, J. Exptl. Med. *121*, 339.

MAURER, P. H., B. F. GERULAT and P. PINCHUCK, 1963a, J. Immunol. *90*, 381.

MAURER, P. H., B. F. GERULAT and P. PINCHUCK, 1966, J. Immunol. *97*, 306.

MAURER, P. H. and M. HEIDELBERGER, 1951, J. Am. Chem. Soc. *73*, 2076.

MAURER, P. H., R. LOWY and C. KIERNEY, 1963b, Science *139*, 1061.

MAURER, P. H., P. PINCHUCK and B. F. GERULAT, 1965, Proc. Soc. Exptl. Biol. Med. *118*, 1113.

MAURER, P. H., D. SUBRAHMANYAM and E. KATCHALSKI, 1959, J. Immunol. *83*, 193.

MCDEVITT, H. O., 1968, J. Immunol. *100*, 485.

MCDEVITT, H. O. and B. BENACERRAF, 1969, Advan. Immunol. *11*, 31.

MCDEVITT, H. O. and M. SELA, 1965, J. Exptl. Med. *122*, 517.

MCDEVITT, H. O. and M. SELA, 1967, J. Exptl. Med. *126*, 969.

MCMASTER, P. R. B., A. L. SCHADE, J. F. FINERTY, M. B. CALDWELL and B. PRESCOTT, 1970, Federation Proc. *29*, 812.

MCPHERSON, J. C., J. R. CLAMP and A. J. MANSTONE, 1971, Immunochemistry *8*, 225.

MEDVECZKY, A. and A. UHROVITZ, 1931, Z. Immun.-Forsch. *72*, 256.

MICHEEL, F. and E. SCHALLENBERG, 1952, Z. physiol. Chem. *291*, 87.

MIHAESCO, C. and M. SELIGMANN, 1968, J. Exptl. Med. *127*, 431.

MILLS, J. A. and E. HABER, 1963, J. Immunol. *91*, 536.

MOZES, E., H. O. MCDEVITT, J.-C. JATON and M. SELA, 1969, J. Exptl. Med. *130*, 493.

MURPHY, T. M. and S. E. MILLS, 1965, Biochem. Biophys. Res. Commun. *18*, 843.

OHTA, Y., T. J. GILL III and C. S. LEUNG, 1970, Biochemistry, *9*, 2708.

OMENN, G. S. and T. J. GILL III, 1967, J. Biol. Chem. *241*, 4899.

OMENN, G. S., D. A. ONTJES and C. B. ANFINSEN, 1970, Biochemistry *9*, 304, 313; Nature *225*, 189.

OSBORNE, T. B., L. B. MENDEL and I. F. HARRIS, 1905, Am. J. Physiol. *14*, 259.

OVARY, Z., 1958, Progr. Allergy *5*, 459.

PAPERMASTER, D. S., T. J. GILL, III and W. F. ANDERSON, 1965, J. Immunol. *95*, 804.

PARISH, C. R. and G. L. ADA, 1969, Immunology *17*, 153.

PAUL, W. E., B. BENACERRAF, G. W. SISKIND, E. A. GOIDL and R. A. REISFELD, 1969, J. Exptl. Med. *130*, 77.

PAUL, W. E., G. W. SISKIND, B. BENACERRAF and Z. OVARY, 1967, J. Immunol. *99*, 760.

PLAYFAIR, J. H. L., 1968, Immunology *15*, 35.

PLESCIA, O. J. and W. BRAUN, 1967, Advan. Immunol. *6*, 231.

PLESCIA, O. J. and W. BRAUN, eds., 1968, Nucleic acids in immunology. New York, Springer-Verlag.

PLESCIA, O. J., W. BRAUN and N. C. PALCZUK, 1964, Proc. Natl. Acad. Sci. U.S. *52*, 279.

PLESCIA, O. J., N. C. PALCZUK, W. BRAUN and E. CORA-FIGUEROA, 1965, Science *148*, 1102.

POLMAR, S. H. and A. G. STEINBERG, 1964, Science *145*, 928.

PRESS, E. M. and R. R. PORTER, 1962, Biochem. J. *83*, 172.

PRESSMAN, D. and A. L. GROSSBERG, 1968, The structural basis of antibody specificity. New York, Benjamin.

QUENG, J. T., C. D. DUKES and J. P. MCGOVERN, 1965, J. Allergy *36*, 505.

RADOVICH, J. and D. W. TALMAGE, 1967, Science *158*, 512.

RAJEWSKY, K. and E. ROTTLANDER, 1967, Tolerance specificity and the immune response to lactic dehydrogenase isoenzymes. *In*: L. Frisch, ed.: Cold Spring Harbor Symposia on Quantitative Biology. New York. Vol. XXXII, pp. 547–554.

RAJEWSKY, K., V. SCHIRRMACHER, S. NASE and N. K. JERNE, 1969, J. Exptl. Med. *129*, 1131.

RAPPORT, M. M. and L. GRAF, 1969, Progress in Allergy *13*, 273.

RAZIN, S., B. PRESCOTT and R. A. CHANOCK, 1970, Proc. Natl. Acad. Sci. U.S. *67*, 590.

REICHLIN, M., E. BUCCI, E. ANTONINI, J. WYMAN and A. ROSSI-FANELLI, 1964, J. Mol. Biol. *9*, 785.

RIMON, A., D. TEITELBAUM, S. BAUMINGER and M. SELA, 1967, Immunochemistry *4*, 505.

ROELANTS, G. E., G. SENYK and J. W. GOODMAN, 1969, Israel J. Med. Sci. *5*, 196.

RÜDE, E., E. MOZES and M. SELA, 1968, Biochemistry 7, 2971.

SAGE, H. J., G. F. DEUTSCH, G. D. FASMAN and L. LEVINE, 1964, Immunochemistry *1*, 133.

SALVIN, S. B. and H.-L. LIAUW, 1967, Int. Arch. Allergy *31*, 366.

SALVIN, S. B. and R. F. SMITH, 1960, J. Exptl. Med. *111*, 465.

SCHECHTER, I., 1965, Biochim. Biophys. Acta *104*, 303.

SCHECHTER, I., 1968, J. Exptl. Med. *127*, 237.

SCHECHTER, I., S. BAUMINGER, M. SELA, D. NACHTIGAL and M. FELDMAN, 1964, Immunochemistry *1*, 249.

SCHECHTER, I., B. SCHECHTER and M. SELA, 1966, Biochim. Biophys. Acta *127*, 438.

SCHECHTER, I., B. SCHECHTER and M. SELA, 1970, J. Biol. Chem. *245*, 1438.

SCHECHTER, I. and M. SELA, 1967, Biochemistry 6, 897.

SCHLOSSMAN, S. F., S. BEN-EFRAIM, A. YARON and H. A. SOBER, 1966, J. Exptl. Med. *123*, 1083.

SCHLOSSMAN, S. F. and H. LEVINE, 1967, J. Immunol. *98*, 211.

SCHLOSSMAN, S. F., A. YARON, S. BEN-EFRAIM and H. A. SOBER, 1965, Biochemistry, *4*, 1638.

SCHNEIDER, C. H. and A. L. DE WECK, 1967, Immunochemistry *4*, 331.

SCHUR, P. H. and M. MONROE, 1969, Proc. Natl. Acad. Sci. U.S. *63*, 1108.

SCHUR, P. H., L. A. MOROZ and H. G. KUNKEL, 1967, Immunochemistry *4*, 447.

SCHWARTZ, E. F. and B. D. STOLLAR, 1969, Biochem. Biophys. Res. Commun. *35*, 115.

SEAMAN, E., L. LEVINE and H. VAN VUNAKIS, 1965, Biochemistry *4*, 1312.

SELA, M., 1966, Advan. Immunol. *5*, 29.

SELA, M., 1969, Science *166*, 1365.

SELA, M., 1970, Ann. N.Y. Acad. Sci. *169*, 23.

SELA, M. and R. ARNON, 1960a, Biochem. J. *75*, 91.

SELA, M. and R. ARNON, 1960b, Biochem. J. *77*, 394.

SELA, M. and R. ARNON 1960c, Biochim. Biophys. Acta *40*, 382.

SELA, M. and S. FUCHS, 1963, Biochim. Biophys. Acta *74*, 796.

SELA, M. and S. FUCHS, 1964, On the role of charge and optical activity in antigenicity. *In*: J. Šterzl, ed.: Molecular and cellular basis of antibody formation. New York, Academic Press. pp. 43–56.

SELA, M., S. FUCHS and R. ARNON, 1962, Biochem. J. *85*, 223.

SELA, M., S. FUCHS and M. FELDMAN, 1963, Science *139*, 342.

SELA, M. and F. HAUROWITZ, 1958, Experientia *14*, 91.

SELA, M. and E. KATCHALSKI, 1956, Science *123*, 1129.

SELA, M. and E. MOZES, 1966, Proc. Natl. Acad. Sci. U.S. *55*, 445.

SELA, M., B. SCHECHTER, I. SCHECHTER and F. BOREK, 1967, Antibodies to sequential and conformational determinants. *In*: L. Frisch, ed.: Cold Spring Harbor Symposia on Quantitative Biology. New York. Vol. XXXII, pp. 537–545.

SELIGMANN, M. and C. MIHAESCO, 1967, Studies on the structure of human IgM globulins. *In*: J. Killander, ed.: Gamma globulins. Nobel symposium *3*. New York, Interscience. pp. 169–185.

SELIGMANN, M., C. MIHAESCO and G. MESHAKA, 1966, Science *154*, 790.

SENYK, G., D. NITEIKI and J. W. GOODMAN, 1971, Science *171*, 407.

SILVERSTEIN, A. M. and P. G. H. GELL, 1962, J. Exptl. Med. *115*, 1053.

SIMONIAN, S. J., T. J. GILL, III and S. N. GERSHOFF, 1968, J. Immunol. *101*, 730.

SINGER, S. J. and F. M. RICHARDS, 1959, J. Biol. Chem. *234*, 2911.

SISKIND, G. W. and B. BENACERRAF, 1969, Advan. Immunol. *10*, 1.

SPITLER, L., E. BENJAMINI, J. D. YOUNG, H. KAPLAN and H. H. FUDENBERG, 1970, J. Exptl. Med. *131*, 133.

STAHMANN, M. A., C. LAPRESLE, D. J. BUCHANAN-DAVIDSON and P. GRABAR, 1959, J. Immunol. *83*, 534.

STAHMANN, M. A., H. TSUYUKI, K. WEINKE, C. LAPRESLE and P. GRABAR, 1955, Compt. Rend. Acad. Sci. *241*, 1528.

STEINBERG, A. D., S. BARON and N. TALAL, 1969, Proc. Natl. Acad. Sci. U.S. *63*, 1102.

STEINBERG, A. D., G. G. DALEY and N. TALAL, 1970, Science *167*, 870.

STOLLAR, D., L. LEVINE, H. I. LEHRER and H. VAN VUNAKIS, 1962, Proc. Natl. Acad. Sci. U.S. *48*, 874.

STUPP, Y., and M. SELA, 1967, Biochim. Biophys. Acta *140*, 349.

SUMMERELL, J. M., and D. A. L. DAVIS, 1969, Transplant. Proc. *1*, 479.

SUSKIND, S. R., M. L. WICKHAM and M. CARSIOTIS, 1963, Ann. N.Y. Acad. Sci. *103*, 1106.

TORII, M., E. A. KABAT and A. E. BEZER, 1964, J. Exptl. Med. *120*, 13.

UNGAR-WARON, H., E. HURWITZ, J.-C. JATON and M. SELA, 1967, Biochim. Biophys. Acta *138*, 513.

VAN VUNAKIS, H., J. KAPLAN, H. LEHRER and L. LEVINE, 1966, Immunochemistry *3*, 393.

VOSS, E. W., JR., K. CORLEY and L. H. HUANG, 1969, Immunochemistry *6*, 361.

WALLACE, S. P., B. F. ERLANGER and S. M. BEISER, 1971, Biochemistry *10*, 679.

WATERSON, R. H., 1970, Science *170*, 1108.

WEBB, T. and C. LAPRESLE, 1964, Biochem. J. *91*, 24.

YANOFSKY, C., 1963, Ann. N.Y. Acad. Sci. *103*, 1067.

YARON, A. and S. F. SCHLOSSMAN, 1968, Biochemistry *7*, 2673.

YOKOYAMA, M., E. G. TRAMS and R. O. BRADY, 1962, Proc. Soc. Exptl. Biol. Med. *111*, 350.

YOKOYAMA, M., E. G. TRAMS and R. O. BRADY, 1963, J. Immunol. *90*, 372.

CHAPTER 2

Molecular size and shape of antigens

FELIX BOREK

Department of Microbiology and Immunology, Albert Einstein College of Medicine, Bronx, New York, N.Y.

2.1. Introduction

In the early days of immunology most of the antigens commonly studied were particulate ones such as bacteria or blood cells. A major group of soluble substances with immunizing properties were toxins of bacterial, animal and plant origin (Zinsser et al. 1940, pp. 78–105) and, eventually some non-toxic bacterial extracts. As the chemical nature of these substances became gradually unravelled, it appeared obvious that the great majority of them were proteins, simple or linked to lipids and/or to carbohydrates, whereas some of them were polysaccharides (ibid., pp. 40–41). These findings gave rise to a generally accepted view that all antigenic substances are of macromolecular (or colloidal) nature and, consequently, that these materials owe their immunogenic properties to their large molecular size. This view, supported by overwhelming experimental evidence, persisted until recently and only in the past decade did it become known that there are certain low-molecular substances which, at least under some conditions, are capable of inducing immunization as well as eliciting immune reactions *in vivo* and *in vitro*.

In this chapter an attempt will be made to review and discuss the findings reported in literature of the past 50 years or so which have a bearing on the question of the macromolecular nature of antigens and, in part at least, on its possible relation to the mechanism of immune response.

2.2. Particulate vs. soluble antigens

Antigens were defined by Landsteiner (1945) as substances 'inciting the formation of and reacting with antibodies'. Studies on alcoholic and ether extracts of erythrocytes and of some bacteria revealed the existence of certain lipoid substances, capable of reacting with antibodies prepared by immunization with whole cells, but incapable of inducing by themselves the formation of antibodies, or capable of this only to a slight extent (ibid., pp. 100–101). Landsteiner (1921) proposed the term 'haptens' for substances of this type. He was able to restore the original immunizing capacity of haptens, such as the heterogenetic substance of Forssman hapten, by mixing them with serum proteins (Landsteiner and Simms 1923). Gonzalez and Armangué (1931) showed that the same objective could be achieved by replacing serum proteins by an inert inorganic adsorbent, kaolin. This finding was confirmed by Landsteiner and Jacobs (1931/32) who also demonstrated that haemolytic antibodies could be produced by injecting a mixture of the Forssman hapten and a suspension of collodion particles. They were also able to produce agglutinins to *Vibrio cholerae* by the injection of the specific lipid substance (obtained by alcohol extraction of the microorganism), adsorbed to charcoal. The immunogenicity of slightly antigenic peptic digest of coagulated sheep serum was markedly increased after its adsorption to charcoal or alum (Jacobs 1934). Similar results were obtained with a brain-derived hapten by Plaut and Rudy (1933). Collodion particles were found by Zozaya (1931) to enhance the immunogenic power of a polysaccharide from *Bacillus anthracis*.

Some information about the possible mechanism of the enhancement of the immune response to weakly antigenic soluble substances by adsorbing the latter to colloidal particles, was supplied by the studies on the immunization with diphtheria toxin. Ramon (1925) observed that the immunizing power of diphtheria toxoid was increased by mixing it with tapioca before injection. He suggested that this improvement was due to slower absorption and possibly slower elimination of the toxoid which prolonged the contact between the antigen and the host, apparently necessary for the proper stimulation of the immunologic system of the latter. Glenny et al. (1926) found that the effectiveness of diphtheria toxin as antigen could be increased in a number of ways including the use of an emulsion of the toxin-antitoxin precipitate, of toxoid precipitated with dilute acetic acid and, most strikingly of all, of toxoid precipitated with alum. Glenny postulated that in all these cases the immunogenic efficiency of the soluble antigen was dependent on its slow dissociation from the insoluble complex in which it had been deposited in the host. Experimental evidence supporting this view was obtained from the experiments of Glenny et al. (1931) in which some guinea-pigs were injected intradermally with toxoid alone and others with alum-toxoid. After three days a portion of the skin containing the injection site was excised from each animal, emulsified and injected into normal guinea-pigs. The recipients of the skin of the alum-toxoid injected guinea-pigs were succesfully immunized, whereas those receiving the skin of the guinea-pigs injected with toxoid alone, were not. The authors conclude that toxoid alone injected into an animal is so rapidly eliminated that very little is available to exert a continuous stimulus. In contrast, the increased antigenic efficiency of alum-toxoid is the consequence of its slow absorption and elimination. The same investigators found that other precipitants such as calcium chloride, colloidal ferric hydroxide or tungstic acid, act in a similar manner to alum. Similar conclusions about the difference in the rates of elimination of free and alum-bound proteins were made by Talmage and Dixon (1953) on the basis of their studies of rabbits injected subcutaneously with ^{131}I-labelled bovine serum albumin.

Consistent with the above findings have been the observations of Uhlenhuth and Remy (1938) on increasing the antigenic power of glycogen and starch by adsorption to alum as well as those of Boyd and Malkiel (1940) on the enhancement of the immunogenicity of haemoglobin by adsorbing it to bacterial cells. The results reported by Mudd and Wiener (1942) showing that intact streptococci produce a better antibody response directed to soluble protein components of these organisms than do the soluble proteins alone, belong to the same category. An additional possibility here is that the presence of adjuvant-like substances in bacterial cells may contribute to the improvement of the immunogenic power of soluble antigens.

Neter et al. (1964) found that intravenous injections of rabbits with soluble antigens from enteric bacteria resulted in minimal antibody formation or none at all. On the other hand, when the immunization was carried out with the same antigens after they had been attached *in vitro* to autologous, isologous or heterologous erythrocytes or to L cells, good antibody response was observed.

Recently there have been interesting applications of the general observation that by increasing the particle size of certain soluble substances it is possible to convert them into more effective immunogens. It has been found, for example, that venoms of certain snakes contain toxic fractions which are poor antigens and as a result the antivenom sera lack the capacity to neutralize the toxic activity of the venom (Piantanida and Muič 1954). This discrepancy has been attributed in part to the low molecular weight of the toxins; attempts to adsorb the latter to aluminum phosphate gel were unsuccessful (Carey and Wright 1960). Kochwa et al. (1959) immunized rabbits with whole venom of *Vipera palestinae* and then tried to boost them with injections of the neurotoxic fraction of the venom; the antitoxin titre was raised but not to a sufficient level. Moroz et al. (1963) utilized the electropositive nature of the neurotoxin by binding the latter to carboxymethylcellulose resin. The soluble form of the toxin-resin complex was found to be non-toxic and highly immunogenic in rabbits giving antisera which neutralized specifically the neurotoxic component of viper venom. The authors interpreted the enhancement of toxin immunogenicity by resin binding as reflecting the increase in molecular weight of the antigen.

Rabbits immunized with human fibrinopeptide B (mol. wt. 1,400), coated on polymethylacrylate particles of $0.6\,\mu$ diameter, produced antibodies against the peptide (Berglund 1965). Olovnikov and Gurvich (1966) obtained a marked enhancement in the production of rabbit antibodies to horse γ-globulin by using for immunization globulin covalently coupled to a particulate cellulose derivative. Rabbits immunized with thyroglobulin bound to acrylic resin particles produced IgM antibody with a titre 20 times higher than animals immunized with thyroglobulin alone (Torrigiani and Roitt 1965). Keyhole limpet haemocyanin (KLH), a protein of 7.5 million molecular weight, was shown by Dixon et al. (1966) to be a powerful antigen in rabbits, but a poor antigen in rats, when injected once in a soluble form. Gallily and Garvey (1968) found that soluble KLH failed to produce measurable anti KLH serum antibody in mice after one injection. However, when KLH coated on bentonite particles was used for immunization, it behaved as a potent immunogen resulting in the formation of antibodies in high titres in mice as well as in rats. The authors compared the uptake of soluble and particulate ^{35}S-KLH by mouse peritoneal macrophages *in vitro*. Both forms of the labelled antigen were taken up by the macrophages, but with a different degree of efficiency. The fraction of ^{35}S-KLH taken up by the cells was four times higher for the particulate than for the soluble form. The authors state that these findings strongly suggest that the enhanced phagocytosis of the particulate antigen might be correlated with increased antibody response.*

On the other hand, immunization of guinea-pigs and rabbits with particulate conjugates containing bovine plasma albumin and diphtheria toxoid covalently bound to polystyrene (Steele 1965), did not result in an enhanced production of antibodies against the proteins used, although studies with ^{125}I-labelled proteins showed that significant amounts of the insoluble protein-resin conjugates persisted at the intramuscular injection sites for considerably longer periods of time than the soluble proteins alone. Steele concludes that 'mere persistence of sizeable amounts of antigen at the injection site does not in itself lead to an

---

* The significance of the phagocytosis of antigen in the induction of immune response is discussed in Chapter 10 of this volume.

augmentation of circulating antibody.' The author suggests that the lack of enhancing effect in this instance of employing particulate instead of soluble forms of antigen, may be caused by a paralysing effect of the large amount of antigen fixed to polystyrene. This interpretation is supported by histological evidence of antigen-antibody reaction at the injection site (Steele and Rack 1965).

Kochwa et al. (1967) studied the effects of adsorbing human γ-globulin (HGG) molecules to polystyrene particles of av. diameter 220 mμ on the molecular structure and immunogenicity of globulin. The authors found that the adsorption process resulted in unfolding of HGG molecules as expressed in an increased number of titrable histidine and amino groups. This structural change of human globulin was accompanied by its increased immunogenicity in rabbits. As the density of the adsorbed protein molecules on the particle surface increased, the number of titrable groups decreased indicating less molecular unfolding. This resulted in a lower capacity of the particulate IgG to induce the formation of anti-light chain antibodies, but the production of anti-heavy chain antibodies was unimpaired and the titre of total anti-HGG antibodies remained unchanged.

Another approach to the modification of the particle size of antigen with the aim of affecting its immunogenic power has been the separation of macromolecular substances into fractions corresponding to different states of aggregation. Dresser (1961) reported that CBA mice could not be immunized by injections of saline solutions of bovine γ-globulin (BGG) which had been freed of all particulate matter by centrifugation at 20,000–30,000 g. The same particulate-free fraction was later shown to induce immune paralysis (tolerance) in CBA mice (Dresser 1962). Fractionation of BGG into paralysing (major) and immunizing (minor) components was also accomplished by the use of DEAE-cellulose column. Studies with ^{131}I-labelled fractions showed that the biological half-life in mice of the paralysing component is longer than that of the immunizing one (Dresser 1963). The author suggests that a component of the particulate antigen not involved in its immunological specificity is responsible for the initiation of immune response. In its absence the aggregate-free antigen is tolerogenic unless supplemented by an adjuvant.* Dresser further argues that assuming the existence of two kinds of antigen receptors on immunocompetent cells, one responsible for the induction of immunity and the other for immune tolerance, it is possible to visualize a competition between receptors of these two kinds

---

* The role of adjuvants in the induction of immune response is discussed in Chapter 4 of this volume.

for antigen. Most antigens apparently have sufficient 'adjuvanticity' to open the path leading to immunization; the paralysing component of BGG seems to be an exception.

Similar results were obtained by Biro and Garcia (1965) who studied the immunological properties of aggregated and aggregate-free fractions of HGG, obtained after heating at 63° and centrifugation at 105,000 g. Rabbits injected intravenously with aggregated HGG produced large amounts of anti-HGG antibodies, whereas those injected with aggregate-free HGG produced no detectable antibodies and became immunologically unresponsive to HGG. ^{131}I-labelled aggregated HGG disappeared from the blood faster than aggregate-free HGG, presumably due to a more rapid phagocytosis. Aggregated HGG accumulated in the spleen, whereas aggregate-free HGG did not. In comparing their results with those of Dresser the authors suggest that the property called by Dresser 'adjuvanticity' may be conferred on γ-globulin by aggregation.

Brown et al. (1970) reported that aggregated HGG, in contrast to soluble HGG, when injected intradermally into guinea-pigs, localized strongly in the germinal centres and in the medullary and sinusoid macrophages of the draining lymph nodes.

Recently a clinical application of the above findings was reported by Butler et al. (1969) in which transplant patients were pretreated with aggregate-free horse γ-globulin and thus made immunotolerant to subsequent injections of horse γ-globulin containing antilymphocyte antibody used in immunosuppressive treatment.

An interesting example of this relation between the size of a particulate antigen and its ability to immunize was provided by the studies of Dietrich and Dukor (1967) in which erythrocytes of several animal species were tested for their immunogenicity in mice. Significant differences in red cell antigenicity were reflected in the dose-antibody response curves in which the antigen dosage was based on *total cell surface* rather than on *total cell numbers*.

The size of the particulate antigen, however, is not always the principal factor which determines whether a primary exposure of the host to that antigen will result in immunization or in another immunological state. This has been clearly shown by Battisto and Bloom (1966a, b) who induced specific immune unresponsiveness to a haptenic substance, picryl chloride and to a protein, BGG, in guinea-pigs by injecting them intravenously with particulate conjugates of picryl or BGG, respectively, covalently coupled to autologous or homologous cells such as spleen cells, peritoneal white cells or erythrocytes. The treatment affected the capacity of the animals to develop delayed type hypersensitivity and to form circulating antibodies to the hapten or antigen in question.

Neither viability nor integrity of the coupled cells was essential to tolerance induction; heat-killed picrylated spleen cells were found to be as effective as live cells and picrylated erythrocyte stromata could be used instead of intact cell conjugates. On the other hand intravenous injections of soluble picrylated plasma proteins or of the particulate picryl-DEAE-cellulose (Battisto, personal communication) were ineffective in the induction of unresponsiveness to picryl chloride. The authors comment that it is not certain whether hapten and antigen must always be associated with cell membranes to induce tolerance, but their persistence in this form during the period of attempted immunization may be important for the maintenance of unresponsive state.

Induction of specific unresponsiveness to a hapten has been recently accomplished by the use of a hapten-carrier conjugate which is not only highly insoluble but also incapable of being phagocytosed in the animal body (Battisto and Borek 1968). When guinea pigs were implanted intraperitoneally with fragments of picrylated polyurethane sponge, they showed no significant immune reactivity to the picryl hapten; most of the animals showed a lack of response, by delayed sensitivity or antibody formation, to a subsequent attempted sensitization with picryl chloride, whereas they could be immunized with an unrelated antigen. Control animals, implanted with uncoupled sponge fragments, responded normally to sensitization with picryl chloride. Available evidence suggests that the tolerogenic activity of the implanted hapten-coupled sponge may be related to the accumulation of peritoneal white cells at the sponge surface (Borek and Battisto 1971). The above results are consistent with the view that interaction of a hapten (or antigen) with the surface of the cells involved in immune response may be sufficient for the induction of immune unresponsiveness, but not for immunization of the host (e.g., see review by Leskowitz 1967).

Thus it is evident that under certain circumstances the use of insolubilized antigen may result in immunological unresponsiveness rather than in an enhanced immunization.

Attempts have been reported aiming at increasing the immunogenicity of tumour cells by coupling them *in vitro* to soluble antigens. The resulting conjugates have been injected into the hosts in the hope of stimulating their immune response to both the new and the old antigenic determinants on the cell surface and thus causing tumour regression. Czajkowski et al. (1967) claimed that malignant tumours regressed in 2 out of 14 patients injected with autologous cancer cells coupled to rabbit globulin. Augustin et al. (1969) coupled Ehrlich ascites cells, before or after x-irradiation *in vitro*, to lysozyme, haemocyanin or R-salt while keeping the cells viable. Experiments on mice and rats showed that x-irradiation of tumour cells had much more effect on increasing the immunogenicity of the latter than coupling them to strong soluble antigens such as haemocyanin. The authors sum up their results by stating that 'even the most excellent surface antigens did not increase protective immunity against cancer cells and in a number of instances tumour enhancement resulted.' Nevertheless it is possible that there may be other ways to stimulate immune response against tumours that have not been tried as yet.*

2.3. *Proteins and proteinoid antigens*

2.3.1. *Molecular size and shape of antigen: factors in immunity and immune tolerance*

Most proteins are distinguished by their relatively large molecular size and by the complexity of their structure. It has been established that the primary structure of proteins determines their most stable three-dimensional configuration and, thereby, their molecular shape (e.g., see Epstein et al. 1963; Anfinsen 1964; Freedman and Sela 1966). It has been also recognized that the specific immunologic reactivity of antigen is located at certain sites of the molecular surface area, known as antigenic determinants. The latter determine also the specificity of the antibody to be formed. Proteins, because of their structural complexity, usually possess more than one type of antigenic determinants and therefore they frequently induce formation of varying amounts of antibodies of different specificities. Sela (1969) uses the term 'immunopotent' for determinants causing the production of specific antibodies in high concentration, in contradistinction to the 'immunosilent' ones which are relatively ineffective under the given circumstances. Conversion of immunopotent into immunosilent determinants and *vice versa* can be accomplished by chemical alteration (Boyd 1956, pp. 117–124).

The relation between the three-dimensional structure of proteins and their immunogenic properties has been shown, for example, in the studies on the immunological consequences of protein denaturation.

Denaturation, whether by physical or by chemical treatment, is known to disrupt the three-dimensional structure of protein molecules, with the unfolding and uncoiling of peptides chains. In globular proteins there is a change to more elongated or fibrous structures. Occasionally dissociation of molecules into smaller units is observed (Putnam 1953).

---

* Various aspects of cancer immunity are discussed in Chapter 16 of this volume.

A number of studies, reported over the past 60 years, involved a comparison between the immunological properties of native and denatured globular proteins such as ovalbumin, for instance. Among the denaturing agents used were heat (Obermayer and Pick 1906; Schmidt 1908; Furth 1925; Muller 1933; Hirata and Campbell 1965), acid, alkali or alcohol (Landsteiner and Barron 1917; Wu et al. 1927; Macpherson and Heidelberger 1940, 1945), sonic vibration (Flosdorf and Chambers 1935), ultraviolet irradiation (Jonesco-Mihaiesti and Baroni 1910; Doerr and Maldavan 1911), photooxidation (Smetana and Shemin 1941), concentrated urea (Erickson and Neurath 1943, 1945; Martin et al. 1943) and nitrous acid (Maurer and Heidelberger 1951). A typical finding in these studies has been that the denaturation of proteins results in a decrease of their immunogenicity and in an alteration of their antigenic specificities, presumably due to the appearance of new determinants on the molecular surface. A correlation was made in some cases between the extent of these immunological changes and the corresponding degree of denaturation (e.g., Macpherson and Heidelberger 1945; Maurer and Heidelberger 1951). Denatured proteins were used to induce the formation of antibodies which reacted well with the immunizing antigens and occasionally equally well (e.g., Obermayer and Pick 1906), but usually not nearly as well with the native antigens. Conversely, no reactions occurred between the denatured antigens and antibodies prepared against the native proteins. A drastic heat treatment of rabbit serum proteins resulted in the loss of their antigenic species-specificity so that they became immunogenic in the rabbit (Uwazumi 1934). Tenbroeck (1914) reported that treatment of ovalbumin with dilute alkali completely abolished its capacity to elicit formation of antibodies, even those with altered specificity. On the other hand, a partial reversal of the denaturation of horse serum albumin yielded a protein antigenically indistinguishable from the native one (Miller 1933). Horse and bovine serum albumins, denatured by treatment with urea and then regenerated by the removal of the denaturing agent, showed a decrease in immunogenicity as compared with the native proteins, but reacted equally well with antibodies formed against the native and the denatured albumin (Erickson and Naurath 1943; Martin et al. 1943). An analogous treatment of horse γ-globulin did not impair the immunogenic power of the latter and even enhanced the immunogenicity of antibody globulin, presumably by making it particulate (Erickson and Neurath 1945). Furthermore, heat-denatured, insolubilized bovine serum albumin (BSA) consisting of particles $1-2\ \mu$ in diameter, was found to produce increased primary and secondary immune responses in rabbits while retaining the original antigenic specificity (Hirata and Campbell 1965; Hirata and Sussdorf

1966).* Less insoluble BSA than soluble BSA was needed to induce a detectable primary response. Moreover, immunization with insoluble BSA resulted in a shorter antibody induction period, the shift from the production of 19S to that of 7S antibody occurring more abruptly and earlier after antigen administration than in the case of soluble BSA (Draper and Hirata 1968). Lindqvist and Bauer (1966) found that aggregated BSA induced in rabbits a consistently higher 19S antibody response than did nonaggregated albumin. Recently Parkhouse and Dutton (1967) observed an unequivocal increase in the immunogenicity of BSA following its physical alteration by heating. This was tested *in vitro* by the antigen-specific stimulation of DNA synthesis in spleen cell suspensions from immunized rabbits. BSA preparations treated with urea of guanidine hydrochloride were at least as stimulating as the native protein and in some cases, more so.

Benacerraf et al. (1956) showed that denaturation of protein by various agents including heat increased the rate of their phagocytosis in the liver and other organs after injection into animals. Lang and Ada (1967) found that ^{125}I-labelled heat-denatured human serum albumin, when injected into the footpads of rats, was trapped in the medullary macrophages of popliteal and aortic lymph nodes to a much greater extent than the unmodified protein.

It is known that the rupture of disulphide bonds in proteins molecules frequently alters their three-dimensional structure and may also result in their fragmentation (see 2.3.2). Reductive cleavage of the disulphide bridges in serum albumin changed drastically the antigenic specificity of the latter (Blumenthal 1936). Alkali-denatured ribonuclease reacted poorly with antibody to the native protein, whereas ribonuclease with disulphide bridges broken by oxidation or reduction did not react at all. The rupture of disulphide bridges also abolished the capacity of this protein to induce antibody formation in rabbits (Brown et al. 1959).

Another interesting aspect of the effect of denaturation on the immunogenicity of proteins is that in some cases, where the denatured protein in question is too weak to induce formation of circulating antibodies, it may still stimulate another type of immune response, notably delayed hypersensitivity. For example, Gell and Benacerraf (1959) found that heat-denatured proteins were as effective as native proteins in provoking delayed response in guinea-pigs, although their capacity to induce antibody formation was lower. Futhermore, immunization of guinea-pigs with gelatin resulted in a state of 'pure' delayed sensitivity

---

* Similar to these observations are the previously discussed findings of Dresser and of Biro and Garcia on aggregated and aggregate-free γ-globulin (2.2).

of low intensity which persisted for 4 months (Benacerraf and Gell 1959). A similar state was obtained in human volunteers by injections with ethylene-oxide treated human serum (Maurer 1961). Phenomena of this type could be responsible for the pathogenesis of certain auto-immune diseases in which a native protein may become immunogenic with respect to the host, due to physical alteration by external agents (e.g. see Burnet 1969, pp. 268–270; Rappaport et al. 1969). In par-ticular, denatured γ-globulin has been postulated to be of critical im-portance in the chain of events leading to rheumatoid arthritis (Franklin et al. 1959; Hollander et al. 1965). Some evidence, supporting this hypothesis, was obtained from rheumatoid patients who developed inflammatory reactions following intra-articular injections with their own γ-globulin (Rawson et al. 1965). Earlier experiments of Milgrom and Witebsky (1960) in rabbits showed that injections of autologous γ-globulin in Freund's adjuvant or precipitated with alum resulted in the formation of antibodies specific to γ-globulin, but reacting much better with heterologous than with homologous material. Similar results were obtained by McCluskey et al. (1962) who induced delayed responses in guinea-pigs and antibody formation in rabbits by injecting autologous γ-globulin, denatured by alkali, urea, ultrasound or heat. Even a more subtle change in the three-dimensional structure of rabbit immune γ-globulin, produced by its complexing with antigen (while maintaining the complex in solution), resulted in its auto-immunogenicity, apparently by exposing new antigenic determinants on the globulin molecule (Henney et al. 1965).

The results of the immunological studies on denatured proteins es-tablished the importance of physical integrity of the three-dimensional structure of antigenic proteins for the induction of immune response and provided a clear evidence against an earlier view that the antibody forma-tion was a consequence of the total destruction of antigen in the host (Vaughan and Wheeler 1907; Heilner 1907).

Consistent with the finding that denaturation of globular proteins results frequently in a decrease of their immunogenicity is the general observation that fibrous proteins such as collagen, fibrin, etc., normally elicit a relatively poor antibody response (e.g., see Waksman and Mason 1949; Steffen 1965; Cathcart et al. 1967; Sri Ram et al. 1968). The im-portance of the triple-helix conformation of collagen for the immuno-logical functions of this protein has not been clearly established. Evi-dence has been obtained showing that the major antigenic determinants of collagen are located in non-helical peptides which can be split off by proteolytic enzymes from the remainder of the molecule but are not affected by thermal denaturation (Schmitt et al. 1964; Timpl et al. 1968;

Michaeli et al. 1968; Michaeli et al. 1969). Nonetheless some determinants which are species-specific are apparently associated with the
triple helix, because following the disruption of the helical conformation
they do not function in *inducing* species-specific antibodies although they
retain the capacity to *react* with the antibodies in the haemagglutination-
inhibition assay (Steffen 1965; for an indirect evidence showing the role
of the triple helix, see Borek et al. 1969).

Another kind of information about the antigenic properties of fibroid
proteins was supplied by Mayer (1957) who reported that the sensitization with haptenic substances, attached to carrier proteins having a
fibrous structure usually results in delayed-type hypersensitivity, whereas the use of globular proteins as carriers leads more often to the immediate-type response. This is in agreement with the previously described observations of Gell and Benacerraf on denatured globular
proteins and on gelatin.

Turning now to the variation of the immunogenicity of proteins with
their molecular size, a striking example of this has been reported recently
by Anderer and Schlumberger (1969) who found that intermolecular
cross-linking of serum proteins by coupling the latter to the diazonium
group of a mixed polycondensate of aromatic amino carboxylic acids,
gave soluble products which induced a greatly enhanced antibody response compared with the original proteins.

A special opportunity for comparing the immunogenic power of
different antigens emerged from the studies on the development of the
immunocompetence of the foetus. Silverstein et al. (1963) showed that
injections of foetal lambs *in utero* at different stages of gestation, from
35 days to full term (150 days), with a mixture of various antigens, resulted in immune responses appearing at a different stage for each antigen. Following antigens were used: bacteriophage ϕX 174, ferritin,
ovalbumin, diphtheria toxoid, BCG and *Salmonella typhosa*. The ability
to reject orthotopic skin homografts was also examined. The foetal lamb
could respond with antibody formation against phage as early in gestation
as it has been technically feasible to carry out the experiment. i.e., at
38–40 days. At that time no immune response could be elicited to a
stimulus by any other antigen used. Later, about the 66th day of gestation, the foetus showed an incipient ability to produce antibodies against
ferritin. The ability to form antibodies against the three antigens at a
given time (late in gestation) followed the same order, the highest titre
being formed against phage and the lowest against ovalbumin. Antibodies to diphtheria toxoid, BCG and *Salmonella* appeared only after
birth. The capacity to reject skin homografts developed at about 80
days gestation. Similar results were obtained in the foetus of Rhesus

monkey where the injection of antigens during the last third of gestation resulted in the production of antiferritin with a titre 16 times higher than that of antiovalbumin antibodies (Silverstein and Kraner 1965). The authors interpret the results as showing that the varying immunological competence of the foetus toward the different antigens may be 'an expression of the differences in "antigenicity" of the agents employed, all acting with greater or lesser success on the same slowly developing cellular elements' (Silverstein et al. 1963). It can be seen that there are marked differences among the physical properties of the antigens involved. For example, the particle weight of ϕ 174 is 6.2×10^6 (Sinsheimer 1959), whereas the molecular weights of ferritin and ovalbumin are 7×10^5 and 4.4×10^4, respectively. It is noteworthy that although both ϕ 174 and *Salmonella* are particulate antigens, they are situated at opposite ends of the spectrum of the immune responsiveness of developing foetus. This finding affirms the view that in addition to the particle size of antigen there are other factors capable of influencing its immunogenic power. These factors may be decisive under certain circumstances including those involving reticulo-endothelial system at early stages of development. At this point it is worth mentioning that Šterzl et al. (1965) found that precolostral germ-free piglets, immunized neonatally with T_2 phage, sheep erythrocytes and killed *Salmonelly paratyphi* B, responded with antibody formation first against the phage, then against the red cells and finally against the bacteria. Differential response to various antigens was also observed following neonatal thymectomy in mice. The capacity to produce antibodies against bovine serum albumin was greatly depressed (Taylor 1963), the response to sheep erythrocytes and *Salmonella typhi* was similarly affected, whereas the response to haemocyanin and ferritin remained unimpaired (Humphrey et al. 1964; Fahey et al. 1965).

The data on differential immune responses to various antigens in immunologically immature animals suggest that it should be possible to induce tolerance to one type of antigen while the animal is producing antibody to another. Such a phenomenon was indeed demonstrated by Miller-Ben Shaul (1962). She injected intraperitoneally neonatal rabbits simultaneously with human serum albumin and bovine fibrinogen, and thereby induced immunological tolerance to the former (still demonstrable in 10 weeks old animals) and active immunization to the latter (precipitins appearing 6 days after injection). Similar results were obtained in neonatal mice (Miller-Ben Shaul 1963) and cats (Miller-Ben Shaul 1965). In the latter case flagella of *Salmonella typhi* and rat collagen also functioned as immunogens. The finding that fibrous proteins are immunogenic at the time when globular proteins are tolerogenic applies apparently only to immature animals. In mature hosts globular proteins are in general better immunogens than fibrous ones – as pointed out earlier in this chapter.

It should be borne in mind that in interpreting the results of at least some experiments in which immune responses of the same animal to two or more antigens are compared, the possibility of antigenic competition ought to be considered. This phenomenon, as originally described by Michaelis (1902), is manifested in the inhibition of the immune response toward one antigen as the result of the injection of another one. There are apparently a number of factors influencing the extent and the direction of competition such as the cross-reactivity between the antigens, their relative amounts, the time interval between their administration, etc. The intrinsic immunogenicity, however, seems to have little effect on the outcome of competition as shown, for example, by the finding that the immune response of mice to ferritin, considered usually a strong antigen, could be readily interfered with the simultaneous injection of a weaker antigen, bovine γ-globulin (Adler 1964). Thus if the antigenic competition is strong enough, it may obscure the contribution of the immunogenic activities of individual antigens.

A difficulty of another kind in interpreting the results of immunization experiments is that of deciding, whether a given immune response is primary or secondary or a combination of both. This difficulty is encountered, for example, when the host had been exposed previously to a cross-reacting antigen, or when the antigen has been administered in complete Freund's adjuvant. The information about the immunogenic power of a given antigen may sometimes depend on the nature of the response studied, because the evidence available shows that the primary and secondary responses differ not only quantitatively, but qualitatively as well (e.g., see Burnet 1969, pp. 194–196).

2.3.2. *Protein macromolecules and their fragments*

One of the questions perplexing immunologists for a long time has been, whether the enzymatic degradation of antigen *in vivo* is a necessary step in the induction of immune response, as expressed in a direct correlation between enzymatic digestibility and immunogenicity. The experimental evidence accumulated over the past 60 years indicates that there is indeed some correlation between these two parameters, but it is not as close and universal as it was once thought to be. Some of the evidence relevant to this problem comes from the comparison between the immunological properties of the molecular fragments of proteins and those of the intact molecules.

An early hypothesis, formulated by Vaughan and Wheeler (1907), stated that the introduction of a foreign protein into the tissues of the body induced the formation of proteolytic enzymes which destroyed and eliminated the foreign substances; the enzymes remaining in excess in the circulation are what we know as antibodies. A similar view was upheld by Heilner (1907) who considered the destruction of the antigenic protein as a prerequisite for the antibody formation. Only two years later, however, Wells (1909) reported on experimental findings quite inconsistent with the above hypothesis. He showed that exhaustive trypsin or pepsin digestion of ovalbumin *in vitro* abolished its ability to sensitize guinea pigs and to evoke systemic anaphylaxis in ovalbumin-sensitized animals. Later Landsteiner (1925/26) reported that peptic digestion products of ovalbumin elicited anaphylactic shock in guinea-pigs sensitized with the same substances, but they did not shock animals sensitive to intact ovalbumin. Similarly, Weil et al. (1938) found that a partial peptic digestion of horse globulin highly impaired its antigenic activity. Cogill and Fell (1940) showed that digestion of horse serum with Taka-diastase resulted in the loss of most of the antigenic specificity of serum proteins as shown by the fact that the protein digest did not elicit anaphylaxis in guinea-pigs sensitive to horse serum.

A general conclusion which can be drawn from the above is that disruption of the primary structure of globular proteins with the consequent molecular fragmentation may lead to alteration of their antigenic properties, presumably through unmasking new determinants at the expense of old ones (see Kaminski 1965). The shape of most determinants of globular proteins is known to depend on the integrity of the major portions of intact molecules (see Crumpton 1967). Thus, with respect to antigenic specificity, the immunological effects of controlled enzymatic digestion are comparable with those of denaturation. However, for example in fibrous proteins consisting of repeating structural units, specificity may be largely retained after fragmentation; here the question remains, how does the immunizing power of the fragments compare with that of the intact molecule.

A partial answer to this question has been provided by the study of the flagellar antigens of certain bacteria. It has been known for some time (see Koffler 1957) that when flagella are treated with heat, dilute acid or detergents, they dissociate into soluble protein subunits, known as flagellins. Flagella, apparently, are highly organized aggregates of flagellin molecules held together by labile, non-covalent bonds. Their size is approximately 20–50 mμ in diameter and up to several microns in length. Below *p*H 3.8 the flagellin molecules behave as monomers, with minimum molecular weight ranging from 14,000 to 20,000, depending on the parent organism; however, above *p*H 3.8 flagellin molecules polymerize, especially in the presence of salts, forming aggregates which are several orders of magnitude smaller than intact flagella (Kobayashi et al. 1959). Immunochemical studies (Koffler 1957) show that, whereas flagellin reacts only with about 15% of the antibodies prepared against intact flagella, flagella react equally well as flagellin with antiflagellin antibodies. This suggests that the flagellin possesses certain antigenic determinants that are absent in the flagellin molecules, but all the remaining determinants are present also in the flagellin. Whatever the interpretation of this discrepancy, the qualitative similarity between the two forms of antigens makes possible a direct comparison of their immunological properties. Such a comparison was made, for example, in the studies of the agglutinin response of rats to injections of flagella and flagellin derived from *Salmonella typhosa* in which antibodies formed against either antigen were used to agglutinate intact flagella (Winebright and Fitch 1962; Fitch and Winebright 1962). Sera of animals immunized with flagella showed a faster rise to peak antibody titre in the primary response than did the sera of animals injected with flagellin. The effect of the route of administration on the magnitude of the response (intra-peritoneal being the most effective, intravenous-intermediate and subcutaneous – the least effective route) was more pronounced in the case of flagella than in that of flagellin. Furthermore, the effect of splenectomy in lowering and delaying the peak titre was more marked when flagella were used as the immunizing antigen than in the case of flagellin. The authors interpret these results as reflecting differences in the distribution of the two forms of flagella antigen among the various antibody-producing organs of the host.

Essentially similar results were obtained by Ada et al. (1963) who compared the immunogenic properties of purified flagella of *Salmonella adelaide* with those of polymeric and monomeric flagellin. Polymeric flagellin, obtained from flagella by acid treatment followed by ammonium sulphate fractionation, was shown by gradient density ultracentrifugation to be physically similar to flagella, containing about 300 subunits, having a length of thickness ratio of 25:1 and visible as rods in the electron microscope. The main structural difference between polymeric flagellin and flagella appeared to be the presence of some acid-insoluble material in the latter. Monomeric flagellin, mol. wt about 30,000, resulted from acid treatment of the polymer. All three forms of flagellar preparations were examined by gel-diffusion against rabbit antisera and found to consist of identical antigens. The three materials were injected into the footpads of several groups of rats in various doses; the sera taken at frequent intervals were assayed for antiflagellar 19S and 7S antibody by the bacterial immobilization method. The results, reported fully by

Nossal et al. (1964), showed that during the first week of immunization flagella as well as polymeric flagellin caused 19S antibody formation, followed by prolonged 7S antibody production. In contrast, monomeric flagellin was almost incapable of inducing a 19S primary response. Moreover, the peak 7S antibody titres resulting from the monomeric injections, were lower than those following the immunizations with the other two antigens. Flagella were 100 times more potent than polymeric flagellin in causing a 19S primary response and 100–1000 times more effective than either polymeric or monomeric flagellin in inducing a 7S primary response. The authors concluded that flagella are somewhat more immunogenic in rats than polymeric flagellin and much more immunogenic than monomeric flagellin. Studies on the cellular distribution of ^{131}I-labelled flagellar antigens aiming at elucidating the above differences (Nossal et al. 1963), among others showed that flagella were trapped and retained in popliteal lymph nodes to a greater extent than monomeric flagellin.

The above studies were recently extended by Parish and Ada (1969a, b) who found that the cleavage of monomeric flaggellin (mol. wt. 40,000) with cyanogen bromide gave four peptide fragments: A, B, C and D, the largest of which, A (mol. wt. 18,000), retained all the antigenic specificities of intact flagellin (Parish, Wistar and Ada 1969). Fragments B, C, and D were non-immunogenic in either rats or rabbits. Fragment A, when administered to rats as a single injection in saline, induced a primary response, but with 20 times less efficiency than flagellin. The same peptide was more effective, though still less so than flagellin, in triggering a secondary antibody response in rats which had been primed with flagellin. Fragment A and flagellin were equally immunogenic when injected in complete Freund's adjuvant. On the other hand, neonatal or adult rats, given daily injections of fragment A for several weeks, acquired a significant degree of immunological tolerance to monomeric and polymeric flagellin. Tolerance had been also induced by repeated injections of newborn rats with monomeric flagellin (Nossal and Ada 1964), but adult rats could not be made tolerant by this means (Parish et al. 1967). The authors correlated their immunological findings with the cellular distribution pattern of ^{125}I-labelled fragment A which, in contrast to flagellin, localized poorly in the medullary macrophages of rat lymph nodes, while it was found at higher concentrations in lymphoid follicles (Ada and Parish 1968). According to the authors' hypothesis, antigen accumulated in the medulla may be involved in the induction of antibody formation and immunological memory, whereas antigen located in the follicles may either trigger primed cells to give a secondary response, or induce tolerance. Fragments B, C, D were poorly localized and retained by rat lymph nodes; the authors conclude that their main contribution to the localization behaviour of flagellin is one of molecular size and/or conformation.*

At this point a related finding of Friedmann and Gaby (1960) may be mentioned; they induced a partial tolerance to *Shigella* antigens in neonatal mice by injecting the latter with an enzymic digest of a crude preparation of the antigens.

Furthermore, it has been found recently (Malley and Perlman 1970) that hypersensitization of patients allergic to timothy pollen was much more effective, when instead of a crude pollen extract, a low-molecular weight fraction was used in the treatment.

Another area where the immunogenic properties of native proteins have been compared with those of their molecular fragments, is that of experimental allergic encephalomyelitis (EAE), an autoimmune process which follows the injection into experimental animals of homologous or heterologous brain tissue (Kabat et al. 1947). Hottle et al. (1949) were the first to report on a dialysable material, obtained from rabbit brain tissue, which induced EAE in guinea-pigs after subcutaneous injection in complete Freund's adjuvant. The active material was protein-free and the authors concluded that it contained only substances of low molecular weight (10,000 or less).

A dialysable peptide with high encephalitogenic activity was obtained also from bovine spinal cord (Robertson et al. 1962), It was pointed out by Kies (1965) that the dialysability of the active material does not necessarily mean that its molecular size is small. However, after testing 17S EAE-active fractions of the spinal cord preparation including proteins, proteolipids, peptides, etc., Lumsden et al. (1966) concluded that the common denominator of EAE activity was a dialysable peptide, released by spontaneous breakdown of larger basic polypeptides and basic protein, itself highly basic and of mol. wt. about 4,400–4,800. The physico-chemical nature of EAE active materials isolated by different investigators was found to be dependent on the solvent system used for the preliminary extraction of nervous tissue. The basis of this variation, according to Carnegie et al. (1967) was that chloroform-methanol inactivated an acid proteinase present in the tissue, whereas

---

* *Added in proof.* In a recent article (J. Exptl. Med. *132* (1970) 31) E. Diener and M. Feldman reported that, unlike in the *in vivo* induced tolerance, fragment A of flagellin failed to induce tolerance *in vitro*, whereas polymerized flagellin was effective under these conditions. The *in vitro* tolerance induction was apparently facilitated by the increased interlinkage of antigen recognition units at the surface of an immunocompetent cell, supplied by the 15,000 A-long polymerized flagellin molecule. The cell is rendered unresponsive once a critical degree of interlinkage is established.

acetone did not. Hydrolysis of basic protein by this proteinase during extraction yielded low-molecular weight encephalitogens.

The immunological relationship between the non-dialysable basic EAE protein and the dialysable basic EAE peptide was studied by Nakao and Roboz-Einstein (1965). Earlier, Bornstein and Appel (1961) demonstrated in the sera of EAE animals, immunized with the basic protein, presence of a demyelinating 'cytotoxic' factor with the characteristics of a γ-globulin. In contradistinction to this, Nakao and Roboz-Einstein found that sera of rats, immunized with the dialysable peptide exerted protective or suppressive effects against EAE when injected into other rats. It was not ascertained, whether the latter effect was the result of a passive transfer of a protective antibody or of immunological unresponsiveness, induced by small quantities of the low-molecular weight antigen still present in the serum.

Recent studies by Eylar and Thompson (1969) elucidated the physicochemical properties of the basic EAE protein ('AI'), isolated in a homogeneous state from bovine spinal cord and myelin. Its mol. wt. is about 16,000 (142 amino acid residues). The molecule exists as a random coil, in a highly unfolded state, with an axial ratio of 10:1. It is resistant to denaturation with heat, urea or alkali and is susceptible to proteolytic digestion *in situ*. Regarding its biological activity, in addition to the strong ability to induce EAE in guinea-pigs, the AI protein is capable of inducing humoral antibody formation in rabbits and guinea-pigs, along with delayed hypersensitivity in the latter (Eyler et al. 1969). Digestion of AI with pepsin, followed by fractionation on a Sephadex column, yielded 11 peptides two of which, 'E' (16 amino acid residues) and 'EI' (26 residues) were more potent in inducing EAE in guinea-pigs than the original AI protein (Hashim and Eylar 1969). Both peptides originate from the same region of the AI molecule. The authors conclude that the 'EAE' determinant, i.e., the molecular site responsible for disease induction, is defined by the primary structure of a small segment of the AI molecule and it may not require a special tertiary conformation. It remains to be established, whether this determinant is identical with that responsible for the delayed-type hypersensitive reaction which is thought to play a causal role in EAE induction (see Paterson 1966).

A rather unusual case of a protein acquiring immunogenic properties only following its fragmentation has been reported recently by Franklin and Pras (1969). It concerns amyloid, an abnormal deposit of insoluble protein with some carbohydrate, found in the tissue of patients with a degenerative disease, known as amyloidosis. Earlier claims about detection of antibodies produced against intact amyloid were disproved by Carthcart et al. (1967) and by Sri Ram et al. (1968) who demonstrated that the antibodies in question were in fact directed against serum proteins, present in amyloid deposits. The major component of amyloid was shown to be a fibrillar protein (Shirahama and Cohen 1967). Pras et al. (1969) isolated pure amyloid fibrils by extracting tissue homogenates with distilled water. Most preparations consisted of a single component with a sedimentation coefficient of 45–50S or as a larger polymer. This material appeared to be non-immunogenic in rabbits; weekly subcutaneous injections in Freund's adjuvant over a period of 9 months did not result in formation of antibodies detectable by complement fixation (Franklin and Pras 1969). Treatment of amyloid fibrils with dilute alkali yielded a soluble material with sedimentation coefficients 1.1–2.8S and mol. wt. of about 35,000–40,000. The degraded amyloid ('DAM'), when injected into rabbits, induced the formation of significant levels of complement-fixing and precipitin antibodies, detected within 2–3 months. Comparison of the antigenic properties of amyloid and DAM suggested that some of the determinants present in the latter are either completely or partially hidden in the polymeric form. The weak immunogenicity of the polymer is consistent with the general observation that fibrous proteins often elicit a poor antibody response. Commenting on the effect of degradation of amyloid on its immunogenicity, the authors state that the reason for this remains obscure though it may be related to the greater susceptibility of DAM to proteolysis *in vivo*.

The immunological properties of insulin have been thoroughly studied and will be discussed later in this chapter (2.3.3). At this point it is pertinent to mention that A and B peptide chains of bovine insulin, obtained by the cleavage of all the disulphide bonds with sulphite, were found to induce in guinea-pigs formation of antibodies. The specificity of the latter showed that the A and B chains differed antigenically from each other; only anti-B antibody cross-reacted with intact insulin (Yagi et al. 1965). Similar results were obtained with S-sulphonated A and B chains of insulin (Varandani 1967). The A chain (21 amino-acid residues) is antigenically stronger than the B chain (30 residues) (Wilson et al. 1962).

Coming back to the studies on globular proteins, enzymatic and non-enzymatic degradation of γ-globulin can be done in such a way as to yield immunogenic molecular fragments. Porter (1959) showed that papain digestion of rabbit γ-globulin (RGG), in the presence of cysteine, gave three chromatographically separable fragments two of which (termed later Fab), of mol. wt. 50,000 each, were antigenically identical and the third one (termed later Fc), of mol. wt. 80,000 was distinct from the other two and contained most of the antigenic determinants of the intact RGG. All the three fragments were at least as effective immunogenically in rats as the original protein. Herd and Ada (1969) have shown that both the intact RGG and its Fc fragment localize preferentially in the follicles of rat popliteal lymph nodes after injection in the footpads, whereas the Fab fragments do not. Similarly to RGG, papain digestion of human γ-globulin (HGG) resulted in three fragments which were immunogenic in rabbits (Franklin 1960).

Reduction of horse, human and rabbit γ-globulins with mercaptoethanol resulted in the dissociation of the globulin molecule into two heavy (mol. wt. 50,000 each) and two light (mol. wt. 20,000 each) polypeptide chains (Fleischmann et al. 1963). Both the heavy and light chains of HGG were capable of inducing antibody formation in rabbits (Cohen 1963).

An interesting example of the way in which molecular fragmentation may affect the immunogenic properties of proteins has been reported recently by Amkraut et al. (1969). The authors used as immunizing antigens haemocyanins obtained from various molluscs and arthropods, with sedimentation coefficients ranging from 12.5 to 107S, as well as their subunits, obtained by the dissociation of haemocyanins with dilute alkali at pH 8.6–10.5, with sedimentation coefficients ranging from 4.4 to 21. The antigens were injected intravenously into rabbits at such time intervals that it was possible to distinguish clearly between primary and secondary responses the intensity of which was measured by the precipitin reaction. The results showed clearly that the primary responses to closely related antigens increased with increasing molecular size. In hyperimmunized animals, on the other hand, the antibody titres were independent of molecular size; they rather showed a dependence on the phylogenetic origin of the material in that mollusc haemocyanins induced higher antibody levels than arthropod haemocyanins both in the intact and in the dissociated form. This underlined the intrinsic difference between primary and secondary responses.

Before ending this part of our discussion it is worth mentioning an observation, made in connection with gastrointestinal disorders ascribed to immune reactions against wheat proteins (Watson 1969). When peptides of mol. wt below 1,500, obtained from acid hydrolysis of gluten, were fed into patients with non-tropical sprue, gastro-intestinal symptoms and mal-absorption were produced (Kowlessar 1967). Watson (1969) interpreted this finding as a result of the reaction of the peptides with previously formed antigluten antibodies assuming that the peptides by themselves were not likely to initiate formation of appreciable amounts of antibody. This conclusion may be correct, but its basis may have to be re-examined, in view of the available evidence of the immunogenicity of certain low-molecular weight substances, presented later in this chapter (2.6).

The enzymatic degradation of protein antigens *in vivo* and its possible significance in the induction of immune response have been discussed in a review of the subject of antigen retention by Campbell and Garvey (1963). The authors have isolated from immunized animals complexes of antigenic fragments of mol. wt. of about 500 with sRNA molecules. They suggest that these complexes carry the information necessary for the synthesis of specific antibodies, although by themselves they are not immunogenic, when injected into intact animals. More recent developments in this field have been reviewed by Gottlieb (1968).

2.3.3. *Some biologically active simple proteins and natural peptides*

Insulin, the first protein with fully determined primary structure, is known to consist of two peptide chains linked with disulphide bonds which together contain 51 amino-acid residues, corresponding to a mol. wt. of 5,734 (Brown et al. 1955). It exists sometimes as a dimer or tetramer (see Prout 1963). The occasional immunogenicity of pork or beef insulin in humans has created a special problem in the therapy of diabetes and has been utilized in the development of the radioimmunoassay for antiinsulin antibodies in human sera (Berson et al. 1956). The peculiarity of insulin as antigen has been its apparent univalent character (Berson and Yalon 1959) which may change under certain circumstances (see Prout 1963). In an attempt to reconcile the low molecular weight of insulin with its immunogenicity, it has been suggested that insulin exists in the body in aggregated form or is partly bound to serum proteins. The available evidence points this out, against the first possibility though not against the second one (Ciba Foundation Coll. of Endocrinol. 1962).

The only known structural difference between pork, human and rabbit insulin is in the C-terminal acid of the B chain which is alanine, threonine and serine, respectively. Dealanylated insulin, containing structure common to that of endogenous insulin in all three species, was found to by immunogenic in man, rabbit and pig (Lockwood and Prout 1962). Moreover, under some conditions, human antibody to insulin may distinguish between whale and pig insulins having presumably identical primary structures (Berson and Yalow 1961). The authors conclude that the tertiary form of insulin, in addition to its primary structure, is important in its antigenicity. This may be in turn related to the polymerization of insulin molecules. The autoimmunogenicity of pork insulin is ascribed to changes in the tertiary structure of molecules which may occur during isolation or crystallization (see Prout 1963).

Another low-molecular weight hormone, glucagon, has been originally isolated as a hyperglycaemia-causing impurity of insulin. It is known to be a single-chain polypeptide containing 29 amino-acid residues, corresponding to a mol. wt. of 3,485 (Staub et al. 1955). Immunogenicity of beef or pork glucagon in rabbits has been demonstrated by Unger et al. (1964), by means of specific binding of the ^{131}I-labelled hormone to immune rabbit sera.

Porcine calcitonin, a peptide hormone with 32 amino-acid residues (mol. wt. 3604) (Bell et al. 1968), has been found to be immunogenic in guinea-pigs (Deftos et al. 1968).

Prolonged immunization of rabbits with the antral peptide hormone gastrin (mol. wt. 2114) in Freund's adjuvant resulted in the production of antibodies, detectable by passive haemagglutination (Schneider et al. 1967).

Subcutaneous injections of rabbits with increasing doses of cobrotoxin, a peptide component of cobra venom (mol. wt. 6,949), in complete Freund's adjuvant over a period of 3 months, induced formation of precipating antibodies (Chang and Yang 1969).

Immunogenicity of biogically active *synthetic* peptides of low molecular weight will be discussed later in this chapter (2.5).

2.4. *Polysaccharide antigens*

Natural polysaccharides constitute a group of substances with the range of molecular sizes comparable with that of proteins, but with much less complex composition and structure. The role of three-dimensional molecular configuration in the immunogenicity of polysaccharides is therefore less important than in proteins. Consequently, the scope of this discussion will be restricted to the consideration of the relation between the molecular size and immunogenicity.

A typical example of polysaccharides with well immunological properties are dextrans, D-glucose polymers produced in nature by the action of certain bacterial enzymes on sucrose and serologically cross-reacting with antisera to pneumococcus of type 2, 20 or 12 (Sugg and Hehre 1942). Native dextrans have molecular weights in the tens of millions. Clinical dextrans, introduced some time ago in Europe as plasma expanders (Gronwall and Ingelman 1944), are prepared by acid hydrolysis of the native dextrans, followed by alcohol fractionation to give products of mol. wt. of about 75,000. Studies of Kabat and Berg (1952, 1953), confirmed by Maurer (1953), have shown that both native and clinical dextrans are immunogenic in man and that injection of 1 mg. of material would induce formation of precipating antibodies and to wheal-and-erythema type skin sensitivity.

The capacity of eight dextran fractions, with average molecular weights ranging from 10,600 to 194,900, to stimulate antibody formation

in man was investigated by Kabat and Bezer (1958). The intensity of
the immune responses in 59 healthy individuals was measured by quantitative precipitin tests of sera (using both the immunizing dextran and
a native dextran preparation as test antigen as well as by skin reactions.
An allowance was made for the possibility of anamnestic response due
to pre-existence of cross-reacting antibodies in some of the subjects
tested. The results showed a clear dependence of the response on the
molecular weight of the dextran preparation used for immunization.
Subjects immunized with dextran fractions having mol. wt. of 51,300 or
lower, showed significantly weaker and less frequent antibody and cutaneous responses than those injected with products having mol. wt. of
90,700 or higher. In the latter case the responses were comparable to
those induced in 12 individuals with two native dextrans having mol. wt.
of about 200,000. The results indicate also that on degradation of native
dextran the capacity to induce skin reaction decreases more rapidly
than the ability to induce antibody production.

In vivo degradation of a long-chained bacterial polysaccharide (Type
III *Diplococcus pneumoniae*) in mice, effected by the injection of the
specific depolymerase, converted immunological paralysis into immune
response (Brooke 1964). This could be probably ascribed to a decrease
in the level of the intact antigen in the body, rather than to an overall
decrease in the molecular weight of the polysaccharide, because the
products of degradation *in vitro* were nonimmunogenic while the antigen
dose below that used for paralysis was found to induce antibody formation.

2.5. *Synthetic polypeptides and other polymeric antigens*

Immunological studies employing synthetic polypeptides as antigens
have been extensively reviewed by Maurer (1964) and by Sela (1966).
Their contribution to the understanding of the molecular basis of antigenicity has been discussed in the preceding chapter by Gill. At this point
only those aspects of the studies will be considered which have a direct
bearing on the possible role of the molecular size and shape of antigen
in immunogenicity.

Most of the antigenic synthetic polypeptides involved in the above
studies have been random linear and multichain (branched) poly-α-
amino acids. A number of physico-chemical parameters related to immunogenicity were examined; provided that most of these were selected
properly, the molecular weight of synthetic antigens could be as low as
4,000–5,000 (Maurer 1964; Sela 1966). Some oligopeptide derivatives

of even smaller molecular size were shown to be immunogenic; these will be discussed later (2.6).

In some cases the molecular size of polypeptides was found to be of importance in determining the type of response to immunization. For example, Brown and Glynn (1968) showed that two preparations of poly-L-proline, one of mol. wt. 14,000 and the other of mol. wt. 40,000, when injected into guinea-pigs in complete Freund's adjuvant, induced a state of immediate-type skin sensitivity, but only the preparation of mol. wt. 40,000 was capable of inducing delayed-type sensitivity. Other examples of this kind will be given later. In general, the immunogenicity of several poly-L-proline preparations was found to increase with increasing molecular weight (Brown and Glynn 1969).

A very important finding related to the role of the molecular shape of antigens in the induction of immune response was based on the studies of synthetic multichain polypeptides with various spatial arrangements of antigenic determinants which could be changed at will depending on the course of polymerization. These studies showed that, in order to induce antibody formation, the immunogenically significant areas of the antigen molecules must be readily accessible and cannot be hidden in the interior of the molecule (Sela and Arnon 1960; Sela et al. 1962; Fuchs and Sela 1963; Fuchs and Sela 1964).

Gill and Doty (1962) did not find any correlation between the extent of α-helical configuration of linear polypeptides and their immunogenicity.

Gill et al. (1968) explored the role of conformation in immunogenicity by comparing the properties of certain synthetic linear polypeptides and their cross-linked derivatives. They concluded that there is no change in the immunogenicity with change in conformation, but they found a marked change in the immunopotency of different antigenic determinants. Linear polypeptides have been found to be more immunogenic (in guinea-pigs) than the multichain copolymers of comparable molecular weights and with similar antigenic determinants, probably because of the greater accessibility of the determinants in the polymers of the first type (Stupp et al. 1966).

Recent application of synthetic polypeptides with defined amino acid sequence to immunological studies helped to elucidate further the role of the conformation of antigen in immune response. For example, the comparative study of a multichain polymer with side-chains consisting of repeating units of the tripeptide L-tyrosyl-L-alanyl-L-glutamic acid, and of a linear, α-helical polymer of the same tripeptide, showed that both polypeptides were good immunogens in rabbits, but almost did not cross-react serologically with each other. Inhibition tests with

                    Felix Borek

a number of peptides of related amino acid sequences have indicated
that in the case of the α-helical polymer, just as in the case of globular
proteins, the antibody specificity originates from the secondary, tertiary
and/or quaternary structure, whereas the specificity of the multichain
polymer is controlled only by the primary structure. Thus the conformational difference between the two polypeptides did not affect their
intrinsic immunogenicity though it was sufficient to make them antigenically distinct (Seal et al. 1967). In another example, an ordered-
sequence polymer (L-Pro-Gly-L-Pro)n, with a collagen-like triple
helix conformation, was found to be immunogenic in guinea-pigs
and rabbits. It produced antibodies which cross-reacted by passive
cutaneous anaphylaxis with a random copolymer of similar composition
(L-Pro^{66}Gly^{34})n, but no delayed-type skin cross-reactions between the
two polypeptides were observed. Apparently the helical conformation
of antigen in this case was more significant in the elicitation of delayed-
type reactions than in determining the antibody specificity. Nonetheless
(L-Pro-Gly-L-Pro)n cross-reacted in the antibody system with collagen
preparations from several species, presumably by virtue of the triple-
stranded conformation, common to the substances involved (Borek
et al. 1969).

Another application of synthetic polypeptides with known amino-acid
sequence was reported by Axelrod et al. (1963) who studied the immunogenicity in guinea-pigs of several polypeptides with structures corresponding to N-terminal portions of ACTH.

The immune responses were measured by (a) delayed skin sensitivity,
(b) systemic anaphylaxis, (c) passive haemagglutination and (d) *in vitro*
inhibition of migration of splenic cells by the antigen. Animals immunized
with a polypeptide consisting of 23 amino acids ('1–23 peptide') gave
a positive response by all four criteria. The immunogenicity of the 1–20
peptide was shown only in two systems: delayed skin sensitivity and
in vitro reactivity of splenic cells, whereas the 1–16 peptide was less
potent than the other two antigens in its ability to induce delayed skin
sensitivity and was incapable of eliciting the activity of spleen cells
in vitro.

Salvin and Liauw (1967) studied the immunogenicity in random-bred
guinea-pigs of synthetic ACTH (1–39 peptide) and its several synthetic
fragments. In addition to the intact molecule, the 1–24 and 11–24
peptides were immunogenic, as shown by delayed-type reactions 6–14
days after a single immunizing injection of antigen in complete Freund's
adjuvant. Sera obtained during the two weeks after sensitization were
devoid of detectable circulating antibodies, as measured by precipitation
in agar, passive cutaneous anaphylaxis, passive haemagglutination and

passive haemolysis. Serum antibodies of γ2 type only were detected by passive haemagglutination in two-thirds of animals after repeated injections of the 1–24 peptide in adjuvant. The smaller C-terminal 17–24 peptide was capable of inducing delayed reactivity to the 1–24 and 11–24 peptides and a questionable reactivity to the immunizing antigen. Still smaller fragments such as the 20–24 or 11–16 peptides were completely non-immunogenic. N-terminal 1–10 or 1–13 peptides induced little or no delayed reactivity, when injected in adjuvant. The authors conclude that most of the immunogenic capacity of the 1–24 peptide is associated with its terminal carboxyl segments (11–24). This capacity 'probably lies in particular amino acid sequences or in the conformation of the molecule, rather than in the presence of a particular type of amino acid or a particular amino acid.'

Dietrich (1966) reported that the synthetic octapeptide, angiotensin II, (mol. wt. 1,031), when injected into guinea-pigs in complete Freund's adjuvant, induced delayed sensitivity in more than 50% of the animals. Intradermal injections of the peptide in saline solution resulted in immediate-type reactivity which could be detected in most cases only by means of angiotensin-protein conjugates. More recently, Dietrich and Rittel (1970) were able to induce in rabbits formation of antibodies against the synthetic human calcitonin M, a peptide hormone with 32 amino-acid residues, after a course of intranodal, intramuscular and subcutaneous injections of the material mixed with charcoal and adjuvant, followed by intravenous injections of the same material in saline. The antibodies were detected by the antigen binding technique and their specificity was studied by binding inhibition.

The above examples suggest that the use of synthetic polypeptides with known amino acid sequence may provide significant information concerning the relationship between the molecular size and conformation of antigen and its immunogenic properties.

Among polymers other than polypeptides which have been studied with regard to their immunogenic properties, polyvinylpyrrolidone (PVP) deserves a special attention. Structurally it is somewhat similar to polypeptides, but it is a non-biological material and there is no evidence that it can be enzymatically degraded. Maurer (1956) reported that among PVP preparations of mol. wts ranging from 10^4 to 10^6, only the polymer of the highest mol. wt. induced formation of precipitin antibodies in humans, injected intramuscularly with PVP doses of approx. 1200 μg/kg of body weight. Rabbits injected with doses of 3000–7000 μg/kg in adjuvant did not respond even to PVP of mol. wt. of 10^6. Recently, Gill and Kunz (1968) were able to induce in rabbits precipitin antibodies by immunization with PVP of mol. wt. of 180,000 but a much lower dose level, within 0.3–100 μg/kg. Higher PVP doses proved to be tolerogenic. Three other vinyl polymers had similar immunogenic properties. Essentially analogous results were obtained in mice by Andersson (1969) who induced formation of antibodies to low doses of PVP preparations of mol. wts of 360,000, 40,000 and 24,000. PVP of mol. wt. of 10,000 was not immunogenic, even when administered over a wide range (10^{-12}–10^4 μg). Gill and Kunz (1968) conclude that the vinyl polymers belong to a class of materials, capable of inducing immune response only at doses lower than those normally used with other antigens. Apparently a macromolecular antigen does not need to be fragmented *in vivo* in order to induce antibody response, but it probably needs to be catabolized so as to maintain its level in tissues below that which causes immune unresponsiveness.

2.6. *Synthetic and natural low-molecular weight antigens*

Certain low-molecular weight compounds have been known for some time to cause allergic reactions in man and in experimental animals. Some of these compounds, such as dinitrochlorobenzene, for example, were found to form covalent bonds with proteins under physiological conditions. Chemical reactions of this type occur *in vivo* and lead to the formation of immunogenic hapten-protein complexes *in situ*. This is considered to be the common mechanism of the induction of allergies by chemical sensitizers (see Eisen 1959). Certain other allergenic compounds, such as derivatives of p-phenylenediamine, for example, though not reactive by themselves, are transformed enzymatically *in vivo* into metabolites capable of reacting with native proteins (see Mayer 1955). There is still another group of low-molecular weight substances with demonstrable allergenic properties which have not been found either to combine covalently with native proteins under physiological conditions or to yield reactive metabolites *in vivo* (see Davies 1958). The immunological properties of the compounds of this class will be discussed below.

2.6.1. *Allergenic chemicals and drugs*
Probably the first instance of experimental immunization recorded in the history of western man has been that of Mithridates, king of Pontus in the first century B.C., who immunized himself against certain poisons by taking them in gradually increasing doses (Guthrie 1958) and by using as antidote the blood of ducks which had been fed with poisonous plants (Meyer-Steineg and Sudhoff 1965). Many centuries later, the

evidence of immunogenicity of low-molecular weight poisons such as arsenous acid and red arsenic disulphide in rabbits was recorded on the basis of the phagocytic reaction leading to the protection of the animals involved and the protective and antitoxic properties of the rabbit sera (Metchnikoff 1894; Besredka 1899).

The potential immunogenicity of trivalent arsenicals acquired clinical significance particularly after the synthesis of arsphenamine (Salvarsan) by Ehrlich in 1909 and its subsequent application in the treatment of syphilis. A number of patients treated with this drug developed allergic skin eruptions such as exfoliative dermatitis and systemic disroders such as serum sickness, granulocytopenia, thrombocytopenic purpura, haemorrhagic encephalopathy and, occasionally, bronchial asthma (see Alexander 1955). The immunological character of the skin reactions to a closely related drug, neoarsphenamine, was established in man by Frei (1928a) and in guinea-pigs by Frei (1928b), Sulzberger (1929) and Sulzberger and Simon (1934/35). Landsteiner and Jacobs (1936) were able to induce systemic anaphylaxis with arsphenamine in experimental animals. Various aspects of the immune responses (including tolerance induction) to neoarsphenamine in guinea-pigs have been described recently by Frey et al. (1966). The authors state that there is no evidence for a covalent binding of this low-molecular weight allergen to proteins *in vivo*. Attempts to prepare immunogenic neoarsphenamine-protein conjugates *in vitro* have failed.

Delayed skin sensitivity to active components of certain plants such as poison ivy is a well-known clinical phenomenon in North-America. It was studied experimentally by Landsteiner and Chase (1939). The ability of purified 3-*n*-pentadecylcatechol, the main active ingredient of poison ivy, and of several related catechols and resorcinols, to induce delayed contact sensitivity in guinea-pigs was reported recently by Baer et al. (1966). The authors suggest that the mechanism of sensitization may involve conversion of catechols to quinones (which are known to react with proteins), but a direct evidence for this is lacking.

Landsteiner and Di Somma (1940) induced contact sensitivity in guinea-pigs to picric acid, a chemical which, unlike picryl chloride, does not bind covalently to proteins under physiological conditions. The authors considered a possibility of the *in vivo* conversion of picric acid to a reactive metabolite, picramic acid, but no evidence was found for the role of the latter in the sensitization process.

Severe allergic reactions provoked by this ingestion of aspirin were reported shortly after the discovery of this drug (Van Leeuwen 1924). The possibility of an immunological basis of these reactions was supported by experiments in which antibodies to aspirin were obtained in rabbits immunized with aspirin-protein complexes, prepared *in vitro* (Butler et al. 1940). In spite of numerous attempts, however, no anti-aspirin antibodies have been isolated from humans with 'aspirin intolerance'. As stated by Samter and Beers (1967), although the symptoms observed simulate allergic reactions in their specificity and timing, there is no convincing evidence that acetylsalicylic acid is either an antigen or an antigenic determinant. It remains to be seen, whether the recently reported ability of aspirin to acetylate serum albumin (Hawkins et al. 1968) is in any way related to 'aspirin intolerance'.

Another antipyretic, aminopyrine, has been found allergenic in some patients; in at least one of them it elicited an anaphylactic shock, when administered orally, as reported by Halpern (1958). The sensitivity could be passively transferred with serum. The author concludes that this drug acts as a complete antigen, because it is chemically only slightly reactive and thus not likely to react rapidly with body proteins *in vivo*.

There is a group of drugs capable of inducing certain blood disorders such as thrombocytopenic purpura which have a demonstrable immuno-logical basis. A typical example of these is Sedormid (allylisopropyl-acetylurea), a sedative capable of binding non-covalently to human blood platelets. This labile complex apparently is immunogenic and induces formation of antiplatelet antibodies which lyse the Sedormid-bound platelets in the presence of complement. Removal of the drug by dialysis abolishes the antigenic character of the platelets (Ackroyd 1958). Among other drugs acting in a similar way are quinine, quinidine and antazoline (ibid.). Quinine has been shown also to induce dermal hyper-sensitivity in guinea-pigs (Landsteiner and Chase 1941).

Immediate-type allergic reactions to four chemically related anti-biotics: chlortetracycline, oxytetracycline, tetracycline and demethyl-tetracycline, have been reported in a nationwide survey in U.S.A. by Welch et al. (1957). Rabbits injected intramuscularly with any of the above substances in complete Freund's adjuvant, produced specific antibodies, detectable by passive haemagglutination though not by passive cutaneous anaphylaxis (Queng et al. 1965). All four analogues were found to bind to some extent (20–47%) to plasma proteins *in vitro* (Kunin et al. (1959), but oxytetracycline, the most immunogenic of the four in rabbits, showed the least protein-binding capacity.

Asthma and rhinitis caused by inhalation of dust containing two water desinfectants, chloramine-T and halazone, were reported in a number of industrial workers exposed to these chemicals. The allergic nature of this sensitization was shown by whealing skin reactions produced by direct tests with both chemicals and after passive transfer with serum (Feinberg and Watrous 1945). One possibility, considered by the authors, was that the chemicals involved act as complete antigens.

A case of contact dermatitis induced by low aliphatic primary alcohols (including methanol and ethanol), even after removing alkehydes and other impurities by chromatography, has been described by Fregert et al. (1963). A possible role for reactive metabolites formed *in vivo* was not excluded by the authors.

Three nitro-olefins, injected into guinea-pigs in complete Freund's adjuvant, induced delayed-type hypersensitivity (Josephson 1966). Since compounds of this type had been shown to react with thiols (Heath and Lambert 1947), the author indicates a possibility that the nitro-olefins in question react with tissue proteins *in vivo*.

Sensitization of guinea-pigs with other low-molecular eight substances such as primulin (Bloch and Steiner-Wourlisch 1930) and tocopherol (Lipton 1965) was also reported.

In some cases the immunogenic properties ascribed originally to certain low-molecular weight compounds, have been found eventually to arise from polymers, spontaneously formed *in situ* and present as contaminants. For example, chlorogenic acid, a low-molecular weight constituent of coffee beans which was once thought to have allergenic properties (Freedman et al. 1964), has been shown to contain a high-molecular weight contaminant, apparently responsible for the allergic reactions to coffee (Layton et al. 1966). Similarly, standard preparations of benzylpenicillin and 6-aminopenicillanic acid have been found to contain high-molecular weight substances, derived from the original compounds by polymerisation under usual storage conditions, which elicited skin reactions in sensitive patients and experimental animals though by themselves were devoid of sensitizing properties (Stewart 1967; Batchelor et al. 1967). Another contaminant, a penicilloylated protein, derived from the fermentation process, possessed also sensitizing power; thus another cause of allergy to penicillin was revealed which had been thought originally to arise only from the *in vivo* penicilloylation of body proteins (e.g., see Schneider and De Weck 1969).

2.6.2. *Other low-molecular weight antigens (of mol. wt less than 2,000)*

It has been found in the past few years that certain oligopeptides, although not immunogenic by themselves, acquire immunogenic properties, when coupled covalently with certain reactive chemicals such as 2,4-dinitrochlorobenzene or diazonium salt of arsanilic acid. Studies on the immune responses to these antigens are reviewed below.

Abuelo and Ovary (1965) found that tri-dinitrophenylated bacitracin A, when injected into guinea-pigs in complete Freund's adjuvant, induced the formation of antibodies specific to the dinitrophenyl (DNP) determinant. Bis-DNP-bacitracin A was non-immunogenic.

Borek et al. (1965) showed that *p*-azobenzenearsonate (Rp) conjugates of hexa-L-tyrosine, tri-L-tyrosine and N-acetyl-L-tyrosine amide were immunogenic in guinea-pigs. Injections of these substances in complete Freund's adjuvant resulted in the induction of delayed sensitivity, followed by the formation of Rp-specific, circulating antibodies. Analogous *p*-azobenzoate and *p*-azobenzenesulphonate conjugates of hexa-L-tyrosine were non-immunogenic.

In order to determine whether or not binding between the Rp-oligotyrosines and guinea-pig proteins may have been responsible for initiating the immune responses to these low-molecular weight substances, incubation mixtures of ^{131}I-labelled Rp-hexa-L-tyrosine and normal guinea-pig serum were fractionated on a DEAE-cellulose column and the fractions analyzed for protein content and radioactivity. Most of the labelled conjugate was eluted in a free form, but a small portion of it was found to be associated with serum fractions, mainly in the pre-albumin and albumin regions. Identical results were obtained with the non-immunogenic hexa-L-tyrosine or its *p*-azobenzoate conjugate. Thus it was concluded that the non-covalent binding to proteins alone could not explain the immunogenic properties of the Rp-oligotyrosine conjugates.

Induction of delayed sensitivity in guinea-pigs with N-acetyltyrosine conjugates of *p*-azobenzene phosphonate and *p*-azobenzenemercurithioglycolate (but not *p*-azobenzoate or *p*-azobenzenesulphonate) was reported by Leskowitz and Zak (1966) and the immunogenicity of the Rp conjugates of N-acetylhistidine, N-acetyltryptophan and N-benzoyltyrosine was shown by Leskowitz et al. (1966) thus confirming and extending the results obtained by Borek et al. (1965). It should be mentioned that the antigens used for testing the response in the experiments of Leskowitz and Zak and Leskowitz et al., were the corresponding conjugates of proteins, whereas Borek et al. used the low-molecular weight antigens for both immunization and testing.

Rabbits could be effectively immunized with Rp-hexa-L-tyrosine though not with Rp-tri-L-tyrosine or Rp-acetyl-L-tyrosine amide (Borek et al. 1967a). The antibody obtained was precipitable with a Rp conjugate of tyrosylated gelatin; it was characterized and purified by means of an immunoadsorbent. Its behaviour on immunoelectrophoresis and DEAE-Sephadex column fractionation indicated its electropositive character. In view of the known correlation between the net charge of an immunogen that of the antibodies formed against it (Sela and Mozes 1966), the authors considered it likely that the negatively charged Rp-hexa-L-tyrosine acts as an antigen in the host independently rather than in combination with body proteins. A direct evidence for this is still lacking.

An interesting observation, made in connection with the studies of the immune responses to Rp-oligotyrosines, was that while high-molecular weight preparations of Rp-poly-D-tyrosine were weak immunogens, Rp-N-acetyl-D-tyrosine amide was as immunogenic in guinea-pigs as its L-isomer (Borek et al. 1967b), a finding consistent with that reported by Leskowitz et al. (1966) for Rp-N-acetyl-D-tyrosine. It is possible that this increase in immunogenicity with decreasing molecular weight in the D-series is a reflection of the relatively poor enzymatic digestibility of the D-amino acid polymers, a difficulty circumvented by the use of the monomer.

Immunogenicity in guinea-pigs of a homologous series of α, N-DNP-oligolysines was studied by Schlossman et al. (1965). They showed that the antigen of the smallest molecular size, capable of inducing both the delayed-type response and antibody formation, was α, N-DNP-octa-L-lysine. α,N-DNP-oligolysines smaller than the heptamer were not immunogenic even after a prolonged course of injections, whereas larger DNP-oligopeptides were excellent immunogens. What could be the possible explanation of this fairly abrupt switch from nonimmunogens to immunogens, when going along the series of DNP-oligolysines in the direction of increasing molecular size?

One possibility considered by the authors is that the immunogenicity of DNP-oligolysines is determined by the relative ease with which these substances can penetrate cellular membranes. In this connection it has been shown by Gilvarg and Katchalski (1965) that the pentamer and higher oligomers of lysine are unable to pass through the cell envelope of *Escherichia coli*. Another possibility is that, in spite of the fact that in the case of high-molecular weight polypeptide the helical configuration was found to be unnecessary for immunogenicity (Gill and Doty 1962), such a structural requirement may hold for low-molecular weight peptide derivatives such as DNP-oligolysines. Indeed octalysine is the first member of the oligolysine series which shows 'helicity' by rotary dispersion measurements. The possibility of a formation of an immunogenic, electrostically-bound complex between the DNP-oligolysines and body proteins *in vivo* was discounted by the authors, in view of the fact that the DNP-D-oligomers have been found to be nonimmunogenic. In fact subsequently it has been shown that even α, N-DNP-nonalysine in which the central lysine has a D-configuration, is non-immunogenic (Yaron and Schlossman 1968). The latter finding indicated also, according to the authors, that the enzymatic digestibility is not a requisite for immunogenicity in this system and that the initial recognition of antigen may involve a stereospecific receptor on the immunocompetent cells.

Subsequent studies on the immune responses to DNP-oligolysines

showed that the heptamer and higher oligomers elicited both immediate
(antibody-mediated) and delayed skin reactions in sensitized guinea-
pigs, whereas oligomers of smaller molecular size were capable of provoking only immediate reactions (Schlossman et al. 1966). This observation that the same requirements exist for a molecule to be immunogenic
and to elicit the delayed response, prompted the authors to put forward
a new hypothesis concerning the nature of delayed-type sensitivity,
according to which the delayed reaction is analogous to a local secondary
response in which an immunogenic molecule reacts with a specific
receptor on an immunologically committed lymphocyte and triggers
this cell to produce antibody or other mediator in the local site (Schlossman and Levine 1967a). Leskowitz (1967) arrived at the same conclusion
on the basis of his experiments with immunogenic and non-immunogenic Rp conjugates.

The findings of Schlossman and his colleagues have been extended by
their subsequent observations that only immunogenic DNP-oligolysines
were capable of: (1) desensitization of animals with delayed sensitivity
(Schlossman and Levine 1967b), (2) inhibiting macrophage migration
in vitro, on incubation with peritoneal exudate cells of sensitized animals
(David and Schlossman 1968) and (3) stimulation *in vitro* of DNA
synthesis in sensitized lymphoid cells (Schlossman et al. 1969). Recently
Spitler et al. (1970) reported that a peptide fragment of the tobacco
mosaic virus protein was capable of stimulating *in vitro* DNA synthesis
in lymphocytes obtained from animals immunized with the whole protein. The peptide involved, though capable of interacting with anti-TMV
antibody, by itself was non-immunogenic. This observation, compared
to that of Schlossman et al. (1969) serves to show, how difficult it is to
draw general conclusions from a study of one particular system as well
as to emphasize once more the fact that a given antigen may be effective
in triggering a secondary response without necessarily being capable of
initiating a primary one.

Another finding, connected with the immunogenicity of DNP-oligolysines, deserves attention at this point. Schlossman et al. (1968) showed
that antibody induced by high-molecular weight preparations of α-DNP-
polylysine was specific for the conformation of these polymers and
differed in its specificity from the antibodies prepared against α-DNP-
oligolysines of small molecular size. An *in vitro* hydrolysis of polymerized α-polylysine yielded fragments which were immunogenic, but no
longer capable of inducing the formation of antibody specific for the conformation of the present molecule, analogously to the situation with
globular proteins and their fragments (see 2.3.2). The authors consider

this as another evidence supporting the view that *in vivo* degradation of larger molecules to smaller ones does not occur prior to the induction of the immune response, at least in the system under study.

De Weck and Schneider (1968) studied the immune responses in rabbits and guinea-pigs to penicilloyl-oligolysines with varying degree of substitution and to mono-substituted penicilloyl-bacitracin. The mono-substituted peptides were immunogenic in animals of both species and some of them elicited antibody-dependent skin reactions in sensitized guinea-pigs. The authors suggest that the latter reactions may have been due to 'specific antibody-polypeptide-non-specific protein' complexes formed *in vivo* by electrostatic interaction and that a similar mechanism may be involved in the induction of immune response to oligolysine derivatives. The formation of polylysine-protein complexes of this type was indeed reported by Papermaster et al. (1965).

Attempts to immunize experimental animals with DNP-amino acids have also been reported. These belong to the class of experiments where the substance used for immunization is not identical with that used to elicit the response. Jansen et al. (1964a, b) reported that pigs, injected intradermally with a mixture of several DNP-amino acids, developed delayed sensitivity to the DNP determinant which, however, was not elicited by the application to the skin of the DNP-amino acids, but only by a challenge with a known sensitizer, dinitrochlorobenzene (DNCB). Similarly, delayed skin sensitivity to nickel was induced with a nickel-alanine complex, but it could be elicited only by the application of nickel sulphate solution. The authors conclude that these hapten-amino acid conjugates, though incapable of covalently binding to proteins and becoming complete antigens, can cause the development of delayed sensitivity. The skin reaction, however, can be triggered only by a high-molecular weight antigen, formed by the coupling of reactive hapten with proteins *in vivo*. Similar observations in guinea-pigs and rabbits were reported recently by De Weck et al. (1966) and Frey et al. (1969). Some DNP-amino acids were regularly immunogenic, whereas others were not. The authors established by chemical analyses and dose-response curves that the activity of most regularly immunogenic DNP-amino acids was not caused by contamination with reactive DNP derivatives, degradation products or DNP-proteins. In some cases (e.g., di-DNP-L-histidine) the immunogenicity was a consequence of an *in vivo* or *in vitro* transfer of the DNP group from the amino acid carrier to proteins. Irregularly immunogenic DNP-amino acids presumably contained highly immunogenic impurities which could not be detected by the methods used.

2.7. *Conclusions*

Most of the studies reviewed in this chapter, indicate that a large molecular size is an important property of a good number of various antigens. It is clear, however, from the data on the immunogenic properties of proteins fragments and of low-molecular weight synthetic antigens that there are substances of molecular weights as low as 500–1,000 (or even lower) which are immunogenic under certain circumstances. It seems to be generally accepted that 'the minimal size requirement for immunogenicity may not always relate to the same chain length or molecular weight in every system. It may rather be related to the three-dimensional structure of the antigen molecule and probably varies from system to system' (Schlossman et al. 1965).

Similarly, the molecular shape of most antigens is important to influencing their immunogenic power only as far as it reflects other properties such as general complexity of the structure*, the number of accessible antigenic determinants, the ability to be transported and/or phagocytosed and/or degraded *in vivo*, and others.

Needless to say, the role in immunogenicity of both molecular parameters discussed in this chapter must be considered in the context of other important factors influencing immune responses the studies on which are reviewed and discussed in this volume.

References

ABUELO, J. G. and Z. OVARY, 1965, J. Immunol. *95*, 113.

ACKROYD, J. F., 1958, Thrombocytopenic purpura due to drug hypersensitivity. *In*: M. L. Rosenheim and R. Moulton, eds.: Sensitivity reactions to drugs. Springfield, Thomas. pp. 28–62.

ADA, G. L. and C. R. PARISH, 1968, Proc. Natl. Acad. Sci. U.S. *61*, 556.

ADA, G. L., G. J. V. NOSSAL, J. PYE and A. ABBOTT, 1963, Nature *199*, 1257.

ADLER, F. L., 1964, Progr. Allergy *8*, 41.

ALEXANDER, H. L., 1955, Reactions with drug therapy. Philadelphia, Saunders. pp. 77–78.

AMKRAUT, A. A., A. MALLEY and D. BEGLEY, 1969, J. Immunol. *103*, 1301.

ANDERER, F. A. and H. D. SCHLUMBERGER, 1969, Immunochemistry *6*, 1.

ANDERSSON, B., 1969, J. Immunol. *102*, 1309.

ANFINSEN, C. B., 1964, On the possibility of predicting tertiary structure from primary sequence. *In*; M. Sela, ed.: New perspectives in biology. Vol. 4. Amsterdam, Elsevier. pp. 42–50.

AUGUSTIN, R., C. R. WEST, S. M. SPARSHOTT, K. D. CHANDRADASA and A. C. BREWER, Proc. Int. Symposium on Tolerance and Immunity in Oncogenesis, Perugia, June 1969 (in press).

---

* The relationship between the structural heterogeneity of antigens and the potential number of responding hosts is discussed in Chapter 11 dealing with the genetic variations of immune response.

AXELROD, A. E., A. C. TRAKATELLIS and K. HOFMANN, 1963, Nature *197*, 146.

BAER, H., J. C. WATKINS and R. T. BOWSER, 1966, Immunochemistry *3*, 479.

BATCHELOR, F. R., J. M. DEWDNEY, J. G. FEINBERG and R. D. WESTON, 1967, Lancet i, 1175.

BATTISTO, J. R. and B. R. BLOOM, 1966a, Federation Proc. *25* (1), 152.

BATTISTO, J. R. and B. R. BLOOM, 1966b, Nature *212*, 156.

BATTISTO, J. R. and BOREK, F., 1968, Federation Proc. *27* (2), 2640.

BELL, P. H., W. F. BARG, JR., D. F. COLUCCI, M. C. DAVIES, C. DZIOBKOWSKI, M. E. ENGLERT, E. HEYDER, R. PAUL and E. H. SNEDEKER, 1968, J. Am. Chem. Soc. *90*, 2704.

BENACERRAF, B., and P. G. H. GELL, 1959, Immunology *2*, 53.

BENACERRAF, B., B. BIOZZI, B. B. HALPERN and C. STIFFEL, 1956, Res. Bulletin *2*, 19.

BERGLUND, G., 1965, Nature *206*, 523.

BERSON, S. A. and R. S. YALOW, 1959, J. Clin. Invest. *38*, 1996.

BERSON, S. A. and R. S. YALOW, 1961, Nature *191*, 1392.

BERSON, S. A., R. S. YALOW, A. BAUMAN, M. A. ROTHSCHILD and K. NEWERLY, 1956, J. Clin. Invest. *35*, 170.

BESREDKA, A., 1899, Ann. Inst. Pasteur *13*, 49, 209, 465.

BIRO, C. and G. GARCIA, 1965, Immunology *8*, 411.

BLOCH, B. and A. STEINER-WOURLISCH, 1930, Arch. Dermatol. Syphilis *162*, 349.

BLUMENTHAL, D., 1936, J. Biol. Chem. *113*, 433.

BOREK, F. and BATTISTO, J. R., 1971, Immunology (in press).

BOREK, F., Y. STUPP and M. SELA, 1965, Science *150*, 1177.

BOREK, F., Y. STUPP and M. SELA, 1967a, J. Immunol. *98*, 739.

BOREK, F., Y. STUPP and M. SELA, 1967b, Biochim. Biophys. Acta *140*, 360.

BOREK, F., J. KURTZ and M. SELA, 1969, Biochim. Biophys. Acta *188*, 314.

BORNSTEIN, M. B. and S. H. APPEL, 1961, J. Neuropath. Exptl. Neurol. *20*, 141.

BOYD, W. C., 1956, Fundamentals of immunology, 3rd Ed. New York, Interscience.

BOYD, W. C. and S. MALKIEL, 1940, J. Bacteriol. *39*, 32.

BROOKE, M. S., 1964, Nature *204*, 1319.

BROWN, H., F. SANGER, and R. KITAI, 1955, Biochem. J. *60*, 556.

BROWN, J. C., J. H. SCHWAB and E. J. HOLBOROW, 1970, Immunology (in press).

BROWN, P. C. and L. E. GLYNN, 1968, Immunology *15*, 589.

BROWN, P. C. and L. E. GLYNN, 1969, Immunology *17*, 943.

BROWN, R. K., R. DELANEY, L. LEVINE and H. VAN VUNAKIS, 1959, J. Biol. Chem. *234*, 2043.

BURNET, F. M., 1969, Self and not-self, Cellular immunology, Book one. Melbourne and Cambridge University Presses. pp. 268–270.

BUTLER, G. C., C. R. HARINGTON and M. E. YUILL, 1940, Biochem. J. *34*, 838.

BUTLER, W. T., R. D. ROSSEN, E. M. HERSH, M. E. DE BAKEY, E. B. DIETHRICH, D. K. BROOKS, D. A. COOLEY, J. J. NORA, R. D. LEACHMAN, D. G. ROCHELLE, J. J. TRENTIN, K. P. JUDD, A. C. BEALL, JR., D. E. JENKINS, R. O. MORGEN and V. KNIGHT, 1969, Nature *224*, 856.

CAMPBELL, D. H. and J. S. GARVEY, 1963, Advan. Immunol. *3*, 261.

CAREY, G. E. and E. A. WRIGHT, 1960, Trans. Roy. Soc. Trop. Med. Hyg. *54*, 50.

CARNEGIE, P., G. LAMOUREUX and B. BENCINA, 1967, Nature *214*, 407.

CATHCART, E. S., F. A. WOLLHEIM and A. S. COHEN, 1967, J. Immunol. *99*, 376.

CHANG, C. C. and C. C. YANG, 1969, J. Immunol. *102*, 1437.

Ciba Foundation Coll. on Endocrinol., 1962, Vol. 14: Immunoassay of hormones, G. E. W. Wostenholme and M. P. Cameron, eds. Boston, Little, Brown Co. pp. 15–16, 43.

COGILL, R. and N. FELL, 1940, J. Immunol. *39*, 207.

COHEN, S., 1963, Nature *197*, 253.

CRUMPTON, M., 1967, The molecular basis of serological specificity of proteins, with particular reference to sperm whale myoglobin. *In*: B. Cinader, ed.: Antibodies to biologically active molecules. Oxford, Pergamon Press. pp. 61–83.

CZAJKOWSKI, N. P., M. ROSENBLATT, P. L. WOLF and J. VASQUEZ, 1967, Lancet ii, 905.

DAVID, J. R. and S. F. SCHLOSSMAN, 1968, J. Exptl. Med. *128*, 1451.

DAVIES, G. E., 1958, Chemical structure and pharmacodynamic action in relation to drug sensitivity. *In*: M. L. Rosenheim and R. Moulton, eds.: Sensitivity reactions to drugs. Springfield, Thomas. pp. 149–172.

DEFTOS, L. J., M. R. LEE and J. T. POTTS, JR. 1968, Proc. Natl. Acad. Sci. U.S. *60*, 293.

DIETRICH, F. M., 1966, Int. Arch. Allergy, *30*, 497.

DIETRICH, F. M. and P. DUKOR, 1967, Immunology *13*, 585.

DIETRICH, F. M. and W. RITTEL, 1970, Nature *225*, 75.

DIXON, F. J., H. JACOT-GUILLARMOD and P. H. MCCOHANEY, 1966, J. Immunol. *97*, 350.

DOERR, R. and J. MALDAVAN, 1911, Wien. Klin. Wschr. *23*, 555.

DRAPER, L. R. and A. A. HIRATA, 1968, Immunology *15*, 23.

DRESSER, D. W., 1962, Immunology *5*, 378.

DRESSER, D. W., 1963, Immunology *6*, 345.

EISEN, H. N., 1959, Hypersensitivity to simple chemicals. *In*: H. S. Lawrence, ed.: Cellular and humoral aspects of hypersensitive states. New York, Hoebner-Harper. pp. 89–122.

EPSTEIN, C. J., R. F. GOLDBERGER and C. B. ANFINSEN, 1963, Cold Spring Harbor Symp. Quant. Biol. *28*, 439.

ERICKSON, J. O. and H. NEURATH, 1953, J. Exptl. Med. *78*, 1.

ERICKSON, J. O. and H. NEURATH, 1945, J. Gen. Physiol. *28*, 421.

EYLAR, E. H. and M. THOMPSON, 1969, Arch. Biochem. Biophys. *129*, 468.

EYLAR, E. H., J. SLAK, G. C. BEVERIDGE and L. V. BROWN, 1969, Arch. Biochem. Biophys. *132*, 34.

FAHEY, J. L., W. F. BARTH and L. W. LAW, 1965, J. Natl. Cancer Inst. *35*, 663.

FEINBERG, S. M. and R. M. WATROUS, 1945, J. Allergy *16*, 209.

FITCH, F. W. and J. W. WINEBRIGHT, 1962, J. Immunol. *89*, 900.

FLEISCHMANN, J. B., R. R. PORTER and E. M. PRESS, 1963, Biochem. J. *88*, 220.

FLOSDORF, E. W. and L. A. CHAMBERS, 1935, J. Immunol. *28*, 297.

FRANKLIN, E. C., 1960, J. Clin. Invest. *39*, 1933.

FRANKLIN, E. C. and M. PRAS, 1969, J. Exptl. Med. *130*, 797.

FRANKLIN, E. C., G. EDELMAN and H. G. KUNKEL, 1959, The rheumatoid factor. *In*: V. A. Najjar, ed.: Immunity and virus infection. New York, J. Wiley and Sons. pp. 92–99.

FREEDMAN, M. H. and M. SELA, 1966, J. Biol. Chem. *241*, 2383.

FREEDMAN, S. O., R. SHULMAN, J. DRUPEY and A. H. SEHON, 1964, J. Allergy *35*, 97.

FREGERT, S., R. HAKANSON, H. RORSMAN, N. TRYDING and P. OVRUM, 1963, J. Allergy *34*, 404.

FREI, P. C., B. BENACERRAF and J. THORBECKE, 1965, Proc. Natl. Acad. Sci. U.S. *53*, 20.

FREI, W., 1928a, Klin. Wschr. *7*, 539.

FREI, W., 1928b, Klin. Wschr. *7*, 1026.

FREY, J. R., A. L. DE WECK and H. GELEICK, 1966, Int. Arch. Allergy *30*, 288; 385; 428; 521.

FREY, J. R., A. L. DE WECK, H. GELEICK and W. LERGIER, 1969, J. Exptl. Med. *130*, 1123.

FRIEDMANN, H. and W. L. GABY, 1960, J. Immunol. *85*, 478.

FUCHS, S. and M. SELA, 1963, Biochem. J. *87*, 70.

FUCHS, S. and M. SELA, 1964, Biochem. J. *93*, 566.

FURTH, J., 1925, J. Immunol. *10*, 777.

GALLILY, R. and J. S. GARVEY, 1968, J. Immunol. *101*, 924.

GELL, P. G. H. and B. BENACERRAF, 1959, Immunology *2*, 64.

GILL, T. J., III and P. DOTY, 1962, The immunological and physico-chemical properties of a group of linear-chain polypeptides. *In*: M. A. Stahmann, ed.: Polyamino acids, polypeptides and proteins. Madison, Univ. of Wisconsin Press. pp. 367–377.

GILL, T. J. III and H. W. KUNZ, 1968, Proc. Natl. Acad. Sci. U.S. *61*, 490.

GILL, T. J., III, D. S. PAPERMASTER, H. W. KUNZ, and P. S. MARFEY, 1968, J. Biol. Chem. *243*, 287.

GILVARG, C. and E. KATCHALSKI, 1965, J. Biol. Chem. *240*, 3093.

GLENNY, A. T., C. G. POPE, H. WADDINGTON and U. WALLACE 1926, J. Pathol. Bacteriol. *29*, 31.

GLENNY, A. T., G. A. H. BUTTLE and M. F. STEVENS, 1931, J. Pathol. Bacteriol. *34*, 267.

GONZALEZ, P. and ARMANGUE, 1931, Compt. Rend. Soc. Biol. *106*, 1006.

GOTTLIEB, A. A., 1968, J. Reticuloendothelial Soc. *5*, 270.

GRONWALL, A. and B. INGELMAN, 1944, Acta Physiol. Scand. *7*, 97.

GUTHRIE, D., 1958, A history of medicine. Philadelphia, Lippincott. p. 70.

HALPERN, B. N., 1958, The immunological character of humoral antibodies in drug allergy. *In*: M. L. Rosenheim and R. Moulton, eds.: Sensitivity reactions to drugs. Springfield, Thomas. pp. 135–148.

HASHIM, G. A. and E. H. EYLAR, 1969, Arch. Biochem. Biophys. *129*, 635.

HAWKINS, D., R. N. PINCKARD and R. S. FARR, 1968, Science *160*, 78.

HEATH, R. L. and A. LAMBERT, 1947, J. Chem. Soc. 1477.

HEILNER, E., 1907, Z. Biol. *1*, 26.

HENNEY, C. S., D. R. STANWORTH and P. G. H. GELL, 1965, Nature *205*, 1079.

HERD, Z. L. and G. L. ADA, 1969, Aust. J. Exptl. Biol. Med. Sci. *47*, 73.

HIRATA, A. A. and D. H. CAMPBELL, 1965, Immunochemistry *2*, 195.

HIRATA, A. A. and D. H. SUSSDORF, 1966, J. Immunol. *96*, 611.

HOLLANDER, J. L., J. MCCARTHY, JR., G. ASTORGA and E. CASTRO-MURILLO, 1965, Ann. Int. Med. *62*, 271.

HOTTLE, G. A., G. A. NEDZEL, J. T. WRIGHT and J. F. BELL, 1949, Proc. Soc. Exptl. Biol. Med. *72*, 289.

HUMPHREY, J. H., D. M. V. PARROTT and J. EAST, 1964, Immunology *7*, 419.

JACOBS, J., 1934, J. Exptl. Med. *59*, 479.

JANSEN, L. H., L. BERRENS and J. VAN DELDEN, 1964a, Naturwissenschaften *16*, 387.

JANSEN, L. H., L. BERRENS and J. VAN DELDEN, 1964b, Dermatologica *128*, 491.

JONESCO-MIHAIESTI, C., and V. BARONI, 1910, Compt. Rend. Soc. Biol. *68*, 393.

JOSEPHSON, A. S., 1966, J. Immunol. *96*, 699.

KABAT, E. A. and D. BERG, 1952, Ann. N.Y. Acad. Sci., *55*, 471.

KABAT, E. A. and D. BERG, 1953, J. Immunol. *70*, 514.

KABAT, E. A. and A. E. BEZER, 1958, Arch. Biochem. Biophys. *78*, 306.

KABAT, E. A., A. WOLF and A. E. BEZER, 1947, J. Exptl. Med. *85*, 117.

KAMINSKI, M., 1965, Progr. Allergy *9*, 79.

KIES, M. W., 1965, Ann. N.Y. Acad. Sci. *122*, 161.

KOBAYASHI, T., T. N. RINKER and H. KOFFLER, 1959, Arch. Biochem. Biophys. *84*, 342.

KOCHWA, S., S. GITTER, B. STRAUSS, A. DE VRIES and M. LEFKOWITZ, 1959. J. Immunol. *82*, 107.

KOCHWA, S, M. BROWNELL, R. E. ROSENFIELD and L. R. WASSERMAN, 1967, J. Immunol. *99*, 981.

KOFFLER, H., 1957, Bact. Rev. *21*, 227.

KOWLESSAR, O. D., 1967, Gastroenterology *52*, 893.

KUNIN, C. M., A. C. DORNBUSH and M. FINLAND, 1959, J. Clin. Invest. *38*, 1950.

LANDSTEINER, K., 1921, Biochem. Z. *119*, 294.

LANDSTEINER, K., 1925/26, Proc. Soc. Exptl. Biol. Med., *23*, 540.

LANDSTEINER, K., 1945, The specificity of serological reactions, 2nd Ed. Harvard Univ. Press. Reprinted in 1962 by Dover Publications, Inc., New York.

LANDSTEINER, K. and C. BARRON, 1917, Z. Immun.-Forsch. *26*, 142.

LANDSTEINER, K. and M. W. CHASE, 1939, J. Exptl. Med. *69*, 767.

LANDSTEINER, K. and M. W. CHASE, 1941, Proc. Soc. Exptl. Biol. Med. *46*, 223.

LANDSTEINER, K. and A. A. DI SOMMA, 1940, J. Exptl. Med., *72*, 361.

LANDSTEINER, K. and J. JACOBS, 1931/32, Proc. Soc. Exptl. Biol. Med. *29*, 570.

LANDSTEINER, K. and J. JACOBS, 1936, J. Exptl. Med. *64*, 717.

LANDSTEINER, K. and S. SIMMS, 1923, J. Exptl. Med. *38*, 127.

LANG, P. G. and G. L. ADA, 1967, Aust. J. Exptl. Biol. Med. Sci. *45*, 445.

LAYTON, L. L., R. PANZANI and J. W. CORSE, 1966, J. Allergy *38*, 268.

LESKOWITZ, S., 1967, Ann. Rev. Microbiol. *21*, 175–176.

LESKOWITZ, S., 1967, Science *155*, 350.

LESKOWITZ, S. and S. J. ZAK, 1966, Nature *211*, 246.

LESKOWITZ, S., V. E. JONES and S. J. ZAK, 1966, J. Exptl. Med. *123*, 229.

LINDQVIST, K. and D. C. BAUER, 1966, Immunochemistry *3*, 373.

LIPTON, M. M., 1965, J. Immunol. *94*, 323.

LOCKWOOD, D. A. and T. E. PROUT, 1962, Clin. Res. *10*, 401.

LUMSDEN, C. E., D. M. ROBERTSON and R. BLIGHT, 1966, J. Neurochem. *13*, 127.

MACPHERSON, C. F. C. and M. HEIDELBERGER, 1940, Proc. Soc. Exptl. Biol. Med. *43*, 646.

MACPHERSON, C. F. C. and M. HEIDELBERGER, 1945, J. Am. Chem. Soc. *67*, 585.

MALLEY, A. and F. PERLMAN, 1970, J. Allergy *45*, 14.

MARTIN, D. S., J. O. ERICKSON, F. W. PUTNAM and H. NEURATH, 1943, J. Gen. Physiol. *26*, 533.

MAURER, P. H., 1953, Proc. Exptl. Biol. Med. *83*, 879.

MAURER, P. H., 1956, J. Immunol. *77*, 105.

MAURER, P. H., 1961, J. Exptl. Med. *113*, 1029.

MAURER, P. H., 1964, Progr. Allergy *8*, 1.

MAURER, P. H. and M. HEIDELBERGER, 1951, J. Am. Chem. Soc. *73*, 2076.

MAYER, R. L., 1955, Progr. Allergy *4*, 79.

MAYER, R. L., 1957, Int. Arch. Allergy *10*, 13.

MCCLUSKEY, R. T., F. MILLER and B. BENACERRAF, 1962, J. Exptl. Med. *115*, 253.

METCHNIKOFF, E., 1894, Ann. de l'Inst. Pasteur *8*, 719.

MEYER-STEINEG, T. and K. SUDHOFF, 1965, Illustrierte Geschichte der Medizin. Stuttgart, Fischer. p. 64.

MICHAELI, D., H. KAMENECKA, E. BENJAMINI, J. R. KETTMAN, JR., D. Y. K. LEUNG and R. C. MINER, 1968, Immunochemistry *5*, 433.

MICHAELI, D., G. R. MARTIN, J. KETTMAN, E. BENJAMINI, D. Y. K. LEUNG and B. A. BLATT, 1969, Science *166*, 1522.

MICHAELIS, L., 1902, Dtsch. Med. Wschr. *28*, 733.

MILGROM, F. and E. WITEBSKY, 1960, J. Am. Med. Ass. *174*, 56.

MILLER, B. F., 1933, J. Exptl. Med. *58*, 625.

MILLER-BEN SHAUL, D., 1962, Bull. Res. Counc. of Israel *10E*, 45.

MILLER-BEN SHAUL, D., 1963, Israel J. Exptl. Med. *11*, 18.

MILLER-BEN SHAUL, D., 1965, Israel J. Med. Sci. *1*, 563.

MOROZ, C., N. GOLDBLUM and A. DE VRIES, 1963, Nature *200*, 697.

MUDD, S. and M. WIENER, 1942, J. Immunol. *42*, 21.

NAKAO, A. and E. ROBOZ-EINSTEIN, 1965, Ann. N.Y. Acad. Sci. *122*, 171.

NETER, E., H. Y. WHANG, T. SUZUKI and E. A. GORZYNSKI, 1964, Immunology *7*, 657.

NOSSAL, G. J. V. and G. L. ADA, 1964, Nature *201*, 580.

NOSSAL, G. J. V., G. L. ADA and C. M. AUSTIN, 1963, Nature *199*, 1259.

NOSSAL, G. J. V., G. L. ADA and C. M. AUSTIN, 1964, Aust. J. Exptl. Biol. Med. Sci. *42*, 283.

OBERMAYER, F. and E. PICK, 1906, Wien. Klin. Wschr. *19*, 327.

OLOVNIKOV, A. M. and A. E. GURVICH, 1966, Nature *209*, 417.

PAPERMASTER, D. S., T. J. GILL, III and W. F. ANDERSON, 1965, J. Immunol. *95*, 804.

PARISH, C. R. and G. L. ADA, 1969a, Biochem. J. *113*, 489.

PARISH, C. R. and G. L. ADA, 1969b, Immunology *17*, 153.

PARISH, C. R., P. G. LANG and G. L. ADA, 1967, Nature *215*, 1202.

PARISH, C. R., R. WISTAR and G. L. ADA, 1969, Biochem. J. *113*, 501.

PARKHOUSE, R. M. E. and R. W. DUTTON, 1967, Immunochemistry *4*, 431.

PATERSON, P., 1966, Advan. Immunol. *5*, 131.

PIANTANIDA, M., and N. MUIC, 1954, J. Immunol. *73*, 115.

PLAUT, F., and H. RUDY, 1933, Z. Immun.-Forsch. *81*, 87.

PORTER, R. R., 1959, Biochem. J. *73*, 119.

PRAS, M., D. ZUCKER-FRANKLIN, A. RIMON and E. C. FRANKLIN, 1969, J. Exptl. Med. *130*, 777.

PROUT, T. E., 1963, Metabolism *12*, 673.

PUTNAM, F. W., 1953, Protein denaturation. *In*: H. N. Neurath and K. Bailey, eds.: The proteins, Vol. 1, Part B. New York, Academic Press. pp. 807–892. ·

QUENG, T. J., C. D. DUKES and J. P. MCGOVERN, 1965, J. Allergy *36*, 505.

RAMON, G., 1925, Compt. Rend. Soc. biol. *93*, 506.

RAPPAPORT, F. T., A. SAMPATH, K. KANO, R. T. MCCLUSKEY and F. MILGROM, 1969, J. Exptl. Med. *130*, 1411.

RAWSON, A. J., N. M. ABELSON and J. L. HOLLANDER, 1965, Ann. Int. Med. *62*, 285.

ROBERTSON, D. M., R. BLIGHT and C. E. LUMSDEN, 1962, Nature *196*, 1005.

SALVIN, S. B. and H-L. LIAUW, 1967, Int. Arch. Allergy *31*, 366.

SAMTER, M. and BEERS, R. F., JR. 1967, J. Allergy *40*, 281.

SCHLOSSMAN, S. F. and H. LEVINE, 1967a, J. Immunol. *98*, 211.

SCHLOSSMAN, S. F., and H. LEVINE, 1967b, J. Immunol. *99*, 111.

SCHLOSSMAN, S. F., A. YARON, S. BEN-EFRAIM and H. A. SOBER, 1965, Biochemistry *4*, 1638.

SCHLOSSMAN, S. F., S. BEN-EFRAIM, A. YARON and H. A. SOBER, 1966, J. Exptl. Med. *123*, 1083.

SCHLOSSMAN, S. F., H. LEVINE and A. YARON, 1968, Biochemistry *7*, 1.

SCHLOSSMAN, S. F., J. HERMAN and A. YARON, 1969, J. Exptl. Med. *130*, 1031.

SCHMIDT, W. A., 1908, Biochem. Z. *4*, 294.

SCHMITT, F. O., L. LEVINE, M. P. DRAKE, A. L. RUBIN, D. PFAHL and P. F. DAVISON, 1964, Proc. Natl. Acad. Sci. U.S., *51*, 493.

SCHNEIDER, C. H. and A. L. DE WECK, 1969, Int. Arch. Allergy *36*, 129.

SCHNEIDER, D. R., G. L. ENDAHL, M. C. DODD, J. E. JESSEPH, N. J. BIGLEY and R. M. ZOLLINGER, 1967, Science *156*, 391.

SELA, M., 1966, Advan. Immunol. *5*, 29.

SELA, M., 1969, Science *166*, 1365.

SELA, M. and R. ARNON, 1960, Biochem. Biophys. Acta *40*, 382.

SELA, M. and E. MOZES, 1966, Proc. Natl. Acad. Sci. U.S. *55*, 445.

SELA, M., S. FUCHS and R. ARNON, 1962, Biochem. J. *85*, 223.

SELA, M., B. SCHECHTER, I. SCHECHTER and F. BOREK, 1967, Cold Spring Harbor Symp. Quant. Biol. *32*, 537.

SHIRAHAMA, T. and A. S. COHEN, 1967, J. Cell. Biol. *33*, 679.

SILVERSTEIN, A. M. and K. L. KRANER, 1965, Studies on the ontogenesis of the immune response. *In*: Molecular and cellular basis of antibody formation. Prague, Czechoslov. Acad. Sci. pp. 341–349.

SILVERSTEIN, A. M., J. W. UHR, K. L. KRANER and R. J. LUKES, 1963, J. Exptl. Med. *117*, 799.

SINSHEIMER, R. L., 1959, J. Mol. Biol. *1*, 37.

SMETANA, H. and D. SHEMIN, 1941, J. Exptl. Med. *73*, 223.

     Felix Borek

SPITLER, L., E. BENJAMIN, J. D. YOUNG, H. KAPLAN and H. H. FUDENBERG, 1970, J. Exptl. Med. *131*, 133.

SRI RAM, J., R. A. DE LELLIS and G. G. GLENNER, 1968, Int. Arch. Allergy *34*, 269.

STAUB, A. L. SINN and O. K. BEHRENS, 1955, J. Biol. Chem. *214*, 619.

STEELE, A. S. V., 1965, J. Pathol. Bacteriol. *89*, 691.

STEELE, A. S. V., and J. H. RACK, 1965, J. Pathol. Bacteriol. *89*, 703.

STEFFEN, C., 1965, Ann. N.Y. Acad. Sci. *124* (Part II), 570.

ŠTERZL, J., L. MANDEL, I. MILLER and I. RIHA, 1965, Development of immune reactions in the absence or presence of an antigenic stimulus. *In*: Molecular and cellular basis of antibody formation. Prague, Czechoslov. Acad. Sci. pp. 351–370.

STEWART, G. T., 1967, Lancet i, 1177.

STUPP, Y., F. BOREK and M. SELA, 1966, Immunology *11*, 561.

SUGG, J. Y. and E. J. HEHRE, 1942, J. Immunol. *43*, 119.

SULZBERGER, M. B., 1929, Klin. Wschr. *8*, 253.

SULZBERGER, M. B. and F. A. SIMON, 1934/35, J. Allergy *6*, 39.

TALMAGE, D. W. and F. J. DIXON, 1953, J. Infect. Dis. *93*, 176.

TAYLOR, R. B., 1963, Nature *199*, 873.

TENBROECK, C., 1914, J. Biol. Chem. *17*, 369.

TIMPL, R., I. WOLFF, G. WICK, H. FURTHMAYR and C. STEFFEN, 1968, J. Immunol. *101*, 725.

TORRIGIANI, G. and I. M. ROITT, 1965, J. Exptl. Med. *122*, 181.

UHLENHUTH, P. and E. REMY, 1938, Z. Immun. Forsch. *92*, 171.

UNGER, R. H., A. M. EISENTRAUT, J. DE V. LOCHNER, J. BAUM. B. E. SIMONS JR., and L. L. MADISON, 1964, Immunological studies of A-cell function. *In*: S. E. Brolin, B. Hellman and H. Knutson, eds.: The structure and metabolism of the pancreatic islets. Oxford, Pergamon Press. pp. 477–487.

UWAZUMI, S., 1934, Arb. Med. Fak. Okayama *4*, 53.

VAN LEEUWEN, W. C., 1924, J. Pharmacol. Exptl. Therap. *24*, 25.

VARANDANI, P. T., 1967, Biochemistry *6*, 100.

VAUGHAN, V. C. and S. M. WHEELER, 1907, J. Inf. Dis. *4*, 476.

WAKSMAN, B. H. and H. L. MASON, 1949, J. Immunol. *63*, 427.

WATSON, D. W., 1969, Gastroenterology *56*, 944.

DE WECK, A. L. and C. H. SCHNEIDER, 1968, Immunology *14*, 457.

DE WECK, A. L., J. R. FREY and H. GELEICK, 1966, Int. Arch. Allergy *29*, 174.

WEIL, A. J., I. PARFENTJEV and K. BOWMAN, J. Immunol. *35*, 399.

WELCH, H., C. N. LEWIS, H. I. WEINSTEIN and B. B. BOEKMAN, 1957, Antibiotic Med. Clin. Therapy *4*, 800.

WELLS, H. G., 1909, J. Infect. Dis. *6*, 506.

WILSON, S., G. H. DIXON and A. C. WARDLAW, 1962, Biochim. Biophys. Acta *62*, 483.

WINEBRIGHT, J. W., and F. W. FITCH, 1962, J. Immunol. *89*, 891.

WU, H., C. TENBROECK and C. P. LI, 1927, Chinese J. Physiol. *1*, 277.

YAGI, Y., P. MAIER and D. PRESSMAN, 1965, Science *147*, 617.

YARON, A. and S. F. SCHLOSSMAN, 1968, Biochemistry *7*, 2673.

ZINSSER, H., J. F. ENDERS and L. D. FOTHERGILL, 1940, Immunity: principles and application in medicine, 5th Ed. New York, Macmillan. pp. 78–105.

ZOZAYA, J., 1931, Science *74*, 270.

CHAPTER 3

Dose, frequency and route of adminstration of antigen

N. A. MITCHISON

National Institute for Medical Research, Mill Hill, London

3.1. Theoretical considerations

3.1.1. Selection theory

As a preliminary to attempting to understand the role of antigen dosage and timing in the immune response it is worth re-stating the clonal selection theory which underlies most modern thinking on the subject. The theory has three principal tenets. (1) One cell produces only one immunoglobulin. (2) A generator of diversity of undefined character operates in such a way that each immunologically active cell produces one among many possible immunoglobulins differing from one another in their variable part. (3) Each antigen-sensitive cell bears receptor molecules which are identical at least in respect of their combining sites with the product of the clone to which the cell will give rise if successfully stimulated. The cellular events of the immune response consist essentially of a cycle in which antigen-sensitive cells pause, then transform and multiply as a result of a combination of antigen with their receptors, then synthesize immunoglobulins, and at the same time generate an expanded population of antigen-sensitive cells with the same receptors, and then eventually return again to a state of pause. Thus, administration of antigen not only initiates the production of antibody but also expands those clones of cells which are capable in the future of initiating further antibody production in response to a second dose of antigen.

Upon entering the body antigen confronts an array of different receptors. Some receptors will fit the determinants of the antigen well (high affinity receptors); others will fit more poorly (low affinity receptors). Because the degree of fit is largely a matter of chance, high affinity receptors will be rare relative to low affinity receptors. Other things being equal the number of receptors which can bind a determinant will depend on its concentration and this in turn will depend on the dose of antigen which has been administered. Consequently large doses of antigen will tend to generate large amounts of antibody of low average affinity, while low doses will generate small amounts of antibody of high average affinity. Furthermore, since each cell which is triggered eventually gives rise to a family of cells sensitive to the same antigen, repeated treatment with antigen will tend to increase the amount of antibody produced. Following a single dose of antigen we can expect two processes to occur. On the one hand, immunological memory will build up in the sense that the ability to make an enhanced secondary response to the antigen will increase as the number of cells sensitive to the antigen increases. On the other hand, antibodies of progressively higher affinity will tend to be produced. ('maturation' of the response). This will be brought about by selection for higher affinity receptors as the concentration of antigen drops as a consequence of elimination and catabolism. This process of selection will be accentuated as antibodies are produced which compete with receptors for the available antigen. Further discussion of the selection theory can be found in recent reviews (Siskind and Benacerraf 1969; Mitchison 1970).

3.1.2. *Factors which alter the simple application of the selection theory*

3.1.2.1. *Signal discrimination*
(a) *Immunological tolerance.*   Large doses of antigen tend to induce immunological tolerance, so that the individual not only produces amounts of antibody smaller than would have been evoked by smaller doses of antigen but also becomes incapable of responding normally to subsequent challenge with the same antigen. There is a fair measure of agreement about the cellular basis of immunological tolerance, which is thought to involve clone loss, i.e., the selective destruction of cells sensitive to the antigen consequent upon binding of antigen to these cells (Dresser and Mitchison 1968; Diener 1970). The mechanism by which cells discriminate between a tolerance-inducing and an immunizing contact with antigen is less clear. One view which rests largely on data concerning the *in vivo* effects of serum protein antigens is that the mode of presentation of antigen is crucial in such signal discrimination. In particular, presentation of antigen *via* macrophages is thought to favour immunization, whereas direct presentation of free antigen is thought to favour tolerance (Frei et al. 1965; Dresser and Mitchison 1968; Mitchison 1968a). Another view which rests mainly on data concerning the *in vitro* effects of flagellin is that signal discrimination depends on the number of contacts with antigen made by the cell, a high number favouring tolerance, a low number favouring immunization (Marchelonis and Gledhill 1968; Diener 1970). A further complication is that immunologi-

cal tolerance can also be induced in a low zone of dosage (Dresser 1962; Mitchison 1968b; Shellam and Nossal 1968). In the immunization of normal adult individuals low-zone tolerance is unlikely to pose a serious problem. Under these circumstances it has been encountered so far only with a limited number of serum protein antigens and with flagellin.

(b) Cellular versus humoral immunity. Certain ways of presenting antigen, e.g., in Freund's complete adjuvant or as antigen-antibody pre- cipitates, and certain routes of immunization, e.g. intradermal, are known to favour cellular as opposed to humoral immunity. The mechanism by which this discrimination operates is not fully understood. One view which in the past has received most attention (Uhr, 1966) is that under these circumstances what would now be called T* cells (Roitt et al. 1969) are selectively attracted to the antigen. Another possibility is that under these circumstances antigenic determinants are presented in a two-dimensional array which fits the distribution of receptors on T rather than B lymphocytes. This possibility is suggested by the recent discovery of a different distribution of immunoglobulin on the surface of T and B** cells (Greaves 1970; Raff 1970).

(c) The choice between immunoglobulin classes. The proportion of antibody belonging to the various immunoglobulin classes varies during the course of the immune response. In addition certain types of antigen and certain routes of immunization favour one immunoglobulin class rather than another. Here there seem to be at least two factors operating. One depends on the intrinsic property of the receptor on the antigen- sensitive cell. For example, a high density of repeating determinants should favour binding to 19S receptors and thus favour a 19S response. Experience with hapten-protein conjugates in which the density of hapten determinants is varied (Mäkelä et al. 1968) and data for blood group determinants with different naturally-occurring densities (Mäkelä et al. 1969) bear out the point. Another factor is that certain regions of the body are particularly rich in antigen-sensitive cells of one immuno- globulin class, so that antigens which enter *via* these regions evoke a selective response. The prime example here is the enteric route which favours IgA production.

(d) Selection in the variable part of the immunoglobulin molecule. Charged antigens tend to elicit antibodies of opposite charge presumably because of electrostatic attraction between the antigen and the receptor (Sela and Mozes 1966; Rüde et al. 1968). A less easily interpretable effect is the selection which certain antigens exercise between immuno-

---

* Thymus-dependent.
** Directly derived from bone-marrow precursors.

globulin molecules containing κ or λ chains (Siskind and Benacerraf 1969).

3.1.2.2. Non-specific mechanisms of antigen concentration and retention

In attempting to interpret the tempo of antibody production and the build-up of immunological memory which follows administration of a dose of antigen it is important to realize that although the major part of the dose is rapidly eliminated from the body a minor part is retained over a long period. Evidence of this comes mainly from experiments with radio-labelled proteins (Campbell and Garvey 1963; Ada et al. 1967). That some at least of the retained antigen is immunogenic is indicated by the following experimental evidence. (i) Extracts of lymphoid organs contain material capable of inducing an immune response when injected into test animals (Campbell and Garvey 1963). (ii) Transfer of intact lymphoid cells into unresponsive (X-irradiated or tolerant) animals injected some time previously with antigen results in antibody production (Mitchison 1965; Britton et al. 1968; Unanue and Askonas 1968). (iii) Antibody passively administered long after antigen injection can block production of antibody (Siskind 1970). (iv) Inter-action of lymphoid cells *in vitro* may release sequestered antigen so that upon transfer the cells spontaneously commence antibody produc-tion (Mitchison 1969a). Fluorescence, auto-radiographic and other data indicate that the bulk of the retained antigen is present in or on macro-phages (Ada et al. 1967; Campbell and Garvey 1963; Roos 1970). That antigen taken up by macrophages is particularly immunogenic, has been shown by two procedures: (i) Macrophages, after exposure to radioactive antigen, are injected into syngeneic mice and the immune response assessed in comparison with that induced by free antigen. (Mitchison 1969b; Unanue and Cerottini 1970; Askonas and Jaroskova 1970). (ii) Antigens and lymphocytes are mixed with or without macro-phages in tissue culture, and the proliferative and/or antibody response of lymphocytes is determined (Shortman et al. 1970). The surface of the macrophage where presentation to the receptor on antigen-sensitive lymphocytes can take place is thought to be the critical site for antigen retention (Unanue and Cerottini 1970).

3.1.2.3. Specific mechanisms of antigen concentration and retention

Whereas the macrophages of an unimmunized individual can function efficiently in the concentration and retention of antigen, other mechanisms of concentration and retention depend on prior immunization. These mechanisms can be regarded as a part of immunological memory;

indeed they may play a role in memory of importance equal to that played by the selection of antibody-forming cell precursors postulated by the basic selection theory. These mechanisms which are specific involve antibodies and can therefore conveniently be classified into mechanisms dependent on humoral antibody and mechanisms dependent on cellular immunity.

(a) Mechanisms dependent on humoral antibody. The presence of humoral antibody induced either by natural or artificial immunization can interfere with the immune response in at least four ways. One is the well known inhibitory effect which has already been referred to in Section 3.1.1. This is thought to operate through competition between humoral antibody and receptors on antigen-sensitive cells for limiting amounts of antigen. A second is the enhancing effect of antibody, particularly of the 19S class (Henry and Jerne 1968; McBride and Schierman 1970) which is thought to operate *via* gross effects on the localization of antigen (Dennert et al. 1971). Although this kind of enhancing effect can be obtained fairly easily with cellular antigens it has not so far been obtained with proteins. A third and more subtle effect of antibody has been described by Feldmann and Diener (1970a, b). This effect which has been obtained with flagellin and other protein antigens *in vitro* using minute doses of antigen and antibody probably operates through the construction of a matrix of antigenic determinants which fit the receptors on the antigen-sensitive lymphocyte. This kind of mechanism has not so far been shown to operate *in vivo*, although Feldman and Diener suggest that certain kinds of 'enhancement' of transplant survival operate centrally in this way. A fourth way in which antibody can interact with the immune response is by promoting the deposition of antigen on the surface of the dendritic cells of the lymph nodes and spleen – 'follicular localization' (Nossal et al. 1964b; Humphrey and Frank 1967). In this reaction the antibody acts as a glue holding antigen (by means of an antigenic determinant) to the cell plasma membrane (by means of the Fc portion of the immunoglobulin). Antigen molecules are thus held extracellularly and can come into contact with passing cells. The purpose of this reaction is not clear. It has been shown for some antigens that antibody formation can occur prior to the follicular localization of antigen. This suggests that the role of antibody in this area may be (i) to sequester antigen so that further antigen activity is inhibited, (ii) to initiate memory and/or trigger memory cells into antibody production, (iii) to react with antigen-sensitive cells in such a way as to cause tolerance. Though these possibilities have been postulated either individually or collectively evidence in favour of any is so far circumstantial.

(b) Mechanisms involving cellular immunity. From a variety of studies on the thymus-marrow interaction, and on the carrier effect obtained with hapten-protein conjugates, the conclusion has been drawn that in certain cellular responses T lymphocytes act as helpers in the stimulation of B lymphocytes which serve as the precursors of antibody-forming cells. Possibly also T lymphocytes can help other T lymphocytes mediate a humoral response. In this type of co-operative response both cells bind antigen specifically, both show immunological memory and both can be rendered tolerant (Miller and Mitchell 1969; Taylor 1969; Boak et al. 1971; Britton et al. 1971; Mitchison 1971a, b, c; Greaves 1970; Mitchison 1971d). Helping is thought to involve the formation of a bridge of antigen between the T and B cells in which one determinant binds to a T cell receptor (almost certainly an immunoglobulin) and another determinant binds to the immunoglobulin receptor of the B lymphocyte (Mitchison et al. 1970). Possibly the formation of a matrix of bridges which permits multi-point binding is of crucial importance (Mitchison 1971e). Whatever the precise mechanism by which help from T cells operates the effect of this help is to alter greatly the reactivity of individuals in whom a population of reactive T cells has been raised by immunization. As a consequence of the presence of helper cells the individual becomes more sensitive to stimulation by the specific antigen, by a factor of the order of one thousand-fold (Mitchison 1971e). Thus, in routine immunization it may be just as important to expand a population of T lymphocyte helpers as to build up a population of specific antibody-producing cells.

More recently it has become clear that T and B lymphocytes have different thresholds of stimulation. This is a fact which needs to be borne in mind in designing schedules of immunization. Low doses of sheep erythrocytes in the mouse tend to stimulate differentially T cells rather than B cells (Möller and Greaves 1971). In the immune response to protein antigens the position is still unclear, but at least in the induction of tolerance T cells clearly respond to much lower concentrations of antigen than do B cells (Mitchison 1971f; Weigle 1971). In general we can expect therefore that low doses of antigen will tend differentially to build up an antigen-concentrating mechanism, whereas high doses will tend differentially to expand the pool of antibody-forming cell precursors.

3.2. Dose of antigen

3.2.1. Dosage with adjuvant

Adjuvants have proved so effective in increasing the amount of antibody produced and so useful in reducing the labour of immunization that they should normally always be used for routine immunization. It is therefore appropriate to consider first findings which have been made with the use of adjuvants. Furthermore, we have a fairly complete picture of the response of rabbits to dinitrophenylated proteins injected in Freund's adjuvant, thanks to the work of Eisen and his school. Representative data are shown in Tables 3.1 and 3.2 taken from Siskind et al. (1968). Table 3.1 shows the average binding affinity of anti-2-4-dinitrophenyl (anti-DNP) antibody synthesized by rabbits with time after immunization. The average affinity of the antibody formed increases progressively with time after immunization. Furthermore, the rate of increase in average affinity is generally slower with higher doses of antigen. These findings are consistent with the selection theory outlined in 1.1. Table 3.2 shows the effect of antigen dose on the amount of anti-DNP antibody formed. The smallest dose of antigen, 0.05 mg, is suboptimal. Maximum antibody production occurs after injection of 0.05 mg. As the dose is further increased antibody is produced initially more rapidly but finally reaches lower levels. This effect of high doses of antigen can be attributed to induction of immunological tolerance. These responses are typical for the rabbit and the guinea-pig, and are little different from those obtained in the mouse (Mitchison 1964; Brownstone et al. 1966).

Very much smaller amounts of antigen are needed for optimal stimulation of T lymphocyte responses. Thus, for induction of delayed hyper-

TABLE 3.1

Effect of antigen dose on the affinity of anti-DNP antibody.*

| | *Affinity* $(-\Delta F^\circ$ *in kcal/mole$)$* | | | |
| | *days after immunization* | | | |
Antigen dose (mg)	13	20	27	41
0.05		9.88	10.0	11.1
0.5	8.72	10.3	11.2	12.7
5.0	8.96	9.70	10.2	11.0
50.0	8.46	8.06	8.52	9.54

* Rabbits immunized with DNP-bovine gamma globulin in complete Freund's adjuvants and bled at the times indicated. Affinities determined by fluorescence quenching of purified antibody with DNP-lysine at 21 °C. Data presented are averages of between 3 and 17 individual animals. (From Siskind 1970.)

TABLE 3.2

Effect of antigen dose on the amount of anti-DNP
antibody formed.*

| Antigen dose | *Antibody concentration (mg/ml)* | | | | | |
| | *days after immunization* | | | | | |
(mg)	4	7	13	20	27	41
0.05			0.02	0.08	0.44	0.54
0.5		0.07	0.26	0.61	2.31	4.23
5.0	0.01	0.07	1.06	1.16	1.80	1.98
50.0	0.04	0.18	1.78	1.14	1.09	1.36

* Rabbits were immunized with DNP-bovine gamma
globulin in complete Freund's adjuvants and bled at
the times indicated. Antibody concentration determined
by quantitative precipitin reaction using DNP-bovine
fibrinogen. Data presented are averages of between 4
and 25 individual animals. (From Siskind 1970.)

sensitivity to diphtheria toxoid and to ovalbumin by specific precipitates incorporated into Freund's complete adjuvant, $2.5 \mu g$ of antigen
is optimal in guinea-pigs (Uhr et al. 1957). Similarly, for optimum induction of helper cells in rabbits and guinea-pigs a dose of $1–50 \mu g$
of bovine γ-globulin in Freund's complete adjuvant is used (Katz et al.
1970). This high sensitivity of T lymphocytes is in line with other findings referred to in 1.2.

There is a vast literature on the use of different adjuvants. In the rabbit
Freund's complete adjuvant is far the most widely used. In the mouse
alum-precipitated protein mixed with *Bordetella pertussis* has advantages (Dresser 1965; Brownstone et al. 1966). Systematic studies have
been made in the rabbit (Weigle et al. 1960) and the mouse (Brownstone
et al. 1966; Spitznagel and Allison 1970).

3.2.2. Without adjuvants

3.2.2.1. Lower threshold of immune response
A single dose of most protein antigens elicits only a slow and feeble antibody response (Figs. 3.1 and 3.2) and few systematic studies have been
made. An exception is flagellin and the related antigens polymerized
flagellin and flagella. These all show a lower threshold of response at
$0.1–0.01 \mu g$ dose (irregularly in the case of flagellin) (Nossal et al. 1964a).
Nossal, Ada and their colleagues have systematically investigated the
immunological properties of these potent immunogens; they are in

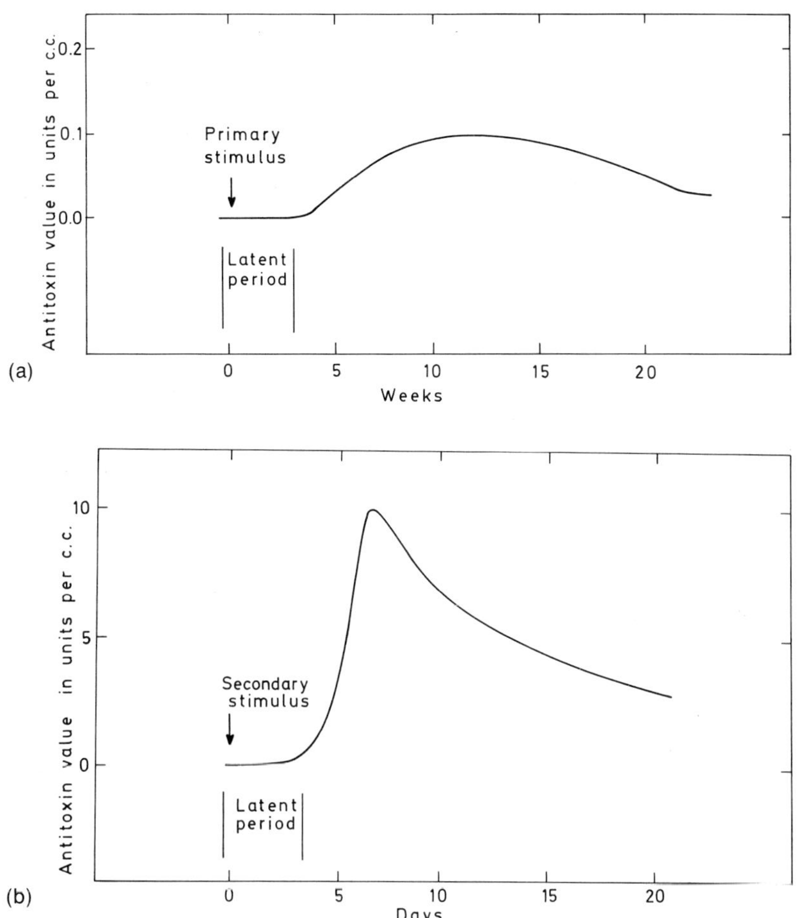

Fig. 3.1. (a) The course of antitoxin production after a single injection in a non-immune animal. (b) The course of antitoxin production after an injection in an immune animal. (From Glenny 1927.)

several ways exceptional, but it is interesting to find that certain preparations of transplantation antigens appear to resemble flagellin (Manson and Simmons 1969; Mitchison 1971d). High levels of antibody can usually be attained by repeated injections of protein antigens. Fig. 3.3 shows the levels of antibody attained after 60 injections spaced 3 times weekly in mice of diphtheria toxoid, ovalbumin, lysozyme and bovine serum albumin (BSA). Clearly there are very different lower thresholds of the immune response; one for diphtheria toxoid is at 0.01–0.1 μg

     N. A. Mitchison

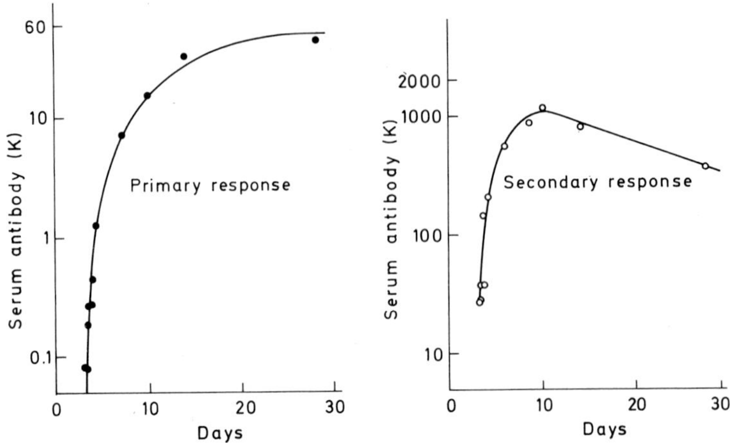

Fig. 3.2. A representative primary and secondary antibody response to intravenous injection of $6 \times 10^8 \, \phi X$. The interval between injections was 3 weeks for the secondary response. (From Uhr et al. 1962.)

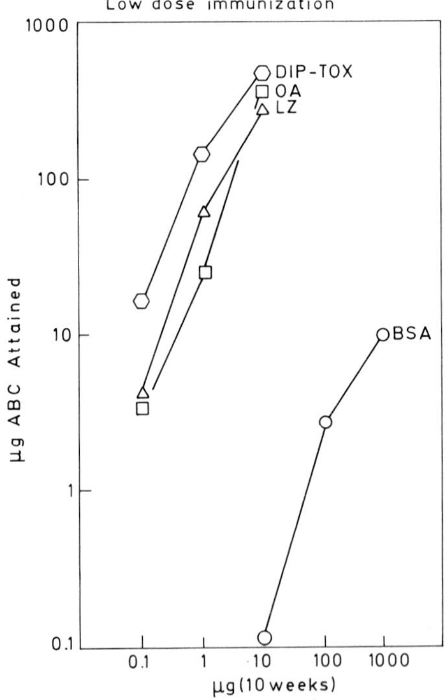

Fig. 3.3. Antibody level attained after prolonged administration of antigen. (From Mitchison 1968a.)

which is lower by a factor of about 1000 times than that for BSA. The response levels off as the doses are increased above the threshold level until the zone of high-dose tolerance is reached.

3.2.2.2. Tolerance effects

Low-zone tolerance can probably be obtained under favourable circumstances with all low and medium molecular weight soluble proteins (oligomeric proteins), e.g., serum protein antigens, ribonuclease, lysozyme, diphtheria toxoid and flagellin (Dresser and Mitchison 1968; Mitchison 1968b; Shellam and Nossal 1968). Furthermore, with the possible exception of flagellin, the minimum dose of antigen needed to induce low-zone tolerance is remarkably constant, at around $1.0\,\mu$g per mouse or proportionately more for larger animals. Repeated doses of antigen are usually needed to induce and maintain low-zone paralysis although one or two injections of certain immunoglobulin antigens are sufficient probably because these proteins are cleared slowly from the circulation. The circumstances under which low-zone tolerance can be obtained vary from one antigen to another according to their immunogenic capacities. Some antigens, exemplified by bovine IgG in the mouse, become entirely non-immunogenic if freed of aggregated material by high speed centrifugation or by *in vivo* passage, and if injected without adjuvant. These proteins will induce tolerance if injected in any quantity above the minimum dose required for tolerance induction. Other antigens, probably the majority, exemplified by diphtheria toxoid in the mouse, are immunogenic over the whole tolerance-inducing range, and in smaller doses as well. These antigens can induce low-zone tolerance only in the immunosuppressed individual, e.g., in animals which have been sub-lethally irradiated or in which specific tolerance of the antigen has already been induced, so that maintaining rather than inducing dosage can be used.

A third category of antigen is exemplified by bovine serum albumin in the mouse. These antigens are immunogenic even when freed of aggregated material by *in vivo* passage, but only at doses higher than the minimum required to induce tolerance. The effect of treating mice with bovine serum albumin therefore varies markedly with the dose. Below the minimum dose needed to induce tolerance nothing happens. At and a little above the dose tolerance is induced. As the dose is increased still further the threshold for immunizing is crossed and the treated animals become immune (as the dose is increased still further a zone of high-dose tolerance is entered – see below). Since the majority of antigens appear to belong to the second category, i.e. the minimum dose required for immunization is well below the threshold for low-zone tolerance,

tolerance of this kind is unlikely to be encountered in the normal course of immunization. After immunosuppression, however, the likelihood of tolerance induction is much increased.

If the aim is to induce low-zone tolerance for mice treatment with 600 r followed by 10 weeks of injection of antigen 3 times a week is recommended (Mitchison 1968b). In other species the immunosuppressive effects of radiation are less certain and treatment with antigen commencing at birth is recommended (Weigle 1967).

The position of flagellin in this scheme is controversial (Shellam and Nossal 1968; Diener 1970). Flagellin certainly shows at least two zones of tolerance (Fig. 3.4). The question is which of these corresponds to

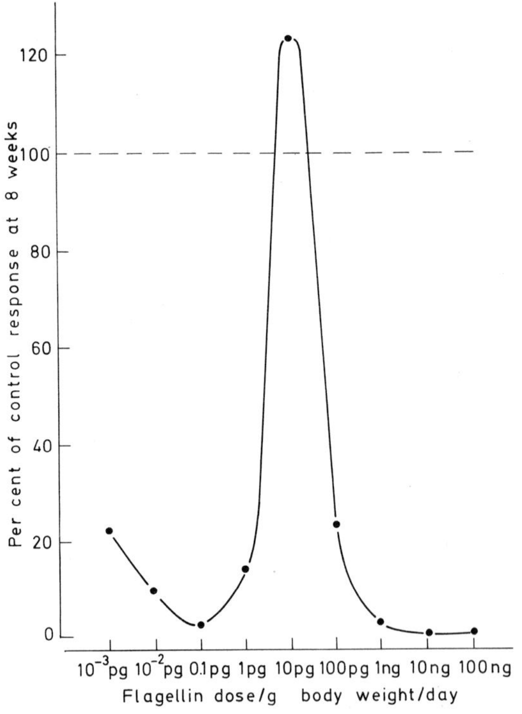

Fig. 3.4. High and low zone tolerance in the rat to flagellin of *S. adelaide* expressed as percentage values of the average control titre. Experimental procedure: $10^{-15} - 10^{-7}$ g of flagellin/g body weight were given to rats, beginning on the day of birth and continuing for two weeks. Control animals received diluent only during this period. All rats were given twice weekly injections of 10 μg of flagellin, beginning the day after daily injections ceased, and continuing until the animals were 10 weeks of age. At 12 weeks of age, all animals were challenged with 10 μg flagellin. (From Diener 1970.)

low-zone tolerance in the sense used here. If the tolerance induced by ultra-low doses (on the left in Fig. 3.4) is regarded as an example of typical low-zone tolerance then the generalization about a constant threshold of low-zone tolerance made above breaks down. If, on the other hand, the right-hand zone in the figure is regarded as low-zone induction then the generalization stands and the tolerance induced by ultra-low doses becomes something altogether exceptional. The matter is of some theoretical importance because a uniform threshold of low-zone induction constitutes a strong argument in favour of the antigen presentation theory (see 3.1.2.1a).

High-zone tolerance is regularly induced when doses of antigen enter the milligram range (Dresser and Mitchison 1968). The effect has been obtained with serum protein antigens in the mouse and the rabbit, but for other antigens there are serious problems of toxicity in this dose range. Our standard procedure for inducing high-zone tolerance of bovine serum albumin in the mouse is to inject 10 mg 3 times a week for 10 weeks, without irradiation (Mitchison 1965, 1971f). High-zone tolerance is thought to be induced when an animal which is already producing antibody is treated with enough antigen to overcome the competitive suppression of induction exerted by the antibody (Dresser and Mitchison 1968). In addition, these high doses of antigen affect B as well as T lymphocytes, instead of T lymphocytes only (Mitchison 1971f), as in low-zone tolerance.

3.3. The response to secondary injection of antigen

3.3.1. Kinetics and quantity of antibody

In comparison with the response to a primary antigenic stimulus a secondary stimulus evokes antibody in larger amounts and more rapidly. This is illustrated in Fig. 3.1 taken from Glenny's classical work on the response of horses to diphtheria toxin. The point is illustrated in greater detail in Figs. 3.2 taken from a recent study of the response of guinea-pigs to bacteriophage ϕX 174 (Uhr et al. 1962). Note that the secondary response evokes about one hundred times as much antibody as the primary response and reaches a peak earlier. Note also that using the very sensitive bacteriophage inactivation assay antibody the 'latent period' is less than three days. An interpretation of these features of the secondary response has been offered in Section 1 in terms of selection by primary immunization of (a) clones of antibody-forming cell precursors (B lymphocytes), and (b) clones of helper cells (T lymphocytes).

                                    N. A. Mitchison

3.3.2. *The timing of secondary immunization*

The capacity to give a heightened secondary response increases slowly after primary immunization. The growth in this sense of immunological memory is illustrated in Fig. 3.5, taken from Fecsik et al. (1964). In this experiment the primary antigenic stimulus was a single injection of diphtheria toxoid. No doubt memory develops over an even longer period after 'primary' stimulation with antigen incorporated in a water

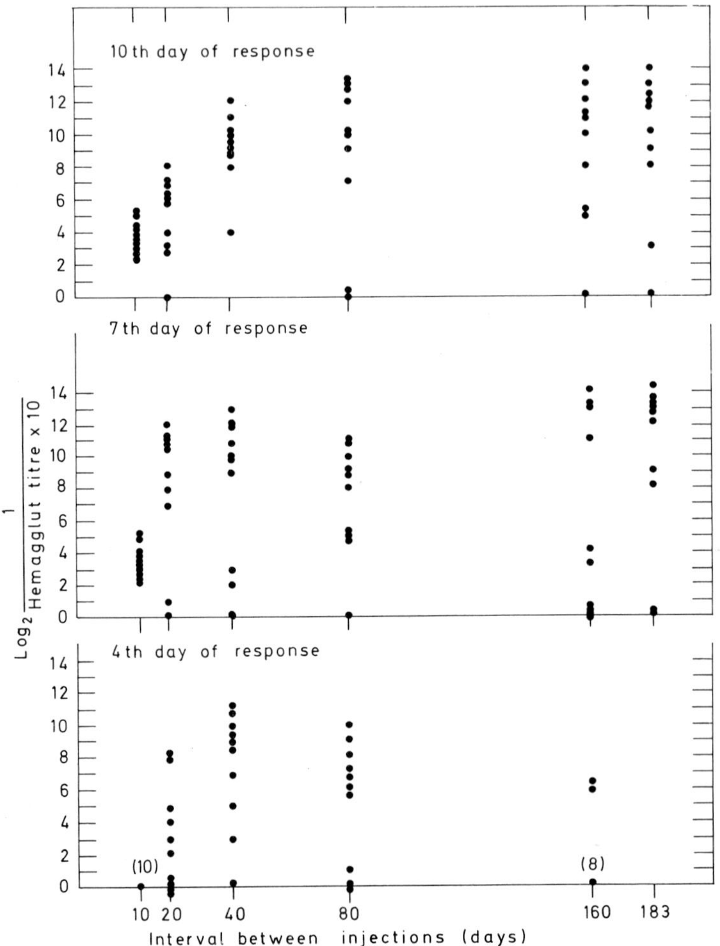

Fig. 3.5. Relation of interval between diphtheria toxoid injections and height of the resultant secondary response. Each dot represents one mouse. Double dose antigen at 183 day interval. (From Fecsik et al. 1964.)

in oil emulsion or in other kinds of depot which leak antigen slowly. Administration of several successive antigenic stimuli can increase the response still further, although less dramatically (see Fig. 3.6, taken from Barr and Glenny 1945).

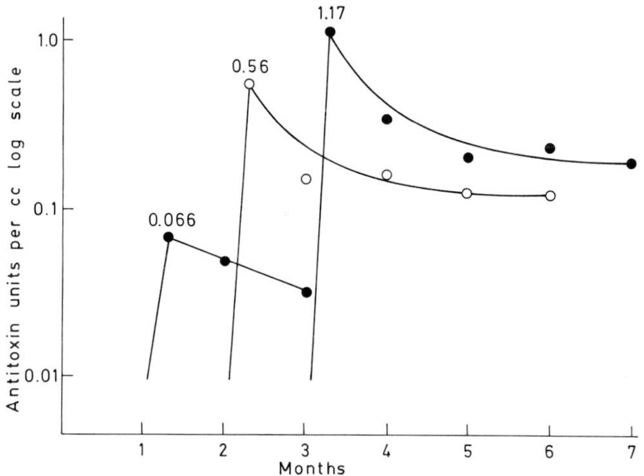

Fig. 3.6. The geometric means of the antitoxic values of the serum of three groups of fifteen guinea pigs given two doses of 0.005 cc (0.25 Lf) of A.P.T. at intervals of 1, 2 and 3 months respectively. (From Barr and Glenny 1945.)

3.3.3.   *Antigen dose in the secondary response*

The secondary response requires smaller doses of antigen than does the primary response. Quantitative studies in mice (Mitchison, 1971a) indicate that with most protein antigens significant responses can be obtained with 0.001 μg of antigen, and that the response reaches a plateau with doses of 0.1–1.0 μg. As in the primary response, however, proteins vary markedly in their intrinsic immunogenic capacity in terms of the dose required to elicit a peak response. This sensitivity of the secondary response can presumably be attributed largely to the activity of helper T lymphocytes. In the light of the considerations outlined in 3.3.1–3 a number of roughly similar standard schedules of immunization have been proposed. In this laboratory we normally immunize rabbits either by a single dose of 0.5–5.0 μg of protein in Freund's complete adjuvant spread among two intramuscular sites, or two successive intramuscular injections two weeks apart (during the interval the emulsion can be stored in its syringe in the refrigerator). After six weeks the rabbits are boosted with 0.1 mg of antigen intraperitoneally, or intravenously, under cover of an anti-histamine such as phenergan. They are bled 9–13 days later. A variant on this sort of schedule which has been much used is to administer the secondary stimulus in Freund's adjuvant (Eisen et al. 1969).

3.3.4. *Affinity*

Antibody evoked in the secondary response tends to have a higher affinity than that evoked in the primary (Steiner and Eisen 1967). Progressive selection among B lymphocytes in the course of primary immunization readily accounts for this finding. As might also be expected, the longer the interval between primary and secondary stimulation the higher the affinity of the final antibodies. This is particularly well illustrated by anti-toxin production in the horse (Barr and Glenny 1945) where avidity grows progressively as the interval is increased up to 12 months. Here again the maximum effect which can be obtained will presumably be determined by the duration of action of the primary antigenic stimulus and this will depend on the use of adjuvants, etc.

'Original sin' is another clear-cut property of the secondary response. Provided that some carrier determinants are held in common (see 3.3.5 below) secondary stimulation can often be obtained with an antigen different from that used for primary stimulation, so long as there is some structural similarity and serological cross-reactivity with the inducing determinant. The antibody which is then evoked tends to have an affinity higher for the primary than the secondary determinant. The phenomenon has been termed 'original antigenic sin' (Fazekas de St. Groth and Webster 1966a, b; Eisen et al. 1969) and can readily be explained in terms of selection of antibody-forming cell precursors by the primary antigenic stimulus. The phenomenon is of some epidemiological importance because, for example, the immune response to a viral infection can in this way yield information about prior infection with related viruses. The point is illustrated for anti-hapten immunization in Table 3.3. Here rabbits which were primed with DNP-bovine γ-globulin (DNP-BGG) made a secondary response to TNP-BGG in which the antibody had a higher affinity for DNP than for TNP.

3.3.5. *The carrier effect*

In raising anti-hapten antibody by immunization with hapten-protein conjugates it is usually necessary to perform secondary stimulation with the same carrier protein as that used for primary immunization (Ovary and Benacerraf 1963; Mitchison 1971a). This effect can readily be explained in terms of a need for helper T lymphocytes elicited by

TABLE 3.3
Secondary response in rabbits primed with DNP-BGG.*

| Second immunogen | Serum antibody level 7 to 9 days after second injection | | Ratio K_0-DNP K_0-TNP |
	Precipitation with DNP-HSA $\mu g/ml$	Precipitation with TNP-HSA $\mu g/ml$	
DNP-BGG	—	100	13
	965	940	1.8
	600	520	2.0
TNP-BGG	415	410	1.4
	1,120	1,170	72
	400	370	—

* Each rabbit received about 1.0 mg DNP-BGG in complete adjuvant in rear footpads. Seven months later, five animals in each of three groups were given a second injection of the indicated immunogen (1.0 mg in complete adjuvant distributed among the four footpads). One day before the second injection, test bleedings showed no precipitating antibodies in any of the 15 rabbits.

the primary immunization (see 3.1.2.3 above). At first sight, there appears to be a contradiction between the carrier effect and the capacity of rather weakly cross-reactive haptens to elicit a secondary response as mentioned in 3.3.4 above. Evidently 'hapten' and 'carrier' determinants behave in different ways. Whether this should be attributed to restrictions on the reactivity of T lymphocytes (Paul et al. 1970) or to polyvalent *versus* oligovalent determinants (Taylor and Iverson 1970) is still the subject of controversy.

3.4. Route of immunization

The literature on the effect of the route of immunization on the immune response is vast and bewildering. There is hardly a medical speciality but claims for its own region of the body a unique reactivity towards antigen. Only major themes will therefore be considered here.

3.4.1. Routes favouring induction of delayed hypersensitivity

Application to the skin is the most effective way of obtaining hypersensitivity to simple chemicals (Chase 1967). The intravenous and parenteral routes are much less effective, and chemicals introduced in this way may induce immunological tolerance, possibly because the conjugates which form with native proteins will then be screened by

                    N. A. Mitchison

the liver (Frei et al. 1965). With protein antigens intradermal immunization favours delayed hypersensitivity, particularly when adjuvants are
not used (Uhr 1966).

3.4.2. *Routes favouring preferential synthesis of various immuno-globulin classes*

The presence of IgA-producing cells in the lymphoid tissue of the gut,
respiratory tract and exocrine glands is well established and these
antibodies play an important role in external secretions (Tomasi and
Bienenstock 1968; Small and Waldman 1969). It is therefore to be
expected that antigens which enter the body, e.g., across the wall of
the gut, should stimulate the local synthesis of IgA antibodies. That this
is indeed the case has been demonstrated by experimental studies with
oral and nasal administration of antigens. This point is illustrated in
Table 3.4, where enteric stimulation (obtained by feeding ferritin in
the drinking water) can be seen to have stimulated local production
of IgA antibodies in the gut and gut-associated lymphoid tissue of mice.

IgE (reagin; homocytotropic antibody) (Bennich et al. 1969) is synthesized preferentially in response to certain types of antigenic stimulation such as from intestinal parasites or pollen, and is produced mainly
in the respiratory tract by patients prone to allergic disorders. The
suspicion is therefore that the respiratory route favours preferentially
production of IgE antibodies.

3.4.3. *Routes favouring induction of immunological tolerance*

Injection of protein *via* a mesenteric vein may be a potent method of
inducing immunological tolerance to protein antigens, possibly for the
reason outlined in 3.4.1 above, but the evidence is incomplete (Battisto
and Miller 1962). A better authenticated example of a route of injection
favouring the induction of tolerance is intrathymic injection (Staples et al.
1966; Horiuchi and Waksman 1968). If rats are sub-lethally irradiated
with a shielded thymus and then injected with bovine γ-globulin the
antigen injected into the thymus induces tolerance in much smaller
quantities than if injected systemically (less by a factor of 100–1000).
The response of mice to this antigen is markedly thymus dependent and
it is likely that in these experiments tolerance is induced in T lymphocytes
while they are still within the thymus prior to their subsequent dissemination to peripheral lymphoid tissue.

3.5. *The production of antisera for radioimmunoassay*

The production of antisera for radioimmunoassay of peptide hormones
constitutes a special problem which merits separate discussion. This is

TABLE 3.4

Anti-ferritin antibodies in serum and lymphoid tissues. C3H mice receiving repeated intraperitoneal stimulation (ferritin intraperitoneally), and enteric stimulation (ferritin in drinking water). (From Crabbe et al. 1969.)

Serum								Antibody-containing cells in lymphoid tissues†			
Concentrations*				Antibody activity**				Spleen	Peripheral lymph nodes	Mesenteric lymph nodes	Intestine
IgG_1	IgG_2	IgA	IgM	IgG_1	IgG_2	IgA	IgM				
Repeated intraperitoneal stimulation											
160	53	8.7	205	18.8	13.2	24.1	—	+++	+++	++++ (+++ in G) (+ in A)	+
34	16.5	7	200	58.8	27.3	—	3.8	++	++	++	++
93	38	7.8	191	18.3	31.6	—	—	+++	+++	+++	++ (++ in A)
58	27	8.2	260	17.2	11.1	—	20.2	+++ (++ in G)	++++ (+++ in G) (+ in M) (+ in A)	+++ (+++ in G) (++ in A)	++ (++ in A)
Enteric stimulation											
5.5	11.5	9.2	124	—	—	32.2		+	—	+ (+ in A)	++++ (++++ in A)
7.5	15	7.5	130	—	—		—	—	—	—	—
15.5	8	8.8	157	—	—	11.4	—	—	—	+ (+ in A)	+++ (+++ in A)
9.5	14	8.5	123	—	—		—	+	+	+	++

* Percentages of values found in a pool of serum from conventional adult C_3H mice.

** Percentages of the immunoglobulin found to combine with ferritin.

† — = no antibody activity or antibody-containing cells detected; + = 1–5 cells/tissue section; ++ = 5–20 cells/tissue section; +++ = 20 – 100 cells/tissue section; ++++ = more than 100 cells/tissue section.

because antibodies of quite exceptionally high avidity are required. In addition there are special problems associated with low immunogenicity due to low molecular weight of some peptides or to their structural similarities with hormones native to the species under immunization. At the same time very great efforts are being made to produce these reagents because of their clinical value and consequent commercial importance. The production of the reagents for radioimmunoassay thus provides an arena in which theories of immunization are subjected to rest.

The dimensions of the avidity problem are specified in Table 3.5. The peptide hormones in plasma occur in a range of concentrations from 1 to 100 times 10^{-12} molar, so that antibodies are needed for their assay which have avidities sufficiently high to bind antigen at these concentrations. Since the assays are performed in a region where the antigen-antibody reaction is bi-molecular, affinities (K_0) of 10^{12} or higher may be required. This falls outside the range of average affinities normally encountered (see e.g., Table 3.1). This is a less serious problem than might be imagined because for the purposes of the assay only a sub-fraction of the total population of antibodies present in a given antiserum need be utilized.

TABLE 3.5

Concentrations of some hormones in plasma.*

Hormone	Molar concentration
Thyroxine	$100,000 \times 10^{-12}$
Hydrocortisone	$100,000$ to $500,000 \times 10^{-12}$
	(p.m.) (a.m.)
Insulin	100×10^{-12}
Glucagon	100×10^{-12}
Growth hormone	60×10^{-12}
Parathyroid hormone	30×10^{-12}
ACTH	1 to 10×10^{-12}
	(p.m.) (a.m.)
Serum proteins	800×10^{-6}

* From Yalow and Berson 1968.

3.5.1. Adjuvant and dosage of immunogen

Antisera are normally produced with the aid of Freund's complete adjuvant (Yalow and Berson 1968; Hurn and Landon 1970). Injection of immunogen without the use of this adjuvant has proved wasted effort (Hurn and Landon 1970). Other adjuvant procedures that have been employed in conjunction with or as an alternative to Freund's are adsorption of immunogen onto microparticulate material such as carbon polystyrene latex or polyacrylamide beads, or onto inorganic salts such as aluminium hydroxide or phosphate (Hurn and Landon 1970). Mixing the peptide with polyvinyl pyrrolidone has also proved effective in the difficult case of glucagon (Assan et al. 1968). Hurn and Landon find that the antibody response is virtually independent of immunogen dosage over a wide range. They recommend doses in the range of 0.1–5.0 mg for primary inoculation in Freund's adjuvant into rabbits, with subsequent injections of approximately half as much. The use of unpurified hormone preparations is recommended so that these doses may contain as little as 1% antigen. The effective dose for guinea pigs is thought not to be much less than that for rabbits.

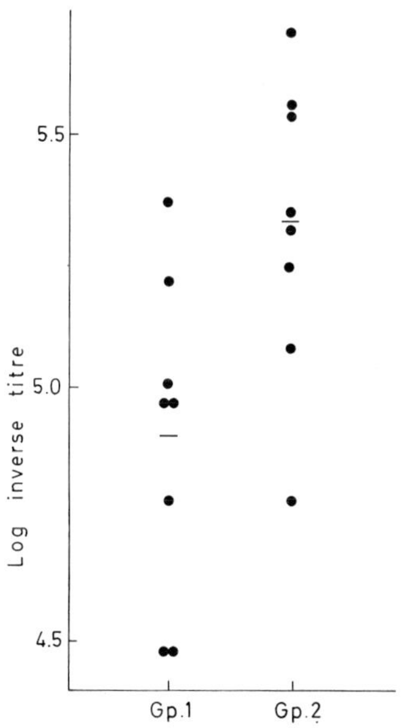

Fig. 3.7. Titres of guinea pig anti-insulin sera, expressed as the log inverse dilution required to bind 40% of 100 pg of ^{131}I-ox insulin. The animals in group 1 received 4 injections at monthly intervals and a fifth injection after a 4-month rest. Those in group 2 received 8 injections at monthly intervals. Each injection comprised 0.5 mg porcine insulin in Freund's complete adjuvant given subcutaneously. The animals in group 2 had a significantly higher mean titre ($p < 0.01$) than those in group 1 who had the rest prior to a final booster injection. (From Hurn and Landon, 1970.)

3.5.2. Route of administration

Normally subcutaneous or intramuscular injections are used (Hurn and Landon 1970; Yalow and Berson 1968). For poor immunogens the available evidence suggests that other sites may be ranked in decreasing order of effectiveness as follows: into the lymph nodes, intraarticular (usually into the knee joints), intradermal, intramuscular, intraperitoneal, subcutaneous, and finally intravenous.

3.5.3. Timing of injections and bleeding

Antibody levels rise slowly after a primary injection of immunogen in Freund's adjuvant, reaching a peak some six weeks later. Booster doses are given not earlier than four weeks after the first injection, nor more frequently than once each month thereafter (Hurn and Landon 1970). Antibody levels rise to a maximum about 10 days after each booster

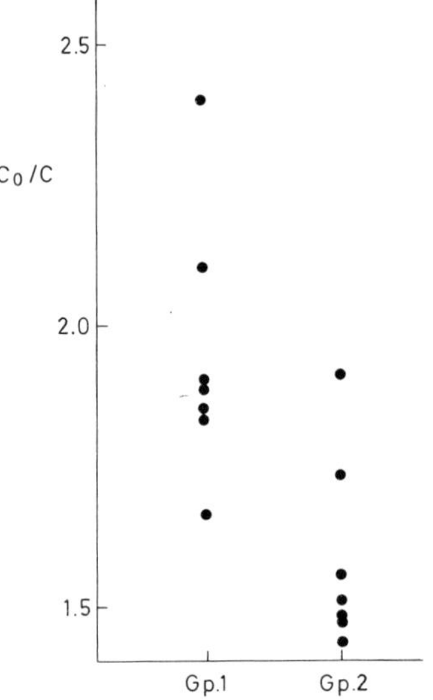

Fig. 3.8. The sensitivity achieved with the anti-insulin sera shown in Fig. 3.7. This was measured in a radioimmunoassay system as:

$$\frac{\text{Counts bound in absence of unlabelled insulin}}{\text{Counts bound in presence of 160 pg unlabelled insulin}} = \frac{C_0}{C}$$

The antisera were used at a final concentration such as to bind approximately 40% of labelled hormone in the absence of unlabelled peptide. The result of one serum from each group was excluded because of marked deviation of the 'zero' binding level from the desired value of 40%. The sensitivity, which is an effective measure of avidity, was significantly higher ($p < 0.05$) in the group 1 guinea pigs who had the lower mean titre. (From Hurn and Landon, 1970.)

injection, and animals should be bled between the 7th and 14th days. Several bleeds may be taken during this time without affecting the amount or quality of the antibody. Hurn and Landon have investigated the question whether a rest prior to boosting enhances the production of highly avid antiserum (Figs. 3.7 and 3.8). Their results seem to confirm the benefit of a long rest period in relation to the avidity of the resultant antiserum. They show also that the group of animals with the antibodies of high avidity have significantly lower titres. These findings conform nicely to the selective theory of antibody induction described above. The theory attributes the higher affinity antibodies to the lower concentration of antigen in the group of guinea pigs which were rested prior to boost.

By way of comment, it is worth noting that in the two areas where well defined antisera are most urgently required for practical purposes, namely radioimmunoassay and antilymphocyte antiserum, there is least agreement on optimum schedules of immunization. Each laboratory and commercial production unit has tended to adopt its own procedure. No doubt in the long run our understanding of the control of the immune response is likely to benefit from all this helter skelter.

References

ADA, G. L., C. R. PARISH, G. J. V. NOSSAL and A. ABBOT, 1967, Cold Spring Harbor Symp. Quant. Biol. *32*, 381.

ASKONAS, B. A. and L. JAROSKOVA, 1970, Macrophages as helper cells in antibody induction. *In*: J. Šterzl and I. Riha, eds.: Proceedings of a symposium on developmental aspects of antibody formation and structure, Prague, 1969, Vol. 2. Prague, Academia. pp. 531–546.

ASSAN, R., G. ROSSLIN and G. TCHOBROUTSKY, 1968, *in*: M. Margouliss, ed.: Glucagon in blood and immunological specificity of glucagon molecule in proteins and polypeptide hormones. Amsterdam, Excerpta Medica Foundation. p. 87.

BARR, M. and A. T. GLENNY, 1945, J. Hygiene *44*, 135.

BATTISTO, J. R. and J. MILLER, 1962, Proc. Soc. Exptl. Biol. Med. *111*, 111.

BENNICH, H., K. ISHIZAKA, T. ISHIZAKA and S. G. JOHANSSON, 1969, J. Immunol. *102*, 826.

BOAK, J. L., N. A. MITCHISON and P. H. PATTISSON, 1971, Eur. J. Immunol., 63.

BRITTON, S., N. A. MITCHISON and K. RAJEWSKY, 1971, Eur. J. Immunol., 65.

BRITTON, S., T. WEPSIC and G. MÖLLER, 1968, Immunology *14*, 491.

BROWNSTONE, A., N. A. MITCHISON and R. PITT-RIVERS, 1966, Immunology *10*, 481.

CAMPBELL, D. H. and J. S. GARVEY, 1963, Advan. Immunol. *3*, 261.

CHASE, M., 1967, Harvey Lectures, 61.

CHASE, P. A., B. R. NASH, H. BAZIN, H. EYSSEN and J. F. HEREMANS, 1969, J. Exptl. Med. *130*, 723.

DENNERT, G., H. POHLIT and K. RAJEWSKY, 1971, Cooperative antibody. A concentrating device. *In*: O. Mäkelä, A. M. Cross and T. U. Kosunen, eds.: Cell interactions in immune responses. New York, Academic Press (in press).

DIENER, E., 1970, The primary immune response and immunological tolerance. *In*: A. Studer and H. Cottier, eds.: Handbuch der allgemeinen Pathologie. Berlin, Springer-Verlag. pp. 250–325.

DRESSER, D. W., 1962, Immunology 5, 378.

DRESSER, D. W., 1965, Immunology 9, 261.

DRESSER, D. W. and N. A. MITCHISON, 1968, Advan. Immunol. 8, 129.

EISEN, H. N., J. R. LITTLE, L. A. STEINER, E. S. SIMMS and W. GRAY, 1969, Israel J. Med. Sci. 5, 338.

FAZEKAS DE ST. GROTH, S. and R. G. WEBSTER, 1966, J. Exptl. Med. *124*, 331 and 347.

FECSIK, A. I., W. T. BUTLER and A. H. COONS, 1964, J. Exptl. Med. *120*, 1041.

FELDMANN, M. and E. DIENER, 1970, J. Exptl. Med. *131*, 247.

FELDMANN, M. and E. DIENER, 1970, Immunology (in press).

FREI, P. C., B. BENACERRAF and G. J. THORBECKE, 1965, Proc. Natl. Acad. Sci. U.S. *53*, 20.

GLENNY, A. T., 1927, J. Hygiene *24*, 301.

GREAVES, M. F., 1970, Transplant. Rev. *5*, 45.

HENRY, C. and N. K. JERNE, 1968, J. Exptl. Med. *128*, 133.

HORIUCHI, A. and B. H. WAKSMAN, 1968, J. Immunol. *100*, 974.

HUMPHREY, J. H. and FRANK, M. M., 1967, Immunology *13*, 87.

HURN, P. A. L. and J. LANDON, 1970, Antisera for radioimmunoassay. *In*: K. E. Kirkham and W. M. Hunter, eds.: Radioimmunoassay methods. Edinburgh and London, E. & S. Livingstone. p. 63.

KATZ, D. H., W. E. PAUL, E. A. GOIDL and B. BENACERRAF, 1970, J. Exptl. Med. *132*, 261.

MÄKELÄ, O., A. M. CROSS and E. RUOSLAHTI, 1968, Similarities between the cellular receptor antibody and the secreted antibody. *In*: Proceeding of the 4th Sanibel Island Conference.

MÄKELÄ, O., E. RUOSLAHTI and C. ENHOLM, 1969, J. Immunol. *102*, 763.

MANSON, L. A. and T. SIMMONS, 1969, Transplant. Proc. *1*, 498.

MARCHELONIS, J. J. and V. S. GLEDHILL, 1968, Nature, Lond. *220*, 608.

MILLER, J. F. A. P. and G. F. MITCHELL, 1969, Transplant. Rev. *1*, 3.

MITCHISON, N. A., 1964, Proc. Roy. Soc. *B161*, 275.

MITCHISON, N. A., 1965, Immunology 9, 129.

MITCHISON, N. A., 1968a, Immunological paralysis as a dosage phenomenon. *In*: B. Cinader, ed.: Regulation of the antibody response. Springfield, C. Thomas. pp. 54–67.

MITCHISON, N. A., 1968b, Immunology *15*, 509.

MITCHISON, N. A., 1969a, Israel J. Med. Sci. *5*, 230.

MITCHISON, N. A., 1969b, Immunology *16*, 1.

MITCHISON, N. A., 1970, Cellular and molecular recognition mechanism prior to the immune response. *In*: A. Studer and H. Cottier, eds.: Handbuch der allgemeinen Pathologie. Berlin, Springer-Verlag. pp. 237–249.

MITCHISON, N. A., 1971a, Eur. J. Immunol., 10.

MITCHISON, N. A., 1971b, Eur. J. Immunol., 18.

MITCHISON, N. A., 1971c, Eur. J. Immunol., 68.

MITCHISON, N. A., 1971d, Transplant. Proc. *3*, 953.

MITCHISON, N. A., 1971e, Cell cooperation in the immune response: the hypothesis of an antigen presentation mechanism. *In*: Proceedings of the VIth International Immuno-pathology Symposium, Grindelwald, 1970. Basel, Schwabe. Immunopathology 6, 52.

MITCHISON, N. A., 1971f, The relative ability of T and B lymphocytes to see protein antigen. *In*: Proceedings of the Third Sigrid Juselius Symposium, Helsinki, 1970. New York, Academic Press. pp. 249–260.

MITCHISON, N. A., K. RAJEWSKY and R. B. TAYLOR, 1970, Cooperation of antigenic determinants and of cells in the induction of antibodies. *In*: J. Šterzl and I. Řiha, eds.: Proof symposium on developmental aspects of antibody formation and structure, Prague, 1969. Prague, Academia. pp. 547–561.

MÖLLER, E., and M. F. GREAVES, 1971, On the thymic origin of antigen-sensitive cells. *In*: Proceedings of the Third Sigrid Juselius Symposium, Helsinki, 1970, (in press).

MCBRIDE, R. A. and L. W. SCHIERMAN, 1970, J. Exptl. Med. *131*, 377.

NOSSAL, G. J. V., G. L. ADA and C. M. AUSTIN, 1964a, Aust. J. Exptl. Biol. *42*, 283.

NOSSAL, G. J. V., G. L. ADA and C. M. AUSTIN, 1964b, Aust. J. Exptl. Biol. *42*, 311.

OVARY, Z. and B. BENACERRAF, 1963, Proc. Soc. Exptl. Biol. Med. *114*, 72.

PAUL, W. E., D. H. KATZ, E. A. GOIDL and B. BENACERRAF, 1970, J. Exptl. Med. *132*, 283.

RAFF, M. C., 1970, Immunology *19*, 637.

ROITT, I. M., M. F. GREAVES, G. TORRIGIANI, J. BROSTOFF and J. H. L. PLAYFAIR, 1969, Lancet *ii*, 367.

ROOS, B., 1970, Makrophagen: Herkunft, Entwicklung und Funktion. *In*: A. Studer and H. Cottier, eds.: Handbuch der allgemeinen Pathologie Berlin, Springer-Verlag. pp. 1–128.

RÜDE, E., E. MOZES and M. SELA, 1968, Biochemistry *7*, 2971.

SELA, M. and E. MOZES, 1966, Proc. Natl. Acad. Sci. U.S. *55*, 445.

SHELLAM, G. R. and G. J. V. NOSSAL, 1968, Immunology *14*, 273.

SHORTMAN, K., E. DIENER, P. RUSSELL and W. D. ARMSTRONG, 1970, J. Exptl. Med. *131*, 461.

SISKIND, G. W., 1970, Antibody binding affinity and the control of the immune response. *In*: J. Šterzl and I. Řiha, eds.: Proceedings of symposium on developmental aspects of antibody formation and structure, Prague, 1969. Prague, Academia. pp. 837–844.

SISKIND, G. W. and B. BENACERRAF, 1969, Advan. Immunol. *10*, 1.

SISKIND, G. W., P. DUNN and J. G. WALKER, 1968, J. Exptl. Med. *127*, 55.

SMALL, P. A. and R. H. WALDMAN, 1969, The secretory immunologic system. *In*: Protides of the biological fluids. Bruges, Elsevier, p. 221.

SPITZNAGEL, J. K. and A. C. ALLISON, 1970, J. Immunol. *104*, 119.

STAPLES, P. J., I. GERY and B. H. WAKSMAN, 1966, J. Exptl. Med. *124*, 127.

STEINER, L. A. and H. N. EISEN, 1967, J. Exptl. Med. *126*, 1185.

TAYLOR, R. B., 1969, Transplant. Rev. *1*, 114.

TAYLOR, R. B. and G. M. IVERSON, 1971, Proc. Roy. Soc. *B176*, 393.

TOMASI, T. B., JR. and J. BIENENSTOCK, 1968, Advan. Immunol. *9*, 1.

UHR, J. W., 1966, Physiol. Rev. *46*, 359.

UHR, J. W., M. S. FINKELSTEIN and J. B. BAUMANN, 1962, J. Exptl. Med. *115*, 655.

UHR, J. W., S. B. SALVIN and A. M. PAPENHEIMER, 1957, J. Exptl. Med. *105*, 11.

UNANUE, E. R. and B. A. ASKONAS, 1968, J. Exptl. Med. *127*, 915.

UNANUE, E. R. and J. C. CEROTTINI, 1970, Fate and immunogenicity of macrophage-associated haemocyanins. *In*: J. Šterzl and I. Řiha, eds.: Proceedings of symposium on developmental aspects of antibody formation and structure, Prague, 1969. Prague, Academia. pp. 521–530.

WEIGLE, W. O., 1967, Natural and acquired immunologic unresponsiveness. Cleveland, World Publishing Co.

WEIGLE, W. O., 1971, The induction and termination of immunological unresponsiveness. *In*: Proceedings of the VIth International Immunopathology Symposium, Grindelwald, 1970. Basel, Schwabe, (in press).

WEIGLE, W. O., F. J. DIXON and M. T. DEICHMILLER, 1960, Proc. Roy. Soc. *B105*, 535.

YALOW, R. S. and S. A. BERSON, 1968, General principles of radioimmunoassay. *In*: Proceedings of Symposium on Radioisotopes in Medicine: *in vitro* studies, Oak Ridge, 1967. U.S. Atomic Energy Commission.

CHAPTER 4

Concepts of the mechanism of action of adjuvants

ROBERT G. WHITE

Department of Bacteriology and Immunology, University of Glasgow, Glasgow, Scotland

4.1. Introduction

The term *adjuvant* finds a widespread application in current immunological literature for substances which (i) convert an apparently non-antigenic substance to an effective antigen, (ii) increase levels of circulating antibody or lead to the production of more effective protective immunity, (iii) increase cell-mediated hypersensitivity and (iv) lead to the production of certain diseases of presumed immunological aetiology, such as allergic encephalomyelitis.

The commonly recognized adjuvants are remarkable for their diversity. Apart from the more obvious such as alum or other aluminium salts (Ramon 1926) bacterial endotoxin (Johnson et al. 1956) and Freund's complete and incomplete mixtures (i.e., water-in-oil emulsions with or without dead mycobacteria (Freund 1956) the following substances also have been described as possessing activity in enhancing the immunogenicity of various antigens when injected at the same time and together with the immunogen: alginate (Amies 1959), saponin (Espinet 1951; Johnson et al. 1963; Richou et al. 1964), lanoline (Ramon et al. 1937), phospholipids (Weiss and Dubos 1956), methylcellulose (Rivensen 1958), quaternary ammonium compounds (Gall 1966), vitamin A (Stark 1966; Dresser 1966), silica (Vigliani and Pernis 1959). In addition to these more or less defined chemical substances, several bacteria have been used without very clear knowledge of the nature of their active principles, e.g., *Bordetella pertussis* (Fleming et al. 1948), *Corynebacterium rubrum* (Crowle 1962a) and *Corynebacterium parvum* (Neveu et al. 1964). Another group of adjuvants from bacteria are the exotoxins of staphylococci (Woods 1937) and diphtheria bacilli (Evans 1967).

This report is not intended to cover comprehensively the available list of adjuvants but an attempt will be made to evaluate some of the possible mechanisms and to stress the common principles of adjuvant activity and to examine a few of the experimental approaches which have been used to study the problem.

4.2. Processing of antigen

A systematic approach based on modes of action is limited by lack of basic knowledge of how an antigen is received into the body or acts to produce an immune response. Much of what is injected appears to by-pass the immunological mechanism and fails to provide an effective stimulus for the biosynthesis of antibody or stimulation of cell-mediated hypersensitivity. Most biochemical studies have indicated that, in the absence of antibody, heterologous mammalian proteins are catabolized within the bodies of other mammals in the same manner as homologous proteins. Current thought involves the macrophage in these events in a variety of ways. Normal catabolism, not relevant to a subsequent immune response is regarded as a rapid sequel to macrophage uptake of most protein immunogens so that 90% is degraded within 3–4 hours (Askonas et al. 1968). However, for some weeks after injection of a protein antigen it is possible to extract from liver and spleen material which still has antigenic properties (in that it can react specifically with homologous antibody) as well as immunogenic properties (in that it is able to induce antibody when injected into other animals (Garvey et al. 1957). This small proportion of the foreign protein is maintained within or on the surface of the cell for long periods of time in what appears to be a bound form, protected from rapid catabolism (White 1963; Nossal et al. 1965). The persisting antigen is localized in macrophages in the medullary areas of nodes or red pulp of spleen, and once a small amount of antibody has been formed, in the dendritic metalophil cells of the germinal centres.

In the case of haemocyanin (*Maia squinado*), Askonas et al. (1968) were able to correlate the immunogenicity of suspensions of macrophages with the small amount of antigen persisting in the cells for prolonged periods of time after an initial uptake *in vivo*. The existence of dendritic cells poses the problem of functional differentiation among macrophages and other immunogen-receiving cells. For instance, it is not clear from the relevant experiments whether antigen is processed and retained in a population of peritoneal macrophages by specialized cells. It is also not clear how the radioactive antigenic material which persists for a long period is bound to cell constituents: this might be the means for protecting antigen molecules against destruction, and also provide a mechanism for an adjuvant which increased this process to enhance immunogenicity. No evidence could, however, be provided by Unanue et al. (1970) that the overall catabolism and retention of ^{131}I-labelled haemocyanin in macrophages was significantly altered in the presence of adjuvants (*Bordetella pertussis* and beryllium sulphate).

Most conventional phenol or sodium dodecyl sulphate methods for preparing RNA extracts of macrophages have failed to yield extracts with significantly increased immunogenicity. However, Askonas and Rhodes (1965) found that an RNA-^{131}I-haemocyanin complex incubated with spleen cells was more immunogenic than equivalent amounts of haemocyanin in the secondary response, thus constituting in effect a 'super-antigen'.

On the basis of these facts, immunogenicity involves processing of antigen by macrophages. Antigen-containing macrophages have been found highly effective in inducing antibody synthesis *in vitro* (Fishman and Adler 1963) and *in vivo* (Gallily and Feldman 1967). The uptake by macrophages of antigens such as *Maia squinado* haemocyanin (MSH) or bovine serum albumin is an effective means for increasing their immunogenicity. The primary response in mice injected with macrophages containing MSH was 3–40 times greater than that observed in mice primed with comparable amounts of soluble material (Unanue and Askonas 1968). However the importance of the macrophage appears to vary with different antigenic systems. Uptake by macrophages of strong immunogens, such as sheep erythrocytes or the high molecular weight haemocyanin from keyhole limpet (Unanue and Askonas 1967) did not lead to increased synthesis of antibody. Particularly in the primary response, the immunogenicity of the native antigen appeared to be greater than that of the macrophage-held protein. In other circumstances macrophage uptake of immunogen appeared to decrease the eventual immune response (Franzl 1966), a result explained on the basis of the more complete degradation of the phagocytosed antigen.

4.3. Role of the antigen carrier

Although the information of the specificity of an immune response resides in the determinants at the surface of the molecule, non-specific factors relating to the whole molecule can determine both the quality and the quantity of the antibody response. The size of the molecule will determine whether antibody is made or not. Possibly the smallest effective immunogenic molecules are about 3000 molecular weight (e.g., a separated chain of insulin [M.W. 2500] or glucagon [M.W. 3600]); above this lower limit the larger the molecular weight the better the antigenicity, so that the snail (*Helix pomatia*) and keyhole limpet haemocyanins (mol. wt 6–8 millions) are among the strongest of antigens. It is also clear that by aggregation a non-antigenic protein can be converted to an effective antigen. Bovine IgG (BGG) loses its immunogenicity when it is spun at high speed to remove any aggregated BGG (Dresser 1961). Heat aggregation of the protein at 70°C can convert a non-immunogenic to an immunogenic preparation.

Several other factors of the carrier determine the level of adjuvanticity which is built into the immunogenic particle. Thus in experiments with hapten-carrier combinations it is found that if the number of haptens attached to the carrier is 3–5, antibodies to the hapten are more likely to be formed than if less haptens are attached. Aggregation might therefore be the means for achieving the optimum number of determinants per particle. Weigle (1962) found that a mixture of two different haptens attached to the same protein were more antigenic than either acting alone. Another similar finding is that a stronger antibody response will develop if the protein carrier comes from an animal species other than that injected.

Some of these findings of built-in adjuvanticity relate to the phenomenon of carrier specificity as it applies to memory. Whereas antibody against a haptenic determinant will usually combine as well with a similar hapten attached to a different carrier, *secondary* stimulation of antibody production does not occur in response to the hapten alone, or hapten on a carrier different from that used in the primary stimulus. When a similar amount of the same determinant on another kind of carrier molecule is used, antibody response to the determinant is characteristic of a *primary* stimulation. The process of antibody formation has recently been suggested to involve interaction of at least two distinct cell types. The experiments involved sheep erythrocytes as immunogen in mice (Davies 1969; Claman and Chaperon 1969; Miller and Mitchell 1969) and they were interpreted to imply that in this system thymus-derived cells are involved in the initial specific interaction with antigen but that the bone-marrow-derived cells actually synthesize the specific antibody. If the thymus-derived cells had the carrier specificity postulated for those involved in cell-mediated immunity whereas the specificity of the bone marrow-derived cells was similar to that of the antibody which they produce, the overall specificity would still show the effect of the carrier. This explanation, if correct, would have very important implications for adjuvant effects due either to the intrinsic qualities of the carrier or of an extrinsic adjuvant. Thus, an efficient stimulation of the thymus-dependent population of lymphocytes might be expected to cause an adjuvant effect on antibody production (see below in relation to the explanation of the mode of action of Freund's complete adjuvant).

4.4. Adjuvant effect of antibody

An important factor influencing the magnitude of an antibody response is the level of specific antibody at the time of antigen injection. Usually this antibody acts to inhibit immunogenicity; occasionally an adjuvant effect is produced. Glenny and Pope (1925) obtained a substantial adjuvant effect by mixing diphtheria toxoid with horse antitoxin as an underneutralized mixture. A similar enhancing effect of small amounts of antibody in the mouse has been described by Terres and Wolins (1961). Similarly, it was found that injection of tetanus or diphtheria toxoid in newborn piglets deprived of colostrum did not lead to detectable antitoxin formation. However, injection of a mixture of toxoid with trace amounts of specific horse antitoxin stimulates specific antitoxin formation in these animals (Segre and Kaeberle 1962). The problem is highly relevant to the prophylaxis of rhesus anti-D immunization in the Rh-negative mother bearing an Rh-positive foetus (and particularly if mother and foetus are ABO-compatible). In these circumstances suppression of primary immunization is required and an adjuvant effect by the injected anti-D would be a disaster. Möller and Wigzell (1965) showed that injection of small amounts of 19S antibody to sheep erythrocytes along with the latter could increase the number of 19S haemolysin-producing cells. The outcome of such experiments would be expected to depend on the ratio of antibody to antigen injected. Barr et al. (1950) found indeed that a critical level of antitoxin could be determined which, if exceeded, would always cause interference with immunization. Other effects may be determined by the avidity of the antibody, its species of origin, its immunoglobulin type and the size of the antigen – all factors which could govern the localization to and fate of the Ag/Ab complex within phagocytic cells. Walker and Siskind (1968) observed that very low concentrations of high-affinity antibody, but not low-affinity antibody, acted as an adjuvant for DNP in rabbits. Stimulation can sometimes be shown to be non-specific; Pearlman (1966) found an increased antibody response in rabbits to *both* determinants of a DNP-sheep erythrocyte conjugate if small doses of antigen were mixed with excess antibody to the sheep erythrocytes. This result may indicate that antibody acts by alteration of the tissue-localization of the antigen. The model for this is contained in the experiments of Jandl (1964) who found that small doses of a non-complement-fixing antibody directed erythrocytes into the spleen; larger doses caused localization in the liver.

Results were obtained by Jenkin and Karnovsky (1967) by use of an immunogenic O-acetylated galactan in mice which support a rather different hypothesis. Addition of antibody under conditions so that the antigen remained in excess led to enhanced catabolism of the acetylated polysaccharide by the lung and, at the same time, an enhanced antibody response. The possibility exists that this effect of antibody is part of the normal mechanism of induction of antibody formation. Thus Boyden (1962) among others has postulated that a natural opsonin may be a necessary recognition factor, able to initiate specific chemotaxis as an Ab/Ag complex, and the absence of which, as in the piglet deprived of colostrum (Segre and Kaeberle 1962) results in decreased capacity to make antibody.

4.5. *Adjuvant action by changing conditions for tolerance induction*

Adjuvants are not only useful for increasing antibody production. Weakly immunogenic proteins which induce tolerance can, by the action of adjuvants, induce antibody production instead. The model used for these experiments is an intravenous injection of 1 mg. of bovine gamma globulin (BGG) into the CBA mouse (Dresser 1961). Particulate BGG which can be centrifuged out of an ordinary solution of dried BGG is immunogenic, whereas the BGG freed from the latter is strongly tolerance-inducing. Similar results have been obtained with BSA in rabbits (Frei et al. 1965).

Various adjuvants can be injected into CBA mice so that a tolerance result is transformed into immunogenicity shown by an immune-type clearance of injected ^{131}I-labelled BGG from the blood stream. This occurs when killed mycobacteria in mineral oil are injected at a subcutaneous site (Dresser 1961) or when vitamin A is ingested (Stark, referred to in White 1966) or injected (Dresser 1966). This type of adjuvant activity by mycobacteria may, of course, activate a different mechanism to that which operates in, say, the guinea-pig and results in higher levels of antibody.

Stark (1970a) found that the action of mycobacteria or peptido-glycolipid extracted therefrom in inducing an immune response in this experimental situation depended upon the level of resting catabolism for BGG – as shown by the half-life of the protein in the pre-immune phase of elimination. When this phase revealed slow catabolism in the controls (half-lives of 4.38–5.0 days) mycobacterial adjuvants failed to induce an immune response. When the half-life in this phase was shorter (3.82–2.96) the mycobacterial adjuvants did induce subsequent immune elimination. Also the adjuvants themselves accelerated the elimination rate in the pre-immune period of elimination. Other strains of mice, with higher normal catabolic rates, frequently gave secondary immune responses in a further exposure to antigen without injection of adjuvant. In a later paper Stark (1970b) showed that thyroxin by mouth predisposed towards an immunological response and mice maintained at a low ambient temperature showed slower catabolism in the pre-immune phase and formed less antibody in the immune elimination phase after mycobacterial adjuvants than controls.

The recent work of Mitchison (1964) has advanced the concept that induction of immunity or tolerance can occur simultaneously at the single cell level, but that the net result in the whole animal is a summation of the individual cellular results. Mitchison (1964) defined the effect of dosage of bovine serum albumin in normal adult mice on these phenomena. Tolerance could be induced in two zones, a high and a low zone; with doses between these, immunity rather than tolerance resulted. It seems that adjuvants can overcome the tolerance inducing effects and secure a change to immunogenicity. This is, however, only true at low dose levels of antigen. Thus mice pretreated with mycobacteria in oil and other adjuvants produced increased responses to a subsequent injection of 1 mg BSA, but decreased, if anything, the response to 10 or 50 mg BSA (Spitznagel and Allison 1970a).

In this system it can be envisaged that the balance between immunogenicity and tolerance-induction depends upon the routing of antigen to the immunologically competent cells, which could be either direct or *via* macrophages. Factors which altered the internal environment of the macrophage could change the balance between tolerance and immunogenicity. It is of interest here that animals which were pretreated with 1 mg of BSA produced reduced responses to a subsequent injection of particulate BSA, suggesting that the soluble BSA had pre-emptied the cells along a tolerance pathway. Spitznagel and Allison (1970b) showed a similar reduction by pretreatment with soluble BSA of the antibody response to macrophage-enclosed BSA. Several agents known to act by labilizing lysosomal membranes have been shown to possess marked adjuvant effects on antibody production in the mouse system; synthetic vitamin A alcohol, beryllium sulphate, silica (Snowit) and bacterial endotoxin (Spitznagel and Allison 1970a). It is of interest and possibly important that vitamin A in previous attempts had failed to act as an adjuvant in either antibody production or induction of delayed-type hypersensitivity in the guinea-pig (Uhr et al. 1963; White 1966) which may represent a quite distinct form of adjuvant activity. The experiments of Spitznagel and Allison provided no evidence that adjuvants increased the uptake of antigen by macrophages, or alter the degradation of antigen in or release of antigen from macrophages.

4.6. Relation of adjuvant activity to surface-activity

A common feature shared by most of the diverse adjuvants listed at the beginning of this article is surface activity. Indeed, as pointed out by Gall (1966) a surprising number of adjuvants feature in a standard list of emulsifying agents such as, for example, that issued by the Pharmaceutical Society of Great Britain in *The Pharmaceutical Pocket Book* (1966). In a systematic search among surface-active agents Gall (1960) found that several of non-ionic surface active agents showed slight activity, notably Span 80 (Sorbitan mono-oleate) and Tween 80 (Polyoxyethylene sorbitan mono-oleate). Anionic surface-active agents appeared to be inactive. Study of a related family of cationic surface-active agents (quaternary ammonium salts) showed clearly the influence of the long alkyl chain. Where a long alkyl chain was absent little or no adjuvant activity was manifest. Where a long alkyl chain was present, hexadecyl, octadecyl and longer chains tended to be more active than their shorter counterparts. As with the quaternary ammonium compounds, both amines and guanidines clearly showed increasing activity with increasing chain length (Table 4.1). With primary amines, high adjuvant activity

TABLE 4.1

Adjuvant activity* in relation to alkyl chain length

	Dose (mg)	*No. guinea pigs reaching titres (diphtheria antitoxin)*						*Score*
		0.001	0.01	0.1	1.0	10		
Primary monoamines general formula alkyl-NH$_2$		> 0.001	0.01	0.1	1.0	10	100	
n-Hexylamine (in 1% Tween 80)	0.5	3	–	2				0.26
n-Decylamine (in 1% Tween 80)	0.5	2	1	1	1			1.46
Cyclohexylamine (in 1% Tween 80)	0.5	1	1	2				1.60
n-Hexadecylamine (in 1% Tween 80)	0.5					2		4.35
n-Hexadecylamine (in 10% dimethyl formamide)	0.1					4	1	4.62
n-Hexadecylamine (in 10% isopropyl alcohol)	0.1				1	3	1	4.42

TABLE 4.1 (continued)

	Dose (mg)	No. guinea pigs reaching titres (diphtheria antitoxin)						Score
n-Octadecylamine (in 1% Tween 80)	0.1					3	2	4.88
n-Octadecylamine					1	8	6	4.76
Dimethyl guanidines general formula N,N'-Dimethyl-N''-alkyl guanidines								
N,N'-Dimethyl-N''-Propyl g. hydriodide	0.1	8	2					0.20
N,N'-Dimethyl-N''-Hexyl g. p-toluene sulphonate	0.1	9	1					0.10
N,N'-Dimethyl-N''-Octyl g. hydriodide	0.1	4	1					0.20
N,N'-Dimethyl-N''-Decyl g. hydriodide	0.1	5	1	–	3	1		1.60
N,N'-Dimethyl-N''-Dodecyl g. hydriodide	0.1			1	3	1	–	3.34
N,N'-Dimethyl-N''-Tridecyl g. hydriodide	0.1				1	4	–	4.00
N,N'-Dimethyl-N''-Tetradecyl. g. hydriodide	0.1			1	1	3	–	3.80
N,N'-Dimethyl-N''-Pentadecyl g. hydriodide	0.1					4	1	4.60
N,N'-Dimethyl-N''-Hexadecyl g. hydriodide	0.1				2	15	3	4.36
N,N'-Dimethyl-N''-Hexadecyl g. methanosulphonate	0.1				2	7	1	4.30
N,N'-Dimethyl-N''-Octadecyl g. hydriodide	0.1					11	9	4.76
N,N'-Dimethyl-N''-Docosyl g. hydriodide	0.1					2	3	4.92

General formula of the N,N'-Dimethyl-N''-alkyl guanidines:

```
           NMe
           ‖
RNHC
           \
            NHMe
```

* Adjuvant activity was tested in the guinea-pig by two injections of diphtheria toxoid (1 Lf in 0.2 ml. subcutaneously). Antitoxin levels at 10 days after second injection. Adjuvants were given with the first dose of antigen at the same site.

is shown by hexadecylamine, a substance which has been extensively studied also by Noll and Younger (1959). In the more complete series of dimethyl guanidines, adjuvant activity clearly begins at 10 carbon atoms, climbs steeply between eight, increases rapidly with twelve carbons and then rises more slowly.

Thus, from Gall's work the requirements for adjuvant activity among the aliphatic nitrogenous compounds appeared as fairly well defined. The compound must be basic and must contain a long aliphatic chain. Neither characteristic was sufficient alone, but providing both were satisfied, a wide range of compounds could show activity. With few exceptions, they were found in tissue culture to cause disruption of cells and were lytic to erythrocytes, although no close correlation was apparent between the severity of action on cells and adjuvant activity.

4.7. Relation of adjuvant activity to a specific lysosome-labilizing effect

If it is accepted that adjuvant activity depends upon surface-active properties, it becomes logical to consider the cell membrane or a specific organelle membrane such as that of the lysosome as a possible site of action. According to some authors (Friedman et al. 1969) there is little evidence to regard any substance as specifically affecting the lysosomal membrane. It is argued that since the cell membrane does not differ essentially from the lysosomal membrane (Thinès-Senpoux 1967), it is to be expected that the cell membrane will suffer the first and more severe attack by any surface active agents – such as vitamin A acid or alcohol, chlorpromazin and dimethyl sulphoxide which some have regarded as specific lysosome labilizers (Allison 1968). However, it seems possible that a relatively insoluble particle of the correct size (such as bentonite or quartz) could act more specifically on the lysosome membrane following phagocytosis and inclusion into phagolysosomes, as suggested by Allison et al. (1966). Nevertheless, Comolli (1967) demonstrated a leakage of ribonuclease, β-glucuronidase and cathepsin from suspensions of rat peritoneal macrophages which had phagocytosed silica into the suspending fluid, clearly suggesting that an important part of the cytotoxic effect of silica is an effort on the plasma membrane.

Several agents which are known to labilize lysosomal membrane with release of there contained enzymes, possess demonstrable adjuvant activity. The main experiences have been with vitamin A derivatives which Fell and Dingle (1963) showed to cause degradation of cartilage matrix *via* the release of lysosomal enzymes. Retinol (synthetic vitamin A alcohol) was found to be more effective as an adjuvant than retinol palmitate, a less biologically active substance (Spitznagel and Allison 1970a). Very high doses of vitamin A, which are toxic, are required for the adjuvant effect, which is increased by its use in an oily vehicle, possibly since degradation *in vivo* is less rapid. Other demonstrated adjuvants which fall into the category of lysosome labilizers are beryllium sulphate, endotoxin, *Bordetella pertussis*, stilboestrol, silica and the polyene antibiotic lucensomycin (Spitznagel and Allison 1970a).

4.8. *The adjuvant effect of water-in-mineral-oil emulsion with added mycobacteria (Freund's complete adjuvant)*

The incorporation of a protein antigen in the watery phase of a simple water-in-oil emulsion results in a marked adjuvant effect. Addition of mycobacteria to the oil phase results in a further marked increase in antibody levels (Fischel et al. 1952). Water-in-oil emulsions (without added mycobacteria) have several effects. First, the local destruction and elimination of the antigen are retarded (Halbert et al. 1946). *Shigella* antigen persisted for 22 weeks after injection when incorporated in water-in-oil. This does not mean that the extra antibody is all made by cells associated with the locally deposited water-in-oil mixture. By immunofluorescence cells containing antibody can be seen in the draining lymph node in greater numbers and over a longer period of time when the antigen is injected as a water-in-oil emulsion than when the same dose of antigen is injected in simple solution. This effect could result from the lengthened contact of immunogen with cells in the node or by virtue of a change in the molecular characteristics of the immunogen – i.e., aggregation of the protein may occur in the preparation of the emulsion. In addition the local granuloma itself becomes the site of large numbers of antibody-containing plasma cells which must contribute appreciably to overall antibody synthesis.

From a practical point of view it is of great importance that the immunogenic stimulus from a water-in-oil emulsion of antigen acts over a very long period of time. From the careful work of Holt (1950) it is clear that with alum-precipitated antigens the antigen although persisting locally, rapidly fails to act as a stimulus to the antibody-producing mechanism. It seems that the escape of antigen to the regional nodes is largely stopped at two weeks after injection by a process of fibrous encapsulation and possibly by the effect of the antibody in forming a surrounding zone of antigen-antibody precipitate within the interstices of the collagen network (Germuth et al. 1959). Water-in-oil emulsions are apparently less affected in this way, possibly since the oil-protected antigen still gets carried through the barrier by macrophages – or circulation of lymphocytes within lymphatics continues to be possible.

The addition of mycobacteria to a water-in-oil emulsion occasions several dramatic changes in the immunological response. These include a striking increase in delayed-type hypersensitivity, synthesis of different immunoglobulins (White et al. 1963), facilitation of the production of diseases such as allergic disseminated encephalomyelitis when brain is the immunogen, or azoospermia when testis is the immunogen, and so-called 'adjuvant disease' when emulsion mixture is injected without added immunogen (Pearson 1956).

Mycobacteria occupy at present a unique role in immunological practice for induction of strong delayed-type hypersensitivity (Raffel 1965; Nelson and Boyden 1964) although the taxonomically-related organisms such as *Nocardia asteroides* or *Corynebacterium rubrum* (Crowle 1962a), which is probably identical with *Nocardia rhodochrous* (Gordon 1966), and taxonomically unrelated organisms such as *Coryne-bacterium parvum* may share this effect. By the same token, it has become accepted that mycobacteria are essential for the production of the disease states resulting from auto-allergic responses, such as allergic encephalitis. These statements, however, are based on the guinea-pig as experimental animal and do not apply to other animal species. In the rat, encephalitis can be induced regularly within two weeks following a single injection of spinal cord in incomplete adjuvant (Paterson and Bell 1962). Mycobacteria fail to increase delayed hypersensitivity in rat (Paterson and Bell 1962) and in the mouse (Crowle 1962b). The claim by Crowle (1962b) to have produced delayed hypersensitivity in mice by an incomplete Freund's adjuvant, has however been challenged by Munoz (1963) who found that the reactions were of the Arthus type which could be duplicated by passive transfer of preformed antibody. In the author's laboratory W. J. Herbert has recently obtained a marked increase in the delayed-type skin response to ovalbumin by use of myco-bacteria in the water-in-oil injection mixture.

In the guinea-pig, use of simple water-oil injection mixture leads to an antibody response to a protein immunogen ovalbumin which at three weeks is entirely, or almost entirely, confined to the fast or γ_1 globulin. But when mycobacteria are added to the emulsion, a new peak of slow or γ_2-immunoglobulin appears (White et al. 1963). The antibody of γ_2 mobility can be clearly separated from the γ_1-antibody by chromato-graphy on DEAE cellulose; both can be split to similar L and different H chains. Since γ_2-immunoglobulin is much more active in complement fixation than γ_1-immunoglobulin (Bloch et al. 1963), the effect of adding mycobacteria to the injection mixture will be shown by higher ratios of antibody determined by complement fixation than by precipitation. Mycobacteria in the immunizing injection will also lead to a striking increase in cytophilic antibody production (Boyden and Sorkin 1961). Moreover, in the guinea-pig this cytophilic antibody is a γ_2-immunoglobulin.

Although it has never been convincingly shown that delayed-type hypersensitivity is in any way dependent upon immunoglobulin, current evidence relating to the guinea-pig seems consistent with the view that adjuvant effect produced on serum antibody levels may be related to the increase in delayed-type or specific cell-mediated hypersensitivity. Indeed, the adjuvant effect on antibody production could depend on the fact that an antigen which is introduced into an animal having delayed hypersensitivity to it yields an increased antibody response (Humphrey and Turk 1963). In the guinea-pig, substantial evidence exists that stimulation of increase in γ_2-immunoglobulins is linked with increase of delayed hypersensitivity. Thus when a wide range of extracted materials from bacteria was tested for adjuvant activity, a direct correlation was apparent between the presence in immunoelectrophoresis of the arc of antibody and the presence of a positive corneal test against the same antigen (White et al. 1963). Secondly, most adjuvants besides mycobacterial peptidoglycolipids are generally regarded as responsible for increasing the biosynthesis of antibody without, at the same time, increasing delayed hypersensitivity. In the guinea pig such adjuvants as aluminium salts, calcium alginate, simple water-in-oil emulsions or silica (Bentonite) act to increase γ_1-immunoglobulin without increasing delayed hypersensitivity.

Nevertheless, occasionally an injection of, for example, ovalbumin plus bentonite intraperitoneally will be followed by delayed hypersensitivity (Wilkinson and White 1966) as shown by a positive corneal test and these exceptional animals are found on immunoelectrophoresis of their serum against antigen, to have a γ_2-antibody precipitin arc. Thirdly, a prior injection of protein antigen will block the ability of a subsequent injection of the same antigen in complete Freund's adjuvant to induce delayed-type hypersensitivity (Boyden 1957). The same animals fail to show γ_2-antibody precipitin arcs (Wilkinson and White 1966; Asherson and Stone 1965; Asherson 1966; Loewi et al. 1966).

A positive adjuvant effect with Freund's complete adjuvant in the guinea-pig is uniformly accompanied by formation of a local necrotic granuloma, whether the mycobacterial component is represented by whole killed virulent or saprophytic mycobacteria, nocardia or their active peptidoglycolipid fractions. The typical cellular components are compact masses of epithelioid cells and giant cells. A similar tissue occupies many of the draining lymph nodes and can occur as subpleural nodules in the lungs (Suter and White 1954). It seems possible that the granuloma formation could also be a consequence of the interaction of persisting antigen with lymphocytes (and secondarily macrophages) activated by delayed-type hypersensitivity. Some support for this is provided by the evidence that deviation of the response by prior injection of protein antigen as described above, causes a great diminution in the size of the local granuloma (Wilkinson and White 1966).

The successful action of mineral oil adjuvants depends on the route of injection. Waksman and Morrison (1951) found that injection into the footpad or intracutaneously into the rabbit was effective for induction of allergic encephalomyelitis but were unable to produce the disease by the intraperitoneal or subcutaneous routes. Presumably the superiority of the footpad and intracutaneous routes depended on the better entry of the oily emulsion into lymphatic channels. Excision of the foot of a guinea-pig as early as one hour after footpad inoculation did not prevent the appearance of the encephalitis, presumably since enough adjuvant and brain tissue has disseminated *via* the lymph channels by this time. Injection of thyroid antigen in mycobacterial oily adjuvant directly into a peripheral lymph node has been claimed by Newbould (1965) to facilitate the production of thyroiditis in the rat. However, Horne and White (1968) found that the footpad of the guinea-pig route was always superior to direct popliteal node injection for both antibody production and induction of cell-mediated hypersensitivity over a wide range of dosage of immunogen and mycobacterial component in complete Freund's adjuvant.

The chemical and physical nature of the active principle of mycobacteria and related organisms has been the subject of extensive investigations. In guinea-pigs, Raffel and Forney (1948) and Raffel et al. (1949) established that the chloroform-soluble wax fraction of a human strain of *M. tuberculosis* would potentiate the development of delayed-type hypersensitivity to egg albumin and picryl chloride. Although a wide variety of mycobacteria of human, bovine, atypical and saprophytic types could be shown to act as adjuvants for increase of both cellular and humoral immunity, only the wax D fractions derived from human and atypical strains (*M. Kansasii*) were found to possess activity (White et al. 1958; White and Marshall 1958). The principal component of wax D is a peptidoglycolipid which is mixed with glycolipid (lipopolysaccharide). The main chemical difference between wax D of human strains of *M. tuberculosis* and wax D from other mycobacteria is the presence in the former of a peptide moiety. Thus an active wax was regarded as possessing the structure of a peptidoglycolipid. Hydrolysis of wax D of human strains yields about half its weight of mycolic acids (branched chain β-hydroxy acids of empirical formula $C_{84-90}H_{176-180}O_4$ which are unique to mycobacteria) and a glycopeptide. The latter contains sugars: arabinose and galactose; three amino sugars, galactosamine, glucosamine and muramic acid; and three amino acids: D- and L-alanine, D-glutamic acid and meso-α-diaminopimelic acid. The three amino acids form a peptide which is linked *via* the L-alanine to the muramic acid, which may be part of a linear polymer of N-acetyl-glucosamine and N-acetyl-muramic acid. The latter links to an arabino-galactamine (Migliore and Jollès 1968).

This peptidoglycolipid has many analogies in its chemical structure with bacterial cell-wall mucopeptide or murein of gram-positive bacteria. All the characteristic hexosamines and amino acids which characterize the latter are found in mycobacterial peptidoglycolipid, which also resemble cell walls in having unnatural amino acids of the D-configuration: D-alanine and D-glutamic acid which are restricted in nature to cell walls, or certain extracellular products of bacteria such as various antibiotics and slime layers. The molecular requirements for surface activity as outlined by Gall (1966) could be satisfied by this molecule.

Possibly the purest peptidoglycolipid fractions of mycobacteria which were tested for biological activity in quantitative comparison with whole mycobacteria were derived by differential ultracentrifugation in ether (Jollès et al. 1962, 1964). This yields material which by negative staining under the electron microscope appears free from bacillary bodies or cell wall fragments, and were shown by J. Gordon to consist of homogeneous, parallel-sided curving filaments 133 Å broad (illustrated in White 1965). By the same negative-staining technique similar filaments were revealed as a multi-layered network of branching 133 Å filaments on the surface of a variety of mycobacterial species (White 1965).

Peptidoglycolipid of this degree of purity was found in a brain-mineral oil mixture to produce encephalomyelitis in half a group of guinea-pigs at a dose of 50 μg. The dose of whole mycobacteria (of the same human strain which was used as a source of the wax) required to produce the same effect was found to be 200 μg (White 1965).

All of this work was done in the guinea-pig. In the chicken, French et al. (1970) found that wax D and peptidoglycolipid fractions which had proved active in guinea-pigs were devoid of adjuvant activity, although whole human or avian mycobacteria were active.

The biological activity of mycobacteria and their extracted peptidoglycolipid fractions is characterized by a very striking stimulation of macrophage proliferation in the tissues (Suter and White 1954; Rupp et al. 1960). This takes the form of a large epithelioid cell-macrophage granuloma at the site of injection, extensive macrophage proliferation in regional lymph nodes and subpleural granulomata. These effects have often been attributed to the direct effect of the wax fractions of mycobacteria and it is of interest that in the chicken peptidoglycolipids and wax D fractions were found to be devoid of either granuloma production or adjuvant activity. However, in all circumstances local granuloma production correlated with adjuvant effect.

Table 4.2 (French et al. 1970) shows the effect of complete and incomplete Freund's adjuvant on antibody production in the chicken. Normally, an intravenous injection of HSA provokes a rapid production of antibody with a peak at 8–10 days.

Use of complete Freund's adjuvant leads to a second, very large and slowly developing wave of antibody. Mycobacterial adjuvant does not increase the first serum peak of antibody. This indicates clearly that activity does not depend on a stimulation of the efferent arc of the immune response, i.e., a population of primed antigen-sensitive cells which are precursors of plasma cells are not caused to synthesize more antibody either as more antibody per cell or by rapid cell-multiplication.

Mycobacterial adjuvants in mice have been shown to induce expansion of the paracortical (thymus-dependent) areas of the draining lymph nodes with appearance of large pyroninophilic blast cells in these areas by the 4th day, following by germinal centre formation and medullary plas-

TABLE 4.2

Serum antibody levels (anti-HSA as ABC_{30} µg/ml) in a chicken (8 weeks) at various time intervals after a single injection of HSA in complete and incomplete Freund's adjuvant mixture compared with controls.

		Average antibody level for group of birds at:						
Antigen and adjuvant	*No. in group*	*10 days*	*18 days*	*21 days*	*35 days*	*40 days*	*49 days*	*59 days*
40 µg HSA in water/ oil emulsion with 5 mg. *M. tuberculosis*	5	5.6	5.9	5.3	152	181	413	258
40 µg HSA in water/ oil emulsion	5	9.6	6.0	3.5	21	16	19	19
40 µg HSA in 0.15 M. NaCl	5	3.0	3.3	1.2	1.6	1.4	0.6	0.7

macytosis at a later stage (Taub et al. 1970). This, coupled with the observations of Hall (personal communication, 1969) in the sheep that the afferent lymphatics of the local granuloma carry large numbers of small and large lymphocytes suggests that a prominent effect of Freund's adjuvant may be in stimulating the thymus-dependent population of lymphocytes, the local anatomical arrangements in the granuloma making for efficient immunogenic liaison with antigen-bearing macrophages. As pointed out previously, it is possible that the adjuvant effect on serum antibody is dependent on a similar primary process.

A variety of processes relevant to adjuvant activity could be involved in influencing the efficiency with which the thymus-dependent population of recirculating, long-lived lymphocytes effect a liaison with the immunogen. Thus, this population of cells has been shown to be strikingly affected by the adjuvant *Bordetella pertussis* (Morse 1964; Morse and Riester 1967). Lymphocytosis in which the numbers of circulating cells rose from 3.7 to more than 10 times the initial value and which was maximal at 4–5 days follows intravenous injection of the bacilli. Histological examination of the spleen, lymph nodes and thymus at this time shows great depletion suggesting that mobilization of cells from extra-vascular sources rather than new formation of cells caused the observed increase in circulating lymphocytes. Use of tritiated thymidine showed that newly-divided cells did not make up a greater proportion of these cells than in a normal mouse.

References

ALLISON, A. C., 1968, Brit. Med. Bull. *24*, 135.

ALLISON, A. C., J. S. HARINGTON and M. BIRBECK, 1966, J. Exptl. Med., *124*, 141.

AMIES, C. R., 1959, J. Pathol. Bact. *77*, 435.

ASHERSON, G. L., 1966, Immunology *10*, 179.

ASHERSON, G. L. and S. H. STONE, 1965, Immunology *9*, 205.

ASKONAS, B. A., I. AUZINS and E. R. UNANUE, 1968, Bull. Soc. Chim. Biol. *50*, 1113.

ASKONAS, B. A. and J. M. RHODES, 1965, Nature *205*, 470.

BARR, M., A. T. GLENNY and K. J. RANDALL, 1950, Lancet *1*, 6.

BOYDEN, S. V., 1962, J. Exptl. Med. *115*, 453.

BLOCH, K. J., F. M. KOURILSKY, Z. OVARY and B. BENACERRAF, 1963, J. Exptl. Med. *117*, 965.

BOYDEN, S. V. and E. SORKIN, 1961, Immunology *4*, 244.

CLAMAN, H. N. and E. A. CHAPERON, 1969, Transplant. Rev. *1*, 92.

COMOLLI, R., 1967 J. Pathol. Bacteriol. *93*, 241.

CROWLE, A. J., 1962a, Antonie van Leeuwenhoek *28*, 183.

CROWLE, A. J., 1962b, J. Allergy *33*, 458.

DAVIES, A. J. S., 1969, Transplant. Rev., *1*, 43.

DRESSER, D. W., 1961, Nature *191*, 1169.

DRESSER, D. W., 1966, Nature *217*, 527.

ESPINET, R. G., 1951, Gac. vet. (B. Aires) *13*, 265.

EVANS, D. G., 1967, *in*: R. H. Regamey et al., eds.: International symposium on adjuvants of immunity. Symposia Series in Immunobiological Standardization, Vol. 6. Basel, Karger. p. 48.

FELL, H. B. and J. T. DINGLE. 1963, Biochem. J. *87*, 403.

FISCHEL, E. E., E. A. KABAT, H. C. STOERK and A. E. BEZER, 1952, J. Immunol. *69*, 611.

FISHMAN, M. and F. L. ADLER, 1963, J. Exptl. Med. *117*, 595.

FLEMING, D. S., L. GREENBERG and E. M. BEITH, 1948, Canad. Med. Ass. J. *59*, 101.

FRANZL, R. E., 1962, Nature *195*, 457.

FREI, P. C., B. BENACERRAF and G. THORBECKE, 1965, Proc. Natl. Acads. Sci. U.S. *53*, 20.

FRENCH, V. I., J. M. STARK and R. G. WHITE. 1970, Immunology *18*, 645.

FREUND, J., 1956, Advan. Tuberc. Res. *7*, 130.

FRIEDMAN, I., A. LAUFER, and A. M. DAVIES, 1969, Brit. J. Exptl. Pathol. *50*, 213.

GALL, D., 1966, Immunology *11*, 369.

GALLILY, R., and M. FELDMAN, 1967, Immunology *12*, 197.

GARVEY, J. S., and D. H. CAMPBELL, 1957, J. Exptl. Med. *105*, 361.

GERMUTH, F. G., JR., A. E. MAUMENEE, J. A. PRATT-JOHNSON, L. B. SENTERFIT, C. E. VAN ARNAM and A. D. POLLACK. 1959, Observations on the site and mechanisms of antigen-antibody interaction in anaphylactive hypersensitivity. *In*: J. H. Shaffer et al., eds.: Mechanisms of hypersensitivity. Henry Ford International Symposium. London, Churchill. p. 155–162.

GLENNY, A. T., and C. G. POPE, 1925, J. Pathol. Bacteriol. *28*, 273.

GORDON, R. E., 1966, J. Gen. Microbiol. *43*, 329.

HALBERT, S. P., S. MUDD and J. SMOLENS, 1946, J. Immunol. *53*, 291.

HOLT, L. B., 1950, Development in diphtheria prophylaxis. London, Heinemann.

HORNE, C. H. W., and R. G. WHITE, 1968, Immunology *15*, 65.

HUMPHREY, J. H. and J. L. TURK, 1963, Immunology *6*, 119.

JANDL, J. H., 1964, Mechanism of immune hemolysis in vivo. *In*: L. Thomas, J. Uhr and L. Grant, eds.: Injury, inflammation and immunity. Baltimore, Williams and Wilkins. p. 339–345.

JENKIN, C. R. and M. L. KARNOVSKY, 1967, J. Immunology *13*, 349.

JOHNSON, A. G., S. GAINES and M. LANDY, 1956, J. Exptl. Med. *103*, 225.

JOHNSON, P., R. A. NEAL and D. GALL, 1963, Nature *200*, 83.

JOLLÈS, P., D. SAMOUR and E. LEDERER, 1962, Arch. Biochem. Biophys. suppl. *1*, 283.

JOLLÈS, P., D. SAMOUR-MIGLIORE, H. DE WIJS and E. LEDERER, 1964, Biochim. Biophys. Acta *83*, 361.

LOEWI, G., E. J. HOLBOROW and A. TEMPLE, 1966, Immunology *10*, 339.

MIGLIORE, D. and P. JOLLÈS, 1968, FEBS Letters *2*, 7.

MILLER, J. F. A. P. and G. F. MITCHELL, 1969, Transplant. Rev. *1*.

MITCHISON, N. A., 1964, Proc. Roy. Soc. *B 161*, 275.

MITCHISON, N. A., 1968, Immunological paralysis as a dosage phenomenon. *In*: B. Cinader, ed.: Regulation of the antibody response. Springfield, Thomas. pp. 54–67.

MÖLLER, G., and H. WIGZELL, 1965, J. Exptl. Med. *121*, 969.

MORSE, S. I., 1964, J. Exptl. Med. *121*, 49.

MORSE, S. I. and S. K. RIESTER, 1967, J. Exptl. Med. *125*, 401.

MUNOZ, J. J., 1963, Bact. Rev. *27*, 325.

NELSON, D. S. and S. V. BOYDEN, 1964, Int. Arch. Allergy *25*, 279.

NEVEU, T., A. BRANELLEC and G. BIOZZI, 1964, Ann. Inst. Pasteur *106*, 771.

NEWBOULD, B. B., 1965, Immunology *9*, 613.

NOLL, H. and J. S. YOUNGER, 1959, Virology *8*, 319.

NOSSAL, G. J. V., G. L. ADA, C. M. AUSTIN and J. PYE, 1965, Aust. J. Exptl. Biol. Med. Sci. *42*, 283.

PATERSON, P. Y. and J. BELL, 1962, J. Immunol. *89*, 72.

PEARLMAN, D. S., 1966, Federation Proc. *25*, 548.

PEARSON, C. M., 1956, Ann. Rheum. Dis. *15*, 379.

Pharmaceutical Society of Great Britain, 1960, The Pharmaceutical Pocket Book, 17th Ed. London, Pharmaceutical Press. p. 29.

RAFFEL, S., 1965, *in*: M. Samter, ed.: Immunological diseases. London, Churchill. p. 146.

RAFFEL, S. and J. E. FORNEY, 1948, J. Exptl. Med. *88*, 485.

RAFFEL, S., L. E. ARNAUD, C. D. DUKES and J. S. HUANG, 1949, J. Exptl. Med. *90*, 53.

RAMON, G., 1926, J. Méd. Franc. *15*, 381.

RAMON, G., R. RICHOU and A. STAUB, 1937, Rev. Immunol. *3*, 389.

RICHOU, R., R. JENSEN and C. BELIN, 1964, Rev. Immunol. *28*, 49.

RIVENSEN, S., 1958, Gac. vet. (B. Aires) *20*, 209.

RUPP, J. C., R. D. MOORE and M. D. SCHOENBERG, 1960, Arch. Pathol., *70*, 43.

SEGRE, D. and M. KAEBERLE, 1962, J. Immunol. *89*, 782.

SHAW, C. M., E. C. ALVORD, JR. and M. W. KIES, 1964, J. Immunol. *92*, 24.

SPITZNAGEL, J. K. and A. C. ALLISON, 1970a, J. Immunol. *104*, 119.

SPITZNAGEL, J. K. and A. C. ALLISON, 1970b, J. Immunol. *104*, 128.

STARK, J. M., 1966, quoted in R. G. WHITE, 1966.

STARK, J. M., 1970a, Immunology *19*, 449.

STARK, J. M., 1970b, Immunology *19*, 457.

SUTER, E. and R. G. WHITE, 1954, Amer. Rev. Tuberc. *70*, 793.

TAUB, R. N., A. R. KRANTZ and D. W. DRESSER, 1970, Immunology *18*, 171.

TERRES, G. and W. WOLINS, 1961, J. Immunol. *86*, 361.

THINÈS-SENPOUX, D., 1967, Biochem. J. *105*, 20.

UHR, J. W., G. WEISSMAN and L. THOMAS, 1963, Proc. Soc. Exptl. Biol. Med. *112*, 287.

UNANUE, E. R. and B. A. ASKONAS, 1967, J. Reticulo-endothelial Soc. *4*, 440.

UNANUE, E. R. and B. A. ASKONAS, 1968, Immunology *15*, 287.

UNANUE, E. R., B. A. ASKONAS and A. C. ALLISON, 1970, J. Immunol.

VIGLIANI, E. C. and B. PERNIS, 1959. J. Occup. Med. *1*, 219.

WALKER, J. G. and G. W. SISKIND, 1968, Immunology *14*, 21.

WEIGLE, W. O., 1962, J. Exptl. Med. *116*, 913.

WEISS, D. W. and R. J. DUBOS, 1956, J. Exptl. Med. *103*, 73.

WHITE, R. G., 1963, Functional recognition of immunologically competent cells by means of the fluorescent antibody technique. *In*: G. E. W. Wolstenholme and J. Knight, eds.: Ciba Foundation Study Group No. 16: The immunologically competent cell; its nature and origin. London, Churchill. pp. 6–16.

WHITE, R. G., 1965, The role of peptido-glycolipids of *M.* tuberculosis and related organisms in immunological adjurrance. *In*: J. Šterzl, ed.: Molecular and Cellular Basis of Antibody Formation. Prague, Czechoslovak Acad. Sciences. pp. 71–83.

WHITE, R. G., 1966, Proc. Roy. Soc. Med. *61*, 1.

WHITE, R. G., L. BERNSTOCK, R. G. S. JOHNS and E. LEDERER, 1958, Immunology *1*, 54.

WHITE, R. G., G. C. JENKINS and P. C. WILKINSON, 1963, Int. Arch. Allergy *22*, 156.

WHITE, R. G. and A. H. E. MARSHALL, 1958, Immunology *1*, 111.

WILKINSON, P. C. and R. G. WHITE, 1966, Immunology *11*, 229.

WOODS, A. C., 1937, Amer. J. Ophthal. *19*, 9 and 100.

CHAPTER 5

The immune response to haptens

SIDNEY LESKOWITZ

Department of Pathology, Tufts Medical School, Boston, Mass.

5.1. Introduction

The importance of haptens in immunology is such as to be obvious to all with the least interest in the subject. Their contribution to our understanding of antibody specificity and structure, to methods of detection and immunoassay of a variety of biologically interesting compounds, and to the thermodynamics of antigen-antibody interaction amongst others are immeasurable. However, a discussion of the role of haptens in such studies is too broad a subject to be encompassed in one chapter and must remain for others to attempt. This chapter will focus on some general aspects of the immune response to haptens and the factors controlling this response.

Although the term hapten is commonly used to refer to low-molecular weight chemical entities, it was originally introduced by Landsteiner (1921) to designate protein-free substances of animal or bacterial origin which, although active *in vitro*, induce no antibody response with the usual methods of immunization. In its strictest sense therefore, the term hapten can be taken to designate any substance, large or small, which does not elicit an immune response by itself but can be demonstrated by appropriate means to react with antibody formed by immunization with a complete antigen.

The range of haptens studied at one time or another is truly phenomenal and covers such diverse substances as simple aromatic chemicals, peptides, oligosaccharides, steroids, drugs, nucleic acids and lipids. It would be well beyond the scope of this chapter to do justice to all these materials despite the considerable interest and importance that attaches to each. An attempt will therefore be made to provide some detail for a selected few haptens in an effort to adduce general principles concerning the nature of immune responses to haptens.

5.2. Methods of conjugation

5.2.1. Covalent binding of haptens

A hapten which by definition is *per se* non-immunogenic, in order to elicit an immune response must first be coupled firmly to a carrier molecule which provides the necessary conditions for immunogenicity (sec later). The ways in which the hapten may be coupled to its carrier depend only on the chemical nature of the hapten and the ingenuity of the investigator, but in general they require either the formation of a covalent bond (for simple chemicals) or very strong ionic interactions (for macromolecules).

One of the most commonly used procedures for coupling simple aromatic compounds to carrier proteins, and one which was magnificently exploited in the protein studies of Landsteiner (1962), makes use of the formation of azo bonds. In general the procedure is applicable to aromatic amines which can be diazotized with cold nitrous acid (Campbell et al. 1963). The diazonium salts formed may then be conjugated directly by addition to the carrier protein in alkaline solution. In practice we have often found it more convenient to isolate the intermediate diazonium salt by addition of fluoboric acid (Wofsy et al. 1963). The dried crystalline fluoborates may be stored indefinitely in a deep-freeze. Repeated conjugations are performed merely by weighing out the required amount of diazonium salt and adding it to the protein carrier dissolved in cold buffer at a pH of 8–9. Specific procedures are described in Williams and Chase (1967) and Campbell et al. (1963).

While the extent of conjugation achieved is often measured by absorption at a wave length characteristic of azotyrosine derivatives, the nature of conjugation with proteins is sufficiently complex to produce highly spurious results with this method. The most likely sites of formation of azo bonds are the aromatic rings of tyrosine and histidine and the ϵ-groups of lysine. Either mono- or di-substituted groups may be formed at all these positions depending on the number of moles of diazonium salt used. In addition, reactions with tryptophan and arginine are possible. The absorption spectra of all these possible conjugates have been determined for model compounds (Tabachnick and Sobotka 1959) and show considerable differences.

With a limiting amount of diazonium salt, preferential conjugation will occur with tyrosine and histidine groups to yield the characteristic orange-red derivatives. However, the nature of the final conjugate formed is to a large degree dependent on the accessibility of reactive groups. Thus the presence of tyrosine and histidine in a particular protein is of little value if they are buried in the interior of the molecule and inaccessible to the diazonium salt. Tabachnick and Sobotka (1960), for example, found that the amount of arsanilic acid conjugated to bovine serum albumin at pH 9 could not usefully be determined by spectral analysis. When all free amino groups were blocked by acetylation, estimate of the extent of conjugation to tyrosine and histidine by spectral analysis could still account for only 50% of bound arsenic determined by direct analysis thus indicating other modes of conjugation. In our own studies we have observed significant differences in spectral properties of conjugates made with arsanilic acid and a series of serum albumins and globulins. In general, when the amount of diazonium salt per weight of protein was kept constant, the azotyrosine absorption for the conjugated globulins was much greater than for the albumins, indicating that while the tyrosine content of these proteins did not differ markedly on a weight basis, the apparent accessibility of these groups for coupling was much higher in globulins than in albumins. Preliminary acetylation of the albumins produced a much more intense azotyrosine spectrum further indicating that much coupling with native albumins took place largely on the ϵ-amino groups. Since the immunogenicity of these various conjugates differed considerably, it is quite apparent that the mode of coupling of haptens to carriers is at least as important as the number of groups coupled.

The utility of the azo coupling method for formation of conjugates is not restricted to simple aromatic amines alone. A number of procedures have been described, for example, in which *p*-aminophenylglycoside derivatives had been prepared, then diazotized and coupled to proteins for use in production of antisera to various oligosaccharides (Goebel et al. 1934; Karush 1957; Allen et al. 1967). The method is widely adaptable for conjugation of many compounds of biologic interest provided a suitable aromatic amine derivative can be synthesized.

One of the most widely used haptens in immunologic research is the 2,4-dinitrophenyl group (DNP). It and the closely related 2,4,6-trinitrophenyl (TNP) group share such highly desirable characteristics as an intense and easily distinguished absorption spectra, stability of the covalent bond formed and high immunogenicity.

The DNP and TNP haptens are attached to protein carriers by a nucleophilic substitution reaction in which the halogen (fluorine or chlorine) in benzene ring position 1 is so activated by the nitro groups in positions 2, 4 and 6 as to be readily displaced by electron-donating groups. Thus in the reaction of a protein with 2,4-dinitrochlorobenzene, the chlorine may be readily displaced by $-NH_2$ groups of lysine, $-OH$ groups of tyrosine and $-SH$ groups of cysteine. It may readily be seen that, when 2,4-dinitrochloro- or 2,4-dinitrofluorobenzene are coupled to proteins, a variety of sites are available for conjugation and the result, as with azo-coupled haptens, is a considerable heterogeneity in hapten determinants.

Some advantage is gained by using the less reactive sulphonic acid. Under the mild alkaline conditions used 2,4-dinitrobenzenesulphonic acid yields conjugated proteins in which only free amino groups are substituted and essentially only DNP-lysine residues are formed. An additional advantage is the water solubility of the sulphonic acids, permitting reaction to take place in homogeneous aqueous solution. Typical conditions for preparation of DNP proteins are given in Williams and Chase (1967). When the sulphonic acid is used for conjugation, the DNP content of conjugates may be readily obtained by spectrophotometric analysis at 360 mμ where the extinction coefficient for ϵ-DNP lysine may be used as a standard.

Although these two methods are the most commonly used for preparation of hapten conjugates, they by no means exhaust the field. A considerable variety of ingenious chemical procedures have been devised for coupling haptens to carriers. These include such diverse procedures as thiolation of the carrier followed by reaction with iodoacetyl haptens (Saha et al. 1966), formation of amide bonds between carboxyl groups on the hapten and ϵ-amino groups on the protein (Erlanger et al. 1957), and polymerizing chains of amino acids on to proteins using N-carboxy-α-amino acid anhydrides (Sela and Arnon 1960). Of particular value for coupling amines or carboxylic acid haptens to proteins is the use of carbodiimide reagents. These compounds with the general formula $R—N{=}C{=}N—R'$ where R and R' represent aryl or alkyl groups react with amines and carboxylic acids to condense them by peptide bond formation with the elimination of a substituted urea $RNHC{=}ONHR'$. Many carbodiimide reagents are water soluble and can be used to couple proteins, peptides and amino acids in aqueous solution under very mild conditions. They have proven especially valuable in coupling such poorly immunogenic peptides as ACTH, bradykinin and angiotensin to protein carriers for antibody formation (Kemp and Woodward 1965; Goodfriend et al. 1966). Several general methods for coupling haptens with carboxyl, amino, hydroxyl or carbonyl functional groups are also available (Beiser et al. 1968).

While most immunologists think of small organic molecules in connection with haptens, another category of naturally occurring macromolecules exists which may also be given this designation. In contrast to the haptens described above which are generally conjugated to carriers by covalent bonds, the macromolecular haptens require only electrostatic binding to carriers for immunization.

5.2.2. Ionic binding of macromolecular haptens

Over the years, a number of antigens were studied which, upon successive purification, were found to lose the ability to immunize while retaining the ability to react with preformed antibodies thus becoming by definition, haptens. One such material, the Forsmann antigen, was shown to lose immunizing activity following removal of all protein from the alcohol extract. Landsteiner and Levine (1928), found that the original immunizing capacity of the purified Forsmann material could be restored by addition of antigenic proteins such as pig serum. These later materials came to be called 'schleppers' presumably for their ability to carry along the hapten through whatever process was required to elicit an immune response, without being covalently bound to it.

Another substance of considerable historical interest is type-specific pneumococcal polysaccharide. While whole pneumococci are excellent antigens for production of huge amounts of antibody in many mammalian species, the purified capsular polysaccharide freed of protein contaminants was found to be poorly immunogenic or non-immunogenic in rabbits (Avery and Goebel 1933) and guinea-pigs (Maurer and Mansmann 1958). Thus they appeared to function as haptens in those species requiring the pneumococcal organisms as carriers or 'schleppers' to achieve complete immunogenicity. In other species such as man and mice the purified polysaccharides behave as complete antigens eliciting active immunity of high degree (Avery and Goebel 1933; Heidelberger 1956).

Intriguing differences exist in the response of various animal species to these polysaccharides which makes a moot question of whether they are to be considered as haptens. Thus humans receiving a single injection of 80 μg of pneumococcal polysaccharide will show a substantial antibody response persisting for many years at a high level without apparent booster effects from further injections of antigen (Heidelberger 1956). Similar results have been obtained with other polysaccharides, such as dextrans, levans and blood group substances. Rabbits, on the other hand, while incapable of responding to the purified polysaccharides, make a response to injections of the whole organisms that resembles that made to protein antigens in that high levels of antibody are reached which tend to decline rapidly without further contact with the antigen. More recently some earlier observations of McLeod were confirmed in showing that rabbits once primed with whole pneumococci would show an anamnestic response nine months later to a second injection of purified polysaccharide (Paul et al. 1967).

It is conceivable that such polysaccharides represent borderline antigens eliciting an immune response unaided in some species and requiring an additional carrier in others. Alternatively it is possible that as haptens they are capable of combining with endogenous carriers to produce complete antigens only in some species and not in others.

Another category of compounds that behave in a similar fashion are the nucleic acids. Early attempts at immunization with nucleic acid rich extracts of bacteria yielded antibodies apparently reactive with DNA as shown by loss of reactivity following DNase treatment (Blix et al. 1954; Phillips et al. 1958). However, as with pneumococcal polysaccharides, progressive purification of DNA lead to material which was decreasingly immunogenic. Stimulated by the clinical observations that patients suffering from lupus erythematosus had in their sera an antibody reacting with purified DNA (Kunkel et al. 1959), a renewed effort was made to define the conditions under which DNA would become immunogenic. A spate of evidence (Plescia et al. 1967; Levine and Stollar 1968) suggested that an appropriate carrier was required. An excellent material for this purpose was found to be methylated bovine serum albumin (Plescia et al. 1964), a protein in which all the carboxyl groups are esterified. The residual amino groups confer a large net positive charge on the molecule making it particularly suitable for complexing to negatively charged nucleic acids by electrostatic interactions. This general method of producing complexes by ionic rather than covalent bonding has proven to be effective for converting not only nucleic acids into complete antigens, but has also worked for other non-immunogenic materials such as certain polypeptides and polysaccharides (Plescia et al. 1964; Maurer 1965). In certain instances when the hapten is positively charged, electrostatic complexes with negatively charged carriers have proved effective (Green et al. 1966). Thus about 40% of random bred Hartley guinea pigs are able to respond to immunization with 2,4-dinitrophenylpolylysine by production of hapten-specific antibodies. When complexes made with this material and acetylated BSA are used for immunization, essentially 100% of the animals respond.

The covalent bonds by which most haptens are bound to carriers (e.g., C–N, C–C) have energies of the order of 40–80 kcal per mole. While the energy of formation of an ionic bond between a carboxyl and amino group is only 4.5 kcal per mole in water (Pauling 1948), the energy of a single ionic bond may be insufficient for the formation of stable complexes, but the multiple interactions occurring between polyanionic and polycationic macromolecules are sufficiently large to make this method applicable to charged macromolecular haptens. It is of interest in this connection that the material used to form the aggregate must in itself be antigenic and complexes of these haptenic macromolecules with such non-immunogens as polystyrenesulphonate or carboxymethyl cellulose were ineffective (Green et al. 1966).

5.3. *Effect of hapten type on immune response*

Probably because of the many variables involved in assaying an immune response to a hapten-carrier conjugate few empirical rules have been found relating the type of hapten and the intensity of the antibody response. Such studies would require conjugates made with the same carrier and containing different haptens coupled in the same ratios by the same type of bonds. Few such studies seem to be available.

The general impression seems to be that haptens coupled by azo linkage to carrier proteins give only slight to modest antibody levels and frequently fail to produce enough antibody, at least without prolonged immunization, to give visible precipitates with antigen (Hoffman et al. 1969). Antigens formed by coupling haptens such as DNP and TNP to free amino groups usually elicit much larger amounts of antibody and are for this reason perhaps the most widely used for studies in antibody structure. In one recent study for example (Brody et al. 1969), a comparison was made of precipitating antibody formation in rabbits immunized with azobenzenearsonate (R) or DNP conjugates of rabbit γ-globulin. Average production of anti-DNP antibody was more than twice that of anti-R. A general experience that we and other investigators have had is the difficulty of detecting antibody-forming cells by the Jerne plaque technique in mice, using azo conjugates for immunization, although this could be done in rabbits (Hraba et al. 1969). However, mice can be readily immunized with DNP conjugates to give large numbers of plaque forming cells (Havas et al. 1969; Yamada et al. 1969). In both cases detection of antibody was attempted with highly coupled proteins attached to red cells so that it seems unlikely that a difference in affinity of anti-R and anti-DNP antibodies produced would account for the results (Pasanen et al. 1969). It is difficult to even offer suggestions as to why such differences might exist. One intriguing possibility lies in the recent observations that 10% of mouse myeloma proteins studied exhibited a measurable binding affinity for DNP conjugates and were also specific for certain purines and pyrimidines (Eisen et al. 1967; Schubert et al. 1968). On the basis of the clonal selection theory one might suggest that the total antibody production elicited is a reflection of the numbers of available clones of cells specific for a given hapten. DNP haptens by virtue of sharing a complementarity with other naturally occurring substances might have a specially large number of clones available for reaction.

In terms of the magnitude of antibody response the group of haptens comprising repeating oligosaccharide units seem to occupy a specially favoured position. It has been known to immunologists for many years that very large amounts of precipitating antibody can be formed by immunizing rabbits (Askonas et al. 1960) and horses (Van Der Scheer et al. 1940) with killed pneumococci. More recently the interesting observation was made that certain rabbits immunized with suspensions of killed streptococci made extremely large amounts of a highly homogeneous antibody specific for the rhamnose disaccharide repeating unit of the group-specific polysaccharide (Osterlund et al. 1966; Braun et al. 1969). This specific globulin which in one instance amounted to about 50 mg per ml. had many of the characteristics of a myeloma protein. The same observation was now been made with type III and VIII pneumococci in rabbits where about 8% of the rabbits immunized respond with extremely high levels of a highly homogeneous antibody (Pincus et al. 1970). Aside from its potential value in the elucidation of antibody structure, the production of such huge amounts of antibody to haptens consisting of simple repeating units such as represented by these bacterial polysaccharides is of considerable interest to concepts of immunogenicity. It suggests that the presence of bacterial bodies somehow causes a restricted number of antibody forming clones to proliferate in a fashion resembling malignancy and producing a progeny that fills much of the available lymphoid space. Unlike multiple myeloma, however, these cells remain under control and cessation of antigen administration produces a prompt fall in antibody production. The alternative proposition that these antigens can simultaneously stimulate many different clones to produce the same antibody provides a severe challenge to strict clonal selection theories and assumes the existence of multipotent clones.

Another measure of the relative immunogenicity of various haptens can be seen in studies involving their competitive interaction. Amkraut et al. (1966) studied the immune response to the azobenzenearsonate (R) and 2,4-dinitrophenyl (DNP) haptens coupled to a variety of carriers. In general they found that the presence of the DNP hapten on the same immunizing molecule bearing the R determinant resulted in a partial or complete suppression of antibody formation to the R group. Such suppression of the R response was found when the ratio of DNP to R group in the carrier molecule was about 1:3. Suppression of the DNP response was much more difficult to effect and required DNP to R ratio of about 1:10. In a similar study the same sort of observation was made (Brody and Siskind 1969) utilizing mixtures of singly conjugated proteins. An immunizing mixture of 0.5 mg. R-rabbit γ-globulin (R-RGG) and 0.5 mg DNP-RGG resulted in a 50% decrease in response to the R determinant compared to that produced by R-RGG alone. No competition was found if the conjugates were injected separately in different feet.

The administration of passive antibody specific for one or other of the haptens one day prior to immunization results in a suppression of antibody formation to that hapten (Brody et al. 1967). Of interest here is the observation that such suppression by passive antibody eliminated the depressive effect of antigenic competition only when immunization was accomplished by haptens administered on separate carrier molecules.

The level at which competition of haptens occurs in the immune response is uncertain, but the available evidence best fits an hypothesis involving some antigen-processing event as the rate-determining step. In any event the ability of DNP hapten to compete favourably with the R hapten for antibody formation is consistent with the above mentioned observations that it gives rise in general to more total antibody, a finding that seems to hold for the competition of more complex systems as well (Adler 1964). While interesting for the insight they shed on immunogenicity of haptens in general, these studies suffer from the disadvantage of the haptens being coupled to the carriers in quite different ways. Therefore, while attempts may be made to utilize the same carrier and to keep the ratio of hapten per carrier molecule constant, the sites of attachment of DNP and R haptens are quite different. Since this produces conjugates in which the molecular environment around each hapten is quite different as is the net charge of the whole conjugate, any conclusions about immunogenicity drawn from such studies remain debatable.

The degree of conjugation of a hapten to a carrier within large limits appears to have little effect on the antibody response. Presumably this may be due to the lack of critical studies on effective doses of the various conjugates. On one extreme several studies indicate that a single DNP hapten on a protein carrier is capable of evoking a measurable antibody response (Eisen et al. 1964; Brenneman and Singer 1968; Little and Counts 1969). In one instance (Brenneman et al. 1968) anti-DNP levels of only up to 100 μg per ml. were produced in rabbits after immunization with mono-DNP-papain in Freund's adjuvant and repeated boosters. On the other hand (Little and Counts 1969), guinea-pigs produced 1–2 mg. anti-DNP per ml. when immunized with mono-DNP-insulin. In general, however, conjugates prepared with few haptens per molecule of carrier are less immunogenic and require either larger doses of antigen or greater periods of immunization to achieve significant antihapten titres of antibody.

At the other extreme of coupling ratio it had been shown sometime ago that R-horse serum was poorly immunogenic if the product contained more than 3% arsenic (Haurowitz 1936). In one confirmation of these studies (Rittenberg and Amkraut 1966) the antihapten response made to conjugates of picrylsulphonic acid (TNP) and keynole limpet haemo-cynin (KLH) was measured in rabbits immunized and boosted without the use of adjuvants. No primary or secondary responses could be elicited with conjugates containing less than 230 or more than 2000 TNP groups per KLH molecule. Optimal hapten to carrier ratios for antibody production were around 900:1. Essentially similar results were obtained with DNP conjugates of polylysine in guinea pigs where progressively larger degrees of coupling produced a lower per cent of responding animals (Kantor et al. 1963). In my own work, serendipity led me to use a lightly coupled R-polytyrosine (Leskowitz 1963) which proved to be immunogenic, whereas a heavily coupled conjugate had previously been reported (Sela and Haurowitz 1958) to be non-immunogenic in rabbits. These results were subsequently confirmed and extended by Borek and Stupp (1966) who showed that maximum responsiveness was achieved with a degree of coupling corresponding to from 5 to 22% of the tyrosine residues being substituted. Above and below that per cent, immunogenicity decreases markedly (Loewi and Nind 1969).

The poor response to lightly conjugated carriers is not difficult to explain in quantitative terms. Almost certainly some minimal number of antigenic determinants is required to provoke an immune response and, if such a determinant is to involve the hapten, it would require very large amounts of carrier to bring a sufficient number of hapten determinants to bear. As the degree of conjugation increases some optimal number of hapten-containing determinants would be reached. The decrease in immunogenicity with increasing degree of hapten coupling requires some explanation and at least two possibilities may be considered. In one the highly substituted conjugate is so altered in physico-chemical properties by changes in ionic charge and surface configuration, that it is cleared by the reticulo-endothelial system in a different fashion. As a corollary of this, 'processing' of the conjugate may occur differently due to interference with enzymatic attack produced by steric inhibition from the many hapten groups present. As an alternative possibility the high degree of substitution may drastically decrease the inherent immunogenicity of the carrier (as will be discussed later). This may play a large role in the response to the attached hapten.

5.4. *Effect of carrier on immunogenicity*

Perhaps even more important than the hapten in determining the magnitude of the immune response, is the nature of the carrier to which the hapten is coupled. In general it would appear that the more foreign (or, to put it another way, the more immunogenic) a carrier protein is to the species being immunized, the higher the antihapten antibody response is likely to be. In one instance in which inbred mice were immunized with DNP conjugates in Freund's adjuvant it was found that anti-DNP antibody levels were highest with bovine γ-globulin, next highest with rabbit and rat γ-globulin and least with mouse γ-globulin conjugates (Fronstin et al. 1967). This was paralleled by the antibody responses made to the carrier proteins themselves. In this particular study the kinetics of all responses measured were the same; only the peak levels achieved were different. A similar study in guinea pigs showed that immunization with DNP-conjugates of bovine γ-globulin, egg albumin, bovine serum albumin and gelatin gave anti-DNP levels averaging 5 mg/ml, 3.5 mg/ml, $<$ 2 mg/ml and $<$ 2 mg/ml respectively (Siskind et al. 1966). It is of some interest in this connection too that the amounts of γ_2 antibody relative to γ_1 antibody varied considerably with the different carriers.

When DNP-polylysine was complexed to anionic foreign proteins such as acetylated bovine serum albumin (BSA) or egg albumin, all guinea-pigs tested made measurable anti-DNP antibody (Green et al. 1966). When acetylated guinea-pig albumin was used for complexing, only a few animals made low levels of antihapten antibody and if non-immunogenic molecules such as carboxymethylcellulose were used, no response was detected.

Another type of difference in response, dependent on the immunogenicity of the carrier, was shown in studies using conjugates of arsanilic acid (Jones and Leskowitz 1965). Conjugates made with non-immunogenic homopolymers of amino acids such as polytyrosine or polyhistidine succeeded in eliciting hapten specific delayed sensitivity but little or no hapten-specific antibody in guinea-pigs. On the other hand R conjugates of highly immunogenic proteins such as insulin, BSA and ribonuclease elicited mainly hapten-specific antibody with little or no hapten-specific delayed sensitivity. An intermediate position was occupied by conjugates of weakly immunogenic materials such as co-polymers of glutamic acid, alanine and tyrosine which produced both hapten-specific delayed sensitivity and antibody. In general, anti-R levels achieved paralleled closely the immunogenicity of the carriers used, but the ability to produce hapten-specific delayed sensitivity did not parallel this efficacy. Thus carriers may control not only the size of the immune response but its quality as well.

Another aspect of the control of antihapten responses exercised by the carrier molecule is seen in the use of isologous proteins for making conjugates. Although frequently advocated as a means of eliciting an anti-hapten response without the attendant complication of antibody to the carrier molecule, such conjugates have the distinct disadvantage of producing only low levels of antibody after persistent immunization (Fronstin et al. 1967; Jones and Leskowitz 1965). This effect of lack of immunogenicity of the carrier stemming from tolerance to one's own proteins can be mimicked by induced tolerance. It has been shown, for example (Paul et al. 1969), that immunization of rabbits with an alum precipitate of DNP-BSA gave an average of 1.08 mg anti-BSA and 0.35 mg anti-DNP antibody. When rabbits were rendered tolerant by prior injection of a total of 1 mg of BSA they produced 0.39 mg anti-BSA and 0.25 mg anti-DNP antibody. If tolerance were induced with a total of 100 mg BSA, average titres of anti-BSA and anti-DNP antibodies were only 0.02 and 0.08 mg/ml respectively indicating that the more profound the tolerance to the carrier, the less the response to the hapten. A more direct comparison of self *versus* induced tolerance to the carrier was made by Nachtigal and Feldman (1964) who studied the antibody response to sulphonic acid in rabbits immunized with sulphanilazo-rabbit γ-globulin and in rabbits made tolerant to human serum albumin and immunized with sulphanilazo-human serum albumin. In both instances comparable but low titres of antihapten antibody were produced. We have made the same observation in guinea-pigs immunized with arsanilic acid conjugates.

An especially interesting example of the effects of tolerance to the carrier on the response to the hapten is seen in the studies on so-called 'non-responder' guinea-pigs in which the conjugate DNP-poly-L-lysine behaves as a hapten, and elicits a response only when complexed electrostatically with an immunogenic carrier such as BSA. It was subsequently shown (Green et al. 1968) that prior induction of tolerance to the BSA carrier effectively suppressed the response to the DNP-poly-L-lysine, despite the fact that it apparently does not contribute to the specificity of the antigenic determinant towards which the antibody is directed. As more quantitative studies appear, the full extent of this phenomenon is beginning to emerge and its eventual explanation must play a central role in our understanding of the concept of immunogenicity. Some attempts at such an understanding will be presented at the end of the chapter.

5.5. *Size of hapten and carrier*

For many years it had been considered axiomatic that antigens were macromolecules of fairly large size, while haptens tended to be simple molecules under 1000 molecular weight. Of late these distinctions have become blurred with the observations that certain very large macromolecules such as pneumococcal polysaccharides and DNA may function as haptens, while very small molecules such as angiotensin (mol. wt 1031) can be immunogenic (Dietrich 1966).

The distinction has been still further blunted by the observation that certain haptens such as arsanilic acid or phosphanilic acid, when conjugated to a single amino acid residue such as N-acetyltyrosine, became immunogenic, albeit only in respect to production of delayed hypersensitivity (Leskowitz and Zak 1966). A critical evaluation of the size of the carrier needed to elicit an immune response to the R hapten was carried out by Borek et al. (1967a) who found that R-hexatyrosine elicited a measurable antibody response in 4 of 4 rabbits by 10 weeks while only 1 in 4 rabbits responded to R-trityrosine and none to R-N-acetyltyrosine-amide. Again only arsanilic acid was effective while p-aminobenzoic acid was not. Thus for a limited number of haptens a curious distinction has arisen between the carrier requirements for a conjugate to elicit delayed hypersensitivity or antibody formation. With arsanilic acid, coupling to a single aromatic amino acid such as tyrosine, histidine or tryptophan (Leskowitz et al. 1966) gives an immunogenic molecule of mol. wt around 400 capable of immunizing for, eliciting and producing tolerance for delayed hypersensitivity (Collotti and Leskowitz 1969). A somewhat larger carrier, six or more tyrosine residues long, is required for antihapten antibody formation. Whether this is due to a clear distinction between the two types of immune response in respect to initiators, or a quantitative effect in which a given amount of a poor immunogen is more capable of eliciting delayed sensitivity than antibody production, is a point of considerable interest.

A somewhat similar case has been made with great elegance for carriers for the DNP hapten. Schlossman et al. (1965) have shown that this hapten coupled to the α-NH_2 group of oligolysines larger than 7 lysine residues are immunogenic in guinea pigs (while any carrier less than 6 lysines is non-immunogenic). This critical size carrier, however, was shown to be necessary for both delayed hypersensitivity as well as antibody formation (Schlossman and Levine 1967) and immunization usually achieved both or neither.

A heroic study of the immunogenicity of DNP coupled to single amino acids was completed recently by Frey et al. (1969) who studied the ability of 39 different conjugates to immunize guinea pigs. They concluded that some conjugates could be shown to participate in 'trans-conjugation' phenomena in which the DNP group was found to transfer to a protein carrier. On this basis the authors counseled caution in evaluating other immunogenicity studies with hapten-amino acid complexes. While especially relevant to those conjugates in which the DNP group is bound to a sulphur, an oxygen or a tertiary amine group, this explanation will not cover those situations in which immunogenicity is lost by a chain reduction of a single lysine residue (Schlossman et al. 1965) or the substitution of a D for an L-amino acid (Schlossman et al. 1969), nor in fact for several immunogenic amino acid conjugates that could not be excluded by the authors themselves on the counts mentioned.

While still a moot point, the progressive reduction in limiting size for at least some hapten conjugates suggests that immunologists may be approaching from two opposite extremes the common denominator of an immunogenic determinant. On the one hand it is quite apparent that large proteins are composed of an unknown but large number of such determinants, while molecules such as R-N-acetyltyrosine may represent the ultimate of a single complete determinant. It is unlikely, however, that size *per se* has more than a secondary effect on immunogenicity. What immunologists must really grapple with, is the ultimate physico-chemical character of a minimal molecular grouping that would suffice to initiate an immune response.

We have seen that while haptens come in a variety of sizes, they have in common an inability to initiate an immune response in the absence of conjugation to a suitable carrier. Similarly there is wide latitude in the size and composition that carrier molecules may take to initiate a response to the attached hapten. It would seem that, if there is to be a guiding principle concerning the nature of effectiveness of carriers, it must concern function and it is towards this concept that the last section will be devoted.

5.6. *Function of carrier molecule*

There are at least three ways in which the role of a carrier in determining the immunogenicity of a hapten may be considered. The first of these has to do with the concept of specificity. Most immunologists now accept as reasonable the notion that the receptor site on an immunocompetent cell is an antibody-like molecule. Initiation of an immune response is considered to result from an effective interaction between this receptor and an immunogenic determinant for which it carries specificity. While the hapten alone may be complementary in structure to this site and bound by it, this interaction is insufficient to initiate a response. This failure might be due to insufficient thermodynamic energy of interaction or inability to effect an allosteric change in such a receptor molecule. The function of the carrier molecule in these terms would be to convert a hapten to a complete determinant by either increasing its energy of interaction with the cell receptor site or rendering it capable of initiating an allosteric effect in the receptor which could be transmitted as a signal throughout the cell. In either event the hapten would be serving as the 'immunodominant tip' towards which much of the specificity is directed but the carrier is required to provide the additional elements of the complete determinant.

A number of observations make this explanation of carrier function unlikely. From the standpoint of energetics it has been shown by Schlossman and Levine (1967) that the non-immunogenic α-DNP-hexalysine is bound by antibody with 96% of the maximum energy of the immunogenic α-DNP-heptalysine. Despite this small difference in energy, immunogenicity is not achieved even by immunization with larger amounts. Similarly the antibody produced following immunization of rabbits with whole pneumococci (Braun et al. 1969) and of non-responder guinea-pigs with DNP-poly-L-lysine BSA aggregates (Green et al. 1968) is completely specific for the polysaccharide or DNP-polylysine haptens respectively and shows no carrier contribution to specificity. It seems highly unlikely, therefore, that the only function of the carrier can be as a contributor to the determinant towards which the cell receptor is directed. Furthermore this interpretation provides little basis for explaining the failure of D-amino acid polymer conjugates to function as immunogens (Benacerraf et al. 1963; Leskowitz 1967) despite the fact that D-amino acids themselves may contribute to the specificity of antibody.

A second and very recent explanation for the role of the carrier was that of Mitchison (1967). Utilizing a hapten-carrier conjugate system to study *in vitro* stimulation of a secondary response he observed that: (1) lymphocyte enriched cell populations proved deficient in susceptibility to *in vitro* stimulation. Restoration of susceptibility could be achieved by addition of peritoneal exudate cells; (2) the carrier protein exercised a large contribution to the stimulation by the hapten-carrier conjugate although making little contribution to the energy of binding by the antibody formed subsequently; (3) stimulation of response could be competitively inhibited by excess carrier. On this basis the suggestion was made that two or more receptors are involved in a co-operative act of recognition necessary for an immune response, one directed to the hapten and the other directed to some determinant on the carrier.

Rajewsky et al. (1969) showed that rabbits stimulated with a sulphanilic acid conjugate of BSA would produce a good secondary response to the sulphanilic acid hapten only if the carrier used in the secondary stimulus was again BSA. However, if the rabbits were also pretreated with another carrier human γ-globulin (HGG), a good secondary response to the hapten could be elicited by sulphanilic acid coupled to HGG. Primary immunization with HGG alone was ineffective. They concluded that the immune stimulus involved the recognition of carrier determinants unrelated to the hapten, and since the receptors to these unrelated determinants are probably on different cells, they further suggested that the immune stimulus for antibody formation requires the interaction of two antigen-bridged cells. In this formulation, therefore, the function of the carrier is again to contribute additional antigenic determinants so that sufficient cell-cell interactions required to produce an immune response may occur.

While this is an intriguing hypothesis attempting to relate several observations on carrier specificity to the recently evolving conception of co-operation between bone marrow- and thymus-derived cell populations in the immune response, certain obstacles to its acceptance remain. Because of its current interest it is worth reviewing objections in some detail.

(1) Several immunogenic conjugates are already known, whose carriers would appear to be too small (on the order of 1 to 7 amino acids) to bridge two cells (Leskowitz et al. 1966; Schlossman et al. 1969). On the other hand large molecules with several antigenic determinants may be non-immunogenic without appropriate carriers (Plescia and Braun 1967; Levine and Stollar 1968). As more is learned about the structure of single antigenic determinants in proteins it is conceivable that some of them will be isolated or synthesized and tested for immunogenicity, providing a critical test for the carrier hypothesis.

(2) A number of instances are known in which a secondary response to the hapten can be elicited following injection of a heterologous carrier conjugate (Rittenberg and Campbell 1968; Steiner and Eisen 1967). These results usually required either a prolonged interval between the first and second stimuli or the use of a highly immunogenic carrier such as keyhole limpet haemocyanin. In any event the responses observed apparently did not require the co-operation of cells produced by preliminary priming with the carrier to effectuate a secondary response to the hapten.

(3) The competitive effects between haptens considered earlier (Amkraut et al. 1966; Brody and Siskind 1969) are difficult to explain with this model; one might expect the presence of two different haptens on a single carrier molecule to produce an enhancing effect since they could collaborate in bridging hapten-recognizing cells of both kinds. Instead the presence of one is found to suppress a response to the other. Similarly the presence of several different haptens on a non-immunogenic carrier might be expected to elicit an antihapten response. Such a result has not to my knowledge been reported yet.

(4) Finally the studies in which apparent co-operation between hapten-specific and carrier-specific cells leads to a secondary hapten response, have all been accomplished by priming with complete Freund's adjuvant. In the absence of experiments in which priming with the carrier was accomplished in such a way as not to produce a simultaneous carrier-specific delayed sensitivity, it is not clear whether the observed response to the hapten followed a possible but not usual pathway. It has been shown previously that prior existence of delayed sensitivity to a carrier may produce an enhanced response to a hapten, without priming to the hapten (Coe and Salvin 1964). Similarly delayed sensitivity to the hapten will produce an enhanced antibody formation to the carrier again without priming to the carrier (Leskowitz 1968). It was suggested that such effects are due to a more efficient utilization of antigen by the cells elicited in a delayed reaction. Since delayed sensitivity plays no role in the initiation of antibody formation by usual methods of immunization, it would be useful to determine whether co-operative effects between hapten-specific and carrier-specific cells can be demonstrated in its absence.

A third hypothesis concerning the function of the carrier in eliciting an immune response to the hapten has to do with antigen 'processing'. Since this topic will be covered in Chapter 10, it will suffice to say here that a good deal of evidence has been adduced to support the concept that antigens must be 'processed' by some type of macrophage before they can elicit an immune response. There is a great deal of uncertainty about the nature of this purported processing step, but at a minimum it would seem to require an enzymatic event. One likely possibility would be the enzymatic linkage of an antigenic determinant to a segment of RNA required for activation of the appropriate immunocompetent cell. Such an event could occur with or without attendant proteolytic breakdown of the rest of the antigen. If this is made an obligatory event in the immune pathway, many of the observations on immunogenicity reported in this chapter become explicable.

Haptens, whether they be simple chemicals or macromolecules, have in common an inability to be enzymatically processed by species in which they are non-immunogenic. Coupling to an appropriate carrier provides the necessary handle by which such processing may be accomplished and it is essential that such carriers be themselves immunogenic, i.e., processable. Hapten-carrier coupling may be by covalent or electrostatic interaction. The carrier in addition may or may not provide some contributed to the total antigenic determinant against which the antibody is directed.

Haptens coupled to non-immunogenic polymers of D-amino acids do not elicit antibody production. As suggested previously (Benacerraf et al.

1963) few enzymes exist capable of processing such carriers in the required manner. It is of interest in this connection that arsanilic acid conjugated to poly-D-tyrosine was found to be non-immunogenic but when coupled to N-acetyl-D-tyrosine was immunogenic (Leskowitz et al. 1966; Borek et al. 1967b). It was almost as if the mono-tyrosine derivative existed already as an antigenic determinant and could be processed, whereas the polymer required and was not susceptible to enzymatic attack. Another interesting example of this sort was reported by Schlossman et al. (1969) who found that a carrier sequence of eight L-lysine residues was required to elicit an immune response to DNP. The interruption of this chain by a single D-lysine residue made the conjugate non-immunogenic.

The behavior of DNP-poly-lysine as a hapten in non-responding guinea-pigs is not due to a lack of cells capable of making antibody of that specificity. Rather it has been suggested that a specific processing event for lysine-containing carriers is missing in these particular animals (Green et al. 1968). Complex protein carriers offer a number of sites for a genetically controlled processing step whereas simple homopolymers offer only one and hence are more likely to allow such genetic control to be manifested as a single dominant trait.

Haptens compete most effectively with each other if present on the same carrier (Amkraut et al. 1966). If injected on separate carriers they must be given in the same injection site (Brody and Siskind 1969). Since clonal selection theory postulates a limited specificity potential for individual lymphoid cells, the competition is best understood at a level, prior to the selection of the specific clone by the antigenic determinant. Antigen processing could be such a rate-limiting step in which certain hapten determinants are favoured for quantitative or qualitative reasons.

Heavily coupled conjugates are poorly immunogenic, despite the fact that they can react quite well with antibody specific for the hapten and presumably an antibody-like receptor on an immunocompetent cell (Rittenberg and Amkraut 1966; Kantor et al. 1963; Borek and Stupp 1966). A possible explanation for this observation was attributed to the steric interference with an enzymatic processing event caused by the numerous hapten molecules blocking access to peptide bonds (Collotti and Leskowitz 1969).

Another possible way of blocking access to sites susceptible of enzymatic processing was reported by Sela (1969). In a study on the role of optical configuration on immunogenicity it was found that a polymer consisting mostly of D-amino acids could be rendered immunogenic by the attachment of 8.5 per cent L-amino acid residues to the outside of the macromolecule. In contrast materials obtained by attachment of short chains of D-amino acids to the outside of a polymer of L-amino acids was non-immunogenic. The results were interpreted to suggest a necessary enzymatic digestibility requirement for immunogenicity made difficult by the outer layer of D-amino acid peptides.

As a last bit of suggestive data bearing on the distinction between a hapten and an immunogen I would like to cite some of my own recent studies on the immunogenicity of R-tyrosine conjugates (unpublished observations). In this case the simple carrier molecule tyrosine was chemically altered in a variety of ways and the dose of resulting conjugate required to immunize was measured. Blocking the ionic groups on the amino acid residue by N-acetylation and amide formation produced no change in immunogenicity. Replacement of the carboxyl group by H resulted in a one log decrease in potency; replacement of the N-acetyl group in a two log decrease and replacement of both groups gave a non-immunogenic conjugate. Charge differences and ability to transfer azo groups to other carriers could not account for these differences. It is tempting to speculate that enzymatic coupling of the amino acid residue *via* the N-acetyl or carboxyl group is a necessary requirement for immunogenicity and in the absence of both the molecule can function only as a hapten.

5.7. *Summary*

Haptens are materials varying enormously in size and composition which have as a common denominator the ability to react with antibody but an inability to elicit antibody formation. When coupled to suitable carriers, they behave as complete immunogens and produce antibody specific for the hapten.

The reasons for the lack of immunogenicity of haptens and the requirements of a good carrier have been explored and the single most likely explanation advanced suggests that an enzymatic processing step is an obligatory event on the pathway to an immune response. Haptens are not susceptible to this enzymatic process and must be attached to carriers which are, before they can elicit an antihapten response.

Bibliography

ADLER, F. L., 1964, Progr. Allergy *8*, 41.
ALLEN, P. Z., I. J. GOLDSTEIN and R. N. IYER, 1967, Biochemistry *6*, 3029.
AMKRAUT, A. A., J. S. GARVEY and D. H. CAMPBELL, 1966, J. Exptl. Med. *124*, 293.
ASKONAS, B. A., C. P. FARTHING and J. H. HUMPHREY, 1960, Immunology *3*, 336.
AVERY, O. T. and W. F. GOEBEL, 1933, J. Exptl. Med. *58*, 730.

BEISER, S. M., V. P. BUTLER and B. ERLANGER, 1968, *in*: P. A. Miescher and H. J. Mueller-Eberhard, eds.: Textbook of immunopathology, Vol. 1. New York, Grune-Stratton. pp. 15–24.

BENACERRAF, B., A. OJEDA and P. H. MAURER, 1963, J. Exptl. Med. *118*, 945.

BLIX, V., C. N. ILAND and M. STACEY, 1954, Brit. J. Exptl. Path. *35*, 241.

BOREK, F. and Y. STUPP, 1966, Immunochemistry *3*, 339.

BOREK, F., Y. STUPP and M. SELA, 1967a, J. Immunol. *98*, 739.

BOREK, F., Y. STUPP and M. SELA, 1967b, Biochim. Biophys. Acta *140*, 360.

BRAUN, D. G., K. EICHMANN and R. M. KRAUSE, 1969, J. Exptl. Med. *129*, 809.

BRENNEMAN, L. and S. J. SINGER, 1968, Proc. Natl. Acad. Sci. U.S. *60*, 258.

BRODY, N. I., G. WALKER and G. W. SISKIND, 1967, J. Exptl. Med. *126*, 181.

BRODY, N. I. and G. W. SISKIND, 1969, J. Exptl. Med. *130*, 821.

CAMPBELL, D. H., J. S. GARVEY, N. E. CREMER and D. H. SUSDORF, 1963, Methods in immunology. New York, Benjamin. p. 79.

COE, J. E. and S. B. SALVIN, 1964, J. Immunol. *93*, 495.

COLLOTTI, C. and S. LESKOWITZ, 1969, Nature *222*, 97.

DIETRICH, F. M., 1966, Int. Arch. Allergy *30*, 497.

EISEN, H. N., J. R. LITTLE, C. K. OSTERLAND and E. S. SIMMS, 1967, Cold Spring Harbor Symp. Quant. Biol. *32*, 75.

EISEN, H. N., E. S. SIMMS, J. R. LITTLE and L. A. STEINER, 1964, Federation Proc. *23*, 559.

ERLANGER, B. F., F. BOREK, S. M. BEISER and S. LIEBERMAN, 1957, J. Biol. Chem. *228*, 713.

FREY, J. R., A. L. DE WECK, H. GELEICK and W. LERGIER, 1969, J. Exptl. Med. *130*, 1123.

FRONSTIN, M. H., H. J. SAGE and J. J. VAZQUEZ, 1967, Proc. Soc. Exptl. Biol. and Med. *124*, 944.

GOEBEL, W. F., O. T. AVERY and F. H. BALARS, 1939, J. Exptl. Med. *60*, 599.

GOODFRIEND, T. L., G. FASMAN, D. KEMP and L. LEVINE, 1966, Immunochemistry *3*, 223.

GREEN, I., W. E. PAUL and B. BENACERRAF, 1966, J. Exptl. Med. *123*, 859.

GREEN, I., W. E. PAUL and B. BENACERRAF, 1968, J. Exptl. Med. *127*, 43.

HAVAS, H. F. and T. HRABA, 1969, J. Immunol. *103*, 349.

HAUROWITZ, F., 1936, Z. Physiol. Chem. *245*, 23.

HEIDELBERGER, M., 1956, Lectures in immunochemistry. New York, Academic Press.

HOFFMAN, D. R., B. L. AALSETH and D. H. CAMPBELL, 1969, Immunochemistry *6*, 632.

HRABA, T. and B. MERCHANT, 1969, J. Immunol. *102*, 229.

JONES, V. E. and S. LESKOWITZ, 1965, Nature *207*, 596.

KANTOR, F. S., A. OJEDA and B. BENACERRAF, 1963, J. Exptl. Med. *117*, 55.

KARUSH, F., 1957, J. Am. Chem. Soc. *79*, 3380.

KEMP, D. S. and R. B. WOODWARD, 1965, Tetrahedron *21*, 3019.

KUNKEL, H. G., H. R. HOLMAN and H. R. G. DEICHER, 1959, *in*: G. E. W. Wolstenholme and M. O'Connor, eds.: Cellular aspects of immunity, Ciba Found. Symp. Boston, Little, Brown and Co. pp. 429–437.

LANDSTEINER, K., 1921, Biochem. *119*, 294.

LANDSTEINER, K. and P. LEVINE, 1928, J. Exptl. Med. *47*, 757.

LANDSTEINER, K., 1962, The specificity of serological reactions. New York, Dover.

LESKOWITZ, S., 1963, J. Exptl. Med. *117*, 909.

LESKOWITZ, S., 1967, Science *155*, 350.

LESKOWITZ, S., 1968, J. Immunol. *101*, 528.

LESKOWITZ, S. and S. J. ZAK, 1966, Nature *211*, 246.

LESKOWITZ, S., V. E. JONES and S. J. ZAK, 1966, J. Exptl. Med. 123, 229.

LEVINE, L. and B. D. STOLLAR, 1968, Progr. Allergy *12*, 161.

LITTLE, J. R. and R. B. COUNTS, 1969, Biochemistry *8*, 2729.

LOEWI, G. and A. P. P. NIND, 1969, Immunology *17*, 175.

MAURER, P. H., 1965, J. Exptl. Med. *121*, 339.

MAURER, P. H. and H. C. MANSMANN, JR., 1958, Proc. Soc. Exptl. Biol. Med. *99*, 378.

MITCHISON, N. A., 1967, Cold Spring Harbor Symposium *32*, 431.

NACHTIGAL, D. and M. FELDMAN, 1964, Immunology *7*, 616.

OSTERLAND, C. K., E. J. MILLER, W. W. KARAKAWA and R. M. KRAUSE, 1966, J. Exptl. Med. *123*, 599.

PASANEN, V. J. and O. MÄKELÄ, 1969, Immunology *16*, 399.

PAUL, W. E., G. W. SISKIND, B. BENACERRAF and Z. OVARY, 1967, J. Immunol. *99*, 760.

PAUL, W. E., G. J. THORBECKE and G. W. SISKIND, 1969, Immunology *17*, 85.

PAULING, L., 1948, The nature of the chemical bond. Ithaca, Cornell Univ. Press.

PHILLIPS, J. H., W. BRAUN and O. J. PLESCIA, 1958, Nature *181*, 573.

PINCUS, J. H., J. C. JATON, K. J. BLOCH and E. HABER, J. Immunol. *104*, 1149.

PLESCIA, O. J. and W. BRAUN, 1967, Advan. Immunol. *6*, 231.

PLESCIA, O. J., W. BRAUN and N. C. PALCZUK, 1964, Proc. Soc. Natl. Acad. Sci. U.S. *52*, 279.

RAJEWSKY, K., V. SCHIRRMACHER, S. NASE, and N. K. JERNE, 1969, J. Exptl. Med. *129*, 1131.

RITTENBERG, M. B. and A. AMKRAUT, 1966, J. Immunol. *97*, 421.

RITTENBERG, M. B. and D. H. CAMPBELL, 1968, J. Exptl. Med. *127*, 717.

SAHA, K., F. KARUSH and R MARKS, 1966, Immunochemistry *3*, 279.

SCHLOSSMAN, S. F., J. HERMAN and A. YARON, 1969, J. Exptl. Med. *130*, 1031.

SCHLOSSMAN, S. F. and H. LEVINE, 1967, J. Immunol. *98*, 211.

SCHLOSSMAN, S. F., A. YARON, S. BEN-EFRAIM and H. A. SOBER, 1965, Biochemistry *4*, 1638.

SCHUBERT, D., A. JOBE and M. COHN, 1968, Nature *220*, 882.

SELA, M. and R. ARNON, 1960, Biochem. J. *75*, 91.

SELA, M., 1969, Science *165*, 1365.

SELA, M. and F. HAUROWITZ, 1958, Experientia *14*, 91.

SISKIND, G. W., W. E. PAUL and B. BENACERRAF, 1966, J. Exptl. Med. *123*, 673.

STEINER, L. A. and H. N. EISEN, 1967, J. Exptl. Med. *126*, 1185.

TABACHNICK, M. and H. SOBOTKA, 1959, J. Biol. Chem. *234*, 1726.

TABACHNICK, M. and H. SOBOTKA, 1960, J. Biol. Chem. *235*, 1031.

VAN DER SCHEER, J., R. W. G. WYCKOFF and F. II. CLARKE, 1940, J. Immunol. *39*, 65.

WILLIAMS, C. A. and M. W. CHASE, eds., 1967, Methods in immunology and immunochemistry, Vol. 1. New York, Academic Press.

WOFSY, L., H. METZGER and S. J. SINGER, 1963, Biochemistry *1*, 1031.

YAMADA, H. and YAMADA, 1969, J. Immunol. *103*, 537.

B. Particulate antigens

CHAPTER 6

Immunogenicity of animal viruses

A. C. ALLISON

*Clinical Research Centre Laboratories, National Institute for Medical Research,
Mill Hill, London*

and

W. H. BURNS

Department of Medicine, Stanford University Medical School, Stanford, Calif.

6.1. Introduction

The science of immunology can be said to have been founded by Jenner's (1798) observations on protection against smallpox by inoculation with cowpox. Since most virus infections cannot yet be treated by chemotherapy, immuno-prophylaxis remains the most effective way to control virus diseases. The important consequences of the introduction of vaccines against smallpox, yellow fever, poliomyelitis and measles are well known, and it seems likely that vaccination will soon reduce the hazard of congenital abnormalities in pregnant women produced by rubella virus. In the veterinary field, vaccines against canine distemper, canine hepatitis, Newcastle disease of chickens and hog cholera have been used with success. With many other viruses the prospects of effective vaccination seem less promising because of antigenic heterogeneity and other problems. Thus the immunogenicity of viruses is of considerable practical importance, and an enormous amount of information has accumulated on antibody production in a wide range of animal forms inoculated with viruses or virus vaccines. In this chapter only a few representative examples can be selected for discussion, to illustrate certain general principles concerning immune responses to animal viruses and in what respects they resemble or differ from responses to other antigens.

As expected, small viruses with small contents of nucleic acid and relatively simple structures, such as poliovirus, have few antigens, while large viruses with much larger contents of nucleic acid and complex structures, such as herpesviruses and poxviruses, have many antigens.

155

With viruses of intermediate size, such as adenoviruses or myxoviruses, the relationship between major antigens and the subunits assembled into intact virions is quite well understood. The best known immune responses to viruses are antibodies of IgM and IgG specificity. The high sensitivity and precision of assays based on neutralization of plaque-forming viruses make this an excellent model system, and much information of general interest has emerged. The antibody responses to a few well studied viruses, and special features such as failure of IgG to suppress IgM formation against poliovirus, are discussed in this chapter. As in other systems, anti-viral antibodies synthesized soon after exposure to antigen may have lower avidity than those synthesized later. This may be associated with a wider range of cross-reactivity of later sera, or after sequential exposure to related antigens. One remarkable feature of such sequential exposure, when stimulation with a related antigen increases the level of antibody to the first viral antigen ('original antigenic sin'), is of theoretical interest and practical importance. Secretory antibodies, largely of IgA specificity, are known to be elicited by several viruses, and are thought to play an important role in protection of the respiratory tract and gut against reinfection. However, since several individuals with severe IgA deficiencies remain healthy, it seems certain that this cannot be the only protective system, and the relationship of IgA with IgE and other antibodies in secretions is discussed.

The most important function of antibody is to neutralize the infectivity of viruses. The mechanism by which this occurs is complex and still incompletely understood. Attachment of antibody to a virus may by itself be insufficient to effect neutralization, and in some cases neutralization can be increased by complement or treatment with specific anti-globulin serum. In many cases the antibody does not prevent attachment of virus to a host cell, and the nature of the host cell itself affects the efficiency of neutralization.

Although soon after Chase made the important distinction between 'immediate' and 'delayed' hypersensitivity it was clear that the response to reinoculation with smallpox vaccine fell into the delayed hypersensitivity class, and similar reactions were observed with other viruses, until recently cell-mediated immune responses to viruses were regarded as little more than curiosities in virology. However, reports that children with severe hypogammaglobulinaemia recover normally from most virus infections, whereas those with defective cell-mediated immunity suffer from severe, progressive infections with vaccinia, measles and viruses of the herpes group, have renewed interest in cell-mediated immune responses against viruses. It is already clear that such responses – analogous to the mechanism bringing about homograft rejection – are of great importance in limiting tumour formation by viruses in experimental animals, and reports of an increased risk of tumour development in renal transplant patients on prolonged immunosuppressive therapy have suggested that the same may also be true in man (see Allison 1970b).

Oncogenic viruses in animals elicit a variety of antibody responses, some directed against virions and others against T(tumour)-antigens. Some can protect the host against virus oncogenesis under certain conditions, whereas others can enhance tumour formation. Thus there is a delicate interplay of cell-mediated and humoral immune responses in virus oncogenesis.

Bound up with the immune responses to tumour-forming viruses is the question whether viruses can under the appropriate conditions induce immunological unresponsiveness or tolerance. Widely held views on this subject have recently been challenged, and available evidence is summarized.

In general studies of immunogenicity, attention has been drawn during the last few years to interactions between three cell types: macrophages, which initially take up antigen (at least in some cases), thymus-derived lymphocytes, which potentiate antibody formation in response to certain antigens, and marrow-derived cells which themselves synthesize antibody. What little is known of the role of these cells in immune responses against viruses is presented, as well as some interesting observations on co-operative effects in which viruses participate.

In the final section some features of immune responses in humans are discussed in relation to the more detailed studies that have been carried out with experimental animals, and reports of anti-viral antibodies producing immunopathological reactions are summarized.

6.2. Virus antigens

Numerous virus antigens have been described. In a few cases their structures have been well characterized and their relationship to components of the corresponding virions have been established, e.g., with adenovirus and influenza virus described below. With small viruses such as the enteroviruses, the antigenic composition is relatively simple. In each of the three types of poliovirus (PV), for instance, two antigens are distinguishable by CF (complement fixation) and immunodiffusion. Infectious virions containing RNA have a D (dense) antigen whereas non-infectious particles have a C (coreless) antigen (Hummeler et al. 1962). The D antigen can be converted to C antigen by denaturation, so that the C antigen can be regarded as a protein that has not attained or retained the D configuration brought about in the complete virion by association with the RNA-containing core. A third antigen, the S antigen, can be obtained by guanidine degradation of the virus and is probably a protein precursor of the virus coat (Scharff and Lewintow 1963). Humans infected with PV develop type-specific antibodies against C and D antigens; only the latter neutralize the virus.

In cells infected with large viruses such as poxviruses and herpesviruses, many antigens can be demonstrated by immunodiffusion and other methods (Watson et al. 1967). Some of these are group-specific, others type-specific. Herpesviruses form a family of enveloped viruses of 1800–2000 Å size and have genomes consisting of double-stranded DNA, the $G+C$ constant ranging for different members from 33 to 72% (Plummer et al. 1969). The herpesviruses infecting man have been divided into four groups which share few common antigens: (1) herpes simplex (HSV), (2) cytomegaloviruses (CMV), (3) varicella-zoster (V-Z) and (4) EB virus. These viruses multiply in the cell nucleus, where the naked icosahedral nucleocapsids can be seen, and acquire their envelopes when budding through the inner lamella of the nuclear membrane, or through cytoplasmic membranes or the plasma membrane (Darlington and Moss 1969). It appears that the nucleocapsids are infectious, but that the envelope increases virus stability and infectivity (Spring and Roizman 1968; Darlington and Moss 1969). Besides morphological similarity, all members of the herpesvirus family tend to produce latent infections and focal cytopathology.

Whereas much progress has been made in correlating the antigens of influenza and adenoviruses with structural components, very little such correlation has been made with the herpesviruses. Until recently HSV, the cause of the common fever blister and·genital lesions, was thought to be of one antigenic type. Several laboratories have now shown that two types can be distinguished by differences in neutralization kinetics (Plummer 1964; Pauls and Dowdle 1967; Plummer et al. 1970), growth characteristics in various cell lines and virulence for laboratory animals (Figueroa and Rawls 1969), and $G+C$ content of DNA (Plummer et al. 1969). Type 1 were facial-oral isolates whereas type 2 were ano-genital isolates.

Myxoviruses, herpesviruses and arboviruses, which develop in relation to host cell membranes, have been shown to incorporate host antigens into the complete virions. Most fully studied in this respect are herpes simplex virus (HSV), Newcastle disease virus (NDV) and influenza virus. HSV can be agglutinated by antisera against the cells in which the virus was grown but not by antisera against heterologous cells (Watson and Wildy 1963). NDV has been shown to contain blood-group substances A or B, Forssmann antigen, or a mononucleosis antigen, depending on the host cells in which it was grown (Rott et al. (1966).

6.2.1. Adenovirus antigens

The adenoviruses are composed of DNA and protein and possess icosahedral symmetry. There are at least 58 types, 33 of them isolated from humans (Blacklow et al. 1969); the latter have been divided into three subgroups according to haemagglutination (HA) characteristics (Rosen 1960). Reviews of the structure and biology of adenoviruses have appeared recently (Norrby 1969a; Schlesinger 1969). The virion has an average diameter of 720 Å and consists of a central nucleoid and an outer capsid. About 18 percent of the virus protein is associated with DNA (Laver et al. 1967); this may represent P antigen (Russell and Knight 1967; Russell et al. 1968) and be produced in cells transformed by oncogenic adenoviruses. The capsid consists of 252 polygonal capsomeres – 240 hexons forming triangular facets, the apices of which are made up of 12 pentons (Figs. 6.1 and 6.2). Each penton consists of a knobbed fibre attached to a vertex capsomere (penton base). Hexons and pentons can be obtained as soluble products of infected cells or by disruption of virions. Originally, 3 antigens were described: a complement-fixing hexon group antigen (A antigen) common to all adenoviruses except the avian GAL virus, a penton group antigen (B antigen) toxic to cells, and a type-specific fibre antigen (C antigen).

The availability of purified capsid subunits and specific antisera has allowed detailed analyses of the antigenic structure of adenoviruses in HA and absorption studies. The subunits have varying capacities for HA: hexons and vertex capsomeres show no such capacity whereas all pentons and the fibres of subgroups II and III show partial HA. The latter is due to the univalency of these particles since dimers of pentons and fibres (at least in the case of subgroup III) show complete HA. Heterotypic sera, which can react with group or subgroup antigens on the fibres or vertex capsomeres can enhance HA by aggregating fibres or pentons into polyvalent complexes; this is termed the haemagglutination enhancement (HE) test. Vertex capsomeres can be identified by their ability to absorb HE antibody and thus decrease the HA normally found when a standard preparation of pentons is subsequently added; this is termed the HE antibody consumption (HEC) test.

Hexons appear to contain several antigens. The α (A) antigen is group-specific and detected in CF tests. The presence of a type-specific antigen, ϵ, was suggested by the surprising finding that only anti-hexon sera contain neutralizing antibody (Wilcox and Ginsberg 1963; Kjellen and Pereira 1968). Antibody to α antigen can be absorbed with hetero-

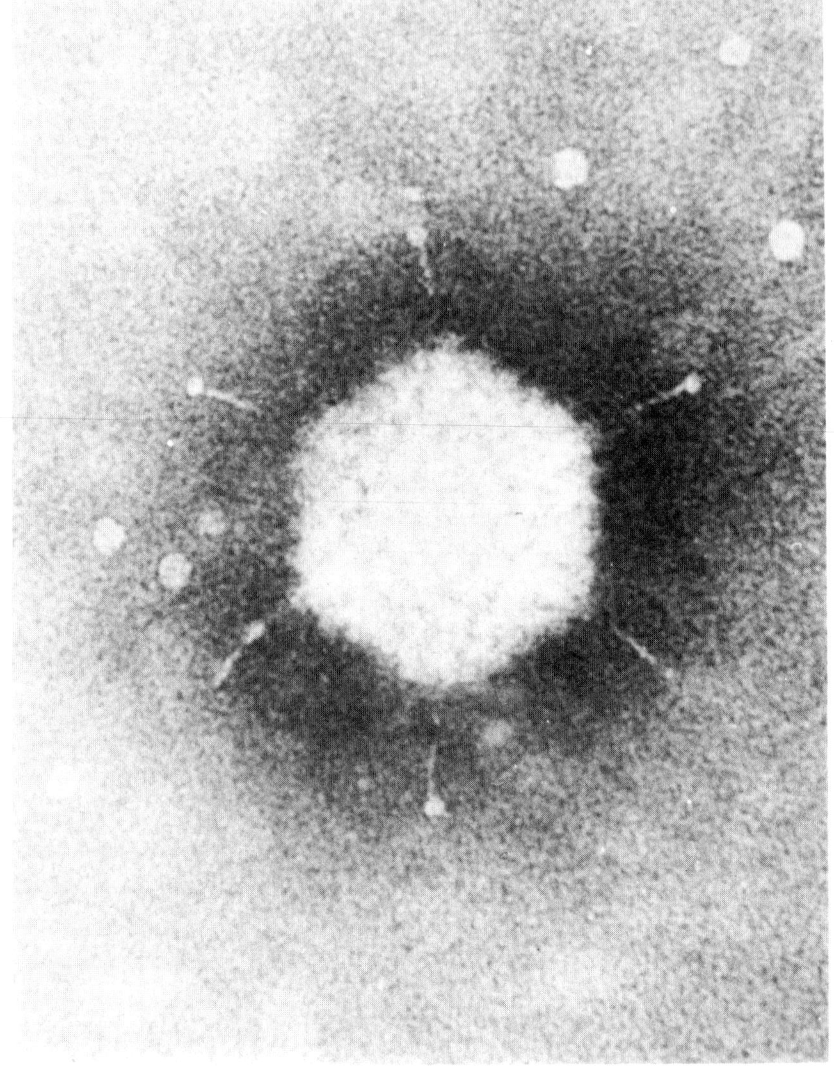

Fig. 6.1. Electron micrograph of adenovirus type 5, negatively stained.

typic virus or hexons, leaving homotypic (anti-ε) antibody which is active in haemagglutination inhibition (HI) and neutralization assays. Using negative staining, this antibody has been shown to attach to the outer surface of hexons in intact virions (Norrby et al. 1969). Agglutination of virions was prominent and might account for the HI activity of this antibody. Another possible mechanism is steric hindrance of the

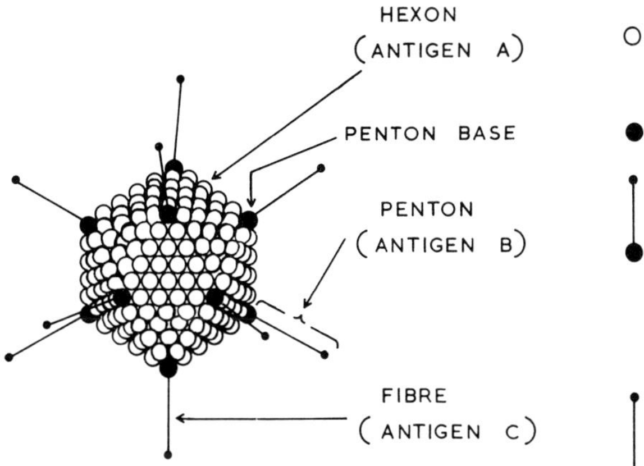

Fig. 6.2. Diagram of the structure of adenovirus showing the position in the virion of various antigens. (Figs. 6.1 and 6.2 by courtesy of Dr. H. G. Pereira.)

fibre haemagglutinin by antibody attached to para-vertex hexons; this is supported by the finding that the HI activity of different anti-hexon sera was inversely related to the fibre length of the viruses tested (Norrby and Wadell 1969). The hexon α antigen appears to be located on the inner aspect of the capsid since antibody to it lacks HI activity and cannot be seen in ultrastructural examination (Norrby et al. 1969); moreover, processes that disrupt the virion result in increased CF activity (Smith 1965). Absorption tests suggest that hexons possess minor intra-subgroup and inter-subgroup antigens as well as α and ϵ (Norrby and Wadell 1969).

Pentons can be separated into their fibres and vertex capsomeres by guanidine treatment. Vertex capsomeres have a group-specific β (B) antigen. Absorption experiments using the HEC test have also shown clear subgroup specificity and some inter-subgroup specificity (Wadell and Norrby 1969). Toxin activity is associated with these capsomeres and its neutralization is group-specific. All fibres contain a type-specific γ (C) antigen which on ultrastructural examination is located at the distal (knobbed) end (Norrby et al. 1969), and can participate in CF and HI reactions. Fibres of subgroups II and III also contain an intra-subgroup specific antigen, δ, located proximally; it cannot react with antibody if the vertex capsomere is attached. It is this antigen which is active in HE tests. Some inter-subgroup specificity has also been detected (Wadell and Norrby 1969).

Wigand and Fliedner (1968) observed that some adenovirus strains react differently in HI and neutralization tests, suggesting they might be intermediate strains. The two type-specific antigens, γ and ϵ, can be differentiated in HI tests using soluble and virion-associated haemagglutinin, respectively. Such analyses have been reported for two strains, and the HI antigen specificity was related to the fibres and the neutralization specificity to the hexons (Norrby 1969b). The latter relationship was not complete, suggesting mutation after a previous recombination between prototypes. Of practical importance, infection with such mosaic viruses might result in HI tests indicating one prototype but neutralizing antibody and protection would be against another type.

6.2.2. *Influenza virus*

Like all myxoviruses, the influenza virus consists of a helical nucleocapsid surrounded by a pleiomorphic envelope which contains projecting spikes of glycoprotein (Fig. 6.4). The virion can be disrupted with lipid solvents and the various components isolated. There are three major antigens determined by the virus genome: haemagglutinin, neuraminidase, and nucleoprotein (Figs. 6.3, 6.5 and 6.6). The influenza viruses are divided into three main types (A, B and C) according to their nucleoprotein, which is termed the 'S' (soluble) antigen. Antibodies against this internal antigen fix C' but have no neutralizing or haemagglutination inhibiting (HI) activities and are unimportant in immunity. Haemagglutinin, or 'V' antigen, is thought to be located on the surface projections of the virion and determines strain specificity; it reacts with neutralizing, CF, and HI antibody. Haemagglutinin can be purified by prolonged ether

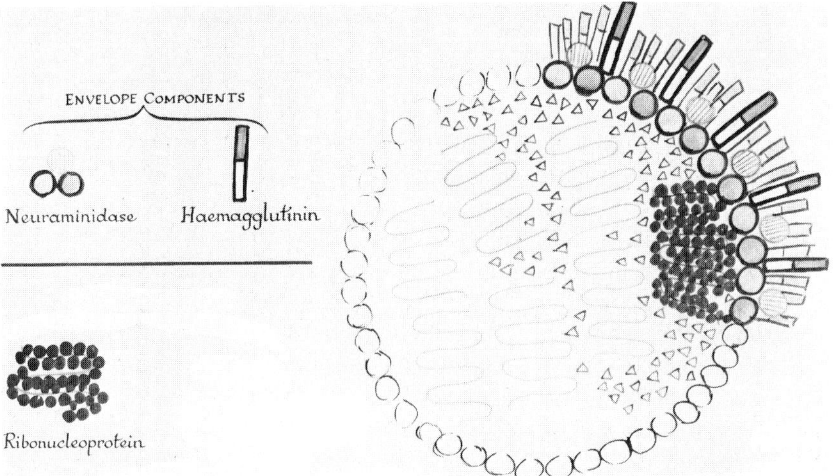

Fig. 6.3. Diagrammatic representation of influenza virus structure.

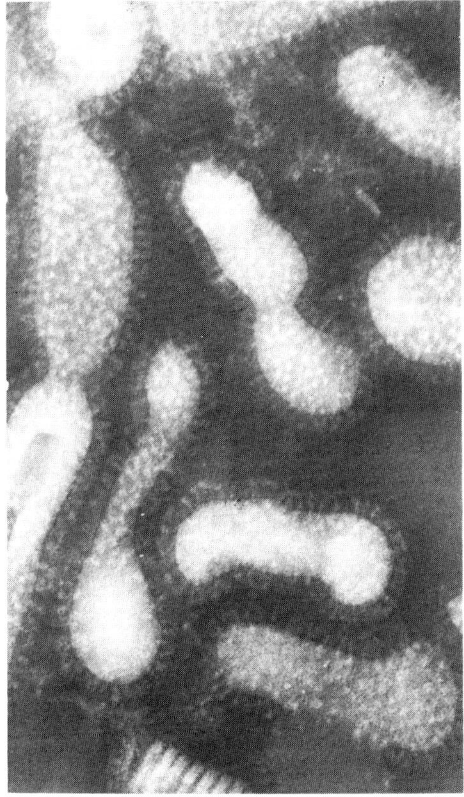

Fig. 6.4. Electron micrograph of negatively stained influenza virus particles (× 250,000).

or detergent treatment (Choppin and Stoekenius 1964; Neurath et al. 1967) and dissociated with urea to give homogeneous subunits which exhibit specific immunogenicity and CF, and can block HA by antibody (Eckert 1966; Laver and Valentine 1969). The neuraminidase is associated with but separable from the haemagglutinin. Neuraminidase brings about elution of the virus from red cells and may function in the release of virus from infected cells (Seto and Rott 1966). The genetic stability of the internal antigen is remarkable while the V antigen, constantly exposed to immunological selection, undergoes frequent changes that result in recurring influenza epidemics. Antigenic changes in neuraminidase also occur and are independent of those affecting the V antigen.

Host antigens are also present in the envelope. The lipid of influenza virus resembles that of the host cell (Kates et al. 1961) and blood-group

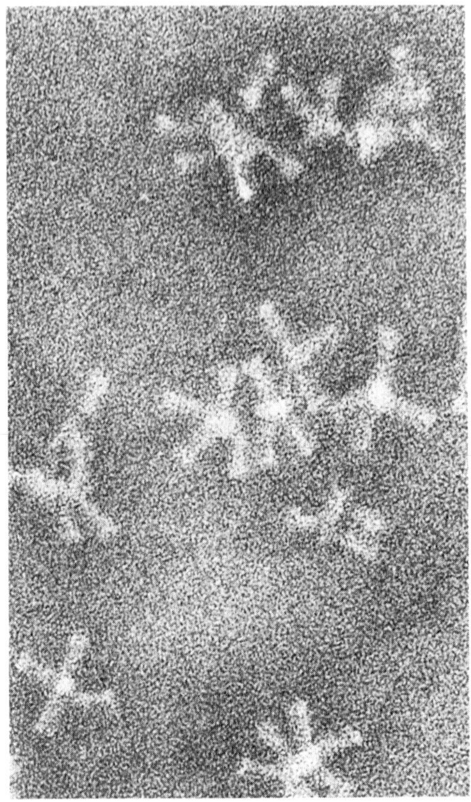

Fig. 6.5. Electron micrograph of negatively stained influenza virus haemagglutinin
(× 500,000).

antigens A and B and Forssmann antigen can be detected in the virions
if grown in cells possessing these antigens (Springer and Schuster 1964).
Virus grown in the chick allantoic cavity has a mucopolysaccharide
antigen (Haukenes et al. 1966) believed to be acquired as the virus grows
in the endodermal cells lining the cavity (Harboe et al. 1966). In adult
chickens, this antigen has been found only in liver and bile (Harboe
and Haukenes 1966).

6.3. Anti-viral antibody responses

6.3.1. Natural antibody

The sera of many normal animals and humans contain low levels of
'natural antibody' against viruses and bacteria. When carefully studied,

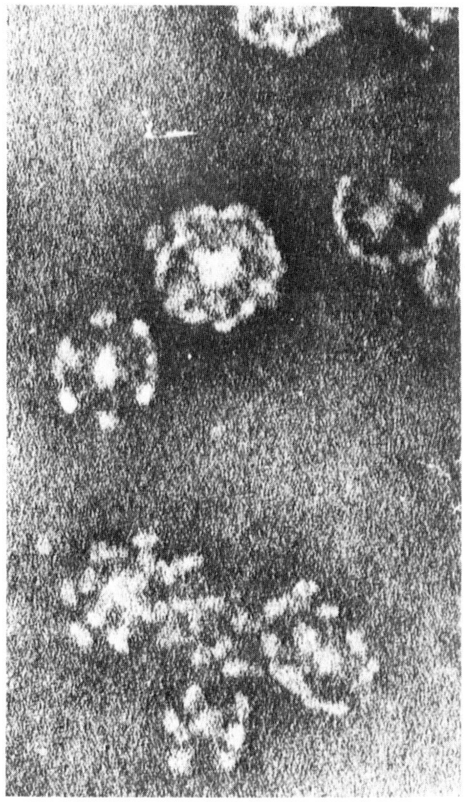

Fig. 6.6. Electron micrograph of negatively stained neuraminidase (× 500,000). (Figs. 6.3 to 6.6 by courtesy of Dr. G. Schild.)

these antibodies have been found to be IgM of low avidity, the biological effectiveness of which is increased by complement (Muschel and Toussaint 1962; Michael and Rosen 1963; Svehag 1964). Svehag has shown that natural antibodies to poliovirus and Coxsackie virus are indistinguishable in physical properties and avidity from early immune IgM. Their presence probably depends on repeated exposure to low levels of specific antigen or cross-reacting antigen. Older animals, with a greater chance of antigenic exposure, have higher titres than young. Animals with and without natural antibody showed identical primary responses to poliovirus; this is consistent with the finding of only short-lived memory for IgM and the fact that the titres of natural antibody were only one tenth of those present when the antigen dose was sufficiently high to elicit a secondary IgM response. Compatible with the postulated origin of natural antibody is the finding that the level of properdin (in this case, probably natural antibody) of germfree animals is lower than normal and increases as the animal is exposed to a conventional environment (Gustafsson and Laurell 1960). Since natural antibody (IgM) does not cross the placenta and its presence in adult animals does not alter the primary response to viruses, it seems to be of limited value in defence against viruses. However, it may increase the immunogenicity of soluble antigens.

6.3.2. *Relationship of IgM and IgG responses*

The responses of rabbits to non-replicating viral antigens have been studied in detail with poliomyelitis type 1 (PV) (Svehag and Mandel 1964a, b; Svehag 1964a, b) and influenza virus (Webster 1965, 1968a, b). In both cases with an adequate antigen dose after a short inductive phase (8–12 hours in the case of PV) IgM antibodies appeared, followed later by IgG antibodies (Fig. 6.7). Small doses of PV produced only a transient IgM response, which after 4 days declined at a rate consistent with the metabolic decay rate of this immunoglobulin. Larger doses of PV elicited both IgM and IgG antibody responses; IgM synthesis continued for 10–14 days, whereas IgG was first detected on the third day and increased until the third week. Thereafter IgG levels remained constant for about 30 weeks and persisted at moderate titres for 2 years. This was not due to chronic infection since UV-irradiated virus gave the same result. Similar findings with antibodies against the bacteriophage ϕX-174 in guinea-pigs had been reported by Uhr and Finkelstein (1963),

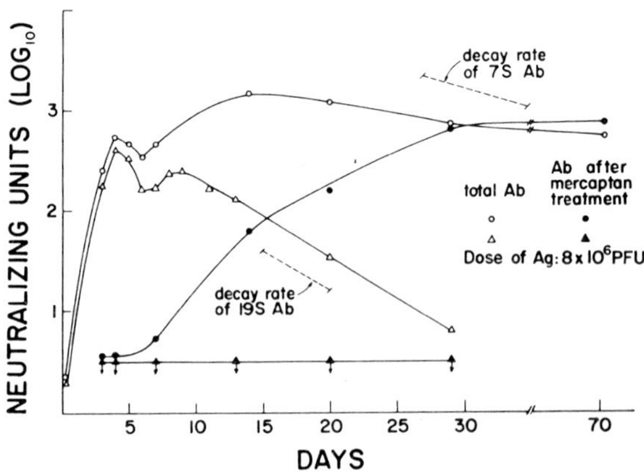

Fig. 6.7. Production of mercaptoethanol-sensitive (19S) and mercaptoethanol-resistant (7S) antibody in rabbits immunized with a large dose of poliovirus. (Svehag and Mandel 1964b, by courtesy of Dr. Svehag.)

although the rate of antibody formation was less antigen-dependent than in the case of PV.

Interesting information on immunological memory has come from the experiments with PV. With low doses of virus eliciting only IgM responses there was no detectable memory; repeated small doses of PV at monthly intervals elicited only transient IgM responses. However, if a second small dose of PV was administered 6 days after the first (2 days after the 19S antibody had begun to decline), a large secondary response consisting exclusively of 19S antibody occurred and the titre rose 100-fold. Again, this secondary response began the day after inoculation of PV and persisted for only 4 days. These results suggest that an immunological memory of IgM antibody production does exist but is very short-lived. The early and large secondary response shows that immunocompetent cells in the primary response do not die after 4 days of antibody release but require further antigenic stimulation for continued antibody production. Similar results have been obtained with the ϕX-guinea-pig system.

The effect of an established 7S antibody response on 19S antibody formation was also investigated. A large dose of PV was given which elicited primary 19S and 7S responses. Forty days later, when the 19S titre was only 1–2% of the peak level but the 7S antibody level was maximal, a second large dose of PV was administered. A large 7S secondary response was found, but the 19S response was the same as the primary response as regards rate of antibody formation, peak titre and time course. Thus the establishment of immunological memory affecting 7S antibody production does not require concomitant establishment of memory for 19S production. Moreover the 19S response of primary type is not affected by pre-existing 7S antibody.

These results are different from those in some other systems, in which 7S antibody has been found to inhibit immunization. Thus, Uhr and Bauman (1961) found that passively administered specific antibody could suppress antibody formation *in vivo*, and other similar observation have been reviewed by Uhr and Möller (1968). Using sheep red blood cells (SRBC) as antigen, Henry and Jerne (1968) found that specific 19S antibody increased the number of cells in the primary response, measured by the plaque technique and mostly producing 19S antibody; in contrast 7S antibody against SRBC suppressed the primary response. An *in vitro* study with polymerized flagellin has suggested that the suppression of antibody formation by specific 7S antibody is mediated through the immunocompetent cell and requires exposure to antibody complexed with antigen (Feldman and Diener 1970). Evidence that 7S feedback regulation occurs physiologically, at least as regards 7S antibody production, has been presented by Graf and Uhr (1969): when antibody against bovine serum albumin was removed from rabbits, a compensatory increase in specific antibody synthesis occurred.

Taken together, these and other experiments suggest that 7S-feedback regulation of antibody production is a real and probably physiological phenomenon. It is therefore surprising that inoculation of PV into animals with large amounts of specific 7S antibody should result in the development of a normal 19S response of primary type. Too little 19S antibody was already present to explain the lack of inhibition by a mechanism analogous to that of Henry and Jerne, and complexes formed would have been in antibody excess, which are inhibitory in Feldman and Diener's system. Antibody avidity does not appear to be relevant since both 19S and 7S antibody at the time the experiments were carried out had high combining strengths with PV. Although it is difficult to suppress an established primary response with specific 7S antibody, in Svehag's experiments the 19S response of primary type had obviously not commenced before the antigen was injected. Hence the relationship between IgM and IgG responses to virus infections has some remarkable and unexpected features. X-radiation before exposure to antigen abolished the 7S but not the 19S response.

The situation in human children in which virus replication is required for immunization is somewhat different. Congenital passive immunity may affect vaccination, especially with live vaccines (Perkins et al. 1959). It had been shown by Plotkin et al. (1966) that antibody in maternal colostrum and milk interferes with 'takes' of orally administered type 1 poliovirus vaccine in newborn children.

Goffe et al. (1966) have found that most human patients with warts produce only IgM antibodies to the human wart virus. They suggest that susceptibility to recurrent attacks of warts may be related to the failure of very small doses of antigen to promote a secondary IgG response.

In congenital rubella, newborn babies have both IgG antibodies, derived from the mother, and their own IgM antibodies. The IgG antibodies decline during the first months of postnatal life but relatively high levels of IgM, including antibody against rubella virus, persist (Alford 1965; Soothill et al. 1966; Sever et al. 1966). In mice congenitally infected with Moloney leukaemogenic virus antibodies appear to be mainly of IgM variety (Hirsch et al. 1969). Since IgM antibodies do not cross the placenta, their presence in the newborn is a useful guide to congenital infection (Stiehm et al. 1966).

In Webster's experiments the route of inoculation of influenza virus in rabbits affected serum antibody levels, intravenous inoculation giving higher titres than intraperitoneal, and these higher than subcutaneous.

By all routes multiple injections of antigen gave higher antibody responses. IgM antibodies were of high avidity and gave high levels of cross-reactivity, whereas the early IgG antibodies were of low avidity and failed to cross-react with related strains of influenza virus. The avidity of the IgG molecules increased during the primary response, and on secondary stimulation the levels of antibody increased greatly although there was only a slight increase in avidity.

With foot-and-mouth disease virus (FMDV) in guinea-pigs, antibodies found 4–8 days after infection are of the 19S class, whereas later antibodies are 7S. The early antibodies have been found to distinguish between three different virus variants and enzyme-treated virus, whereas sera obtained 20 days or later did not. Cowan (1970) has shown that 19S antibodies are specific for distinctive antigenic determinants on the virus particles, whereas 7S antibodies have a single specificity. He suggested that the antigenic determinant site encompassed by 7S antibodies consists of several smaller regions (subdeterminants) each of which can serve as an antigenic determinant site for 19S antibodies.

6.3.3. *Increasing avidity and cross-reactivity of antibodies*

Francis and Shope (1936) noted that sera taken soon after influenza virus immunization showed less cross-reactivity with other influenza strains than did late sera. Many subsequent observations have shown that as the primary immune response progresses and in secondary responses there is an increase in both the avidity and cross-reactivity of the antibody produced. This is true for soluble antigens as well as viruses (Eisen 1966), and the mechanism underlying selection of cells producing high-avidity antibodies has been extensively discussed. In the poliovirus-rabbit system, Svehag (1964b) found that the earliest immune sera contained low-avidity IgM similar to 'natural' macro-globulin antibody. After a few days, the IgM produced was of high avidity, and a similar but slower change was noted for IgG. Following restimulation 40 days later, the IgM produced was again of low avidity, supporting the concept that IgM lacks long-lived memory. Similar results were obtained with influenza virus in guinea-pigs except that highly avid IgM was found in the earliest sera examined; however, since these were taken 5 days after antigenic stimulation, the low-avidity IgM may have been missed (Webster 1968b).

Several explanations have been offered for the observed temporal relationship between increased avidity and cross-reactivity of antibodies. Antibody with high affinity for an antigenic site comprising several determinants should be able to bind with a related antigenic site bearing fewer of these determinants. Increasing cross-reactivity could also result from slowly developing responses to minor antigenic determinants shared with other strains, but this would not necessarily be related to an increased affinity for major antigenic determinants.

Evidence has recently been presented suggesting that the size of the antigenic determinants may determine the cross-reacting patterns with similar strains. Fazekas de St. Groth (1969) compared the ability of eight type A strains of influenza to cross-react with rabbit antisera prepared against each of the other strains. In general, no difference was found between antisera prepared against whole virus or antigenic subunits. Some secondary sera showed a broader specificity than primary sera, while others showed a more limited specificity. Those strains which produced antisera with broader specificities were found to have a more limited capacity to react with heterologous antisera. This suggested that they might possess larger antigenic determinants: binding sites selected for smaller determinants would be unable to bind with larger determinants because of steric factors, but binding sites for larger determinants would be able to encompass and partially bind the smaller determinants. Direct evidence must await analysis of the haemagglutinin structure.

This work may be practically important for two reasons. The antigenic subunit preparations are less toxic than whole virus (Siegerst and Braune 1964a, b), and the demonstration that they are highly immunogenic increases the likelihood that vaccines may be prepared from them. Secondly, as Fazekas de St. Groth remarks, a vaccine with broad cross-reactivity should offer the best protection against unknown virus strains, and the selection of suitable immunizing strains may be aided by the above theoretical considerations.

6.3.4. *Immune responses to antigenically related viruses*

When animals are exposed sequentially to antigenically related viruses, one of two processes can occur. Sometimes the specificity of the antibodies is broadened, as might be expected, and this is useful because it provides wide protection. However, quite often there is a heightened reaction to the original antigen rather than that used for challenge. Examples of the former include observations of Henle and Lief (1963) that repeated exposures of guinea-pigs to the same strain of influenza virus or to serologically related strains elicited antibodies which reacted with antigenically distinct homotypic strains to which the animals had never been exposed. Sequential infection of humans with two group B arboviruses likewise elicited antibodies reacting with a third group B virus to which the subjects had not been exposed (Wissemann et al. 1966). This has been attributed to the high avidity of antibody molecules generated, which are capable of cross-reactions with minor shared antigenic determinants.

The second variety of response to sequential exposure to related viruses results from a particular manifestation of immunological memory which Francis (1953) termed 'original antigenic sin'. Analysis of the serological responses of various age groups to vaccination with influenza virus type A showed that the serological response of a person to this virus is dominated throughout his life by the type of antibody produced as a result of his first exposure to an influenza A virus (see Francis 1953; Davenport and Hennessy 1956). This sort of response occurs in infections of long-lived animals with any virus of which there are cross-reacting antigenic types, e. g., arboviruses (Hearn and Rainey 1963), paramyxoviruses (van der Veen and Sonderkamp 1965) and enteroviruses (Mietens et al. 1964).

Similar effects can be reproduced in laboratory animals by successive exposures to cross-reacting live or killed viruses. From observations of the number and avidity of antibodies produced after secondary exposure to homologous and cross-reacting influenza A viruses, Fazekas de St. Groth and Webster (1964) concluded that there was cross-stimulation of the immunocompetent cells which had been involved in the primary response. Large doses of the second antigen flooded the initially primed cells and the overflow caused a standard primary response in previously unstimulated cells. When the completely unrelated influenza B was given as a second stimulus, there was no change in the antibodies to influenza A and a typical primary response to the B antigens was obtained.

The immunological recall phenomenon termed 'original antigenic sin' is of practical importance in serological epidemiology and vaccination. The former is an attempt to assess the pattern of previous infection by analysing the antibodies in individuals of different ages in a population. This is useful for viruses with single major antigenic types, e.g., measles or the types of poliovirus. With cross-reacting groups such as myxoviruses or arboviruses the pattern of exposure to sub-types is obscured by immunological recall.

When individuals have been previously exposed to influenza A strains, the immunological recall phenomenon imposes restraints on the effectiveness of immunization against a new strain. To overcome the restraint large amounts of antigen, which may be expensive or toxic, are often required for effective protection.

6.3.5. Secretory anti-viral antibodies

For many years it has been suggested that virus infections of the respiratory or alimentary mucous membranes may confer a specific local immunity in addition to producing a systemic immune response. Sabin (1959) pointed out that reinfection is less common, and excretion of virus less persistent, after recovery from infection with live vaccines or wild strains of poliovirus than after vaccination with killed viruses, even though the latter produce high titres of circulating antibody. This has been attributed to antibody in the alimentary tract which can be recovered from the faeces (Kono et al. 1966). The early observations of Francis (1942) suggesting the importance of anti-influenzal antibodies in human nasal secretions were extended by the experiments of Fazekas de St. Groth and Graham (1954) showing that immunity of mice to reinfection with influenza virus was more closely correlated with the presence of antibody in the nasal secretion than antibody in serum.

Following the demonstration that the predominant antibody in sero-mucous secretions is IgA (see Tomasi and Bienenstock 1969) it has become clear that anti-viral antibodies in nasal secretions are mainly of IgA specificity. This is true of antibodies against rhinovirus (Rossen et al. 1966) and parainfluenza 1 virus (Smith et al., 1966). Following natural infections, relatively high titres of IgA antibodies in nasal secretions were found, and there was considerable immunity against reinfection. Intramuscular administration of killed virus vaccines gave high titres of circulating IgG antibody, but this conferred little protection against nasal challenge.

Nevertheless, in assessing the importance of IgA antibodies in protection against respiratory tract infections, it must be recalled that several human subjects with selective IgA deficiency have remained healthy (see Tomasi and Bienenstock 1969); in these subjects there is a compensatory increase in the levels of other immunoglobulins, especially IgM, in secretions. Ammann et al. (1969) have reported that patients with ataxia telangiectasia and IgA deficiency do not suffer from severe recurrent sinopulmonary infections unless they also have a deficiency of IgE. This suggests that IgE can in some measure contribute to protection against sino-pulmonary infection. However, this is not always true: Haddad et al. (1970) have described a hypogammaglobulinaemic boy with severe deficiency of IgG, IgM and IgA, normal cell-mediated immunity, phagocytosis and no detectable deficiency of IgE, who had severe recurrent sino-pulmonary infections. Possibly the antigen-combining capacity of IgE in this patient is restricted. It seems clear that IgA is not alone responsible for protection of the respiratory and alimentary tracts from bacterial and viral infections. Other antibodies, including IgE and IgM, may be effective even in absence of IgA, although further work is required to establish the inter-relationships.

The role of secretory anti-viral antibodies in man is discussed further in the section on immune responses in man.

6.3.6. *Neutralization of viruses by antibody*

Neutralization – the decrease in infectious titre of a virus preparation following exposure to antibodies – is a complex process, the details of which vary from system to system. The first step is the interaction between virus and antibody, which can result in a combination which is at first readily reversible on dilution but with passage of time becomes less readily reversed, e.g., with influenza virus (Lafferty 1963a). Other virus-antibody complexes are more stable initially (e.g., poliovirus – Dulbecco et al. 1956; Mandel 1961; Philipson 1966; adenovirus – Kjellen 1962; NDV – Granoff 1965; and HSV – Yoshino and Taniguchi 1965b). A two-phase aqueous polymer system which distributed free virus and antibody-bound virus in different phases was used by Philipson (1966) to examine poliovirus interaction with various immunoglobulins. Following first-order kinetics, IgG antibody rapidly and irreversibly bound virus. After a short lag, IgM antibody bound virus irreversibly. The Danysz phenomenon, a classical indicator of irreversible antibody-antigen binding, was demonstrated for both, and using counter current distribution with a total dilution factor of 10^{18}, only a minor fraction of the antibody-virus complexes could be dissociated (IgM more so than IgG). Clearly, poliovirus and specific antibody quickly form very stable complexes. The combination can nevertheless be reversed to yield infectious virus by exposure to acid or alkali (Mandel 1961), sonication (Keller 1965), or treatment with fluorocarbons (Ketler et al. 1961), or proteolytic enzymes (Keller 1968).

The Fc part of the antibody molecule, which determines many of its biological properties, is not essential for the neutralization of most viruses since Fab preparations can neutralize influenza virus (Lafferty 1963b), poliovirus (Vogt et al. 1964), HSV (Ashe et al. 1968) and LDV (Notkins et al. 1968). In sufficient quantity, antibody can agglutinate virions or coat them and prevent adsorption to host cells, as shown for NDV (Rubin and Franklin 1957) and poliovirus (Mandel 1962; Keller 1966). Much smaller amounts of antibody can bring about neutralization, and the first-order kinetics of neutralization of poliovirus (Dulbecco et al. 1956) and NDV (Rubin and Franklin 1957) imply that the interaction of a single antibody molecule with a critical site on a virion can neutralize its infectivity. Virus-antibody complexes that are adsorbed to host cells penetrate more slowly and are more susceptible to further neutralization by added antiserum than is adsorbed free virus (Rubin and Franklin 1957; Rubin 1958; Mandel 1962).

The effectiveness of neutralization depends also on the host cells used. Kjellen and Schlesinger (1959) found that the same vesicular-stomatitis-virus-antibody complexes showed different levels of residual infectivity when assayed on chick cells and human cells, and Philipson (1966) reported similar findings with poliovirus-antibody complexes when assayed on monkey and human cells. Thus combination of virus and antibody is not by itself sufficient to bring about neutralization; a host cell factor is also involved, which presumably prevents release of viral nucleic acid in a form that can be replicated. Dales and Kajioka (1964) and Silverstein and Marcus (1964) have suggested that complexes of vaccinia or NDV and antibody are degraded in heterophagic vacuoles rather than being uncoated in the normal fashion (see also Dales 1969). Some virus-antibody complexes are neutralized only in the presence of added complement or specific anti-globulin sera (see below).

The neutralization of adenoviruses has several special features. As with most viruses, neutralization is a two-step process with antibody first binding firmly to virus; this is followed by increasing inactivation (Kjellen 1962). However, neither univalent nor bivalent Fab preparations effectively neutralized adenovirus type 5 (Kjellen 1964, 1965). The bivalent Fab firmly bound virus initially, but inactivation did not follow. Although either Fab preparation blocked HI activity of whole antibody, neither preparation could block the neutralizing activity of whole anti-body. The recent finding that HI and virus neutralization are mediated by two different antigens, the fibre γ antigen and the hexon ϵ antigen, offers a possible explanation for this observation. Fab fragments might be able to bind to γ and prevent HA, but may not bind to ϵ and thus lack neutralizing ability. Experiments with Fab fragments of antisera prepared against the capsid subunits should resolve this question.

Since recent experiments have indicated that antibody directed against type-specific antigens on hexons will neutralize virus (Wilcox and Ginsberg 1963; Kjellen and Pereira 1968; Philipson 1969) whereas antibody directed against fibres will not (Kjellen and Pereira 1968; Pettersson et al. 1968), it seems likely that neutralizing antibody is functioning not to prevent virus-cell attachment, but a later process. Philipson (1969) has reported that ^{32}P-labelled adenovirus, after being treated with anti-sera prepared against purified hexons, pentons, or fibres, attached normally to HeLa and KB cells. Uncoating as indicated by the appearance of DNAase-sensitive DNA followed the normal pattern; however, this is not a good criterion because faulty uncoating could give rise to a DNase-sensitive but non-functional DNA.

Kjellen and Pereira (1968) showed that intra-subgroup heterotypic antisera could combine with adenovirus type 5, but neutralized it only at low *p*H. Adding intra-subgroup heterotypic sera to homotypic sera at neutral pH enhanced neutralization. It was suggested that the low pH and the reaction of homotypic antibody with the outer aspect of the hexons might result in exposure of inner sites with subgroup specificity which then reacted with the heterotypic antibody and enhanced neutralization. These observations, and the fact that only anti-hexon antibodies neutralize, suggest that processes involving changes in hexon conformation and exposure of inner components may be the basis for neutralization. Little is known about the uncoating process but it is reasonable to suppose that altered hexons may give rise to faulty uncoating. Much obviously remains to be learned about neutralization.

6.3.7. *Complement-requiring neutralization*

Muschel and Toussaint (1962) found that normal human sera and early rabbit immune sera contain antibody which neutralizes T coliphages only in the presence of complement (C'), whereas late immune sera of humans and rabbits do not require C'.

Yoshino and Taniguchi (1965a) found that rabbits inoculated with herpes simplex virus (HSV) produce neutralizing antibody as early as 3 days after infection. Sera taken soon after infection differ from those taken later in that C' is required for detection of neutralization by the former. In early (8 day) sera both IgG and IgM antibodies were found to be complement-requiring for neutralization, whereas in late (7 week) sera neutralization was detected in both fractions in the absence of C'. Nevertheless C' increased the neutralizing activity of the late IgM and raised the neutralization rate constant but not the titre of late IgG (Hampar et al. 1968).

The mechanisms by which C' potentiates neutralization are not yet clear. In view of evidence that early antibody is often of low avidity, it was thought that C' might stabilize the virus-antibody complex. However, in the HSV system the virus-antibody complex with early sera is stable, and it is the second step in the reaction, abolition of infectivity, that is facilitated by C' (Yoshino and Taniguchi 1965b). The C'-requiring antibody binds the virus in such a way that the sites required for infection are still exposed, since the infectious complex can be neutralized by late sera. Recent studies with early IgM and pure components of C' have shown that only the activated first component (C1) and high concentrations of C4 (the next component) are required for virus neutralization. Addition of the next two components (C2 and C3) are without effect unless the concentration of C4 is low, in which case neutralization is enhanced by C2 and C3 (Daniels et al. 1969). Similar results have been obtained with early IgM directed against Newcastle disease virus (NDV); the first 4 components of C′ were required for neutralization, but the concentration of C4 may have been suboptimal (Linscott and Levinson 1969).

It is postulated that the C′ reactions result in accumulation of protein on the virion which masks attachment sites, interferes with penetration into the cell or release of viral nucleic acid. The accumulation of proteins of the C′ system at a membrane surface is well established in studies on erythrocytes (Mardiney et al. 1963; Müller-Eberhard 1968). The virus itself appears to be unaltered, since papain treatment reactivates phage neutralized by the early antibody-complement system (Muschel and Toussaint 1962).

Complement-dependent virolysis has been studied by electron microscopy. Avian infectious bronchitis virus is a coronavirus with a complex lipid envelope of host origin with 200 Å projections. Antibody from infected chickens reacted with the projections but not the membrane of virions (Berry and Almeida 1968; Almeida and Waterson 1969). In contrast, antibody from rabbits immunized with chicken-grown virus attached to both membrane and projections, whereas antibody prepared against uninfected chicken cells attached only to membrane. The chickens appeared not to recognize the membrane as foreign. All three antisera neutralized virus more efficiently in the presence of C′. Electron microscopy showed C′ to accumulate on the projections when antibody attached there, and to react with antibody on the membranes to produce 100 Å holes similar to those found in red cells after treatment with activated C′ (Humphrey and Dourmashkin 1965).

6.3.8. *Infectious virus-antibody complexes and their neutralization by anti-globulin sera*

The existence of complement-requiring early antibodies shows that antibody can be firmly attached to a virus without abolishing infectivity. Other evidence of the presence of virus-antibody complexes retaining infectivity has accumulated. In studies of many viruses (herpes, polio, Newcastle disease, influenza, vesicular stomatitis, foot and mouth disease, visna, rabbit pox, vaccinia and encephalitis viruses) a 'persistent fraction' of infectious virus has been found even in the presence of excess neutralizing antibody. This persistent fraction has been shown to consist of virus-antibody complexes by density-gradient centrifugation (Kjellen 1965) and countercurrent distribution (Phillipson 1966). The serum is thought to contain a fraction of antibody that becomes attached to virus without neutralizing it but preventing combination with neutralizing antibody.

The infectious virus in the plasma of mice persistently infected with the lactate dehydrogenase-elevating (LDV) virus was shown by Notkins et al. (1966) to be in the form of non-neutralized virus-antibody complexes. Most of the infectivity was abolished by treating these complexes with heterologous antisera against mouse immunoglobulin. Similar findings with adenoviruses were reported by Kjellen and Pereira (1968). With rabbit antibodies against herpes simplex virus (HSV) Ashe and Notkins (1967) found that the 'persistent fraction' could be markedly reduced by antisera against rabbit immunoglobulin; the latter had no effect in virus not 'sensitized' by the rabbit antibody. Virus sensitized with rabbit immune serum could be neutralized by papain-derived fragments (Fab) of sheep anti-rabbit immunoglobulin, which are univalent and non-precipitating (Ashe et al. 1968). Hence it is unlikely that the anti-globulin sera merely bring about aggregation of virus-antibody complexes.

Aggregates of virus particles, not all of which are accessible to antibody, may however contribute to the persistent fraction. Wallis and Melnick (1967) removed virus aggregates by passage through membrane filters having a pore diameter less than twice that of the virus. The ultrafiltrates were completely neutralized by antisera whereas aggregates obtained by backwashing the filters were not. Recently it was found that treatment of sensitized VEE virus with anti-globulin sera was far more effective in eliminating the persistent fraction of this virus than filtration (Hahon 1970). Thus several factors may contribute to the persistent fraction, and their relative importance may vary in different situations.

6.4. Cell-mediated immune responses to viruses

Evidence is accumulating that many viruses elicit cell-mediated as well as humoral immune responses. This is shown by skin tests with live virus or virus antigen which give rise to delayed hypersensitivity. Such tests must, however, be interpreted with caution because of several sources of ambiguity. One is that reactions can sometimes be elicited by antigens from the foreign cells (e.g., monkey kidney cells or chick cells) or media in which the virus is cultured. If live virus is used, it may have to multiply at the skin test site to build up sufficient antigen to elicit a reaction; under these conditions appearance of serum-mediated hypersensitivity may be delayed for 24 hours or longer. The histology of the reaction site, although useful, cannot be accepted as unambiguous evidence for delayed reactions. When inbred animals are studied, the presence of cell-mediated immunity can be operationally confirmed by transfer of the effect to non-sensitized recipients by injections of viable immunocompetent cells but not by serum. This is readily achieved with sensitivity to vaccinia virus in guinea-pigs (Allison 1967), for example, or in protection of mice against virus oncogenesis (see below).

This technique is not applicable in man, and there is more scope for application of an *in vitro* test for cell-mediated immunity, the generation of macrophage-inhibitory factor (MIF). It has been shown that sensitized human peripheral blood lymphocytes will in the presence of specific antigen inhibit the migration of guinea-pig macrophages (Thor et al. 1968). Inhibition of rabbit macrophages in the presence of sensitized lymphocytes and fibroma virus-infected cells closely paralleled delayed hypersensitivity (Tompkins et al. 1970), and the same authors have been able to demonstrate cell-mediated immunity to vaccinia virus in man by inhibition of migration of rabbit or monkey peritoneal exudate cells mixed with human peripheral blood leukocytes and antigen. In another experiment (Rocklin et al. 1970), human lymphocytes incubated with antigens to which the donor had been immunized, produced MIF capable of acting on guinea-pig peritoneal exudate cells in capillary tubes. Correlation with clinical evidence of cell-mediated immunity (delayed hypersensitivity) to tuberculin, candida and streptokinase-streptodornase antigens was high. This sensitive assay should find use in future work.

6.4.1. *Vaccinia virus*

The first description of delayed hypersensitivity is that of Jenner (1798) who was studying the protection of man against smallpox by inoculation with cowpox. He pointed out that 'It is remarkable that variolous matter, when the system is disposed to reject it, should excite inflammation on the part to which it is applied more speedily than when it produces the Small Pox.' Although von Pirquet (1907) suggested that hypersensitivity contributes to the lesion of primary local vaccinia, it was only later that delayed hypersensitivity was recognized as the dominant feature of the revaccination response. Broom (1947) showed that accelerated revaccination reactions can occur in man in the absence of demonstrable antibody and can be elicited by heated non-infectious virus. Turk et al. (1962) produced in guinea-pigs typical delayed hypersensitivity without demonstrable circulating antibody by injection of virus-antiserum mixtures, following the technique of Uhr et al. (1957) for non-viral antigens. There is little doubt that this is a true cell-mediated immune response. Allison (1967) reported that delayed hypersensitivity against vaccinia virus can be passively transferred in inbred guinea-pigs by peritoneal exudate cells but not by serum. Pincus and Flick (1963) reported that anti-mononuclear cell serum inhibits the development of a local vaccinial skin lesion in guinea-pigs.

There has been a difference of opinion about the role of cell-mediated immunity in recovery from vaccinia virus infections. Friedman et al. (1962) reported that in guinea-pigs administration of methotrexate and X-radiation blocked development of delayed hypersensitivity and antibody to vaccinia virus; nevertheless treated animals recovered from virus infection as rapidly as untreated control animals. It was concluded that antibody and cell-mediated immunity do not play a major role in recovery from virus infection. However, as Allison (1967) has pointed out, the guinea-pig is relatively resistant to vaccinia infection (it is difficult to transfer the virus serially by skin infections in guinea-pigs) so it does not provide a general model. In cortisone-treated rabbits, resolution of vaccinial infection does not take place normally; relatively high titres persist for some time in internal organs and there is a considerable mortality (Bugbee et al. 1960). The most convincing evidence for a role of cell-mediated immunity in recovery from vaccinia virus infections comes from studies of children with immune deficiency syndromes. Children with Bruton-type agammaglobulinaemia usually recover from vaccination normally, despite the presence of very low levels of antibody (or none demonstrable at all), whereas children with impaired cell-mediated immunity develop progressive vaccinial infections (Fulginiti et al. 1968).

6.4.2. Ectromelia (mouse pox) virus

This poxvirus of mice produces a severe and often fatal disease. Fenner (1948) showed that there is an allergic component, as measured by swelling of the foot on challenge with live virus at various times after the primary infection. The allergy was first seen on the seventh day and increased in magnitude thereafter. Since generalized infection of the skin occurs on the sixth day, Fenner considered it unlikely that allergy played an important part in localizing virus in the skin.

6.4.3. Fibroma virus

This virus induces at the site of skin inoculation in adult domestic rabbits tumours which grow rapidly for about nine days and then regress; no tumours are formed on reinoculation of virus. The role of antibody and cell-mediated immunity in this system was analysed by Allison (1966) and Allison and Friedman (1966). Well-marked delayed sensitivity was found after intradermal challenge of the fifth day but circulating antibody was demonstrable only on the seventh day after virus inoculation. The development of cell-mediated immunity on the fifth day after fibroma virus inoculation has also been shown by the *in vitro* macrophage-migration-inhibition technique (Tompkins et al. 1970). In animals given methotrexate, which suppressed delayed hypersensitivity and antibody formation, two differences from controls were seen (Allison and Friedman 1966): tumours developed distant from the original inoculation sites and regression of tumours was markedly inhibited. In methotrexate-treated animals, administration of immune serum prevented the appearance of lesions away from the inoculation site but did not facilitate the regression of the tumour. From these and other observations it was concluded that antibody prevents the dissemination of virus, with formation of secondary tumours, but that the regression of the fibroma is due to a powerful cell-mediated immune response. In newborn rabbits, fibroma virus induces tumours which grow progressively to attain an enormous size and kill the animals. Newborn rabbits were found to produce antibody against the fibroma virus, but no delayed hypersensitivity. It was concluded that the progressive growth of fibromas in newborn animals was due to the slow maturation of the cell-mediated immune response, even though a humoral immune response occurred.

6.4.4. *Herpes simplex virus*

Herpes simplex virus elicits a delayed hypersensitivity reaction in a proportion of adults and a lower proportion of children (Nagler 1944; Rose and Molloy 1947; Anderson and Kilbourne 1961). The skin reaction can also be elicited with a soluble antigen which has not yet been further characterized (Anderson and Kilbourne 1961; Jawetz et al. 1951). The skin test may be useful in diagnosis of primary herpetic and latent carrier infections, and delayed hypersensitivity may be a contributory factor in the pathology of herpetic 'fever blisters'. Delayed hypersensitivity to herpes virus in guinea-pigs has also been described (Brown 1953). The frequency and severity of herpetic infections in immunosuppressed renal transplant patients (Montgomerie et al. 1969) suggests that the virus is normally controlled by an immune reaction, but whether this is mainly cell-mediated is unknown. This problem is discussed further below.

6.4.5. *Influenza virus*

Skin hypersensitivity of the delayed type was demonstrated with influenza virus (Beveridge and Burnet 1944), but the antigen which elicits the reaction was not identified. The same authors stated that live attenuated virus given intranasally was more effective in inducing skin hypersensitivity than killed vaccine injected subcutaneously. Feinstone et al. (1969) have reported that mice infected with mumps and influenza viruses develop cell-mediated immunity as shown by *in vitro* mouse macrophage-migration inhibition tests.

6.4.6. Mumps virus

The existence of dermal hypersensitivity to mumps virus was demonstrated by Enders et al. (1945). The antigen involved is heat-stable, but has not yet been related to a specific viral component. A positive reaction is well correlated with the immune state. Delayed hypersensitivity has also been produced in guinea-pigs infected with mumps, and spleen macrophages isolated from these animals when mixed with mumps antigens become less motile and undergo lysis (Glasgow and Morgan 1957).

6.4.7. Measles virus

Skin testing with measles virus preparations has been described by Isacson (1968). Some of the positive results at 48 hours were apparently virus-specific, whereas others were due to contaminating antigens derived from the cells used to culture the viruses. Lasting delayed sensitivity was observed after repeated administration of measles vaccine. Children with defective cell-mediated immunity have developed lethal giant-cell measles pneumonia (Hoyer et al. 1966; Nahmias et al. 1967), which suggests that cell-mediated immunity may play an important role in protection against this virus which spreads easily from cell to cell.

6.4.8. Poliovirus

Positive reactions obtained on skin testing with poliovirus antigens did not correlate with previous immunization (Lennon et al. 1967). A correlation was found between positive reactions and previous immunization with inactivated measles virus and was probably due to reactions to common cell culture antigens present in the virus preparations.

6.4.9. Lymphocytic choriomeningitis virus (LCM)

The role of cell-mediated immunity in this system has been extensively discussed (Hotchin 1962, 1965; Volkert and Larsen 1965; Lehmann-Grube 1970), and will be considered here only briefly. As shown by Traub (1939), mice infected *in utero* become lifelong carriers of virus, usually without illness. However, when older mice are infected they show more severe effects, including runting and lymphocytic infiltration of the meninges. In such mice suppression of cell-mediated immunity by drugs, neonatal thymectomy or administration of anti-lymphocytic sera greatly reduce the severity of disease produced by LCM. The virus multiplies without cytopathic effects, and it is widely accepted that

LCM disease is due to the pathological effects of the immune response to the virus rather than to virus infection *per se*. Until recently it was thought that the immunopathology was entirely cell-mediated, and what is probably a cell-mediated allergic reaction can be demonstrated by swelling of the foot pad in sensitized mice challenged by virus inoculation (Hotchin 1962). However, the more recent demonstration of immune complexes with virus antigen in LCM-infected mice (Oldstone and Dixon 1969) suggests that renal and other vascular lesions in LCM-infected mice may follow deposition of these complexes. The relative importance of humoral and cell-mediated immunopathological reactions requires further evaluation.

6.4.10. Oncogenic viruses

The oncogenic viruses have been found to give rise to virus-specific antigens in the tumour cells which are demonstrable by transplantation experiments within inbred strains of animals. If an animal has been immunized by exposure to a virus, to graded doses of tumour cells or large doses of irradiated tumour cells, it becomes resistant against transplantation of a syngeneic tumour containing the specific antigen, but not to tumours induced by other viruses. This was discovered by Sjögren et al. (1961) in the case of polyoma virus tumours, and suitable experiments show that the resistance is due to cell-mediated immunity (Sjögren 1964). There is substantial evidence that cell-mediated immunity is of critical importance in limiting virus oncogenesis (see Boyse et al. 1969; Law 1969; Allison 1970a). Thus the resistance of certain strains of newborn mice and all strains of adult mice to oncogenesis by polyoma virus can be overcome by efficient immunosuppression, such as neonatal thymectomy or adult thymectomy and treatment with anti-lymphocytic serum. Transfers of syngeneic lymphoid cells from immune animals can prevent tumour formation in these sensitive recipients, whereas transfers of immune serum after infection do not have any protective effect.

Several studies have shown the cytotoxic effects of immune lymphocytes on virus-induced tumour cells *in vitro*. Recently, the colony inhibition technique has been used to study this phenomenon *in vitro* (Hellström et al. 1969a, b; Heppner 1969), and also the specific inhibition of *in vitro* lymphocyte cytotoxicity by enhancing antiserum.

6.4.10.1. Antibody responses to oncogenic viruses

Apart from eliciting cell-mediated immunity, which is discussed above, oncogenic viruses also stimulate the formation of a variety of antibodies (reviewed by Boyse et al. 1969; Haughton 1969; Habel 1970). Some of these are directed against the virions, and are detectable by neutralization or inhibition of viral haemagglutination, e.g., polyoma virus. Others are directed against virus-specific antigens that have been designated as T(tumour)-antigens and are demonstrable by complement fixation (CF) or immunofluorescence (IF). Antibodies against T-antigens are found in animals bearing primary or transplantable tumours induced by oncogenic DNA viruses such as polyoma, SV40, adenoviruses or adenovirus-SV40 hybrids. Antigens of this type are present also at an early stage in cells undergoing lytic infection with these viruses; they are inactivated at 56°C and are termed 'soluble' because they are not sedimented by centrifugation at 60,000 g. for 2 hours. These properties distinguish the T-antigens from virion antigens, and reactions of different antisera confirm the distinction. Thus hamster sera with high titer CF and IF reactions against T-antigens may show little or no neutralization or CF with virion antigens, and conversely human or monkey sera with high titers of neutralizing and CF antibody against adenovirus usually do not react with T-antigen. Most antibodies against T-antigens in tumour cells induced by oncogenic viruses react with nuclear or cyto-plasmic antigens, although reactions with an antigen or antigens in the cell membrane have also been described (Tevethia et al. 1965; Diaman-dopoulos et al. 1968). The relationship of the latter to the transplantation antigen is not clear; the appearance of antigens not virus-specific, e.g., Forssman antigen, has been reported after transformation of hamster cells with polyoma or Rous sarcoma viruses (O'Neill 1968) and the DNA from SV40 (Robertson and Black 1969).

Antibody responses to the RNA-containing oncogenic viruses – murine and avian leukaemogenic viruses (MLV and ALV) and the mammary tumour virus group (MTV) – have been extensively studied. These antibodies have been demonstrated by *in vivo* cytotoxicity, direct or indirect membrane immunofluorescence, immunodiffusion against virus or soluble antigens, neutralization, indirect haemagglutina-tion and complement fixation (see Boyse et al. 1969).

Relatively high concentrations of some antibodies can protect against transplants of leukaemic cells (or presumably against induced leukaemia), whereas lower concentrations of certain antisera can enhance growth of leukaemic cells. This is discussed by Boyse et al. (1969) and Haughton (1969). Inhibition by serum of the cytotoxic effects *in vitro* of lymphocytes against murine sarcoma virus (MSV)-induced and MTV-induced tumour cells are discussed by Hellström and Hellström (1969) and Heppner (1969). Inhibitory effects of antibody on the induction of MSV tumours, and on growth of transplanted MSV tumour cells are reviewed by Law (1969).

Thus the humoral immune responses to oncogenic viruses are complex.

Neutralizing antibodies, if present before an infection or soon after infection (e.g., acquired from the mother, passively administered or induced by inactivated virus), can prevent oncogenesis by all viruses so far tested (see, for example, Habel 1963, in the case of polyoma virus). Once the virus has infected and transformed a large number of cells, neutralizing antibody is no longer effective in preventing oncogenesis by DNA-containing viruses, although it may play a role in limiting the oncogenic effects of some RNA-containing viruses such as leukaemogenic viruses or MSV. Some antibodies can interfere with cell-mediated immunity and enhance tumour growth. The balance of such effects is delicate and requires careful evaluation in each system under study. Finally, in several systems antibodies are developed against T-antigens, the biological significance of which is still uncertain.

6.5. *Immunological tolerance in virus infections*

Traub (1939) found that mice congenitally infected with lymphocytic chorimeningitis virus (LCM) became lifelong carriers of the virus without symptoms and without demonstrable neutralizing antibody production; in contrast adult animals infected with the virus develop disease and antibodies are formed. This was one of the observations which led Burnet and Fenner (1949) to postulate that, if an immunologically immature animal were exposed to an antigen, tolerance might result. This was obviously not a general phenomenon, since Burnet and Fenner failed to induce tolerance when immature animals were inoculated with bacteriophage or with influenza virus. For many years it was accepted that LCM induces tolerance, both as regards antibody production and cell-mediated immunity, in congenitally or neonatally infected animals, and that cell-mediated immunity makes an important contribution to the disease produced by infection in adult animals (Hotchin 1962; Volkert and Larsen 1965). The amelioration of the disease in adults by immunosuppressive drugs, neonatal thymectomy (Levey et al. 1963) or anti-lymphocyte serum (Hirsch et al. 1967) supported the concept that immunopathological reactions plays an important part in production of disease by LCM infection of adult animals.

Other viruses believed to induce tolerance in congenitally infected animals included the leukaemogenic viruses in birds (Rubin et al. 1962) and mice (Axelrad 1965; Klein and Klein 1966) and the mammary tumour virus in mice (Attia et al. 1965). There is substantial evidence that virus oncogenesis is more easily achieved by inoculating newly born or hatched animals of highly susceptible species (such as the hamster, mouse, rat or chicken) than by inoculation into adults. When it became clear that such tumour cells possess a virus-specific antigen, Habel (1962) suggested that 'the newborn, being immunologically incompetent, tolerates the new antigen and allows tumour growth, whereas the immunologically mature adult rejects the antigen and thus becomes hypersensitive or immune to later challenge with the tumour'.

However, more recent observations have shown that embryos are capable of mounting some immune responses (Sterzl and Silverstein 1967) and have cast doubt on the concept of tolerance induction by viruses. One well-studied example is congenital rubella, in which the infection is contracted in early embryonic life. Neutralizing antibody (maternal IgG) has been detected in the foetus as early as the fifth month of gestation, and at birth the rubella-infected infant has both maternal IgG and its own IgM antibodies. The level of passively transferred IgG falls until about 6 months after birth, when it is replaced by the child's own immunoglobulins, both IgG and often persistent abnormally high concentration of IgM (Alford 1965; Soothill et al. 1966; Sever et al. 1966). Thus rubella infection during the first trimester of pregnancy does not result in tolerance.

Oldstone and Dixon (1968, 1969) have found that mice neonatally infected with LCM are not completely tolerant but make antibodies which are deposited in the renal glomeruli in the form of antigen-antibody complexes. Similar observations on germ-free mice congenitally infected with LCM are presented by Pollard et al. (1968).

Comparable observations on mice neonatally infected with Moloney leukaemogenic virus or murine sarcoma virus were presented by Hirsch et al. (1969). Virus antigen-antibody precipitates were observed in the renal glomeruli and virus-neutralizing antibody could be eluted from the kidneys. Infectious virus in the plasma of these animals could be neutralized by antisera to mouse immunoglobulin (IgM), suggesting that it was present in the form of an infectious virus-antibody complex (see page 28). Thus, newborn animals infected with LCM and murine leukaemogenic viruses are capable of synthesizing some antibody and can no longer be regarded as completely tolerant. Whether there is 'split tolerance' with failure to develop cell-mediated immunity requires further evaluation.

In the case of the DNA-containing oncogenic viruses, it is clear that infection of newborn animals does not result in tolerance either as regards antibody production or cell-mediated immunity (Allison 1969). When newborn mice were infected with polyoma virus, spleen cells taken 6 weeks later were able to protect thymectomized recipients from the oncogenic effects of the virus, showing that in the animals infected as newborns cell-mediated immunity was eventually developed fully.

Two other observations support this interpretation. The first is that suppression of cell-mediated immunity by neonatal thymectomy or administration of anti-lymphocytic sera potentiate oncogenesis by a variety of DNA-containing viruses, including polyoma, adenovirus type 12 and SV40 (see Law 1966; Allison and Law 1968). It follows that under normal conditions the probability of tumour development is reduced by a cell-mediated immune response, even after inoculation of virus in newborns. The second observation is that following inoculation with SV40 or adenovirus type 12 into newborn animals, further inoculations of virus or irradiated tumour cells with the virus-specific antigen diminish tumour development (Eddy et al. 1965; Goldner et al., 1964). Such immunization would not be possible in an animal already tolerant. For these reasons, Allison (1969) has suggested that the high susceptibility of newborns to oncogenesis is not due to tolerance induction but to the relatively slow development of cell-mediated immune responses in newborn as compared to adult animals. It is supposed that by the time an effective cell-mediated immune response is mounted in the newborn animal (three weeks), some of the tumour cell clones have grown to a size beyond immunological control.

There are, however, some filtrable agents of very unusual properties that do not appear to elicit any immune response, cell-mediated or humoral. These are the agents of scrapie in ungulates, kuru and the Creutzfeld-Jacob syndrome in man (see Gibbs and Gajdusek 1970), and mink encephalopathy. The extreme resistance of scrapie to heat, chemicals and ultraviolet and ionizing radiation suggests that it has very little nucleic acid and protein, which would make it unique among viruses. This may contribute to its apparent lack of antigenicity.

6.6. *Interactions of the virus antigens with the immune system*

6.6.1. *Co-operative effects of virus antigens on immunogenicity*
Co-operative effects, in which an immune response to one antigen increases the response to a second antigen coupled with it, have been extensively studied (see Chapters 5 and 10). The most detailed analyses have been of carrier effects, in which a hapten has been coupled to two carrier proteins, but several analogous effects have been described. Thus in chickens the presence of a highly immunogenic isoantigen B on the same cells is required to elicit an immune response to a weaker isoantigen A (Schierman and McBride 1967). Experiments with virus oncolysis have revealed similar phenomena. Thus, Lindenmann and

Klein (1967) immunized mice with preparations of ascites tumour cells infected with influenza virus and found that 11 days later they were resistant to a challenge of 100 lethal doses of uninfected tumour cells. Suitable control experiments showed that direct virus oncolysis was not involved and that simple mixtures of tumour cells and virus did not immunize efficiently. It seems that the immune response to weakly immunogenic tumour cell antigens was increased by association with more immunogenic viral antigens.

These results are of general interest for several reasons. Immune responses to minor antigenic determinants in viruses may be stimulated by responses against major determinants, which could be relevant to the broadening of reactivity in late sera. Virus-infected human tumour cells might be used to stimulate immunity of patients against their own tumours after chemotherapy or surgery. Moreover, co-operative effects might be involved in certain types of autoimmunity. Enveloped viruses such as myxoviruses and herpesviruses are known to contain host cell antigens, which may be structurally modified, and it is conceivable that through co-operative effects the formation of autoantibodies could be elicited. In one of the first examples where the introduction of a virus produces an immune response against an autologous antigen, it has been shown that immunization of chickens with egg-grown influenza will result in the production of antibody against this host antigen (Schoyen et al. 1966). The NZB mice, which show various autoimmune phenomena, carry a leukaemogenic virus serologically related to Gross virus (Mellors et al. 1969), but it is not yet clear what role this virus plays in autoimmunity – apart from deposition of immune complexes with viral antigen in the kidneys, which cannot be regarded as a manifestation of autoimmunity. Interest has been aroused by recent reports of virus-like structures in human patients with lupus erythematosus (Kawano et al. 1969), but confirmation that these are in fact viruses, and are causally related to the disease, is required before the possibility that virus antigens produce such effects by co-operation is taken seriously.

6.6.2. *Role of macrophages in immunogenicity of viruses*

Many proteins in soluble form are less immunogenic than when they are in particulate form, and one factor contributing to this difference is the ease with which particulate antigens are taken up by macrophages; antigen presented in macrophages is more immunogenic than free antigen (see Spitznagel and Allison 1970). Viruses are particulate antigens, although in the course of virus replication soluble antigens are also formed, some of which are constituents of the virions (see above). After intravenous inoculation many particulate antigens are rapidly cleared from the circulation by phagocytosis even in the absence of specific acquired immunity (Rowley 1962). Most viruses are also rapidly cleared from the circulation and are demonstrable in macrophages lining the circulatory spaces (Mims 1964). However, some viruses, e.g., poliovirus type 1 in the mouse (Mims 1964) and bacteriophage ϕX174 in the guinea-pig (Uhr et al. 1962) are removed from the circulation slowly until the onset of immune elimination. With infections of other tissues, e.g., lung and lymph nodes, virus antigen is also rapidly taken up by macrophages where it is demonstrable by immunofluorescence (Mims 1964). Hence macrophages may play an important role in immunogenicity of viruses, presenting antigen in an acceptable form to immunocompetent cells and stimulating proliferation and antibody formation by the latter.

Macrophage uptake can also increase the immunogenicity of soluble viral antigens: intraperitoneal inoculation of viable syngeneic macrophages containing adenovirus hexon antigen has been found to elicit a higher titre of antibody in CBA mice than the same dose of free antigen (P. Sanderson, J. K. Spitznagel and A. C. Allison, unpublished). This is not true of the antibody response to bacteriophage, which is lower when the virus is inoculated after uptake in macrophages than when it is free (Kölsch 1970); perhaps the engulfed particles in macrophages are rapidly degraded. A recent report emphasizes the varying requirements of different antigens to be processed by macrophages for immunogenicity: polymerized bacterial flagellin had no such requirement while sheep red cells, to be immunogenic, required the presence of phagocytic cells *in vitro* and probably *in vivo* (Shortman et al. 1970).

It is also known that the antibody response to virus vaccines is considerably increased by emulsified oil and other adjuvants (Hilleman 1966), and such adjuvants appear to act primarily on macrophages rather than immunocompetent cells (Spitznagel and Allison 1970).

6.6.3. *Role of thymus-derived lymphocytes in immunogenicity of viruses*

There is now substantial evidence that thymus-derived lymphocytes are responsible not only for cell-mediated immunity but also co-operate in certain types of humoral immune response, even though the antibody is synthesized by marrow-derived lymphocytes (Mitchison 1967; Mitchell and Miller 1968). The importance of the co-operative effect of thymus-derived cells is dose-dependent and varies with different antigens. With rather highly immunogenic materials, such as haemocyanin, this effect seems to be relatively slight, whereas with other antigens such as bovine serum albumin and sheep red blood cells the effect is clearly demonstrable.

Although neonatally thymectomized animals, or animals treated with anti-lymphocytic sera show no cell-mediated immunity against virus antigens, the humoral antibody responses so far tested appear to be normal in magnitude, time of appearance and type. This is true, for example, of antibodies against oncogenic viruses and T-antigen demonstrable by haemagglutination inhibition (HI), neutralization, complement-fixation (CF) and immunofluorescence (Allison and Taylor 1967; Allison, unpublished). Hence for these viruses, and perhaps for most highly immunogenic viruses, co-operation of thymus-derived cells in humoral antibody formation may not be important, although for less immunogenic viruses such as LCM this factor could play a much greater role. Thus Volkert and Larsen (1965) reported that in experiments on adoptive transfer of immunity to mice neonatally infected with LCM, injections of hyperimmune serum produced small and transient reductions of virus titres in recipients whereas transfers of lymph-node, spleen or buffy-coat cells markedly reduced virus titres, especially in the liver and spleen, and increased circulating antibody levels in recipients. It is unlikely that with peripheral blood many potential antibody-forming cells were transferred, so that the observed increase in antibody synthesis in the recipients may have been due to a co-operative effect of transferred thymus-derived cells. Further observations are required to establish the point.

6.6.4. *Long-lived immunity to viruses*

Several viruses are known to produce lifelong immunity against re-infection, e.g., the acute exanthemas of childhood, smallpox, poliomyelitis and yellow fever. In some cases the duration of immunity may be increased by repeated subclinical infections. Thus, Krugman et al. (1966) found rises in neutralizing antibody titres in immune subjects exposed to reinfection with measles virus. Even in the absence of re-exposure, immunity may persist for many years. Similar observations have been made on vaccinated subjects exposed to smallpox (Downie and McCarthy 1958). Panum (1847) showed that in the Faroe islands, where successive measles epidemics were separated by intervals of 65 and 31 years, each epidemic infected nearly all those who had not been exposed previously but none of those who had been. Similar reports of antibody persisting in the absence of reinfection include yellow fever for 75 years (Sawyer 1931), poliomyelitis among the Eskimos for 40 years (Paul et al. 1951) and rift valley fever for 12 years (Sabin and Blumberg 1947).

Two explanations for prolonged anti-viral immunity in the absence of reinfection have been offered. Burnet (1959) has suggested that a clone of immunocompetent cells persists, whereas others have suggested that the virus itself may remain in the host. Some viruses are indeed known to persist for many years, e.g., herpes simplex in many humans and measles in subacute sclerosing panencephalitis (Horta-Barbosa et al. 1969; Payne et al. 1969). Enders-Ruckle (1965) recovered measles virus from lymph nodes and spleen some years after measles infection. Adenoviruses are commonly isolated from human tonsillar and adenoidal tissue (Israel 1962; Stohl and Schlesinger 1965), and in rabbits they persist for long periods in splenic and lymph node cells, apparently macrophages (Reddick and Lefkowitz 1969; Allison 1970b). Other viruses also tend to persist in lymphoreticular tissue, apparently in macrophages, and this led Allison (1970b) to suggest that such persistence, with periodic release of antigen to stimulate antibody-forming cells, may contribute to long-lived immunity. A feed-back mechanism could operate, with antibody decreasing the probability of transfer of antigen from macrophages to immunoglobulin-synthesizing cells. When antibody levels fall, compensatory stimulation could follow, and the system could respond rapidly to additional antigen from a subclinical reinfection of the respiratory tract or elsewhere. Evidence has also accumulated that several viruses cannot replicate in untransformed peripheral blood lymphocytes, whereas they replicate readily in lymphocytes transformed by phytohaemagglutinin, anti-lymphocytic sera or antigen stimulation (see Allison 1970b). Persistence of virus genomes with periodic release of antigen might likewise be a factor in long-lived immunity.

Whether persistence of virus or immunological memory, or both, are responsible for prolonged immunity against viruses is at present unknown. Observations of antibody in rabbits two years after inoculation with irradiated poliovirus (Svehag 1964b), and similar observations after administration of killed virus vaccines in man, show that immunological memory exists, but whether it can explain a lifetime of antibody production in the absence of further antigenic stimulation is not yet clear.

6.7. *Immune responses in man*

Immune responses to virus infections in man are important since there is no effective chemotherapy for most virus infections. Most researches have been directed towards measurement of antibodies in the blood, but recently increasing interest has centered on the roles of secretory antibody and cell-mediated immunity and the interplay of these systems in resistance against virus infections. In this section the immune responses of humans to representative viruses will be described, and an attempt made to define the relative importance of various types of immune response. Interferon will not be discussed, although it could play an important contributory role in resistance.

Infections by viruses entering the body through mucous membranes, especially the respiratory viruses which remain there, is greatly influenced by the presence of secretory antibody. After intranasal infection with rhinovirus, neutralizing antibody appeared in serum and nasal secretions (mainly IgA) after 2 weeks (Cate et al. 1966). Antibody did not significantly modify infection or illness, which had usually resolved when antibody appeared; pre-existing antibody was important in preventing infection. In a recent study inactivated rhinovirus 13 was administered intranasally or intramuscularly (Perkins et al. 1969). The former elicited antibody in both serum and nasal secretions, whereas the latter often failed to elicit secretory antibody. On challenge with intranasal live virus, protection was correlated with the presence of secretory but not serum antibody. In natural rhinovirus infections serum antibody does show correlation with protection (Dick et al. 1967; Gwaltney et al. 1967); this may have been due to the simultaneous presence of secretory antibody, especially since immunity was due to natural (intranasal) infection.

Protection against influenza virus depends on the presence of local neutralizing antibody and a mucoprotein in respiratory secretions bearing influenzal receptors which compete with cells for the virus. Nasal neutralizing and HI antibody against influenza virus is largely of IgA type (Rossen et al. 1966; Alford et al. 1967) and protects against reinfection (Waldman et al. 1968b). Intranasal immunization with live or inactivated virus is much more effective in stimulating nasal antibody production than parenterally administered inactivated vaccine (Mann et al. 1968; Waldman et al. 1968a).

Although the only neutralizing antibody against influenza is directed against the V antigen, anti-neuraminidase antibody is found following infections of mice (Schulman et al. 1968) and natural infections of man (Kilbourne et al. 1968). Mice immunized against this enzyme and producing secretory antibody were shown to have markedly decreased pulmonary virus titres if infected with virus having homologous, but not heterologous, neuraminidase (Schulman et al. 1968). What role such antibody plays in human infection is unknown.

Many very different viruses (such as mousepox and poliovirus) depend on a viraemia to establish foci of major infection. Some viruses must multiply locally or in the reticulo-endothelial system before viraemic spread. The delay allows the humoral system time to respond and the antibody formed can diminish the viraemia and protect the host.

Immunity against poliovirus depends largely on the humoral response, which has been well studied and will be considered in some detail.

The importance of antibodies in immunity to poliovirus has long been recognized. Maternal antibody will protect newborns, and natural infection confers homotypic immunity of a high order against both reinfection and disease (Fox et al. 1956; Hammon et al. 1957). Major paralytic disease develops 8–10 days after infection, and the humoral response is already progressing when the patient comes under observation. Studies of natural and experimental infections of humans (using attenuated virus) have largely confirmed the findings in rabbits previously discussed. The level of neutralizing IgM antibody rises rapidly after natural infection, reaches maximum titres in 3–4 weeks, and declines to undetectable levels by 3 months (Svehag and Mandel 1964b; Ogra et al. 1968). IgG titres rise over a prolonged period and may not attain peak levels until after 3 months. IgA antibody is not detectable until 4–6 weeks after infection and rises for at least the ensuing 8 weeks. The early neutralizing antibody is of low avidity (Sabin 1957). Although CF antibody (anti-D and anti-C) attains maximum levels about 2 months and persists for 1–5 years, neutralizing antibody decreases to one-fourth its peak titre by 2 years and persists near that level for decades.

Ogra et al. (1968) have compared the humoral responses to live and inactivated vaccines in infants. Beginning at 2 months of age, 3 monthly doses of trivalent inactivated virus (subcutaneously), or live virus type 1 (at 2 months old) and types 2 and 3 on successive months (orally) were administered; a booster was given at 12 months of age. Poliovirus-binding antibody titres were determined by radioimmunodiffusion and neutralizing antibody assays for type 1 virus were performed on sera and secretions. Maternally derived IgG antibody was detected in low titres in one-fourth of the infants aged 2 months; no sera contained IgM. IgM and IgG were detected 3 days after the first vaccine dose. The IgM titers rose more rapidly than those of IgG and became maximal during the second week before declining to undetectable levels by 8–10 weeks. IgM declined more slowly in recipients of inactivated virus as they had continuous antigenic stimulation (3 doses). IgG titres in both groups continued to rise for 7–10 weeks before leveling off. Serum IgA titres were not detected until 2 weeks after initial immunization; they rose slowly over a 3 month period. After the booster at 12 months, IgM titres showed a transient rise to previous levels, thus duplicating the findings in rabbits. Recipients of live virus had neutralizing IgA in their nasal and duodenal secretions after 16–21 days, which persisted for at least 90 days (duodenal) and 300 days (nasal); recipients of inactivated virus had no secretory antibody to poliovirus. This is in accord with the well established fact that natural infections and (oral) live virus vaccine confer 'gut immunity' whereas inactivated virus vaccine does not. Studies of humans infected with mumps (Brown et al. 1970) and Coxsackie virus (Schmidt et al. 1968) have demonstrated IgM and IgG patterns similar to those following poliovirus infection and suggest this pattern of antibody response is a general phenomenon.

Many viruses that infect man establish persistent or latent infections. Most of these viruses contain DNA (herpesviruses, papilloma virus, adenoviruses), but some are RNA viruses (measles, in subacute sclerosing panencephalitis). It is difficult to discern any common morphological or chemical features in these viruses that might account for persistence. However, it is becoming increasingly clear that control of infection by some of these viruses is particularly dependent on cell-mediated immune responses. Infections by vaccinia and the herpesviruses – HSV, cytomegalovirus (CMV), and varicella-zoster (V-Z) – will be considered.

These infections are disseminated in two ways: local virus multiplication with spread to contiguous cells, and distant spread of virus by blood and lymph. The immune responses primarily responsible for control of these two processes overlap, but the cell-mediated response appears more important in the former while the humoral (antibody) response is more important in the latter.

There are 2 instances in nature where the effect of absent or decreased antibody on infection may be observed – in the newborn who receives no protective antibody transplacentally because the mother lacks immunity, and in the congenital and acquired hypo- or agammaglobulinaemias. The capacity of the late foetus and neonate to make specific antibody varies with the type and dose of antigen (Evans and Smith 1963; van Furth et al. 1965), and increases rapidly with age. For this and other reasons the neonate unprotected by maternal antibody is susceptible to devastating virus infections. Thus, disseminated herpes infection of the newborn is well known and often fatal (MacCallum 1959; Wheeler and Huffines 1965; Nahmias et al. 1969). In a recent survey, disseminated HSV infections of 25 out of 28 neonates were caused by type 2 virus, probably of maternal genital origin (Nahmias et al. 1969). When 6 mothers and their infants were further studied, 3 mothers had no antibody to HSV and their infants had disseminated disease. Of the other 3 mothers, 2 had antibody against type 1 HSV and their infants had encephalitis or disseminated disease. The remaining mother had antibody against type 2 HSV and her infant had mild disease confined to the skin.

Congenital varicella infection is also often fatal. Freud (1958) reviewed 14 cases (3 fatal) and found that either the mother had varicella during the last 2 weeks of pregnancy, or she gave no history of varicella and siblings of the baby had varicella at that time. Cases of congenital vaccinia are exceedingly rare, probably because of the low chance of exposure to the virus.

Among the congenital immune deficiency syndromes, only Bruton's agammaglobulinaemia has decreased humoral response as an isolated immune defect. These patients are not known to be abnormally suscept-ible to virus infections, but at least 1 of these patients had progressive vaccinia (Fulginiti et al. 1968). Chandra (1969) reported 7 infants with significantly lowered serum IgM and IgA levels who developed a generalized but non-progressive vaccinia infection after vaccination. Neutralizing and CF tests for vaccinia were not done but isohaemag-glutinin titres were low. The lymphocytes of 1 patient were tested and responded normally to phytohaemagglutinin stimulation. The lesions were not the progressive, necrotic type seen in deficiencies of cellular immunity and healed normally. More studies of this syndrome are needed before definite conclusions can be drawn, but it appears that the lack of IgM allows viraemic dissemination, while the intact cellular response can limit the lesions locally.

More evidence for the importance of antibody in limiting these infections comes from the partial success in prophylaxis and treatment with immune sera. Kempe (1960) showed that sera from recently vaccin-ated subjects reduced the expected number of smallpox cases in exposed individuals; convalescent sera might prove even more efficacious. Brunell et al. (1969) has shown that gamma globulin from convalescing zoster patients is effective in preventing development of varicella in children recently exposed to varicella, whereas immune gamma globulin is not. Recently, Leonard et al. (1970) showed that sera from con-valescing zoster patients have neutralizing IgG antibody in the electro-phoretically fast fraction that is not present in varicella patients; it appears only when zoster is exacerbated. It was suggested that this fraction might contain the effective antibody.

Although HSV can often be isolated from asymptomatic subjects as well as those with herpetic lesions (Buddingh et al. 1953; Kaufman et al. 1967), the presence of antibody in normal children and adults probably prevents dissemination. The development of this antibody has been well studied. Initial herpetic infection of man usually occurs as a childhood stomatitis. Two to three weeks after infection, neutralizing and CF antibody are present and the virus becomes occult. A large sero–epidemiological study in Japan (Yoshino et al. 1962) showed that during the first 4 months of life, babies often have neutralizing and CF antibody to HSV. There follow several years in which antibody is found in only about 10% of subjects, after which the frequency increases until after age 20 over 80% of subjects have positive sera. Titres varied extensively below age 20, and a heat-labile CF antibody was often detected during this time that was not detected in adults. After age 20 the titres tended to be either high or absent, and neutralizing and CF titres paralleled each other. One interpretation of these observations is that repeated exposure to the virus is required after initial infection before the stable, persisting antibody pattern of the adults is established (Buddingh et al. 1953; Yoshino et al. 1962). In both normal adults and adults with recurring herpetic infections it appears that all serum neutralizing antibody is in the IgG fraction (Deforest and Klein 1968), whereas neutralizing IgA can be detected in the tears of normal adults (Little et al. 1969).

The development of a humoral response does not always eliminate disseminated infection, however, as demonstrated by congenital CMV and rubella infections. Babies may possess maternal IgG, be synthesizing IgM, and continue to excrete virus for years (Hanshaw et al. 1965; McCarthy and Taylor-Robinson 1967).

Evidence for the importance of cell-mediated immunity in controlling infections by these viruses comes mainly from observations on the immunodeficiency syndromes. As mentioned previously, patients with Bruton's agammaglobulinaemia, with normal cell-mediated immunity, have recurrent infections by extracellular pyogenic pathogens but are not abnormally susceptible to virus infections. Congenital conditions in which cell-mediated immunity defects are prominent include ataxia-telangiectasia, Swiss agammaglobulinaemia, and the syndromes of Wiscott-Aldrich, Gitlin, Nezelof, and DiGeorge. In all these syndromes viruses are a recurring and often fatal complication. Fulginiti et al. (1968) described progressive vaccinia in patients with many of these syndromes, particularly in Nezelof's syndrome in which immunoglobulin levels and specific antibody-synthesizing capacity are near normal. Patients with Wiscott-Aldrich syndrome are particularly susceptible to infections by CMV, measles and especially HSV (Cooper et al. 1968).

Patients with short-limbed dwarfism and abnormally fine hair, the cartilage-hair hypoplasia syndrome, frequently have severe varicella infections. Two such patients studied by Lux et al. (1969) illustrate the situation in which humoral responses are intact but cell-mediated responses are faulty. Both patients had normal immunoglobulin levels and had antibody responses to measles (attenuated) vaccine and diphtheria-pertussis-tetanus inoculation. Despite antibody titres to streptokinase-streptodornase and candida, skin testing with these antigens and measles antigen were negative. Dinitrochlorobenzene sensitization was unsuccessful and lymphocyte stimulation with phytohaemagglutinin or allogeneic cells was diminished. A skin graft was rejected more slowly than usual. Both patients had CF antibody to V-Z virus after severe infection. In accord with the other syndromes, the decreased cell-mediated immunity observed predisposed these patients to severe disease after a normally benign V-Z virus infection. As is found in Wiscott-Aldrich syndrome, these patients probably developed their cell-mediated immunity defect after birth since virus infections were not a problem during the first two years of life and one patient was successfully vaccinated.

Debilitating diseases, cancer chemotherapy, and immunosuppressive therapy, which depress cell-mediated and humoral immunity, also lead to increased virus infections, particularly by CMV. Sullivan (1968) reported that most leukaemic children showed sero-conversion within a few months of beginning chemotherapy; this was thought to indicate primary infection. Approximately 65 percent of patients undergoing renal transplantation have antibody to CMV (Craighead et al. 1967; Craighead 1969). After 2–5 months on immunosuppressive therapy, over half of these patients had secondary antibody responses to CMV thought to be a response to activation of the virus.

Treatment with anti-lymphocyte serum (ALS) is sometimes used for immunosuppression in transplant patients and is known to increase the morbidity and mortality of mice peripherally inoculated with several viruses, including vaccinia and HSV (Hirsch et al. 1968; Hirsch and Murphy 1968; Hirsch 1970). A congenital syndrome characterized by recurrent infections, episodic lymphopenia, and impaired humoral and cell-mediated immunity has recently been described in two siblings (Kretschmer et al. 1969). One was found to have a C'-dependent serum lymphotoxic factor only when lymphopenic. At autopsy depletion of small lymphocytes in the thymus-dependent areas of lymph nodes was noted. This condition has many similarities to that found in ALS-treated animals, and it was suggested the lymphotoxic factor might be an antibody. The patient suffered from recurrent herpetic infection and died with herpetic encephalitis. Although some of the cases also had defective humoral immunity, these few examples illustrate the role of cell-mediated immunity in virus infections.

Recent reports of local and systemic reactions in recipients of in-activated measles vaccine when subsequently inoculated with live virus vaccine (Buser 1967; Scott and Bonanno 1967) or experiencing natural infection (Karzon et al. 1965; Raugh and Schmidt 1965; Fulginiti et al. 1967; Nader et al. 1968) suggest the importance of immediate hyper-sensitivity reactions in virus infections. In the former subjects fever, atypical exanthema, and local swelling and erythema developed over 3–8 days. The local reactions could be due to delayed hypersensitivity

(Lennon et al. 1967) or an Arthus-type reaction in which precipitating antibodies are deposited on blood vessel walls, fix C′, and thus attract neutrophils which can produce an injurious inflammatory reaction (Ward and Cochrane 1965). Evidence for the latter mechanism was reported by Bellanti et al. (1969), who described the presence of IgG, measles antigen, and C′ in skin biopsies from the sites of local reaction.

Chanock et al. (1968) have proposed a similar mechanism for the severity of respiratory syncytial virus infection in babies. The lack of secretory antibody would allow establishment of local infection, and circulating maternal IgG antibody could form complexes with virus antigen in the pulmonary tissue and produce an Arthus reaction. Viruses thus elicit many types of immune responses in man – some beneficial and some injurious to the host.

References

ALFORD, C. A., JR., 1965, Am. J. Dis. Children *110*, 455.

ALFORD, R. H., R. D. ROSSEN, W. T. BUTLER and J. A. KASEL, 1967, J. Immunol. *98*, 724.

ALLISON, A. C., 1966, J. Natl. Cancer Inst. *36*, 869.

ALLISON, A. C., 1967, Brit. Med. Bull. *23*, 60.

ALLISON, A. C., 1970a, Proc. Roy. Soc. Med.

ALLISON, A. C., 1970b, *in*: R. van Furth, ed.: Mononuclear phagocytes. Oxford, Blackwell.

ALLISON, A. C. and R. M. FRIEDMAN, 1966, J. Natl. Cancer Inst. *36*, 859.

ALLISON, A. C. and R. B. TAYLOR, 1967, Cancer Res. *27*, 703.

ALMEIDA, J. D. and A. P. WATERSON, 1969, Adv. Virus Res. *15*, 307.

AMMANN, A. J., W. A. CAIN, K. ISHIZAKA, R. HONG and R. A. GOOD, 1969, New Engl. J. Med. *281*, 469.

ANDERSON, W. A. and E. D. KILBOURNE, 1961, J. Invest. Dermatol. *37*, 25.

ASHE, W. K., M. MAGE, R. MAGE and A. L. NOTKINS, 1968, J. Immunol. *101*, 500.

ASHE, W. K. and A. L. NOTKINS, 1967, Virology *33*, 613.

ATTIA, M. A., K. B. DE OME and D. WEISS, 1965, Cancer Res. *25*, 451.

AXELRAD, A., 1965, Progr. Exptl. Tumor Res. *6*, 31.

BELLANTI, J. A., R. SANGA, B. KLUTINIS, B. BRANDT and M. S. ARTENSTEIN, 1969, New Engl. J. Med. *280*, 628.

BERRY, D. M. and J. D. ALMEIDA, 1968, J. Gen. Virol. *3*, 97.

BEVERIDGE, W. I. B. and F. M. BURNET, 1944, Med. J. Aust. *1*, 85.

BLACKLOW, N. R., M. D. HOGGAN, J. B. AUSTIN and W. P. ROWE, 1969, Am. J. Epidem. *90*, 501.

BOYSE, E. A., L. J. OLD and H. F. OETTGEN, 1969, Tumour immunology. *In*: P. A. Miescher and H. J. Müller-Eberhard, eds.: Textbook of immunopathology, Vol. 2. New York, Grune-Stratton. pp. 768–788.

BROOM, J. C., 1947, Lancet, *1*, 364.

BROWN, G. C., J. V. BAUBLIS and T. P. O'LEARY, 1970, J. Immunol. *104*, 861.

BROWN, J. A. H., 1953, Brit. J. Exptl. Pathol. *34*, 290.

BRUNELL, P. A., A. ROSS, L. H. MILLER and B. KUO., 1969, New Engl. J. Med. *280*, 1191.

BUDDINGH, G. J., D. I. SCHRUM, J. C. LANIER and D. J. GUIDRY, 1953, Pediatrics *11*, 595.

BUGBEE, L. M., A. A. LIKE and R. B. STEWART, 1960, J. infect. Dis. *106*, 166.

BURNET, F. M., 1959, A clonal selection theory of acquired immunity. Cambridge University Press, London.

BURNET, F. M. and F. FENNER, 1949, The production of antibodies, 2nd Ed. Melbourne, Macmillan.

BUSER, F., 1967, New Engl. J. Med. *277*, 250.

CATE, T. R., R. D. ROSSEN, R. G. DOUGLAS, W. T. BUTLER and R. B. COUCH, 1966, Am. J. Epidemiol. *84*, 352.

CHANDRA, R. K., B. KAVERAMMA and J. F. SOOTHILL, 1969, Lancet *1*, 687.

CHANOCK, R. M., R. H. PARROTT, Z. KAPIKIAN, H. KIM and C. D. BRANDT, 1968, Perspect. Virol. *6*, 125.

CHOPPIN, P. W. and W. STOEKENIUS, 1964, Virology *22*, 482.

COOPER, M. D., H. P. CHASE, J. T. LOWMAN, W. KRIVIT and R. A. GOOD, 1968, Am. J. Med. *44*, 499.

COWAN, K. M., 1970, J. Immunol. *104*, 423.

CRAIGHEAD, J. E., J. B. HANSHAW and C. B. CARPENTER, 1967, J. Am. Med. Assoc. *201*, 725.

CRAIGHEAD, J. E., 1969, Am. J. Epidemiol. *90*, 506.

DALES, S., 1969, Role of lysosomes in cell-virus interactions. *In*: J. T. Dingle and H. G. Fell, eds.: Lysosomes in biology and pathology, Vol. 2. Amsterdam, North Holland. pp. 69–86.

DALES, S. and R. KAJIOKA, 1964, Virology *24*, 278.

DANIELS, C. A., T. BORSOS, H. J. RAPP, R. SNYDERMAN and A. L. NOTKINS, 1969, Science *165*, 508.

DARLINGTON, R. W. and L. H. MOSS, III, 1969, Progr. Med. Virol. *11*, 16.

DAVENPORT, F. M. and A. V. HENNESSY, 1956, J. Exptl. Med. *104*, 85.

DEFOREST, A. and M. KLEIN, 1968, Federation Proc. *27*, 734.

DIAMANDOPOULOS, G. T., S. S. TEVETHIA, F. RAPP and J. F. ENDERS, 1968, Virology *34*, 331.

DICK, E. C., C. R. BLUMER and A. EVANS, 1967, Am. J. Epidemiol. *86*, 386.

DOWNIE, A. W. and K. MCCARTHY, 1958, J. Hygiene *56*, 479.

DULBECCO, R., M. VOGT and A. STRICKLAND, 1956, Virology *2*, 162.

ECKERT, A. E., 1966, J. Bacteriol. *92*, 1430.

EDDY, B. E., R. D. YOUNG and G. E. GRUBS, 1965, Perspect. Virol. *4*, 209.

EISEN, H., 1966, Harvey Lectures *60*, 1.

ENDERS, J. F., S. COHEN and L. W. KANE, 1945, J. Exptl. Med. *81*, 119.

ENDERS-RUCKLE, G., 1965, Arch. Ges. Virusforsch., *16*, 182.

EVANS, D. G. and J. W. G. SMITH, 1963, Brit. Med. Bull. *19*, 225.

FAZEKAS DE ST. GROTH, S., 1969, J. Immunol. *103*, 1107.

FAZEKAS DE ST. GROTH, S. and D. M. GRAHAM, 1954, Aust. J. Exptl. Biol. Med. Sci. *32*, 369.

FAZEKAS DE ST. GROTH, S. and R. G. WEBSTER, 1964, The antibody response. *In*: G. Wolstenholme and J. Knight, eds.: Ciba Foundation Symp. on cellular biol. myxovirus infections. London, Churchill. pp. 246–271.

FELDMAN, M. and E. DIENER, 1970, J. Exptl. Med. *131*, 247.

FEINSTONE, S. M., E. H. BEACHEY and M. W. RYTEL, 1969, J. Immunol. *103*, 844.

FENNER, F., 1948, J. Pathol. Bacteriol. *60*, 529.

FIGUEROA, M. E. and W. E. RAWLS, 1969, J. Gen. Virol. *4*, 259.

FOX, J. P., H. M. GELFORD, P. R. LE BLANC and D. P. CONWELL, 1956, Am. J. Public Health *46*, 283.

FRANCIS, T., JR., 1942, Harvey Lectures *37*, 69.

FRANCIS, T., JR., 1953, Ann. Internal Med. *39*, 203.

FRANCIS, T., JR. and R. SHOPE, 1936, J. Exptl. Med. *63*, 645.

FREUD, P., 1958, Am. J. Dis. Child. *96*, 730.

FRIEDMAN, R. M. S. BARON, C. E. BUCKLER and R. I. STEINMULLER, 1962, J. Exptl. Med. *116*, 347.

FULGINITI, V. A., J. ARTHUR, D. S. PEARLMAN and C. H. KEMPE, 1962, J. Ped. *69*, 891.

FULGINITI, V. A., C. H. KEMPE, W. E. HATHAWAY, D. S. PEARLMAN, O. F. SIEBER, J. J. ELLER, J. J. JOYNER and A. ROBINSON, 1968, Progressive vaccinia in immunologically deficient individuals. *In*: D. Bergsma and R. A. Good, eds.: Immunologic deficiency diseases in man, Vol. 4. New York, National Foundation Press. pp. 129–151.

FURTH, R. VAN, H. R. E. SCHUIT and W. HIJMANS, 1965, J. Exptl. Med. *122*, 1173.

GIBBS, C. J., JR. and D. C. GAJDUSEK, 1970, Am. J. Trop. Med. Hyg. *19*, 138.

GLASGOW, L. A. and H. R. MORGAN, 1957, J. Exptl. Med. *106*, 45.

GOFFE, A. P., J. ALMEIDA and F. BROWN, 1966, Lancet *2*, 607.

GOLDNER, H., A. J. GIRARDI, V. M. LARSON and M. R. HILLEMAN, 1964, Proc. Soc. Exptl. Biol. Med. *117*, 851.

GRAF, M. W. and J. W. UHR, 1969, J. Exptl. Med. *130*, 1175.

GRANOFF, A., 1965, Virology *25*, 38.

GUSTAFSSON, B. E. and A. LAURELL, 1960, Proc. Soc. Exptl. Biol. Med. *105*, 598.

GWALTNEY, J. M., J. O. HENDLEY, G. SIMON and W. S. JORDON, 1967, J. Am. Med. Assoc. *202*, 494.

HABEL, K., 1962, Cold Spring Harbor Symp. Quant. Biol. *27*, 433.

HABEL, K., 1970, Advan. Immunol. *10*, 229.

HADDAD, Z. H., K. OSGOOD, J. KOROTZER, F. PEETOOM and K. ISHIZAKA, 1970, Lancet *1*, 627.

HAHON, N., 1970, J. Gen. Virol. *6*, 361.

HAMMON, W., E. LUDWIG, G. SATHER and D. S. YOHN, 1957, Am. J. Public Health *47*, 802.

HAMPAR, B., A. L. NOTKINS, M. MAGE and M. A. KEEHN, 1968, J. Immunol. *100*, 586.

HANSHAW, J. B., R. F. BETTS, G. SIMON and R. C. BOYTON, 1965, New Engl. J. Med. *272*, 602.

HARBOE, A. and G. HAUKENES, 1966, Acta Path. Microbiol. Scand. *68*, 98.

HARBOE, A., R. SCHØYEN and A. BYE-HANSEN, 1966, Acta Path. Microbiol. Scand. *67*, 573.

HAUGHTON, G. and D. R. NASH, 1969, Progr. Med. Virol. *11*, 248.

HAUKENES, G., A. HARBOE and K. MORTENSSON-EGNUND, 1966, Acta Path. Microbiol. Scand. *66*, 510.

HEARN, H. J., JR. and C. T. RAINEY, 1963, J. Immunol. *90*, 720.

HELLSTRÖM, I. and K. E. HELLSTRÖM, 1969a, Int. J. Cancer *4*, 587.

HELLSTRÖM, I., C. A. EVANS and K. E. HELLSTRÖM, 1969b, Int. J. Cancer *4*, 601.

HENLE, W. and F. W. LIEF, 1963, Am. Rev. Resp. Dis. *88*, 379. (suppl.)

HENRY, C. and N. JERNE, 1968, J. Exptl. Med. *128*, 133.

HEPPNER, G. H., 1969, Int. J. Cancer *4*, 608.

HILLEMAN, M. R., 1966, Progr. Med. Virol. *8*, 131.

HIRSCH, M. S., 1970, Federation Proc. *29*, 169.

HIRSCH, M. S., A. J. NAHMIAS, F. A. MURPHY and J. H. KRAMER, 1967, J. Exptl. Med., *128*, 121.

HIRSCH, M. S., A. C. ALLISON and J. J. HARVEY, 1969, Nature *223*, 739.

HIRSCH, M. S. and F. A. MURPHY, 1968, Lancet *2*, 37.

HIRSCH, M. S., A. J. NAHMIAS, F. A. MURPHY and J. H. KRAMER, 1968, J. Exptl. Med. *128*, 121.

HORTA-BARBOSA, L., D. A. FUCCILLA, J. L. SEVER and W. ZEMAN, 1969, Nature *221*, 974.

HOTCHIN, J., 1962, Cold Spring Harbor Symp. Quant. Biol. *27*, 479.

HOTCHIN, J., 1965, Natl. Inst. Neurol. Dis. Blindness Monograph *2*, 341.

HOYER, J. R., M. D. COOPER, A. E. GABRIELSEN and R. A. GOOD, 1968, Medicine, *47*, 201.

HUMMELER, K., T. F. ANDERSON and R. A. BROWN, 1962, Virology *16*, 84.

HUMPHREY, J. H. and R. R. DOURMASHKIN, 1965, Electron microscopic studies of immune cell lysis. *In*: G. Wolstenholme and J. Knight, eds.: Ciba Symp. on Complement. London, Churchill. pp. 175–186.

ISACSON, P., 1968, Perspect. Virol. *6*, 141.

ISRAEL, M. S., 1962, J. Pathol. Bacteriol. *84*, 169.

JAWETZ, E., V. COLEMAN and M. F. ALLENDE, 1951, J. Immunol. *67*, 197.

JENNER, E., 1798, An inquiry into the causes and effects of the variolae vacciniae. London, Sampson Low. p. 13.

KARZON, D. T., D. RUSH and W. WINKELSTEIN, JR., 1965, Pediatrics *36*, 40.

KATES, M., A. C. ALLISON and D. A. J. TYRRELL, 1961, Biochem. Biophys. Acta *52*, 455.

KAUFMAN, N. E., D. C. BROWN and E. M. ELLISON, 1967, Science *156*, 1628.

KAWANA, K., L. MILLER and P. KIMMELSTIEL, 1969, New Engl. J. Med. *281*, 1228.

KELLER, R., 1965, J. Immunol. *94*, 143.

KELLER, R., 1966, J. Immunol. *96*, 96.

KELLER, R., 1968, J. Immunol. *100*, 1071.

KETLER, A., Y. HINUMA and K. HUMMELER, 1961, J. Immunol. *86*, 22.

KEMPE, C. H., 1960, Bull. W. H. O. *25*, 41.

KILBOURNE, E. D., W. N. CHRISTENSON and M. SANDE, 1968, J. Virol. *2*, 761.

KJELLEN, L., 1962, Virology *14*, 448.

KJELLEN, L., 1964, Arch. Ges. Virusforsch. *14*, 189.

KJELLEN, L., 1965, Immunology *8*, 557.

KJELLEN, L. and H. G. PEREIRA, 1968, J. Gen. Virol. *2*, 177.

KJELLEN, L. and R. W. SCHLESINGER, 1959, Virology *7*, 236.

KLEIN, E. and G. KLEIŃ, 1966, Nature *209*, 163.

KÖLSCH, E., 1970, *in*: R. van Furth, ed.: Mononuclear phagocytes. Oxford, Blackwell.

KONO, R., S. IKAWA, H. YAOI, JR., C. HAMADA, Y. ASHIHARA and K. KAWAKAMI, 1966, Am. J. Epidemiol. *83*, 14.

KRETSCHMER, R., C. S. AUGUST, F. S. ROSEN and C. A. JANEWAY, 1969, New Engl. J. Med. *281*, 285.

KRUGMAN, S., J. P. GILES, H. FRIEDMAN and S. STONE, 1966, J. Pediat., *66*, 471.

LAFFERTY, K. J., 1963a, Virology *21*, 61.

LAFFERTY, K. J., 1963b, Virology *21*, 76.

LAVER, W. G., J. R. SURIANO and M. GREEN, 1967, J. Virol. *1*, 723.

LAVER, W. G. and R. C. VALENTINE, 1969, Virology *38*, 105.

LAW, L. W., 1969, Cancer Res. *29*, 1.

LENNON, R. G., P. ISACSON, T. ROSALES, W. R. ELSEO, D. T. KARZON and W. WINKELSTEIN, JR., 1967, J. Am. Med. Assoc. *200*, 275.

LEONARD, L. L., N. J. SCHMIDT and E. H. LENNETTE, 1970, J. Immunol. *104*, 23.

LEVEY, R. M., N. TRAININ, L. W. LAW, P. H. BLACK and W. P. ROWE, 1963, Science *142*, 483.

LINDENMANN, J. and P. A. KLEIN, 1967, J. Exptl. Med. *126*, 93.

LINSCOTT, W. and W. LEVINSON, 1969, Proc. Natl. Acad. Sci. U.S. *64*, 520.

LITTLE, J., Y. CENTIFANTO and H. E. KAUFMAN, 1969, Am. J. Ophthal. *68*, 898.

LUX, S. E., R. B. JOHNSTON, JR., C. AUGUST, B. SAY, U. B. PERCHASZADEH, F. S. ROSEN and V. A. MCKUSICK, 1970, New Engl. J. Med. *282*, 234.

MACCALLUM, F. O., 1959, Acta Virol. (suppl.) *3*, 17.

MCCARTHY, K. and C. H. TAYLOR-ROBINSON, 1967, Brit. Med. Bull. *23*, 185.

MANDEL, B., 1961, Virology *14*, 316.

MANDEL, B., 1962, Cold Spring Harbor Symp. Quant. Biol. *27*, 101.

MANN, J. J., R. H. WALDMAN, Y. TOYO, G. C. HEINER, A. T. DAWKINS and J. A. KASEL, 1968, J. Immunol. *100*, 726.

MARDINEZ, M. R., H. J. MÜLLER-EBERHARD and J. D. FELDMAN, 1968, Am. J. Pathol. *53*, 253.

MELLORS, R. C., T. AOKI and R. J. HUEBNER, 1969, J. Exptl. Med., *129*, 1045.

MICHAEL, J. G. and F. S. ROSEN, 1963, J. Exptl. Med. *118*, 619.

MIETENS, C., K. HUMMELER and W. HENLE, 1964, J. Immunol. *92*, 17.

MIMS, C. A., 1964, Bacteriol. Rev. *28*, 30.

MITCHELL, G. F. and J. F. A. P. MILLER, 1968, Proc. Natl. Acad. Sci. U.S. *59*, 296.

MITCHISON, N. A., 1967, Cold Spring Harbor Symp. Quant. Biol. *32*, 431.

MONTGOMERIE, J. Z., D. M. O. BECROFT, M. CROXSON, P. B. DOAK and J. D. K. NORTH, 1969, Lancet, *ii*, 867.

MÜLLER-EBERHARD, H. J., 1968, Advan. Immunol. *8*, 1.

MÜLLER-EBERHARD, H. J., A. P. DALMACCO and M. A. CALCOTT, 1966, J. Exptl. Med. *123*, 33.

MUSCHEL, L. H. and A. J. TOUSSAINT, 1962, J. Immunol. *89*, 35.

NADER, R. P., M. HORWITZ and J. ROUSSEAU, 1968, J. Ped. *72*, 22.

NAGLER, F. P. O., 1944, J. Immunol. *48*, 213.

NAHMIAS, A. J., D. GRIFFITH, C. SALISBURY and K. YOSHIDA, 1967, J. Am. Med. Assoc. *201*, 729.

NAHMIAS, A. J., W. R. DOWDLE, W. E. JOSEY, Z. N. NAIB, L. M. PAINTER and C. LUCE, 1969, J. Ped. *75*, 1194.

NEURATH, A. R., RUBIN, B. A. and W. A. PIERZCHALA, 1967, Z. Naturforsch. *22b*, 850.

NORRBY, E., 1969a, J. Gen. Virol. *5*, 221.

NORRBY, E., 1969b, J. Virol. *4*, 657.

NORRBY, E., H. MARUSYK and M. HAMMASKJOLD, 1969, Virology *38*, 477.

NORRBY, E. and G. WADELL, 1969, J. Virol. *4*, 663.

NOTKINS, A. L., M. MAGE, W. K. ASHE and S. MAHAR, 1968, J. Immunol. *100*, 314.

NOTKINS, A. L., S. MAHAR, C. SCHEELE and J. GOFFMAN, 1966, J. Exptl. Med. *124*, 81.

OGRA, P., D. T. KARZON, F. RIGHTHAND and M. MACGILLIVRAY, 1968, New Engl. J. Med. *279*, 893.

OLDSTONE, M. B. A. and F. J. DIXON, 1969, J. Exptl. Med. *129*, 483.

O'NEILL, C. H., 1968, J. Cell Sci. *3*, 405.

PANUM, P. L., 1847, Virchows Arch. Pathol. Anat. Physiol. *1*, 492.

PAUL, J. R., J. T. RIORDAN and J. L. MELNICK, 1951, Am. J. Hyg. *54*, 275.

PAULS, F. P. and W. R. DOWDLE, 1967, J. Immunol. *98*, 941.

PAYNE, F. E., J. V. BAUBLIS and H. H. ITABASHI, 1969, New Engl. J. Med. *281*, 585.

PERKINS, F. T., R. YETTS and W. GAISFORD, 1959, Brit. Med. J. *1*, 1083.

PERKINS, J. C., D. N. TUCKER, H. KNOPF, R. D. WENZEL, A. Z. KAPIKIAN and R. M. CHANOCK 1969, Am. J. Epidemiol. *90*, 519.

PETTERSSON, U., L. PHILIPSON and S. HOGLUND, 1968, Virology *35*, 204.

PHILIPSON, L., 1966, Virology *28*, 35.

PHILLIPSON, L., 1969, International Virology *1*, 90.

PINCUS, W. B. and J. A. FLICK, 1963, J. Infect. Dis. *113*, 15.

PIRQUET, C. VON, 1907, *in*: Klinische Studien über Vakzination und vakzinale Allergie. Leipzig, Deuticke.

PLOTKIN, S. A., M. KATZ, R. E. BROWN and J. S. PAGANO, 1966, Am. J. Dis. Children *111*, 27.

PLUMMER, G., 1964, Brit. J. Exptl. Path. *45*, 135.

PLUMMER, G., C. R. GOODHEART, D. HENSON and C. BOWLING, 1969, Virology *39*, 134.

PLUMMER, G., J. L. WANER, A. PHUANGSAB and C. R. GOODHEART, 1970, J. Virol. *5*, 51.

POLLARD, M., M. KOJUMA and N. SHARON, 1968, Perspect. Virol. *6*, 193.

RAUGH, L. W. and R. SCHMIDT, 1965, Am. J. Dis. Child. *109*, 232.

REDDICK, R. A. and S. S. LEFKOWITZ, 1969, J. Immunol. *103*, 687.

ROBERTSON, H. T. and BLACK, P. H., 1969, Proc. Soc. Exptl. Biol. Med. *130*, 363.

ROCKLIN, R. E., O. L. MEYERS and J. R. DAVID, 1970, J. Immunol. *104*, 95.

ROSE, H. M. and E. MOLLOY, 1947, Federation Proc. *6*, 432.

ROSEN, L., 1960, Am. J. Hyg. *71*, 120.

ROSSEN, R. D., R. H. ALFORD, W. T. BUTLER and W. E. VANNIER, 1966, J. Immunol. *97*, 369.

ROSSEN, R. D., R. G. DOUGLAS, JR., T. R. CATE, R. B. COUCH and W. T. BUTLER, 1966, J. Immunol. *97*, 532.

ROTTO, O., DRZNIEK, R., SABER, M. S. and REICHERT, G., 1966, Arch. Virusforsch. *19*, 273.

ROWLEY, D., 1962, Advan. Immunol. *2*, 241.

RUBIN, H., 1958, Virology *4*, 533.

RUBIN, H., L. FANSHIER, A. CORNELIUS and W. F. HUGHES, 1962, Virology *17*, 143.

RUBIN, H. and R. FRANKLIN, 1957, Virology *3*, 84.

RUSSELL, W. C. and B. E. KNIGHT, 1967, J. Gen. Virol. *1*, 523.

RUSSELL, W. C., W. G. LAVER and P. J. SANDERSON, 1968, Nature *219*, 1127.

SABIN, A. B., 1957, Special Publications, N.Y. Acad. Sci., *5*, 113.

SABIN, A. B., 1959, *in*: V. A. Najjer, ed.: Immunity and virus infection. New York, Wiley. p. 211.

SABIN, A. B. and R. W. BLUMBERG, 1947, Proc. Soc. Exptl. Biol. Med. *64*, 385.

SAWYER, W. A., 1931, J. Prevent. Med. *5*, 413.

SCHARFF, M. D. and L. LEWINTOW, 1963, Virology *19*, 491.

SCHIERMAN, L. W. and R. A. MCBRIDE, 1967, Science, *156*, 658.

SCHLESINGER, R. W., 1969, Advan. Virus Res. *14*, 1.

SCHMIDT, N. J., E. H. LENNETTE and J. DENNIS, 1968, J. Immunol. *100*, 99.

SCHØYEN, R., A. HARBOE and L. WANG, 1966, Acta Pathol. Microbiol. Scand. *68*, 103.

SCHULMAN, J. L., M. KHAKPOUR and E. D. KILBOURNE, 1968, J. Virol. *2*, 778.

SCOTT, T. F. M. and D. E. BONANNO, 1967, New Engl. J. Med. *277*, 248.

SETO, J. T. and R. ROTT, 1966, Virology *30*, 731.

SEVER, J. L., R. J. HUEBNER, A. FABIYI, G. R. MONIF, G. CASTELLANO, C. L. CUSUMANO, R. G. TRAUB, A. C. LEY, M. R. GILKESON and J. M. ROBERTS, 1966, Proc. Soc. Exptl. Biol. Med. *122*, 513.

SHORTMAN, K., E. DIENER, P. RUSSELL and W. D. ARMSTRONG, 1970, J. Exptl. Med. *131*, 461.

SIEGERST, R. and P. BRAUNE, 1964a, Virology *24*, 209.

SIEGERST, R. and P. BRAUNE, 1964b, Virology *24*, 218.

SILVERSTEIN, S. and P. MARCUS, 1964, Virology *23*, 370.

SJÖGREN, H. O., 1964, J. Natl. Cancer Inst. *32*, 661.

SJÖGREN, H. O., I. HELLSTRÖM and G. KLEIN, 1961, Exptl. Cell Res. *23*, 204.

SMITH, C. B., R. H. PURCELL, J. A. BELLANTI and R. M. CHANOCK, 1966, New Engl. J. Med. *275*, 1145.

SMITH, K. O., 1965, J. Immunol. *94*, 976.

SOOTHILL, J. F., K. HAYES and J. A. DUDGEON, 1966, Lancet *i*, 1385.

SPITZNAGEL, J. K. and A. C. ALLISON, 1970, J. Immunol. *104*, 128.

SPRING, S. and B. ROIZMAN, 1968, J. Virol. *2*, 979.

SPRINGER, G. F. and R. SCHUSTER, 1964, Klin. Wschr. *42*, 221.

ŠTERZL, J. and A. M. SILVERSTEIN, 1967, Advan. Immunol. *6*, 337.

STIEHM, E. R., A. J. AMMANN and J. D. CHERRY, 1966, New Engl. J. Med. *275*, 971.

STROHL, W. A. and R. W. SCHLESINGER, 1965, Virology, *26*, 208.

SULLIVAN, M. P., J. B. HANSHAW, A. CANGIR and J. J. BUTLER, 1968, J. Am. Med. Assoc. *206*, 569.

SVEHAG, S., 1964a, J. Exptl. Med. *119*, 225.

SVEHAG, S., 1964b, J. Exptl. Med. *119*, 517.

SVEHAG, S. and B. MANDEL, 1964a, J. Exptl. Med. *119*, 1.

SVEHAG, S. and B. MANDEL, 1964b, J. Exptl. Med. *119*, 21.

TEVETHIA, S. S., M. KATZ and F. RAPP, 1965, Proc. Soc. Exptl. Biol. Med. *119*, 896.

THOR, D. E., R. E. JUREZIZ, S. R. VEACH, E. MILLER and S. DRAY, 1968, Nature *219*, 755.

TOMASI, T. B., JR. and J. BIENENSTOCK, 1969, Advan. Immunol. *9*, 1.

TOMPKINS, W. A. F., C. ADAMS and W. E. RAWLS, 1970, J. Immunol. *104*, 502.

TRAUB, E., 1939, J. Exptl. Med. *69*, 101.

TURK, J. G., A. C. ALLISON and M. N. OXMAN, 1962, Lancet *i*, 405.

UHR, J. W. and J. B. BAUMAN, 1961, J. Exptl. Med. *113*, 935.

UHR, J. W. and M. S. FINKELSTEIN, 1963, J. Exptl. Med. *117*, 457.

UHR, J. W., M. S. FINKELSTEIN and J. B. BAUMANN, 1962, J. Exptl. Med. *115*, 655.

UHR, J. W. and G. MÖLLER, 1968, Advan. Immunol. *8*, 81.

UHR, J. W., S. B. SALVIN and A. M. PAPPENHEIMER, JR., 1957, J. Exptl. Med. *105*, 11.

VAN DER VEEN, J. and H. J. A. SONDERKAMP, 1965, Arch. Ges. Virusforsch. *15*, 721.

VOGT, A., R. KOPP, G. MAASS and L. REICH, 1964, Science *145*, 1447.

VOLKERT, M. and J. H. LARSEN, 1965, Progr. Med. Virol. *7*, 160.

WADELL, G. and E. NORRBY, 1969, J. Virol. *4*, 671.

WALDMAN, R. H., J. A. KASEL, R. V. FULK, R. B. HORNICK, G. C. HEINER, A. T. DAWKINS and J. J. MANN, 1968a, Nature *218*, 594.

WALDMAN, R. H., J. J. MANN and P. A. SMALL, 1968b, Clin. Res. *16*, 336.

WALLIS, C. and J. L. MELNICK, 1967, J. Virol. *1*, 478.

WARD, P. A. and C. G. COCHRANE, 1965, J. Exptl. Med. *121*, 215.

WATSON, D. H. and WILDY. P., 1963, Virology *21*, 1000.

WATSON, D. H., P. WILDY, B. HARVEY and W. SHEDDEN, 1967, J. Gen. Virol. *1*, 139.

WEBSTER, R. G., 1965, Immunology *9*, 501.

WEBSTER, R. G., 1968a, Immunology *14*, 29.

WEBSTER, R. G., 1968b, Immunology *14*, 39.

WHEELER, C. and W. HUFFINES, 1965, J. Am. Med. Assoc. *191*, 455.

WIGAND, R. and D. FLIEDNER, 1968, Arch. Ges. Virusforsch. *24*, 245.

WILCOX, W. C. and H. S. GINSBERG, 1963, Proc. Soc. Exptl. Biol. Med. *114*, 37.

WISSEMAN, C. L., JR., M. KITAOKA and T. TAMIYA, 1966, Am. J. Trop. Med. Hyg. *15*, 588.

YOSHINO, K. and S. TANOGUCKI, 1965a, Virology *26*, 44.

YOSHINO, K. and S. TANIGUCHI, 1965b, Virology *26*, 61.

YASHINO, K., S. TANIGUCHI, R. FURUSE, T. NAJIMA, R. FUJII, M. MINAMITANI, R. TADA and H. KUBOTA, 1962, Japan. J. Med. Sci. Biol. *15*, 235.

CHAPTER 7

Immune responses to bacterial antigens

D. M. WEIR

Department of Bacteriology, University of Edinburgh Medical School, Edinburgh, Scotland

7.1. Introduction

Bacterial antigens have the distinction of being the first antigenic substances to attract the attention of biologists. This interest arose with the realization at the end of the last century that bacterial vaccines could be used to afford protection against infectious diseases.

Much effort has since then been expended by microbiologists at elucidating the immunochemical characteristics, genetics, environmental determinants and prophylactic use of bacterial antigens. Systems of identification and classification have been built up on knowledge of the antigenic characteristics of micro-organisms and some success has been achieved in the isolation and use of protective antigens extracted from bacteria and potent vaccines are in wide use against a large variety of infectious diseases.

The borders of immunology today extend far beyond the fields which nurtured its development and the emphasis has shifted into the highly complex biological problems of the relationship between cells and their environment and the molecular biology of the processes affected by such interaction.

Bacterial antigens are of importance in immunology today because they offer a readily available source of homogeneous, immunochemically defined material which allows the study of the relationship between the cells of the immune system and foreign antigenic materials that can in certain circumstances affect the survival of the individual.

7.2. The interaction of bacterial antigens with the immune system

7.2.1. Specific and non-specific effects

The effectiveness of an antigen, bacterial or non-bacterial is dependent on two characteristics of the potential antigen: (1) the specific immunochemical nature of the antigenic determinants and their phylogenetic relationship to the immunized animal – the more foreign the better the antigen – and (2) the non-specific effects on the lymphoid tissues of structures associated with the immunizing material which potentiate the immunogenicity of the antigen – this is sometimes called the 'built-in adjuvanticity' of the antigen molecule. This latter characteristic is a well recognized property of bacterial antigen and is an important immuno-logical phenomenon which has provided much insight into the workings of the immune system. Furthermore, these non-specific effects probably have important implications in situations where abnormal reactions of the immune system arise as in, for example, various autoimmune states. The non-specific effects of bacterial antigen on the immune system have been studied in detail in a number of instances including, for example, *Bordetella pertussis*, bacterial endotoxin, various corynebacteria, and lipid antigens of acid fast bacteria which are considered in Chapter 4.

The end result of an antigenic stimulus in terms of the level of circulating antibody or cell-mediated immunity is a reflection of two opposing processes – tolerance induction and immunity. One of the important factors determining the outcome of the stimulus is the presence of built-in adjuvanticity of the antigen molecule. It is well known that serum protein antigens such as bovine serum albumin (BSA) or bovine gamma globulin (BGG) can induce tolerance if presented to mice or rabbits in aggregate-free form (Dresser 1962; Pinckard et al. 1968). In contrast the same antigen in aggregated form will induce immunity. The aggregated material has added built-in adjuvanticity. This effect is not necessarily the same as that brought about by depot adjuvants such as Freund's adjuvant which act by means of slow release, granulomata formation and probably increased numbers and mobility of antibody-producing cells. Adjuvanticity in the form discussed here may act simply as a 'physiological switch' which directs a cell in contact with antigen to synthesize specific antibody rather than become tolerant (Dresser 1969). In the case of aggregated *versus* aggregate-free BSA, the adjuvanticity of the aggregated antigen in CBA mice is associated with a decrease in the lysosomal enzyme, acid phosphatase, of lymphocytes which in turn is associated with cell proliferation and antibody production (Jacob and Weir 1971) and the effect of aluminium phosphate injected intraperitoneally might be through an effect on macrophage lysosomes as proposed by Dresser (1969).

The effect of pertussis vaccine has for some time been recognized to be associated with a profound increase in the number of circulating leucocytes. The lymphocytosis is attributed to alteration in the patterns of circulation and not to increased production of these cells (Morse and

Riester 1967). The granulocytosis in contrast is partly due to increased production. Dresser has reported that after i.v. or i.p. injection of pertussis there is evidence for increased cell division in lymphoid organs and increase in weight and number of cells in the spleen but not in peripheral lymph nodes. The possibility that the dividing cells are non-circulating lymphocytes cannot be ruled out. These cells may be the non-circulating thymus-independent population of lymphocytes. If mice are neonatally thymectomized, the leucocytosis produced by pertussis vaccine is clearly reduced and this is associated with a marked decrease in the thymus-dependent population of lymphocytes in blood and peripheral lymphoid tissue (Kalpaktsoglou et al. 1969). It thus seems possible that the effect of pertussis vaccine is on both thymus-dependent and thymus-independent lymphocytes and would affect both cell-mediated and humoral immune responses. Further evidence is required on the effects of pertussis vaccine on these two expressions of immunity in both thymectomized and normal animals. The effects appear to be independent of increased phagocytotic activity of the reticulo-endothelial system. Elucidation of the cellular mechanisms involved probably requires extension to pertussis vaccine of the studies cited above on built-in adjuvanticity of serum protein antigen on lymphocyte and lysosome activity.

Certain Gram-positive organisms of the genus *Corynebacteriaceae* and in particular *C. parvum* seem capable of activating the immune system and of disturbing the balance between tolerance and immunity. Rabbits which are injected with a tolerogenic dose of aggregate-free BSA become hyperresponsive to the antigen if pretreated with *C. parvum* (15 mg. of a heat killed suspension injected intravenously). This immune response is associated with a rapid increase in the relative binding affinity of the antibody produced, comparable to the injection of alum-precipitated BSA (Pinckard et al. 1967, 1968). A similar effect has been noted in mice (McBride, unpublished results) using 5 mg. of killed organism and the stimulus to the immune system has been found to result in a transient haemolytic anaemia with the production of an immune response detected by both the immunocytoadherence technique and the Jerne plaque method. An even more marked effect has been noted with a 'corynebacterium-like' organism isolated from rheumatoid joint material. As little of 0.1 mg. dry weight of the organism stimulated an anti-mouse red cell response in CBA mice, with peak activity between 5 and 7 days (McCracken et al. 1971). This anti-red cell response could have significance as an explanation for the unexplained anaemia associated with rheumatoid arthritis.

Both the latter organism and *C. parvum* at these dose levels unlike pertussis vaccine lead to a blood leucopenia. This effect on the redistribution of the mobile cell population may account directly or indirectly for the observed adjuvant effects of these organisms. Increases in the activity of the reticulo-endothelial system, as judged by the usual criteria of clearance of colloidal carbon or radio-labelled antigen, and distribution changes as noted by autoradiographic examination cannot be equated directly with the adjuvant activity of *C. parvum* (McBride, unpublished results). The effects however may contribute along with other activities of the adjuvant to the altered reactivity of mice to tolerogenic doses of antigen. Preliminary evidence, using a cell transfer technique, shows that a glass-bead-column-purified lymphocyte population (taken from *C. parvum*-treated animals), as well as the macrophage population may be capable of transferring the altered responsiveness to BSA in mice (McBride, unpublished results). If these results can be confirmed, at least part of the activity of this adjuvant material would appear to be due to an effect on lymphocytes.

Another extensively studied bacterial derived substance with built-in adjuvanticity is the lipopolysaccharide of Gram-negative organisms referred to as bacterial endotoxin. The material has been implicated in activating cells of the reticulo-endothelial system and has effects on vascular permeability, probably involving activation of the complement system and anaphylotoxin (Lichtenstein et al. 1969). Endotoxin has been shown to alter lysosomal membranes causing release of β-glucuronidase and cathepsin (Weissman and Thomas 1962). The expression of the adjuvanticity properties of the material is in its ability to alter tolerance thresholds so that induction of unresponsiveness is prevented by, for example, aggregate-free bovine gamma globulin (BGG) (Claman 1963). The enhancement of RES phagocytic activity appears to be independent of the effect on tolerance induction (Golub and Weigle 1967). However, recent work by Spitznagel and Allison (1970) shows that macrophages from mice treated with endotoxin are more effective in inducing an immune response to BSA than macrophages from untreated animals. These workers were unable to show any demonstrable effect on the uptake or degradation of antigen by macrophages. Endotoxin treatment of lymphocytes in contrast to these results failed to alter their response to BSA. The *in vitro* effect of endotoxin on lymphoid cells in culture in facilitating priming of the cells may enable the elucidation of the mechanisms whereby the material alters cellular activity.

In studies performed with *Salmonella* flagellin from *S. adelaide* (Parish and Ada 1969) separation of the immunogenic fraction of the molecule from the components carrying the built-in-adjuvanticity has been achieved using a cynanogen bromide digest of flagellin. Fragment A with a molecular weight of about 18,000 contains most if not all of the antigenic determinants of the molecule. This fragment had altered *in vivo* properties compared to the whole molecule showing, for example, different patterns of localization in the lymph nodes. In order to express its full immunogenicity it required to be combined with the other lower molecular weight fragments B, C and D which enabled fragment A to be taken into the medullary macrophage.

These important observations, it is hoped, will lead to further studies of the *in vivo* biological properties of bacterial antigen with a view to localizing the immunogenic and adjuvant structures of the bacterial cell antigens. At present there is a remarkable lack of information of this type.

In considering the effects of these bacterial substances on the interaction of the cells of the immune system with the environment there are 3 levels at which they may act:

(1) They may act at the level of the cell membrane, perhaps by altering the effects of exoenzymes present at the cell surface which might be considered normally to serve as a sensing mechanism to explore and react to environmental changes. Another possible effect at the cell membrane is on transport enzymes or permeases thus altering the passage of antigen molecules from the environment into the interior of the cell. The observation in this laboratory of increased lymphocytic acid phosphatase levels and an increase in its density on gradient centrifugation when CBA mice are given tolerogenic doses of aggregate-free BSA suggests a passage of antigen into the cell (Jacob and Weir 1971). This could conceivably be altered in the presence of an appropriate stimulus such as that provided by bacterial endotoxin or other source of adjuvanticity. In this experimental situation heat-aggregated BSA (with built-in-adjuvanticity) has the opposite effect to the aggregate-free material and results in decrease in acid phosphatase levels of splenic lymphocytes at 48 hrs after stimulation. It might thus be suggested that this difference is due to alteration in cell permeability associated with aggregated antigenic stimulus.

(2) The stimulus might alter intracellular processing of antigen either in a cell which might respond directly to an antigen or alternatively in a co-operating cell such as a macrophage. In the case of aggregate-free antigens which can readily induce tolerance (perhaps by direct contact with the lymphocyte membrane), more efficient uptake and degradation by macrophages would be likely to protect lymphocytes from direct contact with the tolerogenic antigen.

(3) Recent evidence on the effect of localized injection of adjuvant material on the draining lymph node (Taub et al. 1970) indicates that paracortical expansion and hyperplasia are characteristic histological accompaniments to the injection of substances with adjuvanticity. These

findings have led to the suggestion that these changes may be partly due to augmented cellular traffic which would facilitate contact between immunocompetent cells and trapped antigen and lead to blast transformation. Such an interpretation would be consistent with the effects of pertussis organisms in increasing blood lymphocyte levels and decreasing the numbers in the thymus and peripheral lymph nodes. In the experiments cited above, the contralateral nodes did indeed show a slight decrease in cellularity.

7.2.2. Tolerance induction and bacterial antigens

Immunological tolerance is the subject of a vast literature describing the dose requirements, duration, specificity and abrogation of the phenomenon. The precise cellular mechanisms underlying tolerance induction remain even today a matter of speculation. In general terms an antigen which is able to diffuse freely in the body fluids is more tolerogenic than immunogenic. In comparison an antigen which is readily taken up on the surface of cells of the reticulo-endothelial system or taken into such cells, is more immunogenic than tolerogenic. Particulate bacterial antigens fall into the latter category.

The now classical report of Mitchison (1964) describing low- and high-zone tolerance with an intermediate immunizing zone has attracted much attention and many immunological phenomena are now interpreted in terms of this idea. Like many studies on tolerance, use was made of relatively weak serum protein antigens phylogenetically close to the host, injected in soluble form. Weak immunogens can be converted to powerful immunogens by combination with adjuvants. This added adjuvant effect prevents tolerance induction to the antigen. Thus in the case of bacterial antigens phylogenetically distant to the host, capable of inducing a strong immune response and able to be readily phagocytosed, induction of tolerance is a very difficult matter which appears to involve very large doses of antigen.

Low-zone tolerance is understandably readily induced by weakly immunogenic antigens which can remain in contact with lymphocytes sufficiently long to induce paralysis without at the same time inducing immunity. As immunity can be induced by a very small number of molecules of antigen (e.g., 100 ng of *Salmonella* flagellin) a role has been suggested for the dendritic macrophages in concentrating the antigen molecules in a small area and allowing intimate contact with a mobile population of lymphocytes in the spleen and lymph nodes. In the situation where tolerance is induced, either this concentration mechanism (perhaps dependent on antibody on the surface of macrophages) is affected by the presence of higher concentrations of antigen, or is not operative because of the absence of appropriate antibody on the surface of macrophages. It would seem possible that weakly immunogenic antigens have this property because of the absence of macrophage localization (normally due either to specific or perhaps cross-reacting antibody). This is borne out by the work of Ada et al. (1964) who found that weakly immunogenic antigens were only weakly localized in the lymphoid follicle by dendritic macrophages, whilst highly immunogenic material such as *Salmonella* antigens were readily localized. With this type of explanation in mind it is thus of considerable interest to show if low zone tolerance can be induced to highly immunogenic *Salmonella* antigen. This has recently been achieved by Shellam and Nossal (1968) using the soluble flagellin antigen of *Salmonella adelaide* (100 μg in neonatal rats) and even more significantly by the *particulate* antigen, polymerized flagellin of the same bacterium, $10^{-3} - 10^{-5}$ pg/g body weight daily for 2 weeks from the day of birth in rats. Two zones of tolerance were noted, the higher zone requiring doses ten times larger than the low doses.

The response to polymerized flagellin is qualitatively and quantitatively different from other models. The antigen concentration required for low zone induction is extremely small (about 10^{-20} M), much lower than soluble flagellin (about 10^{-14} M) or BSA (about 10^{-8} M). Shellam (1969) points out that the effectiveness of these extremely low concentrations of polymerized flagellin defies detailed interpretation. It seems likely that the absence of follicular localization that occurs in newborn rats is partly responsible for this phenomenon and it can be predicted that tolerance induction in adults to these antigens would follow an entirely different pattern in view of the known follicular localization that occurs. In general, it can be concluded that low-zone tolerance induction in adult animals with highly immunogenic bacterial antigens is an unlikely possibility.

In contrast to this view, linking absence of follicular localization with tolerance induction is the approach of Parish and Ada (1969) who propose that antigen located in the medulla of lymph nodes may be concerned with antibody formation and immunological memory, whereas antigen localized in the follicles may either trigger primed cells or induce tolerance. This idea is supported by their observation with cyanogen bromide digests of *Salmonella* flagellin. Fragment A, which appeared to be the immunologically active ingredient of the digest, was the fragment which was capable of inducing tolerance and which localized strongly in the lymphoid follicles.

This type of work with bacterial antigens is of considerable value in elucidating the parameters of tolerance induction with antigens of different types and is useful groundwork required for example in the possible future of strong and weak histocompatibility antigens in transplantation immunology.

Studies on tolerance induction by bacterial endotoxin have been made possible by alkali detoxication thus allowing the administration of large quantities of material which would in normal circumstances kill the recipient and with such detoxified endotoxin it proved possible to give sufficient material to produce complete paralysis by a single injection into adult mice (Britton 1969). The range between a paralysing and an immunizing dose was narrow and between 1 and 3 mg. was found to immunize whilst 8 mg induced paralysis. Like heterologous protein antigens, the lower immunizing doses of this antigen resulted in the highest number of antibody-producing cells and the highest antibody titres. This is considered to be due to the higher doses inducing an increasing degree of paralysis and thus less immunization. No distinct low-zone paralysis was found with this antigen in contrast to the work of Shellam and Nossal (1968) discussed above. However, the work with endotoxin was performed in adult animals and no definite conclusion can be drawn yet in the light of the need to use newborn animals which would not be expected to show follicular localization of the antigen and thus to be more readily rendered tolerant by low doses of antigen.

This study provided some interesting information on the mechanisms of maintenance of the tolerant state which is generally considered to be dependent on persistence of antigen or its fragments. The tolerant state to endotoxin was found to be remarkably short (about 36 days) despite the fact that the lipopolysaccharide persists in an immunologically active form for at least 45 days in mice. Britton offers the explanation that in view of the fact that an intact thymus is required for recovery from immunological paralysis, any increased activity of the thymus would be likely to hasten the process. It is known that bacterial endotoxin causes cellular depletion of the thymus (Rowlands et al. 1965) and Britton tentatively suggests that this results in an increased rate of repopulation of the thymus by bone marrow precursors, thus augmenting the rate of formation of immunocompetent clones and thus breaking paralysis. On the other hand the observations on the effects of endotoxin on the thymus were made using a non-detoxified material (likely to exert a toxic effect on thymus cells) and thus cannot necessarily be compared directly with work using detoxified material. It seems more likely that the observation might be simply explained by suggesting a direct stimulatory effect of detoxified endotoxin on an intact thymus with resulting enhanced thymic influence on the peripheral lymphoid tissues. The precise mechanism underlying this interesting observation will clearly require further investigation.

Tolerance induction as discussed above is thought to be the end result of a process of concomitant immune stimulation and paralysis of lymphocytes, the antigen being presented in such a way that the final outcome is tolerance rather than immunity.

Bacterial endotoxin, as has been noted, can be used after detoxification in large doses to bring about tolerance in adult mice. Mice which have been pre-immunized with *E. coli* can be paralysed 24 hrs later with a large dose of endotoxin (Britton 1969). However before paralysis developed there was a normal exponential increase in the number of IgM producing plaque-forming cells for 70–90 hrs. No serum antibodies were detected presumably because of the large excess of circulating endotoxin. The conclusion drawn from these data is that once antigen-sensitive cells are triggered by antigen to transform and divide for antibody production, they are insensitive to antigen. The cells which can be suppressed are limited to those that are uncommitted and sensitive to antigen. Similar observations have been made with respect to tolerance induction in non-bacterial systems. One of the major difficulties of explanations of this type is that no account is taken of one of the probable pathways taken by triggered transforming lymphocytes towards memory cells (probably small lymphocytes). If committed cells are insensitive to paralysis by antigen, then memory cells would be expected to survive for later reactivation by antigen. This would be inconsistent with a state of true tolerance.

Unfortunately, in the experiments just described, the evidence for paralysis was based on the final falling off of the numbers of plaque-forming cells and the animals were not challenged again with endotoxin which would have shown if memory cells had persisted. It had, however, previously been shown (Britton 1969) that paralysis by endotoxin (without pre-immunization) was present 8–21 days later when the animals were challenged.

It is possible that antigen-sensitive cells when exposed to a tolerogenic stimulus do actually differentiate to antibody-producing cells but what is responsible for tolerance is that the cells fail to proliferate in the usual manner at the time when blast transformation occurs. Perhaps the trigger for proliferation depends upon interaction with the macrophage. Thus, as in the experiments just cited, antibody-forming cells may be found but these would not show the exponential increase in numbers associated with the development of immunity. This phenomenon has been described after a tolerogenic dose of pneumococcal polysaccharide antigen in mice (Howard et al. 1969). Whether this antigen is a special case in view of its persistence in the host or if this phenomenon is true of antigen in general, has not yet been established. Work with other antigens such as sheep red blood cells whilst showing that during tolerance induction plaque-forming cells are initially formed, is complicated by the possibility that the responding cells are directed at a minor antigenic component of the red cell membrane and that tolerance only develops to such antigen on repeated exposure. Preliminary experiments with a tolerogenic dose of aggregate-free BSA in the author's laboratory failed to show in CBA mice more than a very few spleen cells making anti-BSA using the immunocytoadherence technique.

7.2.3. Interaction of bacterial antigens with cells of the immune system
The possibility has received much attention in the last few years that lymphocytes interact directly with antigen leading either to transformation to immunoblasts or perhaps to tolerance induction. It is known that lymphocytes appear to be coated with immunoglobulins, or fractions thereof, on the basis of the ability to induce transformation with various specific anti-immunoglobulin sera (Sell and Gell 1965) or by the uptake of labelled antisera (Raff et al. 1970). That this immunoglobulin is specific antibody is suggested by the work of Byrt and Ada (1969) who found that a labelled bacterial protein, flagellin of *Salmonella adelaide* was taken up by lymphocyte-like cells of the mouse and rat spleen, thoracic duct, peritoneal exudate and bone marrow by autoradiography. The reaction of antigen with cells from all tissues examined was inhibited by specific antisera to mouse immunoglobulins except in the case of bone marrow. The uptake of labelled antigen could be inhibited by pretreatment of the cells with excess unlabelled material. The authors calculated that under the conditions of the test about 17,000 molecules of flagellin were taken up by each cell – this occupied less than 0.1% of the cell surface. Whilst various types of cell took up antigen on their surface – macrophage of peritoneal exudates and polymorphs of spleen and bone marrow – the cells which reacted most strongly were clearly mononuclear cells with a very high nuclear-cytoplasmic ratio, $6–12\ m\mu$ in diameter. These cells resembling lymphocytes were tentatively termed lymphocyte-like cells. It is not possible to decide if all the reactive cells are precursors of cells which will go on to make specific antibodies to the bacterial antigen. That this is unlikely is suggested by comparisons of the numbers of spleen cells reacting with labelled flagellin ($400–900$ labelled cells$/10^6$ spleen cells) with only 10 to $50/10^6$ spleen cells reacting in response to sheep red blood cells. The latter estimate is however obtained in the *in vivo* situation and may not be directly comparable. The authors favour the view that the reacting cells represent a virgin population which have synthesized small amounts of specific anti-flagellin antibody and are attempting to resolve the question further

by studies in tolerant, thymectomized and immune animals. One of the difficulties of studies of this type is that they say very little about what is likely to happen in the *in vivo* situation when antigen is presented to the lymphoid organs and involving complex inter-relationships between macrophages and lymphoid cells, between 'antigen-reactive' lymphocytes and bone marrow-derived immunoglobulin-producing cells. Their value lies in elucidating the nature of the lymphocyte surface membrane and how it can interact with its environment. The question of the steps leading to immunoglobulin production either in the cell which comes in direct contrast with antigen or as a result of intercellular co-operation will probably only be elucidated in intact lymphoid organs.

7.3. *Genetic control of the immune response and bacterial antigens*

The immunogenicity of bacterial antigens has been discussed in relation to the interaction of the antigens with the lymphoid tissues taking into account both non-specific and specific effects. Consideration of these interactions is usually a reflection of interest in elucidating the cellular mechanisms of antibody production, immune tolerance and the important question of initiation of the immune response by selective, genetically determined, cell responses. Less often considered is the problem of the genetic control of the immune response with respect to patterns of inheritance of the ability of particular strains of animals to respond to certain antigens.

Genetic variations are considered by Dr. Battisto in Chapter 11 of this volume. The ability of only certain guinea-pigs to respond to the dinitrophenyl hapten attached to a poly-L-lysine carrier has been known for some time. This Mendelian dominant trait is thought possibly to be effective at the antigen-processing stage of the immune response. In the context of a discussion on bacterial immunogenicity mention should be made of a report by Auzins and Rowley (1969) indicating strain differences in mice in their ability to respond to O-somatic anti--gens of *Salmonella typhimurium*. BALB/C mice, injected with a standard dose of *S. typhimurium* C5 vaccine, were found to be less responsive than Swiss white strain mice. The BALB/C mice failed to respond to antigen 5 and their response to the 1, 4 and 12 O-somatic antigens, whilst reaching the same magnitude as Swiss mice, was less prolonged. The susceptibility of BALB/C mice to the organisms is thought to be related to their failure to respond to antigen 5. Why the BALB/C mice fail to respond to antigen 5 is not clear but their ability to phagocytose and process the organism is indicated by the response to the other somatic antigens. Auzins and Rowley propose that the difference may be in the requirement of a larger dose of antigen 5 to induce immunity. BALB/C mice can be protected against *S. typhimurium* infection by immunization with large doses of O-acetylated galactan which cross-reacts with antigen 5.

This phenomenon can be distinguished from the overall hyper-reactivity of some strains of mice to protein antigen, e.g., BSA in NZB mice compared to CBA, DBA/2 and C57 Bl strains (Weir et al. 1968) or BGG (Staples and Talal 1969).

These latter observations appear not to be selective for particular antigens as is found in Auzins and Rowley's experiments but are more likely to be due to an overall over-reactivity of the lymphoid tissues involving both macrophage uptake and processing, and lymphocyte reactivity.

7.4. Bacterial antigens and the heterogeneity of the immune response

The immune response to bacterial antigens has several characteristics which led to the view that this form of response was different from that to soluble protein antigens. Amongst the differences are those related to the particular class or classes of immunoglobulin stimulated by these antigens. IgM antibodies can readily be detected after immunization of various species with the somatic-O antigen of *Salmonella*. These antibodies appear within a few days after immunization whilst in contrast IgG antibodies take more than a month before they can be detected in the blood.

This widely held view of the immune response to bacterial antigens has had to be modified since it was shown that purified IgM anti-*Salmonella typhimurium* O antibody had as much as 1000 times the agglutinating, bactericidal and opsonizing activity of its IgG counterpart when compared on a molar basis (Robbins et al. 1965). Furthermore, hyperimmune sera yielded much more IgG antibody than IgM. Clearly then, the greatly exaggerated serological activity of IgM antibodies can result in a very false impression as to the molar content of the different classes of immunoglobulin in immune serum. These difficulties illustrate well the dangers in drawing conclusions from tests which depend on secondary phenomena which arise following primary antibody-antigen union. Such tests, as is now recognized, are subject to the differing biological activities of the different immunoglobulin classes. Only when tests designed to detect primary binding of antigen and antibody are used, can valid conclusions be drawn. An even more direct approach is to examine the production of individual immunoglobulin classes by individual cells.

By means of specific antiglobulin sera to rabbit IgG and IgM Altmeier et al. (1966) have been able to characterize the primary and secondary response to the O-somatic antigen of *Salmonella typhimurium*. These workers were able to establish that IgG antibody could be increased to 17 times the concentration of the IgM agglutinating antibody without changing the end point of the IgM titre in the antiglobulin test. Anti-globulin tests carried out on whole sera would thus give titres representing only the activity of the specific immunoglobulin class being examined. IgG antibody was found to appear as early as 5 to 8 days after immunization and exhibited an initial increase in concentration roughly parallel to IgM antibody. After secondary stimulation IgG activity rapidly reached levels 10 to 100 times those noted in the primary response. The authors conclude that there remains little reason to consider the antibody response to somatic antigens to be very different from that induced by soluble protein antigens.

Again using an antiglobulin test with specific antisera for human IgG, IgA, IgM and IgD, Kerr et al. (1967) were able to show that in addition to IgM agglutinating antibodies in human brucellosis, non-agglutinating IgG and IgA also existed specific for the *Brucella* antigen. This confirmed and extended earlier work in which non-agglutinating complement-fixing IgG was found to be characteristic of chronic brucellosis (Kerr et al. 1966; Coghlan and Weir 1967). These observations give added support to the view that bacterial antigens behave in much the same way as soluble protein antigen in the immune response.

A primary binding method utilizing radio-iodinated diphtheria toxoid in antigen excess has been applied to the study of the immunoglobulin classes in human sera with activity against this antigen. The complexes of antibody and antigen were precipitated with rabbit antibody specific for IgG, IgA or IgM and the radioactivity in the precipitate converted to the binding value for antibody (Newcomb and Ishizaka 1967).

Following immunization with 0.5 ml. alum-precipitated diphtheria toxoid, 8 of 10 humans had a measurable IgG response and 5 of these also produced IgA antitoxin. The ratio of the IgG to IgA was about 6:1, but the magnitude of the IgA response bore no simple relationship to the size of the IgG response. The subject with the highest IgG response had one of the lowest IgA responses. None of the sera had any detectable IgM antitoxin. Four patients with dysgammaglobulinaemia, with IgM levels as high as 10 times normal, also failed to produce any IgM antitoxin after immunization, producing only IgG and IgA.

This unexpected result is interpreted as suggesting that any IgM antibodies produced to diphtheria antigens are directed towards antigen lacking in highly purified toxoid preparations. These data contrast with other reports suggesting the presence of IgM antibodies in humans and rabbits able to combine with diphtheria toxin but significantly, unable to neutralize its toxicity (Robbins 1965). As the IgM antibody was detected by passive haemagglutination, it seems very likely that the IgM was directed at non-toxoid impurities. Bauer et al. (1963) noted that IgM anti-diphtheria antibodies required prolonged contact at 0°C with diphtheria toxin before neutralization occurred. It thus seems likely that IgM antibodies in the *in vivo* situation play no part in the neutralization of the toxigenic properties of diphtheria exotoxin. Another interesting finding, arising from the work of Newcomb and Ishizaka, was that polymers of IgA had greater toxoid-binding activity than monomer IgA and this is in line with the greater efficiency of polymeric IgA in haemagglutination tests.

The IgA antitoxin has a poorer neutralizing ability than IgG and it has been suggested that IgA is directed at fewer determinants on the toxin molecule (Raynaud 1967).

It can thus be seen that in general there is no difference between bacterial antigens and protein antigens in the characteristics of the immune response which they call forth. There are however differences within each group which can determine the final expression of the immune response. Some of these characteristics have already been considered, e.g., the phylogenetic relationship to the host with its effect on the immunogenicity of the antigen – tolerance or immunity, whether an antigen can directly transform the lymphocyte for antibody production or if it requires the help of the macrophage. Another feature determining the host response is the physical state of the antigen – whether it be particulate (as are many bacterial antigens) or soluble. The particulate flagellar antigen polymerized flagellin of *Salmonella adelaide* appears to preferentially stimulate an IgM immune response (Ada et al. 1965) in the same way as the protein antigen thyroglobulin which when coated onto acrylic particles results in a prolonged IgM response (Torrigiani and Roitt 1965). The same appears to be true of particulate subcellular tissue antigens (Weir 1967). In contrast, little or no IgM antibody was detected in the sera of rats injected with soluble flagellin antigen (Ada et al. 1965).

A bacterial antigen which has been extensively studied with respect to its selective effect on immunoglobulin production is the endotoxin of *E. coli*. This antigen preferentially stimulates synthesis of IgM, and IgG antibodies have not been detected even after several months of immunization in mice.

The question of whether or not there are two cell lines responsible for IgG and IgM synthesis is at the moment a highly controversial one and how these cells are regulated is very uncertain. Feedback inhibition by both IgM and IgG antibody may occur but is probably concerned more with the intensity of the response than in the control of which particular class of immunoglobulin is produced. However, it is conceivable that should an antigen be able for some reason to stimulate a high and rapidly appearing IgM response, then the remaining antigen might be diverted from those cells capable of initiating IgG antibodies. Such a situation might be envisaged in the presence of an existing degree of immunity to an antigen, shared perhaps between the immunizing antigen and another material with which the animal had had previous contact. This would fit with the finding that whilst low doses of IgM antibody passively administered can increase the immune response to sheep erythrocytes, higher doses cause suppression. Bacterial endotoxin after one injection results in a first peak of IgM antibody within a few days. The antibody by combining with antigen interferes with stimulation of further immunocompetent cells and as the antibody level falls off suppression would end, thus leading in the presence of persisting antigen to a further stimulation of IgM antibody. This pattern would repeat itself until the antigen had disappeared (Möller 1969).

A consequence of such a mechanism would be that higher doses of antigen should be able to overcome this selective formation of IgM antibodies. In the case of bacterial endotoxin, this cannot normally be tested because of its toxic effects in high doses (the appropriate experiments have not been performed using detoxified material). However, experiments with sheep red blood cells injected, mixed with antiserum, support this possibility. As the ratio of cells to antiserum was increased, IgG antibody was formed. The conclusion drawn from these experiments was that for the appearance of IgG precursors, an intensive proliferation and selection process is needed involving the presence of antigen (Šterzl 1969). The question may be asked as to the participation of thymus-derived antigen-reactive cells and marrow-derived antibody producing cells. Is it possible that the thymus-derived cells are IgM producing and that these co-operate with the marrow-derived cells for a complete immune response? The restriction described above would depend on a failure to involve the marrow-derived population.

The relationship of the dose of antigen to the quality of the antibody produced is difficult to study with bacterial antigens. It might be predicted, however, on the basis of studies with hapten conjugates, that low doses of bacterial antigens would be likely to produce higher-affinity antibody than would higher doses of antigen. The smaller quantity of antigen stimulating only those cells which, by virtue of having higher-affinity receptors, could capture the available antigen. Such a response would also result in the late appearance of antibody as the fewer cells stimulated would take some time to proliferate and produce immunoglobulins in quantity.

Consideration of this type would have implications for the type of immunization schedule desirable to produce effective levels of high-quality antibody and argues for a small initial stimulus with an interval of some weeks to allow the development of a large population of cells producing high-affinity antibody followed by a larger secondary stimulus to increase this cell population further.

7.5. *The cell-mediated immune response and bacterial antigens*

Cell-mediated immunity was first recognized in chronic bacterial disease and was known as bacterial allergy or allergy of infection. The classical example of this form of immune reactivity is the response to the antigen of the tubercle bacillus known as delayed hypersensitivity to distinguish it from the rapidly appearing or immediate form of hypersensitivity due to humoral antibodies. The delayed hypersensitivity reactions in experimental animals have been shown to depend on the activity of living cells (lymph node, spleen and peripheral white blood cells) which can be transferred to a normal animal. The lymphocyte has been identified as the important cell in this transfer process. It is now clearly established that for the development of cell-mediated immunity an intact thymus is required and that thymus-dependent lymphocytes can be found in the white pulp of the spleen around the central arteries and in the paracortical areas of the lymph nodes. Furthermore, there is a recirculation process from these areas which enables competent lymphocytes to pass through the body tissues and come in contact with any foreign material which has entered the tissues. Despite many years of effort the detailed mechanisms of an interaction of the lymphocyte and antigen in cell-mediated immunity are far from being understood. In part, this has been due to the absence of a quantitative assay of cell-mediated immunity with only the development of a skin reaction to injected antigen in a sensitive individual as the available test.

A step forward was the *in vitro* test of macrophage migration inhibition of George and Vaughan (1965). This developed from earlier observations using spleen, bone marrow and buffy coat explants from sensitized animals in which macrophage migration could be inhibited by various

                    D. M. Weir

bacterial antigens, including those from tubercle bacilli, streptococci, and brucellae (see Turk 1967).

The relationship of migration inhibition to cell-mediated immunity was shown by the correlation between inhibition and delayed hypersensitivity reactions to diphtheria toxoid and ovalbumin and the absence of inhibition in the presence of precipitating antibody in the absence of a delayed component (David et al. 1964). Migration inhibition was found to depend on the presence of a small percentage of lymphocytes in the macrophage suspension and normal macrophages could be rendered sensitive to inhibition if mixed with a small proportion of sensitized lymphocytes.

Trypsin treatment of the cells was found to prevent migration inhibition *in vitro*, but if trypsin-treated lymphocytes were transferred to a normal animal, delayed hypersensitivity reactions could be induced in the recipient. This has been explained as a recovery by the lymphocytes from the effects of trypsin, supported by the finding that puromycin and actinomycin D could inhibit the effect of lymphocytes on macrophages, suggesting that the cells require intact protein synthetic mechanisms (Turk 1967).

An active material has been extracted from the supernatant of 24 hr cultures of lymphocytes and PPD antigen (25 μg) and the material has been found to be associated with a Sephadex G100 peak of molecular weight of 67,000 (Bennett and Bloom 1968). This study, although in the main performed in non-inbred Hartley guinea-pigs, was also carried out using an inbred strain (strain XIII) with the same results, thus ruling out the possibility that the results depended on histocompatibility differences between lymphocytes and macrophages of different animals.

In a recent comprehensive study, Dumonde and his colleagues (1969) have described assays on MIF and three other factors, generated by activated guinea-pig lymphocytes exposed to antigen *in vitro*: an inflammatory factor (probably equivalent to lymph node permeability factor) assayed by permeability changes leading to the accumulation in the skin of radio-labelled protein previously injected into the animal's circulation, a cytopathic factor active against mouse fibroblasts estimated by ^{51}Cr release and a mitogenic factor assayed by ^{3}H thymidine uptake of lymphocytes exposed to the supernatant material. It was concluded from purification procedures that the soluble factors were not retained antigen, intact antibody or complexes of antigen and antibody. It is not yet clear, however, if the different cell-free activities can be attributed to a single molecule or multiple molecular entities.

The chemical nature and mechanisms of activation and action of these lymphocyte-generated substances awaits elucidation, but their role as possible regulators of lymphocyte proliferation and macrophage concentration in cell-mediated responses is of considerable interest. Of particular importance is the role of different populations, antigen reactive thymus-derived cells and marrow-derived antibody-producing lymphocytes in participating in the generation of these factors. Do these factors assist, as suggested by Dumonde and his colleagues, in facilitating co-operation between compartments of the lymphoid system? What features of the antigen determine the expression of this form of immunity? Is it possible to distinguish between the effects of different antigenic forms in the stimulation of different aspects of the cell-mediated response as is the case in humoral immunity? Are tolerance mechanisms in the cell-mediated immune system similar to those in antibody-mediated immunity or is only the immunologically specific 'antibody-like receptor' on the lymphocyte involved? What is the chain of events following contact of antigen with a sensitized lymphocyte? What is the explanation of the fact that vaccination with BCG leads to delayed hypersensitivity and provides protection, yet development of delayed hypersensitivity to the Wax D fraction of the tubercle bacillus is not associated with protection of animals from challenge with virulent organisms? What is the relationship between the extent of the allergic response and protection in bacterial infections? Only when answers to some of these questions are available, will it be possible to assess with any certainty the mechanisms and role of cell-mediated immune reactions in bacterial allergy. The situation at the moment allows only uninformed guesswork.

7.5.1. *Lymphoid cells and macrophage activity in bacterial immunity*

The microbicidal properties of macrophage are a well recognized phenomenon and that this can be enhanced in an immunologically non-specific manner has been established by the extensive studies of Mackaness and his colleagues on *Listeria monocytogenes* infections in mice (see Mackaness and Blanden 1967). Recent evidence from these workers show that adoptive transfer of both protection against *L. monocytogenes* and delayed hypersensitivity can be achieved by filtered (macrophage-deficient) spleen cell suspensions obtained from *Listeria*-infected mice (Mackaness 1969). The cells concerned are inactivated by anti-lymphocyte globulin (which appears not to react with macrophages) and are devoid of protective activity when transferred to X-irradiated recipients suggesting that radio-sensitive cells, probably macrophages, are influenced by the transferred lymphocytes. Thus the protective effect is not directly brought about by the lymphocytes themselves.

An important point with wider implications which emerges from these studies is that anti-lymphocyte globulin can only suppress immune mechanisms if the committed cells recirculate and that extravascular cells are not readily inactivated (Mackaness and Hill 1969). This conclusion supports the observations of Denman and Frankel (1968) and means that differences in susceptibility of various states of immunity to suppression can be explained by their anatomical location rather than inherent differences in the cells themselves.

The mechanism of activation of host macrophages by immune lymphoid cells remains to be established, but Mackaness (1969) considers that the macrophage migration inhibitory factor (MIF) may be involved. This is supported by the slower development of resistance in the liver than in the spleen where the lymphoid cells are more abundant. Whether or not MIF is responsible for all the functional and morphological changes in macrophage activity remains at the moment a matter of speculation and a possible role of cytophilic antibody, elaborated by immune lymphocytes, cannot be excluded.

7.6. *Summary and conclusions*

The interaction of bacterial antigens with the immune system can be seen to consist of (1) specific effects depending on the nature of the antigenic determinants carried by the micro-organism and (2) non-specific effects which can be thought of as adjuvant-like activity. Some recent success has been achieved in the separation of these two effects in *Salmonella* flagellin, the fragments containing the adjuvanticity, altering the pattern of localization of the antigenic fragment. Follicular localization of bacterial antigen appears likely to be of importance in deciding whether tolerance or immunity develops and has wide implications in immunology. Another effect which may occur in parallel is an augmentation in cellular traffic facilitating contact between immunocompetent cells and the trapped antigen.

Studies with bacterial antigens have thrown light on the interaction of the lymphocyte with its environment showing that some 17,000 molecules of flagellin are taken up by individual cells occupying less than 0.1% of the cell surface. Further work is required to ascertain what proportion of reactive cells go on to make antibody and whether inter-cellular co-operation is required for this. Low-zone tolerance in adult animals to highly immunogenic bacterial antigens seems an unlikely possibility.

Bacterial antigens despite earlier doubts appear to behave like other non-bacterial antigens with respect to their ability to stimulate the various aspects of the immune response.

The relationship between bacterial antigens and the cell-mediated immune response presents at the moment an extremely complex and ill-defined picture. The role of lymphocyte factors in facilitating co-operation between compartments of the lymphoid system is an area wide open to investigation and the importance of this is indicated by the apparent ability of lymphocytes to influence macrophages to resist infective agens.

References

ADA, G. L., G. J. V. NOSSAL and C. M. AUSTIN, 1964, Aust. J. Exptl. Med. Sci. *42*, 331.

ADA, G. L., G. J. V. NOSSAL and C. M. AUSTIN, 1965, Studies on the nature of immunogenicity employing soluble and particulate bacterial proteins. *In*: J. Šterzl, ed.: Molecular and cellular basis of antibody formation. Prague, Czechoslovak Acad. Science. p. 31.

ALTEMEIER, W. A., J. B. ROBBINS and R. T. SMITH, 1966, J. Exptl. Med. *124*, 443.

AUZINS, I. and D. ROWLEY, 1969, Immunology *17*, 579.

BAUER, D. C., M. J. MATHIES and A. B. STAVITSKY, 1963, J. Exptl. Med. *117*, 889.

BENNETT, B. and B. R. BLOOM, 1968, Proc. Natl. Acad. Sci. U.S. *59*, 756.

BRITTON, S., 1969, Immunology *16*, 527.

BYRT, P. and G. L. ADA, 1969, Immunology *17*, 503.

CLAMAN, H. N. J., 1963, J. Immunol. *91*, 833.

COGHLAN, J. D. and D. M. WEIR, 1967, Brit. Med. J. *2*, 269.

DAVID, J. R., S. AL-ASKARI, H. S. LAWRENCE and L. THOMAS, 1964, J. Immunol. *93*, 264.

DENMAN, A. M. and E. P. FRANKEL, 1968, Immunology *14*, 107.

DRESSER, D. W., 1962, Immunology *5*, 378.

DUMONDE, D. C., R. A. WOLSTENCROFT, G. S. PANAYI, M. MATTHEW, J. MORLEY and W. T. HOWSON, 1969, Nature *224*, 38.

GEORGE, M. and J. H. VAUGHAN, 1962, Proc. Soc. Exptl. Biol. Med. *111*, 514.

GOLUB, E. S. and W. O. WEIGLE, 1967, J. Immunol. *98*, 1241.

HOWARD, J. G., J. ELSON, G. H. CHRISTIE and R. G. KINSKY, 1969, Clin. Exptl. Immunol. *4*, 41.

JACOB, K. H. A. and D. M. WEIR, 1971, Changes in acid phosphatase levels in liver and spleen after antigenic stimulation in mice. Immunology, in press.

KALPAKSTOGLOU, P. K., E. J. YUNIS and R. A. GOOD, 1969, Clin. Exptl. Immunol. *5*, 91.

KERR, W. R., J. D. COGHLAN, D. J. H. PAYNE and L. ROBERTSON, 1966, Lancet *2*, 1181.

KERR, W. R., D. J. H. PAYNE, L. ROBERTSON and R. R. A. COOMBS, 1967, Immunology *13*, 223.

LICHTENSTEIN, L. M., H. GEWURZ, N. F. ADKINSON, H. S. SHIN and S. E. MERGEN-HAGEN, 1969, Immunology *16*, 327.

MACKANESS, G. B., 1969, J. Exptl. Med. *129*, 973.

MACKANESS, G. B. and R. V. BLANDEN, 1967, Progr. Allergy *11*, 89.

MACKANESS, G. B. and W. C. HILL, 1969, J. Exptl. Med. *129*, 993.

MCCRACKEN, A., W. H. MCBRIDE and D. M. WEIR, 1971, Clin. Exptl. Immunol. *8*, 949.

MITCHISON, N. A., 1964, Proc. Roy. Soc. *B161*, 275.

MÖLLER, G., 1967, *in:* M. Landy and W. Braun, eds.: Immunological tolerance. New York, Academic Press. p. 220.

MORSE, S. I. and S. K. REISTER, 1967, J. Exptl. Med. *125*, 619.

NEWCOMB, R. W. and K. ISHIZAKA, 1967, J. Immunol. *99*, 40.

PARISH, C. R. and G. L. ADA, 1969, Immunology *17*, 153.

PINCKARD, R. N., D. M. WEIR and W. MCBRIDE, 1967, Clin. Exptl. Immunol. *2*, 331.

PINCKARD, R. N., D. M. WEIR and W. H. MCBRIDE, 1968, Clin. Exptl. Immunol. *3*, 413.

RAFF, M. C., M. STERNBERG and R. B. TAYLOR, 1970, Nature *225*, 553.

RAYNAUD, M., 1967, Heterogeneity of diphtheria antibodies. *In:* B. Cinader, ed.: Antibodies to biologically-active molecules. London, Pergamon Press. pp. 197–251.

ROBBINS, J. B., 1965, Studies on the interaction of immunoglobulins towards protein antigens with biological activity. *In:* J. Šterzl, ed.: Molecular and cellular basis of antibody formation. Prague, Czechoslovak Acad. Sci., pp. 241–251.

ROBBINS, J. B., K. KENNY and E. SUTER, 1965, J. Exptl. Med. *122*, 385.

ROWLANDS, D. T., H. N. CLAMAN and P. D. KIND, 1965, Amer. J. Path. *46*, 165.

SELL, S. and P. G. H. GELL, 1965, J. Exptl. Med. *122*, 432.

SHELLAM, G. R. and G. J. V. NOSSAL, 1968, Immunology *14*, 273.

SPITZNAGEL, J. K. and A. C. ALLISON, 1970, J. Immunol. *104*, 128.

STAPLES, P. J. and N. TALAL, 1969, J. Exptl. Med. *129*, 123.

ŠTERZL, J., 1967, *in:* M. Landy and W. Braun, eds.: Immunological tolerance. New York, Academic Press. p. 247.

TAUB, R. N., A. R. KRANTZ and D. W. DRESSER, 1970, Immunology *18*, 171.

TORRIAGIANI, G. and I. M. ROITT, 1965, J. Exptl. Med. *122*, 181.

TURK, J. L., 1967, Delayed hypersensitivity. Amsterdam, North-Holland.

WEIR, D. M., 1967, Lancet *2*, 1071.

WEIR, D. M., W. MCBRIDE and J. D. NAYSMITH, 1968, Nature *219*, 1276.

WEISSMAN, G. and L. THOMAS, 1962, J. Exptl. Med. *116*, 433.

CHAPTER 8

Immunity in the systemic mycoses

S. B. SALVIN*

Department of Microbiology, School of Medicine, University of Pittsburgh, Pittsburgh, Pa.

8.1. Introduction

Immunity in an individual animal to a given pathogen is defined classically as the capacity of that animal to destroy and eliminate all the cells of that pathogen from the host tissues. Thus, a mouse immune to a given strain of virulent pneumococcus is able to survive because of this power to destroy all cells of the pathogen, and therefore avoid acute disease and death.

Not all enhanced resistance, however, is that absolute. In chronic diseases, as exemplified by tuberculosis and the deep-seated or systemic mycoses, resistance, either natural or laboratory-induced, does not measure up to this degree. Apparently, the host-parasite relationships are such that the pathogen exhibits a relatively low grade of virulence and/or that the host has an innate partial immunity or resistance to invasion. Therefore, an increase in resistance by a given individual would tend to restrict growth and dissemination of the pathogen, although viable organisms may still remain in the host tissues.

This enhanced resistance, or partial immunity, has been demonstrated in the systemic mycoses in varying degrees. In coccidioidomycosis, enhanced resistance has been well illustrated, while in a disease such as sporotrichosis, enhanced resistance is, if present at all, of a low grade. In this paper, enhanced resistance, or partial immunity, is discussed for the following systemic mycoses: (1) aspergillosis, (2) candidiasis, (3) cryptococcosis, (4) N. American blastomycosis, (5) histoplasmosis, (6) coccidioidomycosis, and (7) sporotrichosis.

---

* Supported in part by the United States-Japan Cooperative Medical Science Program administered by the National Institute of Allergy and Infectious Diseases of the National Institutes of Health, Department of Health, Education, and Welfare (AT 08528).

8.2. Aspergillosis

Human infections with *Aspergillus* have been reported, with much of the disease due to such species as *A. fumigatus*, *A. flavus*, or *A. niger*. Such infections seldom are encountered, except in persons who are chronically ill or, more particularly who have been treated with corticosteroids or ACTH, or with broad spectrum antibiotics (Sidransky and Friedman 1958, 1959; Mankowski and Littleton 1954). In this regard, mice that inhaled large doses of *A. flavus* spores showed increased mortality on treatment with cortisone acetate, but not with antibiotics bicillin and tetracycline, whereas control mice were highly resistant to fatal pulmonary aspergillosis. Inhaled spores rapidly germinated into hyphae which grew throughout the lung tissue of mice treated with cortisone, but did not germinate into hyphae in the lungs of normal mice. The greater the number of spores that were inhaled and the longer the duration of cortisone treatment, the higher was the mortality rate. Amphotericin B was ineffective as a therapeutic agent in cortisone-treated mice exposed to spores.

Mice receiving 1.5 mg alloxan either 2 or 7 days before inhalation of spores also became highly susceptible to fatal pulmonary aspergillosis (Sidransky and Verney 1962). Whereas control mice developed only a mild nonfatal bronchitis and pneumonitis, the lungs of alloxan-treated mice after 3 days showed a bronchopneumonia with hyphal invasion from bronchi and bronchioles into the surrounding soft tissues.

Further studies with exposure of mice to aerosols of dry, viable spores of *A. flavus* indicated that a variety of agents or conditions, singly or in combination, can enhance host susceptibility (Sidransky et al. 1965). Thus, when mice were administered single doses of 200, 400, or 600 r total-body irradiation one day before exposure to fungal spores, a mortality of 20%, 55%, and 94% respectively resulted, whereas only 11% of control mice died. Mice pretreated with immunosuppressive drugs that produced a high degree of leucopenia had a high mortality on subsequent exposure to spores, namely, 63–100%. In this category were cyclophosphamide, fluorouracil, chlorambucil, mitomycin C, and mechlorethamine hydrochloride.

Mice were inoculated with various forms of transplantable lines of lymphoid leukaemia and four days later exposed to spores. A total of 61% to 84% of the dying mice had mild to moderate hyphal bronchopneumonia, while only 4% of the control mice had such signs.

The mechanism of the enhanced susceptibility of such treated mice was examined by light and electron microscopy (Epstein et al. 1967, 1968; Merkow et al. 1968). Spores phagocytosed by alveolar macrophages were partly or wholly enveloped in thin empty spaces inside phagocytic membranes. Lysosomes of control alveolar macrophages were densely aggregated in regions around the phagocytosed spores and were fusing with the phagocytic membranes. In contrast, alveolar macrophages from cortisone-treated mice that had phagocytosed spores, had lysosomes equally distributed through the cell cytoplasm. Also, fusion of the lysosomes into the phagocytic membranes was seldom observed. Thus, corticosteroids seem to have the property of stabilizing phagocytic membranes, and thereby of permitting rapid intracellular spore germination.

Although man and most laboratory animals are resistant to pulmonary infection with species of *Aspergillus*, birds are highly susceptible (Clark et al. 1954; Ainsworth and Rewell 1949). Among wild birds, aspergillosis is typically a disease of recently-captured water birds, although sporadic cases do appear in birds of all types after long periods of captivity. Possibly, the disease exists in the wild state far from contact with other animals. In one study of 68 cases, 45 yielded pure cultures of *A. fumigatus*, three of *A. flavus*, and one of *A. nidulans* (Ainsworth and Rewell 1949). For some weeks before death, the birds showed signs of emaciation and respiratory distress, in addition to loss of appetite and poor plumage. The high incidence of disease in captive penguins was reduced by rapid transportation under sanitary conditions from their native habitat and by their subsequent maintenance in an environment at low temperature and with filtered air.

Toxins have been isolated from cultures of *A. fumigatus* and *A. flavus* (Bodin and Gautier 1906; Henrici 1939; Tilden et al. 1961), and shown to be haemolytic, antigenic, and lethal in rabbits, guinea pigs and mice. When they are obtained from washed mycelium and from concentrated culture fluids, they act as powerful nephrotoxins and cause a characteristic necrosis in the kidney cortex. Immune sera, prepared in rabbits against the toxins, prevented all the toxic effects. Precipitation titres of these antisera were closely related to their neutralizing capacity.

The toxin from *A. fumigatus* was concentrated and purified by acetone precipitation, chromatography, and electrophoresis (Rau et al. 1961; Tilden et al. 1963; Wynston and Tilden 1963). Although the haemolytic and toxic properties were associated during migration in an electric field, they seemed to be two separate substances. Also, the nephrotoxin from *A. fumigatus* was different electrophoretically from the *A. flavus* toxin, although both toxins contained large amounts of carbohydrates.

Aspergillosis has also been implicated in cases of chronic asthma. The main features of the syndrome were periods of wheezing with low-grade fever, transient pulmonary infiltrates, and eosinophilia of blood and sputum. The sputum contained small plugs, which consisted of clumps of mycelia of *A. fumigatus* (Hinson et al. 1952). Such patients with allergic aspergillosis frequently had immediate-type skin reactions and precipitins to antigens from *A. fumigatus*. Hypersensitivity to the fungus may be the basis for the pulmonary eosinophilia, and precipitating antibody may be the basis for Arthus-like reactions in the lungs (Pepys et al. 1959; Campbell and Clayton 1964; Agbayani et al. 1967). One-month old culture filtrates, cell sap from mycelial mats, and saline extracts of dried mycelium were active in the order of decreasing potency in the detection of skin hypersensitivity. Such reactive patients also responded to a wide variety of extracts from other species of the genus.

References

AGBAYANI, B. F., P. S. NORMAN and W. L. WINKENWERDER, 1967, J. Allergy *40*, 319.

AINSWORTH, G. C. and R. E. REWELL, 1949, J. Comp. Pathol. Therap. *59*, 213.

BODIN, E. and L. GAUTIER, 1906, Ann. Inst. Pasteur *20*, 209.

CAMPBELL, M. J. and Y. M. CLAYTON, 1964, Am. Rev. Resp. Dis. *89*, 186.

CLARK, D. S., E. E. JONES, W. B. CROWL and F. K. ROSS, 1954, J. Am. Vet. Med. Assoc. *124*, 116.

EPSTEIN, S. M., T. D. MIALE, J. MOOSSY, E. VERNEY and H. SIDRANSKY, 1968, J. Neuropathol. Exptl. Neurol. *27*, 473.

EPSTEIN, S. M., E. VERNEY, T. D. MIALE and H. SIDRANSKY, 1967, Am. J. Pathol. *51*, 769.

HENRICI, A. T., 1939, J. Immunol. *36*, 319.

HINSON, K. F. W., A. J. MOON and N. S. PLUMMER, 1952, Thorax *7*, 317.

MANKOWSKI, Z. T. and B. J. LITTLETON, 1954, Antibiotics Chemother. *4*, 253.

MERKOW, L., M. PARDO, S. M. EPSTEIN, E. VERNEY and H. SIDRANSKY, 1968, Science *160*, 79.

PEPYS, F., R. W. RIDDELL, K. M. CITRON, Y. M. CLAYTON and E. I. SHORT, 1959, Am. Rev. Resp. Dis. *80*, 167.

RAU, E. M., V. L. KOENIG and E. B. TILDEN, 1961, Mycopathol. et Mycol. Appl. *14*, 347.

SIDRANSKY, H. and L. FRIEDMAN, 1958, Am. J. Pathol. *34*, 585.

SIDRANSKY, H. and L. FRIEDMAN, 1959, Am. J. Pathol. *35*, 169.

SIDRANSKY, H. and E. VERNEY, 1962, Lab. Invest. *11*, 1172.

SIDRANSKY, H., E. VERNEY and H. BEEDE, 1965, Arch. Pathol. *79*, 299.

TILDEN, E. B., S. FREEMAN and L. LOMBARD, 1963, Mycopathol. et Mycol. Appl. *20*, 253.

TILDEN, E. B., E. H. HATTON, S. FREEMAN, W. M. WILLIAMSON and V. L. KOENIG, 1961, Mycopathol. et Mycol. Appl. *14*, 325.

WYNSTON, L. K. and E. B. TILDEN, 1963, Mycopathol. et Mycol. Appl. *20*, 272.

8.3 Candidiasis

Infections with species of the genus *Candida* are caused primarily by *C. albicans*, although other species, such as *C. parakrusei*, *C. tropicalis*, and *C. krusei*, may also assume a pathogenic role (Benham 1931; Wikler et al. 1942; Wolfe and Henderson 1951; Mankowski 1957; Salvin 1963).

A variety of laboratory animals are susceptible to such infections, especially on intravenous challenge (Mankowski 1957; Meyer and Ordal 1946; Fuentes et al. 1952; Hasenclever 1959; Winner 1960). Swiss white mice are more susceptible than albino rabbits to intravenous inoculation with *C. albicans*, while *C. tropicalis* is lethal for mice, but not for rabbits (Hasenclever 1959; Hasenclever and Mitchell 1961a). The addition of 5% gastric mucin to an inoculum markedly reduced the resistance of mice to lethal infections, and increased the extent and rapidity of infections with weakly pathogenic isolates (Strauss and Kligman 1951; Salvin et al. 1952).

A very striking transformation occurs in the yeast cell of *C. albicans* after injection into a susceptible laboratory animal (Hill and Gebhardt 1956; Young 1958). Yeast-like cells of other members of the genus *Candida* fail to exhibit these same alterations under the same conditions. A majority of the organisms develop short filaments, and apparently thereby resist phagocytosis. Yeast-form cells thus are observed intracellularly, with evidence of digestion, while the filaments seem to invade host cells and do not show signs of deterioration. Thus, in contrast to other dimorphic fungi, the mycelial form, not the yeast-like form, seems to grow in the animal tissues. The host cells that act as phagocytes are monocytic, with few polymorphonuclear leucocytes being involved. Intraperitoneal inoculation may result in invasion of all the abdominal organs, with the pancreas and kidney usually yielding the greatest numbers of *C. albicans* cells (Evans and Winner 1954). The rapid elimination of the pathogen form the circulation suggests that proliferation of the fungus occurs primarily in the tissues. The growths may become very dense, with short filaments developing into long, intertwined mycelium. With the exception of *C. stellatoidea*, yeast-like cells of other species of *Candida* fail to develop the filamentous form under the same experimental conditions. In experimentally-infected mice, the organism may survive in the kidney for relatively long periods of time without resulting in death of the host. In a study of possible differences in pathogenicity between antigenic groups A and B of *C. albicans*, about the same degree of virulence was found in strains belonging to one or the other of the two groups (Hasenclever and Mitchell 1961b).

When non-lethal suspensions of *C. albicans* organisms were mixed with therapeutic doses of aureomycin and injected intraperitoneally into mice, the mixture was found to be fatal (Seligmann 1952). A similar effect was obtained when aureomycin was administered from 24 hours before to 4 hours after inoculation with *C. albicans*. This virulence-enhancing activity of aureomycin paralleled its antibiotic activity, since chemical or physical agents that destroyed one also eliminated the other. When aureomycin was included in a broth culture medium in concentrations greater than 0.1 mg. per ml, the growth of *C. albicans* was significantly stimulated. Penicillin, chloramphenicol, erythromycin, or streptomycin did not show a similar *in vitro* effect (Huppert et al. 1953; Huppert and Cazin 1955; Huppert et al. 1955). When methyl and propyl parabens were mixed with the aureomycin, the enhanced growth of *C. albicans* which appeared with pure aureomycin was eliminated. When aureomycin was administered to mice via the oral route, *C. albicans* tended to become well established in the microbial flora of the intestinal tract. In a comparison of the direct stimulation of *in vitro* growth of *C. albicans* by a variety of antibiotics and the presence of superinfection with this organism, no direct correlation was observed. The explanation for such a superimposed fungal infection during antibiotic therapy probably lies in a biological mechanism different from direct stimulation of fungal growth by the antibiotic.

Patients treated with broad spectrum antibiotics also may show an increased incidence or severity of infection with *C. albicans* (McVay and Spruntz 1951; Robinson 1954). Organisms which normally inhabit the body may restrain the growth of *C. albicans* by their overwhelming capacity to use nutritive substances present. The development of candidiasis may also be the result of lowered resistance of the host to the invasion of the aetiologic agent.

Since conventional mice could be infected only with difficulty, if at all, *per os* with *C. albicans*, oral administration of the fungus to germ-free animals was carried out to determine whether infection with *C. albicans* would occur in the absence of other microorganisms (Phillips and Balish 1966). Conventional ND-1 mice fed 10^6 viable *C. albicans* cells per animal did not show signs of infection in the gut wall, and only yeast forms of *C. albicans* were found in the contents of the alimentary tract. In contrast, within 48 hours of oral challenge, fecal samples from germ-free individuals had many hyphal elements. Lesions developed in the mucosal area of the stomach, and contained large numbers of hyphae and mycelia with blastospores. Thus, increased susceptibility to infection seemed associated with absence of intestinal microorganisms and with the conversion of the yeast cells into hyphal elements.

Treatment of mice with cortisone leads to systemic spread of the fungus, and ultimately to death. Histiocytes of cortisone-treated mice frequently contain *Candida* cells, while such phagocytosis is not seen in untreated animals (O'Grady et al. 1964). It is difficult to explain this observation, especially since phagocytosis seems directed solely against the yeast form and the filamentous phase is responsible for the destructive effects of the infection.

Alloxan diabetes decreased survival times of mice with experimental candidiasis, in comparison to the survival times of non-diabetic mice (Andriole and Hasenclever 1962). The kidney seemed to be the primary tissue in which progressive infection appeared after intravenous administration of *C. albicans* to alloxan-diabetic and normal mice. The numbers of *C. albicans* cells, however, were significantly higher in the kidneys of the alloxan-diabetic mice, and histologically the lesions developed earlier, were more severe, and persisted longer. Apparently, the metabolic changes induced by alloxan diabetes influence important factors associated with host resistance to *C. albicans*.

Chronic candidiasis may also occur in patients with defects in cellular immunity. For example, one patient with chronic mucocutaneous candidiasis showed defective cellular immunity by (a) failure to develop delayed skin reactions to a variety of antigens, (b) prolonged survival of skin homografts, and (c) decreased stimulation of peripheral blood lymphocytes by phytohaemagglutinin (Buckley et al. 1968). Chronic oral candidiasis, accompanied by cellular anergy, prolonged homograft survival, and growth retardation, may also be associated with thymic aplasia.

Another case of disseminated candidiasis was characterized by the inability of the patient's neutrophils to kill *C. albicans* cells (Lehrer and Cline 1969). This condition was associated with absence of detectable levels of the lysosomal enzyme myeloperoxidase, although other granule-associated enzymes were present at normal levels. Polymorphonuclear leucocytes from patients with chronic granulomatous disease of childhood phagocytose *C. albicans* normally, but are unable to kill the fungus cells intracellularly (Oh et al. 1969). Polymorphonuclear leucocytes from normal human adults and newborn infants phagocytosed and killed approximately 30% of intracellular organisms in 60 min.

A significantly increased carrier rate of *C. albicans* occurs among children with malignant disease (Winter and Foley 1956). As the condition of the patient declines, the carrier rate rises. Although it seems clear that candidiasis is a disease of the debilitated patient, true evaluation of the primary predisposing factors is difficult because of treatment of many of the patients with antibiotics and/or cortisone. Analysis of sera from patients with advanced lymphoma or leukaemia did not indicate a specific decrease of antibody titre to *C. albicans* (Brody and Finch 1960). Thus, the suggestion is that decline in tissue defense mechanisms rather than in humoral antibody forms the basis for the increased incidence of disseminated candidiasis in patients with leukaemias or lymphomas.

Chronic experimental infection of Swiss mice induced by intravenous injection of *C. albicans* was reported to have produced profound and prolonged pathologic changes in the thymus gland (Mankowski 1968a). Since such thymic damage also occurred in adrenalectomized animals infected with this yeast, the changes were concluded to have been due to the particular infection. *C. albicans* organisms entered the thymus readily. An increase in the number and size of Hassall's corpuscles was directly related to the number of injected *C. albicans* cells. PAS (periodic acid-Schiff)-positive material, presumably from the invading micro-organisms, was frequently found inside the corpuscles. Dilatation of the thymus vessels was most characteristic of the disease, with the degree of distention being proportional to the number of injected fungal cells. The medulla of the thymus was also heavily invaded by lymphocytes, many of which were pyknotic, with a wrinkled appearance, and seemingly in a degenerating state. Observation of the presence of germinal centers in the thymus of infected mice is pertinent to the reported occurrence of changes resembling human myasthenia gravis in the course of experimental *C. albicans* infection (Mankowski 1963). Thymus extracts from young rats or rabbits also were reported to have a beneficial effect on the course of the infection in mice (Mankowski 1968b).

Laboratory animals have been actively immunized against *C. albicans*. Mice were inoculated subcutaneously with multiple doses of living, merthiolate-killed, or sonically-disrupted fungal cells, and then challenged intravenously with 10^4 to 10^5 viable organisms. Some resistance was induced, since fewer deaths occurred among the vaccinated than the control animals (Mourad and Friedman 1961b). Mice immunized subcutaneously with cell walls of *C. albicans* were protected against intravenous challenge, in that their lives were prolonged in comparison to those of the controls (Dobias 1964). Higher mortalities have resulted when living cells were used as the immunizing agent prior to challenge (Fischer and Horbach 1958). Doubt therefore exists as to whether living cells can induce added resistance in laboratory animals, especially when the exact role of an endotoxin-like substance in the *C. albicans* cells is in doubt. The substance may enhance the growth of organisms in a succeeding inoculation and thereby cause a higher death rate, or it may increase non-specific host resistance to later challenges.

Endotoxins have been found in isolates of *C. albicans*, although their exact role in the pathogenesis of the disease is not completely understood (Salvin 1952; Mourad and Friedman 1961a; Dobias 1957). Young mice could be killed by intraperitoneal injection of dead yeast cells, or by intravenous inoculation of a soluble substance obtained by sonic oscillation.

Endotoxin injected subcutaneously in Freund's adjuvant in mice did not seem to stimulate the development of acquired resistance against chronic lethal candidiasis. Protection by lipopolysaccharide against acute toxicity of *C. albicans* lasted for 10–14 days (Hasenclever and Mitchell 1963a). A bimodal manifestation of tolerance or resistance to the toxicity of *C. albicans* was apparent after administration of lipopolysaccharide. Thus, endotoxin given 1 or 6 days before intravenous challenge with 10^7 yeast cells of *C. albicans* resulted in extended survival time. Mice that received endotoxin at the same time as the intravenous challenge showed increased susceptibility in comparison to the control group (Hasenclever and Mitchell 1963b). In mice injected intraperitoneally with single doses of lipopolysaccharide, tolerance to *C. albicans* toxicity reached a high level one day later, receded to a point at 3 days after injection where little resistance was measured, and then returned at 6 days to about the same level as with a one-day interval. There was then a gradual return to normal at 10–14 days after the initial injection (Hasenclever and Mitchell 1962).

Rabbits inoculated intravenously with 10^9 dead yeast cells developed a febrile response indistinguishable from that induced by Gram-negative bacterial endotoxin. The rise in body temperature began about 30 minutes after injection, peaked once or twice or formed a small plateau, then gradually disappeared by about 10 hours. When viable *C. albicans* cells were injected, the febrile response did not return to normal, but remained elevated for several days, usually until the death of the animal (Kobayashi and Friedman 1964).

In a study of immunologic and toxic differences between mouse-avirulent and mouse-virulent strains, differences in cell-surface materials were detected which could be extracted with solvents such as ethanol-ethyl ether and phenol (Isenberg et al. 1963). The extracts are complex haptens which behave like endotoxins in rabbits and mice. In the virulent strains, the complex seems to be polysaccharide in nature, whereas in the avirulent strains fats and lipids are substituted for some polysaccharides on the cell surface.

References

ANDRIOLE, V. T. and H. F. HASENCLEVER, 1962, Yale J. Biol. Med. *35*, 96.

BENHAM, R. W., 1931, J. Infect. Dis. *49*, 183.

BRODY, J. I. and S. C. FINCH, 1960, Blood *15*, 830.

BROWN, C., JR., S. PROPP, C. M. GUEST, R. T. BEEBE and L. EARLY, 1953, J. Am. Med. Assoc. *152*, 206.

BUCKLEY, R. H., Z. J. LUCAS, B. G. HATTLER, JR., C. M. ZMIJEWSKI and D. B. AMOS, 1968, Clin. Exptl. Immunol. *3*, 153.

DOBIAS, B., 1957, Am. Med. Assoc. J. Dis. Child. *94*, 234.

DOBIAS, B., 1964, Arch. Med. Scand. Suppl. *421*, 1.

EVANS, W. E. D. and H. I. WINNER, 1954, J. Pathol. Bacteriol. *67*, 531.

FISCHER, G. W. and L. HORBACH, 1958, Arch. Hyg. u. Bakteriol. *142*, 14.

FUENTES, C. A., J. SCHWARZ and R. ABOULAFIA, 1952, Mycopathol. et Mycol. Appl. *6*, 176.

HASENCLEVER, H. F., 1959, J. Bacteriol. *78*, 105.

HASENCLEVER, H. F. and W. O. MITCHELL, 1961a, Sabouraudia *1*, 16.

HASENCLEVER, H. F. and W. O. MITCHELL, 1961b, J. Bacteriol. *82*, 578.

HASENCLEVER, H. F. and W. O. MITCHELL, 1962, J. Bacteriol. *84*, 1325.

HASENCLEVER, H. F. and W. O. MITCHELL, 1963a, J. Bacteriol. *86*, 401.

HASENCLEVER, H. F. and W. O. MITCHELL, 1963b, J. Bacteriol. *85*, 1088.

HILL, D. W. and L. P. GEBHARDT, 1956, Proc. Soc. Exptl. Biol. Med. *92*, 640.

HUPPERT, M. and J. CAZIN, JR., 1955, J. Bacteriol. *70*, 435.

HUPPERT, M., J. CAZIN, JR. and J. SMITH, JR., 1955, J. Bacteriol. *70*, 440.

HUPPERT, M., D. A. MACPHERSON and J. CAZIN, JR., 1953, J. Bacteriol. *65*, 171.

ISENBERG, H. D., J. ALLERHAND, J. I. BERKMAN and D. GOLDBERG, 1963, J. Bacteriol. *86*, 1010.

KOBAYASHI, G. S. and L. FRIEDMAN, 1964, J. Bacteriol. *88*, 660.

LEHRER, R. I. and M. J. CLINE, 1969, J. Clin. Invest. *48*, 1478.

MANKOWSKI, Z. T., 1957, Trans. N.Y. Acad. Sci. *19*, 548.

MANKOWSKI, Z. T., 1963, Mycopathol. et Mycol. Appl. *19*, 1.

MANKOWSKI, Z. T., 1968a, Mycopathol. et Mycol. Appl. *36*, 233.

MANKOWSKI, Z. T., 1968b, Mycopathol. et Mycol. Appl. *36*, 247.

MCVAY, L. V. and D. H. SPRUNT, 1951, Proc. Soc. Exptl. Biol. Med. *78*, 759.

MEYER, E. and J. Z. ORDAL, 1946, J. Bacteriol. *52*, 615.

MOURAD, S. and L. FRIEDMAN, 1961a, J. Bacteriol. *81*, 550.

MOURAD, S. and L. FRIEDMAN, 1961b, Proc. Soc. Exptl. Biol. Med. *106*, 570.

O'GRADY, F., R. E. COTTON and R. E. M. THOMPSON, 1964, Brit. J. Exptl. Pathol. *45*, 656.

OH, M. K., G. E. RODEY, R. A. GOOD, R. A. CHILGREN and P. G. QUIE, 1969, J. Ped. *75*, 300.

PHILLIPS, A. W. and F. BALISH, 1966, Appl. Microbiol. *14*, 737.

ROBINSON, H. M., JR., 1954, A.M.A. Arch. Dermatol. *70*, 640.

SALVIN, S. B., 1952, J. Immunol. *69*, 89.

SALVIN, S. B., 1963, Progr. Allergy *7*, 238.

SALVIN, S. B., J. C. CORY and M. K. BERG, 1952, J. Infect. Dis. *90*, 177.

SELIGMANN, E., 1952, Proc. Soc. Exptl. Biol. Med. *79*, 481.

STRAUSS, R. E. and A. M. KLIGMAN, 1951, J. Infect. Dis. *88*, 151.

WIKLER, A., E. G. WILLIAMS, E. D. DOUGLASS, C. W. EMMONS and R. C. DUNN, 1942, J. Am. Med. Assoc. *119*, 333.

WINNER, H. I., 1960, J. Pathol. Bacteriol. *79*, 420.

WINTER, W. D. and G. E. FOLEY, 1956, Pediatrics *18*, 595.

WOLFE, E. I. and F. W. HENDERSON, 1951, J. Am. Med. Assoc. *147*, 1344.

YOUNG, G., 1958, J. Infect. Dis. *102*, 114.

8.4. Cryptococcosis

Cryptococcus neoformans, which may cause infections in man and animals, has a special affinity for the central nervous system (Stoddard and Cutler 1916; Cox and Tolhurst 1946; Barron 1955; Pounden et al.

1952). After analyses of human material, the respiratory tract was considered as the main portal of entry, with possible haematogenous dissemination of the organism to other tissues such as skin, mucous membranes, bones and joints. In studies on experimental cryptococcosis induced in mice by inoculation subcutaneously, intraperitoneally, or intracerebrally, infection of the brain was characterized by proliferation of the yeast cells to form large lesions with minimal infiltration. This predilection for the brain in disseminated infection is believed related to the minimal inflammatory response in cerebral tissue (Littman and Zimmerman 1956).

Although the organism has an obvious capsule, correlation does not exist between the size of this capsule and either the immunogenicity or virulence of the fungus. Although the weakly encapsulated strains were more immunogenic in rabbits than the strongly encapsulated strains, antisera of reasonably high potency were consistently produced by either type (Neill et al. 1950). Antibody titres were determined by agglutination of cells grown on agar cultures, "Quellung" reactions with cells from infected mice, and precipitation tests with polysaccharide from a weakly encapsulated strain as antigen. In tests wherein yeast cells were injected intracerebrally into white Swiss mice, thinly encapsulated cells were equally as virulent as heavily encapsulated cells (Littman and Tsubura 1959). Thus, although strains may vary in their virulence in mice, it is not the size of the capsule alone that determines this difference.

Although the organism was considered to be weakly antigenic, high-titred sera have been obtained both from experimentally infected animals and naturally infected humans (Salvin 1950; Evans 1949; Kaufman and Blumer 1968; Bloomfield et al. 1963; Gordon and Jedder 1966; Walter and Jones 1968). *C. neoformans*, instead of being a poor antigen, may under certain conditions produce an excess of antigen from its polysaccharide capsule during the period of infection. In the presence of this excess polysaccharide antigen, antibodies, although present, might not have the opportunity to function or to express themselves. Accordingly, the sera of patients suspected of having cryptococcosis should be tested both for antibody and antigen.

Three serotypes, A, B, and C, have been described for *C. neoformans* by means of agglutination tests and capsular reactions (Evans 1950). These serotypes are not, however, related to the virulence of the strains. Serologic classification of the organism is based on differences in a pentosan located in the capsule (Evans 1950; Evans and Kessel 1951).

C. neoformans may form a capsule and grow on a variety of media at 37°C. On repeated cultivation on bacteriological peptone culture media, a decline in the amount of capsular substance may occur. The organism can be stimulated to synthesize abundant capsular substance by transfer to a special synthetic culture medium and further incubation at 37°C for 48–72 hours (Littman 1958). That temperature is also an important factor in growth of the organism is indicated in that, although *C. neoformans* grows abundantly on a variety of media at 37°C, saprophytic cryptococci do not grow well on artificial media at 37°C and are not virulent for mice. At higher temperatures such as 103°F, the viability of the yeast cells decreases greatly and the virulence of the organism also declines (Kuhn 1939, 1949; Littman and Borek 1968). Thus, mice maintained at elevated room temperatures (35°–36°C) survived longer than control mice maintained at regular room temperatures (24°–27°C), after each group had been inoculated intravenously, intraperitoneally, or intracerebrally with lethal doses of the yeast. A direct effect of temperature therefore could explain the natural resistance of some species of animals, such as pigeons or rabbits, to cryptococcsis. Also, artificial fever therapy might be helpful in the treatment of human cases.

Increased resistance to experimental cryptococcosis has been induced in mice (Louria 1960; Abrahams and Gilleven 1960; Louria et al. 1963). Death following a lethal intravenous challenge was delayed by prior intraperitoneal or intravenous injection of living high-virulence or low-virulence strains. The size of the capsule was not correlated with the degree of protection. Immunization with heat-killed cells did not produce any protection against lethal challenge. The enhanced resistance was species-specific and did not manifest itself after challenge with such heterologous microorganisms as *Mycobacterium tuberculosis*, *Staphylococcus aureus*, or *Klebsiella pneumoniae*. Similar delay in death following lethal intravenous challenge occurred after administration of *Salmonella* endotoxin. This resistance is obviously non-specific and has been demonstrated after challenge with a variety of heterologous microorganisms (Landy 1956).

Enhanced resistance has also occurred following vaccination of mice with formalin-killed cryptococcal cells (Abrahams and Gilleven 1960). This protection was demonstrable after lethal intravenous challenge in (a) the prolonged median survival time, (b) the increased number of survivors, and (c) the reduced numbers of viable yeast cells recoverable from the tissues of the immunized animals. In the demonstration of this protection, emphasis was placed on careful execution of test procedures, such as route and dose of vaccine administration, time of challenge, and virulence of challenge strain.

A factor has been described in cell-free human serum which can inhibit growth of *C. neoformans* (Baum and Artis 1961, 1963). This factor is resistant to heating at 65°C for 30 minutes, is most active at pH 7.4 to 7.5, and achieves a maximum effect after 4–5 days contact with the yeast cells. Exactly what role, if any, this substance plays in resistance to human cryptococcosis has not yet been elucidated.

Cryptococcosis has frequently been associated with Hodgkin's disease and other syndromes with reticulo-endothelial pathology (Collins et al. 1951; Zimmerman and Rapaport 1954). In a study of 60 cases of cryptococcosis, 30% occurred in patients with Hodgkin's or related diseases. Although cryptococcal infections are thought usually to start in the lungs, the possibility arises that an individual with a malignancy of the reticulo-endothelial system has weakly pathogenic strains of cryptococcus on his skin, in his gastrointestinal tract, or in his lungs. Such organisms may become infectious in hosts where resistance has been decreased by altered physiology of the reticulo-endothelial system. Thus, extensive dissemination may be expected and does occur in patients with Hodgkin's disease, lymphosarcoma, and leukaemia.

C. neoformans has been established as being present in certain environments in the soil and in association with pigeon droppings. The organism was found to multiply rapidly in moist pigeon excreta extracts, reached counts up to 6×10^6 per ml within a few weeks, and remained viable for more than two years at room temperature. Accordingly, man must have frequent exposure to air or soil containing the pathogen, yet does not develop frequent severe progressive infections. Mild infections do occur (Muchmore et al. 1968; Salvin and Smith 1961). He must therefore have a high degree of innate resistance to progressive infection with *C. neoformans*, – a resistance which may be overcome on exposure to high numbers of yeast cells (Muchmore et al. 1963) or after the host resistance deteriorates with internal degenerative disease.

References

ABRAHAMS, I. and T. G. GILLEVEN, 1960, J. Immunol. *85*, 629.

BARRON, C. N., 1955, J. Am. Vet. Med. Assoc. *127*, 125.

BAUM, G. L. and D. ARTIS, 1961, Am. J. Med. Sci. *241*, 97.

BAUM, G. L. and D. ARTIS, 1963, Am. J. Med. Sci. *246*, 87.

BLOOMFIELD, N., M. A. GORDON and D. F. ELMENDORF, JR., 1963, Proc. Soc. Exptl. Biol. Med. *114*, 64.

COX, L. B. and J. C. TOLHURST, 1946, Human torulosis: a clinical pathological and microbiological study with a report of thirteen cases (Melbourne University Press, Melbourne, Australia).

COLLINS, V. P., A. GELLHORN and J. R. TRIMBLE, 1951, Cancer *4*, 883.

EVANS, E. E., 1949, Proc. Soc. Exptl. Biol. Med. *71*, 644.

EVANS, E. E., 1950, J. Immunol. *64*, 423.

EVANS, E. E. AND J. F. KESSEL, 1951, J. Immunol. *67*, 109.

GORDON, M. A. and D. K. JEDDER, 1966, J. Am. Med. Assoc. *197*, 961.

KAUFMAN, L. AND S. BLUMER, 1968, Appl. Microbiol. *16*, 1907.

KUHN, L. R., 1939, Proc. Soc. Exptl. Biol. Med. *41*, 573.

KUHN, L. R., 1949, Proc. Soc. Exptl. Biol. Med. *71*, 341.

LANDY, M., 1956, Ann. N.Y. Acad. Sci. *66*, 292.

LITTMAN, M. L., 1958, Trans. N.Y. Acad. Sci., Series II, *20*, 623.

LITTMAN, M. L. and R. BOREK, 1968, Mycopathol. et Mycol. Appl. *35*, 329.

LITTMAN, M. L. and E. TSUBURA, 1959, Proc. Soc. Exptl. Biol. Med. *101*, 773.

LITTMAN, M. L. and L. E. ZIMMERMAN, 1956, Cryptococcosis. New York, Grune & Stratton.

LOURIA, D. B., 1960, J. Exptl. Med. *111*, 643.

LOURIA, D. B., T. KAMINSKI and G. FINKEL, 1963, J. Exptl. Med. *117*, 509.

MUCHMORE, H. G., F. G. FELTON, S. B. SALVIN and E. R. RHOADES, 1968, Sabouraudia *6*, 285.

MUCHMORE, H. G., E. R. RHOADES, G. E. NIX, F. G. FELTON and R. E. CARPENTER, 1963, New England J. Med. *268*, 1112.

NEILL, J. M., I. ABRAHAMS and C. E. KAPROS, 1950, J. Bacteriol. *59*, 263.

POUNDEN, W. D., J. M. AMBERSON and R. F. JAEGER, 1952, Am. J. Vet. Res. *13*, 121.

SALVIN, S. B., 1950, J. Immunol. *65*, 617.

SALVIN, S. B. and R. F. SMITH, 1961, Proc. Soc. Exptl. Biol. Med. *108*, 498.

STODDARD, J. L. and E. C. CUTLER, 1916, Torula infection in man. Monograph of the Rockefeller Institute for Medical Research, Vol. 6.

WALTER, J. E. and R. D. JONES, 1968, Am. Rev. Resp. Dis. *97*, 275.

ZIMMERMAN, L. E. and H. RAPPAPORT, 1954, Am. J. Clin. Pathol. *24*, 1050.

8.5. North American blastomycosis

North American blastomycosis is primarily a pulmonary disease caused by *Blastomyces dermatitidis*. This granulomatous disease produces a primary lesion at the point of entry, from which involvement of the regional lymph nodes occurs regularly, and from which dissemination to the skin and other organs may occur. Pulmonary blastomycosis may be found without skin manifestations, or may become arrested even in the presence of active extrapulmonary pathology, such as cutaneous, osseous, or prostatic. The disease probably spreads to a large extent *via* the haematogenous route, since the double-walled single-budding yeast cells have been repeatedly seen in blood vessels (Baum and Schwarz 1959; Blastomycosis, Cooperative Study 1964). Although direct cutaneous inoculation of the fungus into the skin of man is extremely rare, such cases have been reported and show a clinical picture of an indurated, ulcerative primary lesion at the site of inoculation with lymphadenopathy limited to the involved limb (Wilson 1955).

The fungus is pathogenic for mice, with the virulence varying from strain to strain (Hitch 1942; Marcus et al. 1960), and being parallel to the lipid content of the yeast cells (DiSalvo and Denton 1963). Disseminated blastomycosis can also be induced in adult hamsters after intraperitoneal, intramuscular, or subcutaneous injection (Landay et al. 1968). Generally, an abscess is formed at the site of injection, and caseous lesions develop in regional lymph nodes and in the lungs. Other species, such as the dog and monkey, are also susceptible to the disease (Smith 1966).

Mice have been made more resistant to subsequent intravenous challenge by previous sublethal intravenous inoculation with living organisms (Hill and Marcus 1959). All animals were found to be infected, although the extent of disease was less in mice that had been previously infected. Injection of formalin-killed yeast-phase cells did not reveal any enhanced resistance in mice subsequently challenged intravenously.
(Guidry and Bujard 1964). At 37°C, the yeast-phase cells penetrated chorioallantoic (CA) membrane of embryonated hen eggs was compared
The capacity of the cells of the yeast and mycelial phases to invade the into the mesoderm, where they proliferated and produced abscesses. In order for the mycelial phase not to be confined to the ectoderm but to penetrate into the mesoderm, the hyphae first had to convert to the yeast phase.

In man, the development of disease is related to the immunologic status of the patient (Smith 1949). Some patients acquire delayed hypersensitivity as indicated by a positive skin reaction to the antigen blastomycin, and others develop humoral antibodies which are detectable by complement-fixation tests. Four groups have been described with different combinations of immunologic reactions.

The first group included patients with recent pulmonary involvement, with or without cutaneous invasion. The disease was apparently not extensive, since humoral antibodies could not be detected. Delayed hypersensitivity, and presumably cellular immunity, was present since the patients developed skin reactions on intradermal testing.

The patients in the second group had more extensive infections, and were not only skin positive, but also had complement-fixing antibodies in their sera. The humoral antibodies were no longer detectable after clinical recovery, although the skin tests remained positive for extended periods of time.

In the third group of patients, humoral antibodies were present, but skin tests with blastomycin were negative. These individuals had a poor prognosis, in that the complement-fixation results indicated progressive disease, while the absence of responses to intradermal testing suggested terminal anergy.

The final group with negative skin tests and absence of detectable circulating antibodies included patients in the terminal phase of disease, or more likely individuals with recent infections who had not had time to develop delayed allergy or detectable humoral antibodies. Chemotherapy in this latter group has a good chance for success in the prevention of dissemination.

References

BAUM, G. L. and J. SCHWARZ, 1959, Am. J. Med. Sci. *238*, 661.

Blastomycosis. Cooperative study of the Veterans Administration, 1964, I. Am. Rev. Resp. Dis. *89*, 659.

DISALVO, A. F. and J. F. DENTON, 1963, J. Bacteriol. *85*, 927.

GUIDRY, D. J. and A. J. BUJARD, 1964, Am. J. Trop. Med. *13*, 319.

HILL, G. A. and S. MARCUS, 1959, Bacteriol. Proc. 87.

HITCH, J. M., 1942, J. Invest. Dermatol. *5*, 41.

LANDAY, M. E., E. P. LOWE, J. MITTEN and F. X. SMITH, 1968, Sabouraudia *6*, 318.

MARCUS, S., G. A. HILL and R. A. KNIGHT, 1960, Ann. N. Y. Acad. Sci. *89*, 193.

SMITH, C. D., J. W. BRANDSBERG, L. A. SELBY and R. W. MENGES, 1966, Sabouraudia *5*, 126.

SMITH, D. T., 1949, Ann. Int. Med. *31*, 463.

WILSON, W. J., E. P. CAWLEY, F. D. WEIDMAN and W. S. GILMER, 1955, A.M.A. Arch, Dermatol. *71*, 39.

8.6. Histoplasmosis

The respiratory tract is generally considered to be the route of entry of the fungus, *Histoplasma capsulatum*. Both animals and man are believed to acquire a primary pulmonary infection by inhalation of air-borne conidia as part of the growth of the saprophytic phase in the soil. After becoming lodged in the lung tissue, the conidia soon convert to the invasive yeast-like phase. Dissemination of the small, budding yeast-like cells occurs haematogenously, with a tendency toward concentration in tissues containing many reticulo-endothelial cells.

Early development of the disease was examined after injection of conidia into the anterior chamber of the rabbit eye (Day 1949). During the first week of infection, an exudate appeared consisting of polymorphonuclear leukocytes, lymphocytes, and a few macrophages containing the pathogen. As the infection progressed, granulomatous lesions could be detected microscopically; yeast cells were more common within macrophages and giant cells.

Observations after subcutaneous injection of one of the growth phases of *H. capsulatum* into guinea-pigs, gerbils, or white mice revealed that the cells of the yeast phase tended to remain extra-cellular for about 24 hours, before an accumulation of macrophages resulted in the phagocytosis of the pathogen (Brandt 1950b). After an injection of a chlamydospore suspension, many degenerate, or are phagocytosed by the large multinucleate giant cells before some of the spores show changes within the nucleus that lead to production of yeast cells and to their liberation into the host tissues.

After intranasal administration of a saline suspension of viable tuberculate chlamydospores to mice, dissemination of the yeast phase from the lung to the liver and spleen was found by culture to occur within four days (Procknow 1960). Microscopically, the inflammatory reaction in the lung was discernible in 3 to 6 hrs, with polymorphonuclear leucocytes being the prominent cell type. By 36 hrs post infection, the polymorphonuclear leucocytes had started to degenerate and to be replaced by epithelioid cells. The amount of exudate was increasing, with many macrophages appearing therein. Internal segmentation of the spore then became apparent, followed by the development of defects in the spore wall. Rupture of the wall at this point caused escape of yeastlike cells through the defects into the lung parenchyma. Usually, this release of yeast cells with subsequent disintegration of the remaining wall was accomplished before the seventh day.

At this time, focal granulomatous infiltrates clogged many alveoli. Macrophages filled with yeast phase cells of *H. capsulatum* were numerous and scattered throughout the exudate. By ten days post infection, pulmonary invasion was characterized by diffuse foci of dense exudates throughout both lung fields. Lesions were present and enlarging in other organs of the reticulo-endothelial system, and mice were beginning to die of disseminated disease. The blood became increasingly positive by culture for the yeast-like cells.

The intravenous route requires very few organisms to establish an experimental infection in mice. In fact, a single viable aggregate of the yeast phase is sufficient to infect a mouse (Rowley and Huber 1954, 1955), while systemic infections can be regularly induced with an inoculum of about 100 aggregates of one of several strains per mouse. The dose of yeast phase cells that can produce extensive infection and death is greater and more variable than that which can produce a chronic infection. The histopathology after inoculation *via* any one of several routes is comparable in that conversion to yeast phase occurs within the tissues exposed and a prompt local response is marked by proliferation of cells of the reticulo-endothelial system and engorgement of macrophages with the yeastlike cells. During the first two weeks after intravenous injection, small infiltrates of mononuclear cells increase in size within the liver and spleen. The Kupffer's cells of the enlarged liver become heavily parasitized, sometimes to the point of compression and necrosis. This infiltration by cells of the monocytic or macrophagic line, containing many phagocytosed yeastlike cells, has been noted in almost all of the body tissues.

Inoculation of mice with cells of the yeast phase *via* the intraperitoneal route resulted in lesions mostly in the inoculation site, liver, spleen, and pancreas (Grayston et al. 1956; Kipkie and Howell 1951). Lesions occurred occasionally in the heart, lungs, and gastro-intestinal tract, but typically not in the brain. After insertion of single spores into the peritoneal cavity, the fungus was recovered by culture techniques from the liver, spleen, or adrenal glands (Ajello and Runyon 1953). The optimum period for isolation of the organism from the tissues was about eight weeks.

The intracerebral route of inoculation is effective in production of high mortality in mice, but is obviously unnatural (Kipkie and Howell 1951; Grayston and Salvin 1956; Howell and Kipkie 1950, 1951). Within two days, a cellular infiltration of mononuclear cells, with some polymorphonuclear infiltration, can be detected, with cells of the yeast phase present within the exudate. The cellular infiltrate in the meninges tends to extend along the perivascular spaces into the brain. After an extended period of time, depending on the size of the inoculum, abscesses with necrotic centers develop surrounded by mononuclear cells or macrophages. The cells of the pathogen may be free within the necrotic material or phagocytosed within the macrophages. Dissemination from the brain occurs early, sometimes within 48 hours after infection, with focal collections of lymphocytes and subsequently granulomas appearing in the liver and spleen.

Experimental systemic histoplasmosis can also be induced in rabbits by intraperitoneal or intravenous inoculations, and is characterized by the development of granulomas and the presence of macrophages engorged with yeast cells (Salvin and Hottle 1948; Hazen and Tahler 1950; Scheff and Pfeifer-Scheff 1950). After intraperitoneal inoculation, lesions on the omentum are found to contain large numbers of macrophages and epithelioid cells, with occasional giant cells. Hamsters also develop disseminated histoplasmosis after intraperitoneal or subcutaneous inoculations, with the typical involvement of macrophages and the reticulo-endothelial system (Drouhet and Segretain 1952; O'Hern 1961).

Study of the disease in dogs was stimulated by the many cases of naturally occurring histoplasmosis. In spontaneous canine disease, although lesions were found in a variety of tissues, the gastro-intestinal tract was considered the main portal of entry (Robinson and McVickar 1952). The microorganism, after ingestion by the host, produced lesions in the intestine, from which the yeastlike cells presumably spread haematogenously to the lungs, lever, spleen, bone marrow, and other organs.

Other studies of natural histoplasmosis in the dog suggested that the lung was the portal of entry (Rowley et al. 1954; Schwarz and Bingham 1956). Intrapulmonary lesions associated with regional lymph nodes, both with macrophages containing numerous *H. capsulatum* cells, resembled typical primary complexes which result from inhalation of the saprophytic spores of the fungus. Progressive fatal histoplasmosis in all of nine dogs developed after intratracheal inoculation of the yeast-like phase, with death occurring 11 to 42 days later (Farrell et al. 1953). *H. capsulatum* was isolated in all nine animals from both antemortem blood cultures and from tissues collected at autopsy, primarily lung, spleen, and liver, and less extensively from mesenteric and bronchial nodes.

Dogs were also infected after intratracheal inoculation with spores of the mycelial phase (Procknow 1960). Whether the infection resulted in uncomplicated primary disease or in fatal disseminated disease depended on the challenge dose.

Severe histoplasmosis was produced in monkeys by inoculation of the yeast phase intravenously or intratracheally (Saslaw et al. 1960). A more mild disease developed after intranasal administration of the yeastlike cells, while clinical signs of illness were not observed in monkeys inoculated via the gastric route. Experimental infections with a pathogenesis essentially similar to the foregoing species have been reported in rats (Middleton et al. 1950), chickens (Menges and Haberman 1955), and guinea-pigs (Reid et al. 1942).

H. capsulatum was found to be infectious for the developing chick embryo (Larsh et al. 1958). The tuberculate macroconidium, the micro-conidium, and the mycelial fragment were all active pathogens, with the latter the most infectious. In addition, HeLa cells growing as a monolayer in a medium containing 20% fresh guinea-pig serum were capable of being infected with as few as 3 to 20 yeast phase organisms (Larsh and Shepard 1958). *H. capsulatum* was also grown in mammalian histiocytes maintained in culture (Howard 1965). The intracellular generation time was about 11 hours, and did not vary with different isolates of the fungus, in guinea-pig cells *vs.* mouse cells, in mouse cells in the presence of specific hyperimmune serum, or in cells from normal or immunized animals.

The course of primary histoplasmosis was also studied with the aid of the rabbit ear chamber (Farid and Barclay 1953; Procknow and Ray 1962). Within one hour after infection of the tissue with tuberculate macroconidia, leucocytes began to accumulate on the vascular endo-thelium. During the next 2–3 hrs, leucocytes were attracted toward the spores and then became packed about the fungal elements. Macrophages completely engulfed a small proportion of the spores before they were disrupted; the rest of the spores were surrounded by host phagocytosing cells, their cell walls disintegrated, and cells of the yeast phase liberated. Remnants of spore walls were phagocytosed and carried away by macrophages. A second inflammatory reaction started at this point, tended to be progressive, and was characterized by vascular dilatation and massive exudation of fluid and cells. Thrombosis of the vessels set in at the site of infection, spread peripherally, and was followed by necrosis and abscess formation.

Strains may vary greatly in their virulence to mice and other laboratory animals (Howell et al. 1950; Anderson and Marcus 1968). This difference has been demonstrated after intracerebral or intravenous inoculation by determination of the LD_{50} thirty days later. In addition, filamentous primary isolates and their subcultures have been separated into two distinct colonial types (A and B), which have different microscopic characteristics. The yeastlike forms of the two types are, however, indistinguishable. Since A rapidly overgrows B, the possibility exists that such types may differ in virulence or antigenicity (Daniels et al. 1968). The basis for variations in virulence is not understood, especially since a capsular substance is not present (Ribi and Salvin 1956), and injurious extracellular enzymes or exotoxins have not been demonstrated.

Resistance to infection has been induced or demonstrated in laboratory animals and man. Such enhanced resistance was expressed as decreased death rates after lethal challenge, as a lowering in pathologic tissue changes after sublethal or lethal challenge, and as an inhibition of multiplication of the yeastlike cells of *H. capsulatum* within host tissues.

Increased resistance may develop after a sublethal infection. Rabbits in which the anterior chamber of one eye had been infected 2 to 14 weeks previously and in which the previously uninfected eye did not show clinical signs of disease were reinoculated in the uninfected eye (Day 1949). Eyes in rabbits which had received their initial infection only 2 to 4 weeks earlier developed iritis and general signs resembling primary infection. Eyes in rabbits which had been originally infected 6 to 14 weeks previously had an initial inflammatory reaction after reinfection but failed to develop iritis. Thus, some immunity was conferred after 4 to 6 weeks of ocular or systemic infection.

In dogs which did not develop signs of clinical disease after intratracheal inoculation with mycelial phase, increased resistance to subsequent challenge with mycelial phase was noted (Farrell et al. 1953).

Young male mice previously infected with *H. capsulatum* were more resistant to a lethal challenge than normal mice of the same age and sex (Salvin 1955b). In one group of experiments, for example, of 246 mice that were infected and later challenged, only 22% died within 21 days.

On the other hand, 92% of 259 similarly challenged control mice died during that period. Neither the size of the sublethal infection nor the route of administration was of importance in the induction of resistance, since mice infected intraperitoneally, intracerebrally, intravenously or subcutaneously all showed resistance to lethal intracerebral challenge. This enhanced resistance was relatively specific, in that it was not apparent in animals previously infected intraperitoneally with 10^6 cells of *B. dermatitidis* or *C. albicans*. Marked reduction of yeastlike cells in various tissues was characteristic of reinfected mice, as compared to the numbers in the corresponding tissues of control animals. For example, in spleens of control mice and guinea-pigs that had been infected with sublethal doses, the number of cells of *H. capsulatum* increased for the first 2 to 3 weeks after inoculation, and then gradually decreased. In the reinfected animals, in contrast, the number of fungus cells remained at the same relatively low levels in the spleen during the 8 post-challenge weeks of observation. Thus, an immunizing infection merely reduces the number of pathogenic cells and the amount of pathologic responses in the host, but does not eliminate the *H. capsulatum* completely from the host tissues.

Evidence exists that resistance to reinfection also occurs in man. This conclusion is based on the location, incidence, and nature of epidemics of histoplasmosis in relation to prevalence of histoplasmin sensitivity (Grayston and Furcolow 1953; Lehan and Furcolow 1957). Of the many epidemics, a small minority occurred in the area of greatest endemicity according to histoplasmin sensitivity. Most of them were reported from areas of low to moderate sensitivity. In addition, the soldiers at the Camp Crowder, Mo., and Camp Gruber, Okla. outbreaks came from states with low incidence of histoplasmin reactors. The probability is then that epidemics involved individuals who had not had previous exposure to the microorganisms and therefore were susceptible to infection.

The involvement of children in many of the epidemics would confirm the opinion that people involved in epidemics of histoplasmosis have not had previous exposure to the aetiologic agent. The number of reactors to histoplasmin among children has been found to be lower than among the adult population.

Personnel in laboratories actively engaged in studies on histoplasmosis, especially such studies wherein the mycelial phase is involved, are skin-test positive. Such individuals do not develop clinical disease, although they are repeatedly exposed to the fungus. Primary infection, therefore, seems to confer increased resistance to reinfection. When these individuals inhale large quantities of conidia, the resistance may be overwhelmed. Here, the incubation period is shorter and clinical disease lasts for a shorter period than in previously uninfected individuals.

Increased resistance to challenge with *H. capsulatum* has been achieved after injection of killed cells of the yeast phase (Salvin 1953, 1955a, 1956, 1960; Schaefer and Saslaw 1954; Hill and Marcus 1959). Mice resisted lethal intracerebral challenge after cells of the yeast phase grown in a liquid medium and killed by exposure to 1:5000 merthiolate for 5 days at 37°C had been injected intraperitoneally two weeks previously. Mice immunized with heat-killed cells showed increased resistance to lethal intraperitoneal challenge with the pathogenic cells in 5% mucin. Mice injected with formalin-killed yeast-like cells once a week for 3 weeks resisted lethal intravenous challenge.

In this process of immunization and subsequent lethal challenge, cultures of the tissues usually revealed the presence of viable cells of *H. capsulatum*. Although the pathogen was not eliminated completely, the host tissues contained fewer fungal cells than controls. Such cells remained in the mouse tissues for long periods of time without causing death or increased disease.

Mice immunized and subsequently challenged intracerebrally had fewer pathologic findings than control mice, which had parenchymal abscesses and extensive meningitis (Grayston and Salvin 1956). The immunization process did not prevent dissemination of the pathogen from the challenge site, probably because of the predilection of the fungus for cells of the reticulo-endothelial system.

Living cells of the yeast-like phase seemed to be better immunogens than dead cells. Introduction of a sublethal dose of living cells into host tissues was followed by a brief period of fungus multiplication, before enhanced resistance developed. The amount of immunogenic material was thereby increased. Also, since the specific substance has not been identified, it is not known what immunologically deleterious effect killing of the yeastlike cells has.

Fractions of the yeast phase have been prepared for immunization of mice. After exposure of cells of the yeast phase to vibration in a Mickle tissue disintegrator, a cell-wall and a protoplasmic fraction were obtained (Salvin and Ribi 1955). Since the protoplasm of merthiolate-killed cells was released in a fine, dispersed state, the cell walls were readily separated by centrifugation and filtration. Intraperitoneal injection of the cell-wall material increased resistance of mice to lethal intraperitoneal or intracerebral challenge. The protoplasmic fraction, in contrast, had little or no protective properties. The cell-wall fraction, like whole cells, inhibited the growth of the fungus sufficiently to prevent death, but not to eliminate the *H. capsulatum* from the mouse tissues.

Purifications of the immunogenic or resistance-inducing fractions have been attempted. A fraction was obtained after the yeast phase had been grown in broth for 3 to 7 days under constant rotation at 37°C; after addition of merthiolate to a final concentration of 1:5000, the resulting broth culture was maintained at 37°C for 5 to 7 days (Salvin and Smith 1959). After purification, an active component was obtained which gave a single symmetrical boundary in the ultracentrifuge and by immunodiffusion, but had an electrophoresis pattern with two or more components. The fraction contained both carbohydrate and protein components. Injection of appropriate doses of this fraction into 21-day-old mice enhanced their resistance to subsequent lethal intracerebral challenge.

A polysaccharide-rich fraction, containing 4% nitrogen, was also effective in increasing resistance in mice to intravenous challenge with the yeast phase of *H. capsulatum* (Knight et al. 1959). Mice inoculated with the whole yeast cell, however, showed greater resistance than those immunized with the polysaccharide fraction.

Although it is well established that enhanced resistance to infection may be induced with *H. capsulatum*, the mechanism is not understood. A correlation does not exist between the presence of precipitins and resistance to dissemination. Precipitins tend to develop early in the disease, but their presence or titre is not correlated with restriction or spread of the infection. The antigen typically used in such tests is a filtrate of the broth in which yeast or mycelial phase has been grown.

Complement-fixing antibodies do not indicate the degree of resistance of the animal to the disease. In fact, since dissemination usually is accompanied by an increase in the titre of complement-fixing antibodies, they obviously do not act in restriction of the pathogen.

Serum was assayed for its capacity to induce passively specific enhanced resistance in non-immunized mice or guinea-pigs (Salvin 1960). When serum from a resistant animal was passively transferred to a normal recipient before, during, and after challenge, changes in the course of infection could not be detected. Such antisera from resistant guinea-pigs were also unable to inhibit the growth of the yeast phase *in vitro*. Pertinent to the role of humoral antibody is the apparent situation whereby progressive infections of *H. capsulatum* do not occur with relatively high frequency in agammaglobulinaemic individuals who have permanent residence in endemic areas. A case of idiopathic hypogammaglobulinaemia was reported wherein characteristic X-ray changes were present, a positive skin test of the delayed type developed to histoplasmin, and complement-fixing antibodies to *H. capsulatum* could not be detected (Seltzer et al. 1955). Apparently, the patient had histoplasmosis, but the disease was of a non-progressive nature. Although the possible role of humoral antibody should not be abandoned, the basis of resistance probably is associated with a cellular mechanism involving delayed hypersensitivity.

That delayed hypersensitivity may be associated with resistance in histoplasmosis is further indicated by studies on *in vitro* activity of mononuclear cells in the presence of specific antigen. Leukocytes from guinea-pigs experimentally infected with *H. capsulatum* were more sensitive to inhibition of migration in the presence of 1 : 1000 dilution of histoplasmin than those from normal guinea-pigs (Johnson and Scherago 1960). This inhibition of migration was specific to the degree that leucocytes from animals with histoplasmosis migrated in the presence of brucellergen to the same degree as did leucocytes from normal animals.

Blastogenesis of lymphocytes from patients with various clinical types of histoplasmosis was studied in the presence of the antigen, histoplasmin (Newberry et al. 1968). Herein, the incorporation of tritiated thymidine into DNA was used as the indicator of blastogenesis. The uptake of thymidine was greater for the healthy histoplasmin-positive donors than for the histoplasmin-negative donors. Also, the group of patients with acute histoplasmosis reacted similarly to the healthy histoplasmin-positive donors. Patients with chronic histo-plasmosis, on the other hand, reacted more like the donors who were histoplasmin-negative. Generally, the more severe the illness, the greater was the depression of blastogenesis. Information was not available as to whether the lymphocytopenia was the result of the disseminated infection or the cause of the chronic disease.

Infection with *H. capsulatum* may have a non-specific effect on resistance to other organisms. For example, prior intraperitoneal injection of the yeast phase of *H. capsulatum* has a striking modifying effect upon the course of infection following a subsequent intraperitoneal challenge with *Rickettsia typhi* (Salvin and Bell 1955). This antagonistic action of one infectious agent on another was apparently not due to specific antibodies. The time and dose relationships between *H. capsulatum* and *R. typhi* were of importance in showing the inhibitory effect. The antagonism or interference was highly specific in the sense that six other species of fungi did not influence infection of *R. typhi*. The exact mechanism is unknown.

Resistance to infection with *H. capsulatum* in man may also be influenced by the presence of other conditions or diseases. A patient with Hodgkin's disease, leukaemia, or lymphoma is more likely to develop severe histoplasmosis (Cawley and Curtis 1948). Whether these conditions enhance the severity of primary disease or whether they facilitate dissemination from a previously localized primary lesion is not known. The debilitating influence of other fungal diseases on the course of histoplasmosis is indicated by coexistence of histoplasmosis with cryptococcosis or blastomycosis.

Although a degrading effect of cortisone on the course of infection with *C. albicans* is well established, treatment of mice or guinea-pigs with cortisone has little influence on the dissemination of experimental histoplasmosis (Baum et al. 1954; Vogel et al. 1955). X-irradiation, on the other hand, seems to increase the severity of disease in mice or guinea-pigs subsequently challenged with *H. capsulatum* (Brandt 1950a).

References

AJELLO, L. and L. C. RUNYON, 1953, J. Bacteriol. *66*, 34.

ANDERSON, K. Z. and S. MARCUS, 1968, Am. Rev. Resp. Dis. *99*, 608.

BAUM, G. L., S. M. ADRIANO and J. SCHWARZ, 1954, Am. J. Clin. Pathol. *24*, 903.

BRANDT, F. A., 1950a, S. Afr. J. Med. Sci. *15*, 1.

BRANDT, F. A., 1950b, J. Pathol. Bacteriol. *62*, 259.

CAWLEY, E. P. and A. C. CURTIS, 1948, J. Invest. Dermatol. *11*, 443.

DANIELS, L. S., M. D. BERLINER and C. C. CAMPBELL, 1968, J. Bacteriol. *96*, 1535.

DAY, R., 1949, Am. J. Ophthalmol. *32*, 1317.

DROUHET, E. and G. SEGRETAIN, 1952, Ann. Inst. Pasteur *83*, 381.

FARID, Z. and W. R. BARCLAY, 1953, A.M.A. Arch. Pathol. *68*, 413.

FARRELL, R. L., C. R. COLE, J. A. PRIOR and S. SASLAW, 1953, Proc. Soc. Exptl. Biol. Med. *84*, 51.

FURCOLOW, M. L., 1963, New England J. Med. *268*, 357.

GRAYSTON, J. T. and M. L. FURCOLOW, 1953, Am. J. Pub. Health *43*, 665.

GRAYSTON, J. T., P. L. ALTMAN and G. C. COZAD, 1956, Experimental histoplasmosis in mice. A preliminary report. Pub. Health Monogr. No. 39, pp. 99–105.

GRAYSTON, J. T. and S. B. SALVIN, 1956, A.M.A. Arch. Pathol. *61*, 422

HAZEN, E. L. and E. D. TAHLER, 1950, J. Invest. Dermatol. *15*, 205.

HILL, G. A. and S. MARCUS, 1959, J. Infect. Dis. *105*, 26.

HOWARD, D. H., 1965, J. Bacteriol. *89*, 518.

HOWELL, A., JR. and G. F. KIPKIE, 1950, Proc. Soc. Exptl. Biol. Med. *75*, 121.

HOWELL, A., JR. and G. F. KIPKIE, 1951, Am. J. Trop. Med. *31*, 33.

HOWELL, A., JR., G. F. KIPKIE and N. C. DURHAM, 1950, J. Lab. Clin. Med. *36*, 547.

JOHNSON, R. W. and M. SCHERAGO, 1960, Am. Rev. Resp. Dis. *81*, 96.

KIPKIE, G. F. and A. HOWELL, JR., 1951, A.M.A. Arch. Pathol. *51*, 312.

KNIGHT, R. A., G. HILL and S. MARCUS, 1959, Proc. Soc. Exptl. Biol. Med. *100*, 356.

LARSH, H. W. and C. C. SHEPARD, 1958, J. Bacteriol. *76*, 557.

LARSH, H. W., V. E. SCHOLES, A. HINTON and S. SILBERG, 1958, Proc. Soc. Exptl. Biol. Med. *98*, 570.

LEHAN, P. H. and M. L. FURCOLOW, 1957, J. Chron. Dis. *5*, 489.

MENGES, R. W. and R. T. HABERMAN, 1955, Am. J. Vet. Res. *16*, 314.

MIDDLETON, J. G., D. L. MCVICKAR and J. C. PETERSON, 1950, Proc. Soc. Exptl. Biol. Med. *75*, 164.

NEWBERRY, M. W., JR., J. W. CHANDLER, JR., T. D. Y. CHIN and C. H. KIRKPATRICK, 1968, J. Immunol. *100*, 436.

O'HERN, E. M., 1961, J. Immunol. *87*, 728.

PROCKNOW, J. J., 1960, The pathogenesis of histoplasmosis in animals. *In*: H. C. Sweany, ed: Histoplasmosis. Springfield, Ill., Thomas. pp. 246–267.

PROCKNOW, J. J. and G. C. RAY, 1962, J. Lab. Clin. Med. *59*, 496.

REID, J. D., J. H. SCHERER, P. A. HERBUT and H. IRVING, 1942, J. Lab. Clin. Med. *27*, 419.

RIBI, E. and S. B. SALVIN, 1956, Exptl. Cell Res. *10*, 394.

ROBINSON, V. and D. L. MCVICKAR, 1952, Am. J. Vet. Res. *13*, 214.

ROWLEY, D. A. and M. HUBER, 1954, J. Infect. Dis. *96*, 174.

ROWLEY, D. A. and M. HUBER, 1955, J. Infect. Dis. *97*, 27.

ROWLEY, D. A., R. T. HABERMAN and C. W. EMMONS, 1954, J. Infect. Dis. *95*, 98.

SALVIN, S. B., 1953, J. Immunol. *70*, 267.

SALVIN, S. B., 1955a, Am. J. Hyg. *61*, 72.

SALVIN, S. B., 1955b, J. Immunol. *74*, 214.

SALVIN, S. B., 1956, Trans. N.Y. Acad. Sci. *18*, 462.

SALVIN, S. B., 1960, Resistance of animals and man to histoplasmosis. *In*: H. C. Sweany, ed: Histoplasmosis. Springfield, Ill. Thomas. pp. 99–112.

SALVIN, S. B. and E. J. BELL, 1955, J. Immunol. *75*, 57.

SALVIN, S. B. and G. A. HOTTLE, 1948, J. Immunol. *60*, 57.

SALVIN, S. B. and E. RIBI, 1955, Proc. Soc. Exptl. Biol. Med. *90*, 287.

SALVIN, S. B. and R. F. SMITH, 1959, J. Infect. Dis. *105*, 45.

SASLAW, S., H. N. CARLISLE and J. SPARKS, 1960, Proc. Soc. Exptl. Biol. Med. *103*, 342.

SCHAEFER, J. and S. SASLAW, 1954, Proc. Soc. Exptl. Biol. Med. *85*, 223.

SCHEFF, G. J. and I. M. PFEIFER-SCHEFF, 1950, Am. Rev. Tuberc. *62*. 374.

SCHWARZ, J. and E. L. BINGHAM, 1956, J. Am. Vet. Med. Assoc. *128*, 611.

SELTZER, G., S. BARON, and M. TOPOREK, 1955, New England J. Med. *252*, 252.

VOGEL, R. A., M. MICHAEL JR. and A. TIMPE, 1955, Am. J. Pathol. *31*, 535.

8.7. Coccidioidomycosis

Coccidioidomycosis, caused by the dimorphic fungus *Coccidioides immitis*, is endemic to arid southwestern United States, and to parts of Argentina, Bolivia, and Paraguay. The fungus grows in the soil, from where arthrospores are blown about by winds. The infectious particles enter the body typically via the respiratory tract, or possibly also via the gastrointestinal route. On very rare occasions, the organism may invade host tissues via the skin (Wilson et al. 1953). The disease usually appears as an acute, self-limiting respiratory infection, and more rarely as a chronic disseminating infection involving many of the host tissues. With coccidioidin as the antigen in intradermal testing, the aetiology of the primary acute 'valley fever' was determined and extensive studies on the nature of coccidioidomycosis followed (Smith et al. 1948).

The development of delayed hypersensitivity to coccidioidin during the early phases of an acute upper respiratory infection was of importance in establishing the diagnosis of the disease. The incubation period for development of delayed allergy typically was from 10 to 14 days, with a range of 7 to 28 days (Smith et al. 1948; Smith 1940). The capacity to react was acquired during an infection with *C. immitis*, although the infection itself could be subclinical. This reactivity lasts for many years after the onset or arrest of the disease. Occasionally, a patient may develop little or no hypersensitivity to coccidioidin, in which situation the chronic disseminated form of the disease usually follows. This anergy may be common in fatal cases. The basis of this anergy or low level of hypersensitivity may be associated with excessive amounts of antigen present and the accompanying desensitization, or an immune deficiency of the host resulting in a failure to react sufficiently to antigenic stimulation.

Persons who are coccidioidin-positive are considered resistant to reinfection. Individuals with 'erythema nodosum' are highly reactive to the skin-testing antigen and are also highly resistant to dissemination of the fungus.

The specific hypersensitivity probably persists for a long time. Thus, 80 to 90% of long-time residents of an endemic area react intracutaneously to the antigen, although possibly this persistence of hypersensitivity may be due to repeated exposure to *C. immitis*. Nevertheless, only 2 of 78 reactors residing in a nonendemic area for a year converted to nonresponders (Smith et al. 1946). This long-lasting hypersensitivity may be associated with the presence of antigens within host tissues, since spherules or endospores have been found in healed calcified lesions in the lungs of coccidioidin reactors (Butt and Hoffman 1945).

Although skin tests with coccidioidin are useful in establishing past infection, they are not helpful in determination of concurrent infection unless active conversion is seen. Serologic tests provide a useful aid in prognosis and diagnosis.

With coccidioidin as antigen in precipitation and complement-fixation tests, antibodies are not detected in extremely mild inapparent infections (Smith and Saito 1957; Smith et al. 1950, 1957, 1956). As the infection becomes more severe and extended, the serologic tests tend to become positive. Serologic tests become positive only after the appearance of delayed hypersensitivity. Precipitins, which usually appear before complement-fixing antibodies, may be detected in clinically inapparent primary infection, and are low or absent in most disseminated infections. Half of the patients with primary disease develop discernible precipitating antibodies within the first week of disease, while 91% become positive within the first three weeks. None become positive after the fourth week of illness. By then, precipitins have started to decrease, so that by the sixth month of illness, most precipitins have disappeared.

Complement-fixing antibodies, which develop much more slowly, may develop during the first three months of illness. A peak in the number of positives is reached during the second month, after which a decline occurs. Complement-fixation titres increase with the severity of the disease. According to the procedure of C. E. Smith, 97% of positive sera from individuals with nondisseminating disease had titres less than 1:32 (Smith et al. 1950). Precipitins do not initially occur or increase in titre as complement-fixing antibodies are declining.

In more recent years, modifications of this procedure have appeared. Whereas Smith et al. (1948, 1950) prepared the antigen from stationary growth of many strains of C. immitis on an asparagine synthetic medium at 37°C for one or more months, a technique for more rapid production of coccidioidin has been introduced (Pappaglanis et al. 1961a). Herein, a multi-strain inoculum is grown in a glucose-yeast extract medium on a shaker at 30–33°C for three days. The filtrate from the fungus growth is used as the complement-fixation antigen. The remaining mycelial mat is washed, suspended in distilled water plus 3% toluene, and incubated at 37°C for three days. The resulting solution from filtration is the crude precipitation antigen.

The agar gel immunodiffusion procedure with the broth filtrate as antigen has been adapted as a screening procedure for the detection of positive antisera (Huppert and Bailey 1963, 1965a, 1965b). A latex particle agglutination test has been substituted for the tube precipitin test (Huppert et al. 1968). Although no single test is adequate for the detection of all positive specimens from diagnosed cases, a combination of the foregoing two procedures can detect 93% of the specimens. Both tests are simple, highly reproducible, and effective.

Of the various laboratory animals employed in the study of coccidioidomycosis, probably mice and rats have been most extensively used. These species may be readily infected with C. immitis by one of a variety of routes. Intranasal inoculation under anesthesia led to pulmonary infection with dissemination absent or minimal (Tager and Liebow 1942). Mice that had been inoculated intraperitoneally with mycelial phase showed a high susceptibility to many strains of the fungus (Friedman et al. 1955, 1956). The relative virulence of 100 particles grown on solid media ranged from 100% survival through 90 days. Subcutaneous inoculation of 100 arthrospores of a virulent strain resulted in localized abscesses, which developed a necrotic purulent or caseous center, a zone of mononuclear and polymorphonuclear cells and, a rim of spongy epithelioid cells, all surrounded by a fibrous capsule and granulation tissue (Pappagianis et al. 1959). Viable *C. immitis* could be cultured from some of these local abscesses, but not from others, while with the aid of the periodic acid-Schiff stain, many degenerate fungal cells or fragments were shown to be present. The administration of cortisone acetate just prior to or at the time of challenge did not enhance dissemination from the local lesions to the viscera.

Albino mice were also highly susceptible to intracerebral challenge (Karrer 1953). Of two strains assayed, between 1–9 particles produced 50% mortality.

The resistance of mice to subsequent intraperitoneal challenge with 100 viable spores has been increased by prior subcutaneous inoculations with suspensions of killed mycelial particles (Friedman and Smith 1956). The enhanced resistance was evoked both by homologous and heterologous strains, by formalin- or acetone-killed organisms, and by vaccines grown in submerged culture in liquid medium or on the surface of solid medium. The protection was illustrated in that 95 to 100% of the vaccinated animals were still alive at 60 days post-challenge, whereas only 20% of the controls survived that length of time. Nearly all survivors, however, were infected with the fungus.

Substantial resistance was also indicated in mice with a subcutaneous administration of a highly virulent strain of *C. immitis* (Friedman et al. 1955) or with intraperitoneal inoculation of a low virulence strain, followed by intraperitoneal challenge (Converse et al. 1962). Increased resistance to intranasal challenge was also induced in mice by prior immunization with mycelium or arthrospores (Levine et al. 1960).

When spherules were able to be grown in artificial culture in large quantities, the opportunity presented itself to examine and compare the immunogenicity of the cells which normally exist as a pathogen in host tissues (Levine et al. 1960; Converse 1955, 1956, 1957; Converse and Besemer 1959; Baker and Braude 1956). Thus, repeated intramuscular injection of a heat-killed, saline suspension of spherules into guinea-pigs increased their resistance to an aerosol of living arthrospores (Vogel et al. 1954). When mice were challenged with arthrospores via the intranasal route, greater protection was induced by subcutaneous or intramuscular vaccination with multiple doses of the spherule-endospore phase grown *in vitro* than with either the mycelial or arthrospore phases (Levine et al. 1961). Mycelial vaccine doses totaling 6.0 mg were not as efficaceous as one-third this dose of the spherule-endospore vaccine. Most of the mice immunized with spherule-endospore vaccine survived for observation periods up to six months after intranasal challenge with arthrospore doses that greatly exceeded those lethal to control mice. Although the vaccinated survivors seemed to be in good health, a high percentage were culturally positive on autopsy. The immunogenicity of the spherules and endospores was associated primarily with the particulate fraction of sonically disrupted cells. Apparently, the spherule wall is the primary site of the immunogenic substances (Kong et al. 1961). The importance of the spherule wall thus parallels the situation in *H. capsulatum*, where the wall fraction of the yeast phase is also most immunogenic (Salvin and Ribi 1955).

The immunogenicity of the tissue phase as a vaccine varied with its stage of development (Levine et al. 1965). Unreleased endospores were non-immunogenic, but naturally-released ones were. Seemingly, the immunogens were developed approximately at the time of endospore emergence from the spherule. The synthesis appeared to be associated with the development of the wall in the growing endospore, since the wall of the resulting spherule accounted for almost all of the immunogenicity. The change of the endospore to a mature spherule was paralleled by an increase in immunogenicity. When the spherule finally ruptured and released endospores, the preparation showed less immunogenic potency. At this time, very few spherule walls were observed, probably having been lysed very rapidly.

The spherule vaccine seemed to be specific to the extent that it did not protect mice against challenge with *Cryptococcus neoformans* or *Pseudomonas pseudomallei* (Kong et al. 1968). The protective antigen, however, was not strain specific, since spherules of one strain of *C. immitis* increased resistance in mice to challenge with a variety of other strains of the same species (Levine et al. 1965; Kong et al. 1964).

A coccidioidin, derived from the spherule phase grown *in vitro*, was examined for its activity as a skin-testing antigen in mice and guinea pigs, in comparison with the conventional coccidioidin derived from growth of the mycelium (Kong et al. 1966; Levine et al. 1969). The spherule coccidioidin elicited stronger reactions at a lower dose, and produced reactivity in a higher percentage of animals for a longer period of time.

Although intramuscular injection of killed spherules enhanced the resistance of mice and resulted in survival after intranasal challenge doses of arthrospores as high as 200 LD_{50}, introduction of the vaccine via the intravenous route failed to protect the mice against a challenge of 5 LD_{50}. This suppression of enhanced resistance occurred either with spherules or with endospores, but was not induced by a weakly immunogenic soluble cell fraction (Levine and Kong 1966). The protective properties of the spherule vaccine were also decreased in male mice by treatment with testosterone, and in mice of both sexes by treatment with oestradiol (Levine and Madin 1962).

Vaccination of cynomolgus monkeys (*Macaca irus*) with killed spherule-endospore suspensions of *C. immitis* resulted in increased resistance to intranasal challenge with 200 arthrospores (Levine et al. 1962). During a 265-day period after challenge, 5 of the 10 control monkeys died, and two others were moribund. In contrast, none of 8 vaccinated animals succumbed to the challenge during this interval. Roentgenographic examination and subsequent autopsy findings indicated far less pulmonary pathology in the vaccinated group. The spherule vaccine did not stimulate production of detectable circulating antibodies, although a weak delayed hypersensitivity developed. This combination of the presence of delayed hypersensitivity and the absence of complement-fixing or precipitating antibodies occurs in mild or subclinical infections in man. After challenge, however, the vaccinated monkeys developed high complement-fixation titres, in a situation which in humans indicates a poor prognosis.

Since symptomatic reinfections are almost non-existent in endemic areas of coccidioidomycosis, strong and lasting immunity seems to be acquired in man after infection with *C. immitis*. After viable arthrospores had been introduced intranasally into mice, they showed marked resistance to subsequent intranasal challenge. This resistance was especially striking, since little protection was apparent after similar immunization with formalin-killed arthrospores and subsequent intranasal challenge (Pappagianis et al. 1961b). This increased resistance of mice occurred whether the viable arthrospores came from strains of *C. immitis* of high or low virulence.

Viable arthrospores were also effective in increasing resistance of monkeys (*Macaca mulatta*) to *C. immitis* (Converse et al. 1963; Blundell et al. 1961). Animals vaccinated in the forearm with as little as 10 viable arthrospores were challenged 6 months later via the respiratory route with about 7000 viable arthrospores. Enhanced resistance obviously had developed after vaccination, since the monkeys remained healthy after respiratory challenge, their chest X-rays were negative, lung cultures were mostly negative, and only minor histopathologic changes were observed on autopsy at 120 days. In contrast, control monkeys or monkeys that had previously received up to 10^9 nonviable arthrospores showed severe clinical disease, positive chest X-rays, positive lung cultures, massive pulmonary destruction, and death in over half the animals. Apparently, the development of enhanced resistance depended on the conversion of the arthrospores and the subsequent growth of spherules in the monkey tissues.

Although living arthrospores appear to be effective as a vaccine in monkeys, it is extremely unlikely that such a vaccine would ever be used to enhance resistance of man to *C. immitis*. Killed spherules, or

 S. B. Salvin

a purified antigen therefrom, seem to present the more logical choice because of their non-infectivity and their capacity to increase resistance.

References

BAKER, O. and A. I. BRAUDE, 1956, J. Lab. Clin. Med. *47*, 169.

BLUNDELL, G. P., M. W. CASTLEBERRY, E. P. LOWE and J. L. CONVERSE, 1961, Am. J. Pathol. *39*, 613.

BUTT, E. M. and A. M. HOFFMAN, 1945, Am. J. Pathol. *21*, 485.

CONVERSE, J. L., 1955, Proc. Soc. Exptl. Biol. Med. *90*, 709.

CONVERSE, J. L., 1956, J. Bacteriol. *72*, 784.

CONVERSE, J. L., 1957, J. Bacteriol. *74*, 106.

CONVERSE, J. L. and A. R. BESEMER, 1959, J. Bacteriol. *78*, 231.

CONVERSE. J. L., M. W. CASTLEBERRY, A. R. BESEMER and E. M. SNYDER. 1962, J. Bacteriol. *84*, 46.

CONVERSE, J. L., M. W. CASTLEBERRY and E. M. SYNDER, 1963, J. Bacteriol. *86*, 1041.

FRIEDMAN, L. and C. E. SMITH, 1956, Am. Rev. Tuberc. and Pulm. Res. *74*, 245.

FRIEDMAN, L., C. E. SMITH and L. E. GORDON, 1955, J. Infect. Dis. *97*, 311.

FRIEDMAN, L., C. E. SMITH, W. G. ROESSLER and R. J. BERMAN, 1956, Am. J. Hyg. *64*, 198.

HUPPERT, M. and J. W. BAILEY, 1963, Sabouraudia *2*, 284.

HUPPERT, M. and J. W. BAILEY, 1965a, Am. J. Clin. Pathol. *44*, 364.

HUPPERT, M. and J. W. BAILEY, 1965b, Am. J. Clin. Pathol. *44*, 369.

HUPPERT, M., E. T. PETERSON, S. H. SUN, P. A. CHITJIAN and W. J. DERREVERE, 1968, Am. J. Clin. Pathol. *49*, 96.

KARRER, H. E. 1953, Proc. Soc. Exptl. Biol. Med. *82*, 766.

KONG, Y. M., H. B. LEVINE and C. E. SMITH, 1961, Sabouraudia *2*, 131.

KONG, Y. M., H. B. LEVINE, S. H. MADIN and C. E. SMITH, 1964, J. Immunol. *92*, 779.

KONG, Y. M., D. C. SAVAGE and L. N. L. KONG, 1966, J. Bacteriol. *91*, 876.

LEVINE, H. B. and Y. M. KONG, 1966, J. Immunol. *97*, 297.

LEVINE, H. B. and S. H. MADIN, 1962, Sabouraudia *2*, 47.

LEVINE, H. B., J. M. COBB and G. M. SCALARONE, 1969, Sabouraudia *7*, 20.

LEVINE, H. B., J. M. COBB and C. E. SMITH, 1960, Trans. N.Y. Acad. Sci. *22*, 436.

LEVINE, H. B., J. M. COBB and C. E. SMITH, 1961, J. Immunol. *87*, 218.

LEVINE, H. B., Y. M. KONG and C. E. SMITH, 1965, J. Immunol. *94*, 132.

LEVINE, H. B., R. L. MILLER and C. E. SMITH, 1962, J. Immunol. *89*, 242.

PAPPAGIANIS, D., H. B. LEVINE, C. E. SMITH, R. J. BERMAN and G. S. KOBAYASHI 1961b, J. Immunol. *86*, 28.

PAPPAGIANIS, D., C. E. SMITH, R. J. BERMAN and G. S. KOBAYASHI, 1959, J. Invest. Dermatol. *32*, 589.

PAPPAGIANIS, D., C. E. SMITH, G. S. KOBAYASHI and M. T. SAITO, 1961a, J. Infect. Dis. *108*, 35.

SMITH, C. E., 1940, Am. J. Publ. Health *30*, 600.

SMITH, C. E. and M. T. SAITO, 1957, J. Chronic Dis. *5*, 571.

SMITH, C. E., M. T. SAITO and S. A. SIMONS, 1956, J. Am. Med. Assoc. *160*, 546.

SMITH, C. E., R. R. BEARD, H. G. ROSENBERGER and E. G. WHITING, 1946, J. Am. Med. Assoc. *132*, 833.

SMITH, C. E., M. T. SAITO, R. R. BEARD, R. M. KEPP, R. W. CLARK and B. Y. EDDIE, 1950, Am. J. Hyg. *52*, 1.

SMITH, C. E., M. T. SAITO, C. C. CAMPBELL, G. B. HILL, S. SASLAW, S. B. SALVIN, J. E. FENTON and M. A. KRUPP, 1957, Public Health Reports *72*, 888.

SMITH, C. E., E. G. WHITING, E. E. BAKER, H. G. ROSENBERGER, R. R. BEARD and M. T. SAITO, 1948, Am. Rev. Tuberc. *57*, 330.

TAGER, M. and A. A. LIEBOW, 1942, Yale J. Biol. Med. *15*, 41.

VOGEL, R. A., B. F. FETTER, N. F. CONANT and E. P. LOWE, 1954, Am. Rev. Tuberc. *70*, 498.

WILSON, J. W., C. E. SMITH and O. A. PLUNKETT, 1953, Calif. Med. *79*, 233.

8.8. Sporotrichosis

Sporotrichosis is a chronic disease generally characterized in man by the development of nodular lesions or abscesses in the skin, subcutaneous tissues, or lymph nodes. Chronic progressive sporotrichosis of an extremity was induced in white mice by a single injection into the paw of a suspension of spores and mycelium of *Sporotrichum Schenckii* (Baker 1947). In some of the animals, sporotrichosis of the foot and later of the ankle developed, with the mice recovering spontaneously. In other mice, the disease was fatal, with abundant proliferation of the organism. This situation differs from that in man, in whom fungal cells are so few in number that they are difficult to find on direct examination. Mouse macrophages engulfed large quantities of yeast-like cells. Lesions appeared which were suppurative, necrotizing and fibrosing, as well as macrophagic. Pathogenicity of strains varied somewhat, with cigar-shaped and round cell forms, as well as asteroid bodies, typically developing in the tissues (Mariat et al. 1962). The disease also has been induced experimentally in hamsters, guinea-pigs, rats and rabbits (Mariat and Drouhet 1954; Negroni and Prado 1951; Norden 1951). When rats were inoculated in the tip of the tail, the lesions could be observed as they spread up the tail (DuToit 1942). Male rats developed scrotal reactions after intraperitoneal inoculation with sporotrichotic material. The scrotum became swollen and inflamed, the testes enlarged, with small abscesses present.

Sporotrichosis in man does not seem to be followed by a period of highly increased resistance (DuToit 1942). In fact, individuals with sporotrichosis were infected experimentally while they actually were recovering from the disease (Brown et al. 1947).

Enhanced resistance to reinfection was reported in rats that had been originally infected subcutaneously and cutaneously with spores of *S. Schenckii* and then reinfected cutaneously (Jessner 1922). When rats were initially infected by cutaneous inoculation and then subsequently challenged intracardially, the period during which the fungus could be cultured from the blood was shortened (Kesten and Martenstein 1929). While control animals yielded organisms from their blood for an average of 25 days after challenge, the blood of reinfected rats became culturally negative on an average of eleven days after intracardial reinfection.

Mice have been protected against lethal intravenous challenge of *S. Schenckii* yeast-like cells either by vaccination with formalin-killed cells or by sublethal preinfection with living cells (Hasenclever and Mitchell 1959). Although the death rate was slightly reduced in mice receiving formalin-treated cells, the fungus was still present in the liver and spleen. The rate of survival was also slightly greater in previously infected mice, in comparison with controls. The length of the initial immunizing infection seemed to have little influence upon the rate of survival after challenge. Attempts at passive immunization with serum from rabbits immunized against *S. Schenckii* or with serum from previously infected mice did not modify the course of subsequent challenge.

References

BAKER, R. D., 1947, Am. J. Trop. Med. *27*, 749.

BROWN, R., D. WEINTRAUB, M. W. SIMPSON, F. W. SIMSON, M. A. F. HELM, J. W. BOWEN, F. A. BRANDT and C. BERMAN, 1947, Sporotrichosis infection on mines of the Witwatersrand. Johannesburg, Transvaal Chamber of Mines.

DU TOIT, C. J., 1942, Proc. Transvaal Mine Medical Officers Assoc. *22*, 111.

HASENCLEVER, H. F. and W. MITCHELL, 1959, J. Invest. Dermatol. *33*, 145.

JESSNER, M., 1922, Klin. Wschr. *1*, 2428.

KESTEN, B. and H. MARTENSTEIN, 1929, Arch. Dermatol. *20*, 441.

MARIAT, F. and E. DROUHET, 1954, Ann. Inst. Pasteur *86*, 1.

MARIAT, F., P. LAVALLE and P. DESTOMBES, 1962, Sabouraudia *2*, 60.

NEGRONI, P. and J. M. PRADO, 1951, An. Soc. Cient. Argent. *151*, 32.

NORDEN, A., 1951, Acta Pathol. et Microbiol. Scand. Suppl. *89*, 1.

8.9. Summary and conclusions

Severe disease resulting from internal dissemination of the systemic fungi is not frequent in man, although many of the potentially pathogenic mycotic agents may be common in the environment. Man therefore must be able to resist the penetration into, or the multiplication, or growth of these agents in vital tissues. To survive and thrive in areas heavily contaminated with such potential pathogens as *C. immitis* or *H. capsulatum*, man not only must have innate or nonspecific resistance, but also must be able to acquire enhanced resistance to a specific organism. Antibodies have not been demonstrated to be capable of developing or enhancing resistance to the systemic mycoses.

The basis to resistance, therefore, probably lies in a *cellular mechanism* associated with macrophages and lymphocytes. Procedures which alter mononuclear activity in an individual are likely to alter his resistance to the ubiquitous fungi. Patients with diseases leading to anaemia or leucopenia or after prolonged treatment with drugs leading to bone marrow changes seem to develop more serious mycotic diseases. Other factors, such as the phagocytic capacity of the cells, the amount and activity of lysosomal enzymes, and the serum components relating to phagocytosis, may be influential in maintaining resistance to the invasive fungi.

Acquired resistance has been enhanced by mild infection with fungal species or by immunization with dead cells. Although previous infection seems to produce more effective and longer lasting resistance in laboratory animals than immunization with dead cells, such a procedure is too hazardous for application in man. Enhanced resistance to a specific fungus has been produced by immunization with killed cells of the specific agent. For example, injection of dead yeastlike cells of *H. capsulatum* or of killed spherules of *C. immitis* has definitely increased the resistance of laboratory animals to subsequent challenge. In other mycoses, such as cryptococcosis, inoculation of the host animal with dead cells has produced an enhanced degree of resistance, but one which is less obvious. Although purified components of cell walls have been isolated, such as from the yeastlike phase of *H. capsulatum*, and although such components have been found to increase resistance of laboratory animals, little is known of the chemical nature of the active moiety. Generally, such active fractions are more effectively isolated from the tissue phase than the saprophytic phase of a dimorphic fungus. In man or animals which have been rendered more resistant by virtue of previous exposure to living organisms or by hyperimmunization with dead cells, increased resistance is not absolute, in that living cells of the pathogen are not completely eliminated from the host tissues. Such cells, however, do not multiply or disseminate to the degree that they do in normal, non-immune animals.

CHAPTER 9

The immunogenic
properties of mammalian cells

DAVID FRANKS

Department of Pathology, University of Cambridge, Cambridge

9.1. Introduction

In earlier chapters in this book it will probably have been shown that
it is not always easy to distinguish immunogenic functions of the antigen
from functions of the host. When mammalian cells are considered it is
often impossible to make this distinction. Nevertheless, the aim of
this chapter is to discuss the various types of mammalian cell antigens
that exist and what kind of immunological response they evoke, without
considering extensively the way in which the host responds to these
antigens. The response to one particular form of mammalian cell –
antigen-transplantation immunity – is discussed in a later chapter, but
is must be clear that much that can be written about histocompatibility
systems is also true of the response to other mammalian cell antigens,
certainly to blood group antigens, and also to cellular antigens of other
mammalian species.

One of the most interesting aspects of immunogenicity which is
relevant to the consideration of mammalian cells is the concept of antigen
strength: why some antigens readily provoke a response, while the
immunogenicity of other antigens is much feebler. It is necessary,
however, to distinguish what is purely a laboratory artefact: the difficulty
of detecting a response to certain antigens. It is frequently difficult, for
example, to detect antibodies to certain blood group antigens by direct
agglutination, but it is irrational to regard such antigens as 'weak' antigens. Indeed as far as mammalian cells are concerned, the only sensible
course is to consider immunogenicity in relation to the detection system
which is being used. Immunogenicity is usually quantitated, if at all, in
terms of titre or strength of the maximum response; although it is possible
to assay immunogenicity in terms of weight of antibody produced or
number of allergic lymphoid cells, this is seldom done, nor indeed does it
add very much to our understanding. It is also possible to discuss, as

will be done later for the human rhesus blood group antigens, the question of the likelihood of an individual responding to an antigen. This is governed by the host's genetic constitution, particularly by the blood group antigens present and by previous exposure to the same and related antigens.

9.2. *Variation in antigen strength: features of the individual, the cell and the detection systems*

Many cellular antigen systems in mammals show variations in antigen strength between different cells in the same individual, and between the same cell from different individuals of the same species. Where such differences occur between individuals they are most likely to be due to genetic effects. One very typical blood group system which shows this effect is the G system in rabbits (Heard 1955; Joysey 1955; Cohen 1958). This system contains three allelic genes, W, Y and Z, each of which produces an antigen, and Joysey showed that the reaction of, for example, anti-Y with the YW heterozygote's cells was considerably weaker than with the YY homozygote. This distinction was seen only when direct agglutination of the red cells was used to detect the antigen and such distinctions were not seen if anti-globulin tests were used. An even more marked form of this variation was found in a blood group system in the horse (Franks, 1962a) where the presence of an antigen could be detected in some horses by both anti-globulin test and by techniques involving complement fixation, such as lysis or conglutination, whereas in others the antigen would be detected only by anti-globulin tests and not by lysis. It was suggested that this variation in the horse was due to a complex system of gene interaction (Franks 1962b). In the rabbit system, Heard (1955) suggested that the strongly agglutinating cells had many more antigen sites than did the poorly agglutinating cells, an hypothesis which was suggested by the observation that fewer absorptions with strongly agglutinating cells were required to remove all antibody than were needed with poorly agglutinating cells, and this hypothesis was further strengthened by the demonstration (Boursnell et al., 1955) that strongly agglutinating cells took up about six or seven times as many antibody molecules labelled with ^{131}I than did poorly agglutinating cells.

Many such examples of variation in 'antigen strength' are now known. Initially all of these examples of quantitative variation are given simple explanations, like the one above, but further investigation invariable discloses further complexity. For example, in the rabbit WYZ system, YW heterozygous cells were the least agglutinable with anti-Y, and YY homogozygous cells were the most agglutinable. The other heterozygote, YZ cells gave intermediate reactions, and overlapped the range of the YW cells. Similar investigations were made by Cohen (1955), who like Joysey, estimated the 'strength' of agglutination by a modified scoring system, and who showed that there was considerable scatter in the scores obtained with cells of rabbits with the same WYZ genotypes, and in particular when animals of different breeding strains were compared, which suggests that differences in agglutinability are not simply the result of interactions between the genes producing the three antigens.

Other examples of differences in 'antigen strength' are known which are due not to variation in the amount of antigen present, but to the presence of absence of chemical groupings on the cell surface which affect the ability of antibody either to combine with the antigen or to produce agglutination. The well known variation in the J blood group antigen in cattle is due to variations in the amount of a material sensitive to neuraminidase on the surface of the red cells (Uhlenbruck et al. 1967).

Although quantitative variation in antigen or variation in availability of antigen might very easily effect its ability to provoke a response, because of the well known relationship between antigen dose and immunogenicity, it is much more important to realize that such variations may very easily affect the assessment of response.

9.3. *An inventory of mammalian cell antigens*

The factor which is most likely to affect an immunological response to a mammalian cell antigen is the presence or absence of that antigen in the animal itself. It is worthwhile considering, therefore, what kinds of mammalian cell antigens there are. These antigens may vary tremendously in distribution, from antigens, such as heterophil antigens, present in all members of several very diverse species, to antigens like the TL (thymus-leukaemia) antigens which are restricted to certain cells of a small number of inbred strains of one species, the mouse.

9.3.1. *'Species' antigens*

It is customary to begin a discussion of the types of cellular antigens with 'species' antigens, although it is difficult to give a rigorous definition of what is meant by this term. If it means anything, it ought to mean an antigen present in all members of the same species, but absent from all other species. It is usually used, however, for a collection of antigens with which an uncharacterized polyvalent serum reacts. This antiserum may also contain heterophil antibodies and antibodies to allo-antigens. Antibodies to species antigens may be of practical value, but they are of little fundamental interest.

9.3.2. Heterophil antibodies

There exists a large group of antibodies which although stimulated by an antigen on one cell, are found to react with another cell, often from a widely different species. Strictly speaking, therefore, it is the antibody which is heterophil, not the antigen. The best known of these heterophil antibodies is the antibody to the Forssman antigen (Forssman 1911). This 'antigen' is now known to be a complex of related antigens and it is best to restrict the description 'Forssman antibody' to that originally described by Forssman as an antibody which is stimulated by the injection of autoclaved guinea-pig kidney, and which also reacts with sheep red blood cells, although it is probably a good idea to add that it is not present on bovine red cells, to distinguish it from another heterophil antibody, the Paul-Bunnell antibody. The Forssman antigen is a complex of related antigens, and although considerable effort has been made to analyse and characterize these antigens, it cannot be said that this has been either successful or profitable. It is important, however, to realize that not all of these related antigens may be present in a species broadly characterized as Forssman-positive, and that it is perfectly possible to produce a Forssman antibody (as defined above) in a Forssman-positive species, such as the chicken. For years there has been a controversy about whether there is a cross-reaction between the Forssman antigen and the human blood group A antigen. This controversy was started because Schiff and Adelsberger (1924) did not know that there are 'A' antigens present in both sheep and guinea-pigs, and the confusion was made worse because later investigators were unaware that the A antigen is an allo-antigen in sheep. Recently however, Flory (1968) and Rose (1968, personal communication) have clarified this problem, and shown that although it may be important from a practical point of view to decide whether an antibody is anti-Forssman or anti-A, such a distinction is ultimately meaningless, since A, like Forssman, is a complex antigen, and in the end, whether a particular antibody is called anti-A or anti-Forssman may be a matter of personal taste. It should be stressed, however, that there are anti-A antibodies which are *not* Forssman antibodies (do not react with sheep or guinea-pig kidney cells) just as there are anti-Forssman antibodies which do not react with human A red cells or red cells of one of the related A allo-antigen systems in other species.

Anti-A is similar to anti-Forssman in another respect, in that some of the anti-A antibodies in man are heterophil antibodies. It seems likely that the naturally occurring antibodies are provoked by exposure to microorganisms (Springer et al. 1959) and that antibodies to these microbial antigens happen to react with identical or similar antigens on the red cells of some human beings, so that anti-A is a heterophil antibody which is also an antibody to an allo-antigen. The evidence which suggests that this is so is provided by experiments on germ-free chicks. Normal chickens have antibodies which react with the human blood group B antigen. Germ-free chicks do not, but if they are fed on a particular strain of *E. coli* (081), they do produce anti-B antibodies. It must be admitted that this evidence is suggestive rather than definite. The human B blood group antigen is not an allo-antigen in chickens, and anti-B in chickens does not have the characteristic properties of the naturally occurring anti-B in man (see later), and there is plenty of scope for those who prefer to believe the bizarre alternative hypotheses that have been put forward.

Another well known heterophil antibody is the Paul-Bunnell antibody, (see Carter and Penman 1961, for review) which occurs in individuals suffering from infectious mononucleosis. It may be recognized by its reaction with cattle red cells, but not with guinea-pig kidney cells; its stimulus is unknown but it is at least possible that it is provoked by the agent which causes infectious mononucleosis.

These considerations have little to do with mammalian cells as immunogens, but it must be obvious that the study of mammalian cell antigens as immunogens could be complicated by the fact that the reaction being investigated may be a heterophil reaction rather than the reaction provoked by the cell itself. For example, the sheep red cell has been widely used in studies on rosette formation by allergized cells: at least part of the response to the injection of sheep red cells may be a secondary response to antigen present on microbes as well as on sheep cells.

One of the features of human 'naturally occurring' anti-A and anti-B which is unusual is the persistence of the antibody, its titre unchanged for months or even years. It seems that this is a feature of polysaccharide antigens which are being continually recycled, rather than of antigens which provoke heterophil antibodies, although such antigens frequently are polysaccharides. One of the best demonstrations of this was by Britton et al. (1968), who showed phases of production of antibodies for *E. coli* 055:B5 lipopolysaccharide in mice for up to 70 days, and prolonged production of IgM antibodies. It is well known that even when individuals are injected deliberately with human A or B red cells to stimulate the appearance of anti-A or anti-B 'immune' IgG, the anti-A or anti-B IgM continues to be produced at the same titre as before; another piece of evidence which suggests that the anti-A and anti-B IgG and IgM antibodies may be directed against different antigens.

9.3.3. Blood group allo-antigens

The mammalian cell antigens whose immunogenicity has been most extensively studied are the allo-antigens, that is antigens present in some but not all, members of the same species. These antigens may also be present in other, usually closely related species (like the human MN) blood group antigens in other primates), they may also react with heterophil antibodies (like the A antigen) and they may also be auto-antigens, or at any rate react with auto-antibodies, like the human rhesus e antigen which reacts with an antibody produced in auto-allergic haemolytic anaemia of the warm antibody type (see later). Some allo-antigens, like the human I antigen, may react with all three types of antibody.

Because of their importance in blood transfusion and haemolytic disease of the newborn, a certain amount of information is available about the immunogenicity of blood group antigens in man. The most extensively studied is the human rhesus D antigen. It is now well established that only in a proportion of women at risk (rhesus-negative with a rhesus-positive foetus) are anti-D antibodies produced. One reason for this is the 'protection' conferred when mother and foetus are incompatible on the ABO blood group system (Levine 1958; Cohen 1960), where the mother is for example O, and therefore has anti-A in her serum, and the foetus is A. Here the foetal red cells which pass into the mother are coated with a macroglobulin antibody which does not fix a complement, and because of this are sequestered in the liver, an organ which contains little lymphoid tissue, rather than the spleen, where they might be expected to stimulate antibody formation. It was because of this that Clarke (1967) and Clarke et al. (1958) suggested that anti-D should be given to rhesus-negative mothers at risk. However, anti-D IgG has been generally used, *postpartum*, because it was thought too dangerous to run the risk of intravascular agglutination by anti-D IgM. It seems probable that passively administered anti-D IgG exerts its effect by some form of central inhibition, and therefore specific for the D antigen, rather than the way in which anti-A IgM works, which is non-specific as far as the protection is concerned, by sequestration of the antigen away from lymphoid tissues (see Woodrow 1970, for review).

However, even when the anti-A protective mechanism is taken into account, there still remains a significant group of rhesus-negative women 'at risk' who never produce anti-D, just as only a proportion of rhesus-negative men will make anti-D when injected with D-positive cells. One ingenious suggestion which has been put forward to account for this is that the individuals who fail to produce these antibodies are those who have been rendered tolerant in foetal life by exposure to maternal D antigen. This idea was put forward independently by Brambell and N. A. Mitchison in 1950 (see Race and Sanger 1968), and by Owen et al. (1954) and was investigated by Booth et al. (1953), who showed that there was no evidence to support this hypothesis, a finding subsequently confirmed by Ward et al. (1957) and by Mayeda (1962). In an investigation of the production of 'immune' anti-A by mothers based on the same hypothesis, Konugres (1964) found some suggestions that some degree of tolerance to A or B can be developed *in utero*.

There remains, therefore, a proportion of individuals who do not produce anti-D antibodies, and it must be acknowledged that it is not known why this is.

Anti-D is the most important cause of haemolytic disease of the newborn, that is, it is the most frequent cause, and it is also the antibody most frequently found in human sera, other than anti-A and anti-B, during routine typing or cross-match. It is therefore frequently described as a 'strong' antigen. Other antibodies are found less frequently, and the corresponding antigens are therefore loosely described as 'weaker', although part at least of the infrequent occurrence of some antibodies, such as anti-Kell results from the rareness of the antigen in the population. It is hardly necessary to point out that the severity of haemolytic disease of the newborn or of a transfusion reaction is no more a guide to the strength of the antigen than is the titre of antibody or whether it produces agglutination or lysis. All these are as much results of the physicochemical properties of the antibody as anything to do with the antigen, or are secondary results of the antigen-antibody interaction. There has been some discussion recently of the concept of strong and weak antigens in relation to histocompatibility antigens, and in my view, these terms, although widely used, cannot be given any meaningful definition.

The concept of antigen strength in relation to histocompatibility antigens has also been extensively discussed by Hildemann (1970) who suggests that donor 'antigen strength' for histocompatibility antigens can be rigorously defined only in relation to recipient genotype, discusses many of the features of 'antigen strength' and tries to draw some general conclusions from the wide variety of observations that have been made. He contends that it is the allelic combination rather than the histocompatibility locus which determines the strength of the antigenic difference (Hildemann 1970, and Hildemann and Cohen 1967). The evidence is compelling for histocompatibility antigens in the mouse, but is less so for ABO antigens acting as histocompatibility antigens in man, where Hildemann quotes the conclusion of Cepellini et al. (1969) that the incompatibility of an A_1 graft is very much stronger than an A_2 graft in an O recipient. This assessment would seem to be so complicated by the quality, frequency and physico-chemical properties of the respective antibodies, as to make it impossible to assess the inherent strength of the A_1 and A_2 antigens. Indeed it is not really known whether the ABO antigens are histocompatibility antigens in the normally accepted sense of the word, since 'naturally occurring' anti-A and anti-B will inevitably damage cells through various antibody-mediated mechanisms.

It is also well established that pre-immunization is more likely to shorten graft survival or strengthen graft-*versus*-host reactions for 'weak' histocompatibility systems than for 'strong' systems.

Simonsen (1970) puts forward the view that the relative strength of transplantation antigens is a function of the number of antigen-sensitive cells which can react with the antigen. He quotes Brent and Medawar's (1966) work on the normal lymphocyte transfer reaction in guinea-pigs which showed that a lymphoid cell essentially either responds or does not respond (the 'quantal theory of immunity'), and hence that the number of cells responding determines the strength of the reaction. This may be true for the inherently simple model of the normal lymphocyte transfer reaction, but in other situations, such as graft rejection, it seems almost inevitable, as suggested by Hildemann, that features of the host will modify the reaction. However Simonsen's hypothesis puts the problem firmly in the second part of this book as a role of the host, and so outside the scope of this chapter.

Of course, the postulate that a larger number of antigen-sensitive cells exist to some antigens than to others is in itself a puzzling thing. Can we believe that it has nothing to do with the chemical nature of different antigens, and the ease with which proliferation of cells is produced by chemically different antigens?

Many attempts have been made to produce allo-antibodies to red cell antigens in species other than man, and independent investigators frequently find that antibodies to certain antigens are very readily made, while antibodies to other antigens can perhaps only be produced by one investigator on one occasion. In the horse, the only species besides man in which haemolytic disease of the newborn occurs spontaneously, it was found that antibodies to one antigen (antigen 6 or A) account for about 50% of all cases of the disease. Antibodies to this antigen are readily produced by injection. Another group of antigens (the 1-2-5 group of antigens) is responsible for a further 40% of cases in the horse (Franks 1962a).

A very interesting species from this point of view is the guinea-pig. Attempts have been made to produce antibodies to red cell allo-antigens in the guinea-pig, but this was unsuccessful (Mynors et al. 1950). These attempts were made by injection of red cells, and it is interesting to note that attempts to produce allo-antibodies to tissue cell antigens in the guinea-pig by injection were also unsuccessful, although such antibodies were produced following skin grafting (Brummerstedt and Franks 1970).

The picture however emerges of a certain amount of uniformity in the type of blood group systems present. Many species have an allo-antigen system of the A type, to which antibodies occur naturally in the serum of 'A'-negative individuals of that species. (In some species A or B antigens may be present in all members of the species.) There is also one or two antigen systems to which antibodies may be readily produced, and which may give rise to serious transfusion reactions or haemolytic disease of the newborn. Other systems may be known to which antibodies can be produced less readily. Too much should not, perhaps, be made of this pattern, since it may easily reflect the pattern of the activities of blood group investigators, rather than anything of immunological significance.

9.3.4. *Cell-restricted antigens*

Some antigens are restricted in their distribution, being present on some cells but not on others in the same individual. They may be detected as antibodies produced in other species (xeno-antibodies or 'hetero-antibodies') which have been absorbed appropriately, or they may be detected by antibodies produced in the same species, either in an animal in which the cells occur, or in other animals of the same species. Those antigens which can be studied with antibodies produced in the same species are, in general, more rewarding than those studied with absorbed xeno-antibodies, since with the latter antibodies there is always the possibility that antigen differences between cells may be quantitative rather than qualitative.

Examples of cell-restricted antigens are the Theta (θ) antigens (Reif and Allen, 1964), restricted, so it is claimed, to the thymus cells, thymus-derived and brain tissue cells of mice of θ-positive strains, the thymus-leukaemia (TL) antigens and a group of antigens of tumour cells, variously described as neoantigens or tumour-specific trans-plantation antigens (TSTAs). There are many puzzling features of these cell-restricted antigens: some of these problems are discussed in a fascinating review by Boyse and Old (1969).

9.3.5. *Auto-antigens*

Auto-allergy (auto-immunity) is the production of antibodies or allergic cells which react with an individual animal's own antigens. It is helpful perhaps to distinguish between auto-antibodies (or auto-allergic cells) which are auto-reactive but stimulated by some extraneous antigen, and antibodies which are stimulated by the animals own cells. An example of an auto-reactive situation would be the reaction of antibody produced against streptococcal cell wall antigens which react with heart muscle (Kaplan 1967). It is less easy to give an example of the second type of antibody with confidence, since it is always possible that some extraneous antigen may be discovered to account for any idiopathic auto-allergic disorder. However, a good illustration would be the auto-antibodies which are responsible for increased red cell breakdown in auto-allergic haemolytic anaemia.

A great deal has been written about auto-allergy, but little is relevant to the present consideration of the function of mammalian cell antigens in immunogenicity. However, there are certain features of the antigens which may be involved in auto-allergic processes which are of general interest.

One such feature is the frequency with which antibodies to allo-antigens are produced, for example the high frequency with which antibodies to the rhesus antigen e are produced in auto-allergic haemolytic anaemia of the warm antibody type. Other examples of this kind are known, for example many Donath-Landsteiner antibodies (biphasic haemolysins) are anti-P + P$_1$ in blood group specificity, (Levine et al., 1963; Worlledge and Rousso, 1957; Marsh, 1961) while auto-antibodies in auto-allergic haemolytic anaemia of the cold antibody type are usually anti-I in specificity (Wiener et al., 1956). It is perhaps not the fact that these auto-antibodies are specific for an allo-antigen which is surprising (after all, an antigen might be quantitatively more prominent, or more readily available), but the fact that each disorder seems to have its 'own' allo-antigen. It is necessary to inject a note of caution here, however, since there is an undoubted tendency once antibody specificity has been ascribed to an auto-antibody, for other investigators to find further examples of the same specificity, and, perhaps, to neglect those which do not 'fit in'. Donath-Landsteiner antibodies can be anti-i in specificity (Weiner et al., 1964), as well as anti-P + P$_1$ as mentioned above.

From the point of view of this book, it would have been valuable to discuss whether the type of allergic response may be restricted for any of the types of antigens. Reluctantly, however, one is forced to admit that the information is simply not available.

 David Franks

References

BOOTH, P. B., I. DUNSFORD, J. GRANT and S. MURRAY, 1953. Brit. Med. J. *ii*, 41.

BOURSNELL, J. C., D. H. HEARD and V. RIZK, 1955, J. Hygiene *53*, 420.

BOYSE, E. A. and L. J. OLD 1969, Ann. Rev. Genet. *3*, 269.

BRENT, L. and P. MEDAWAR, 1966, Proc. Roy. Soc. *B165*, 281.

BRUMMERSTEDT, E. and D. FRANKS, 1970, Transplantation *10*, 137.

BRITTON, S., T. WEPSIC and G. MÖLLER, 1968, Immunology *14*, 491.

CARTER, R. L. and H. G. PENMAN, 1969, Infectious mononucleosis. Oxford, Blackwell Scientific Publications.

CEPELLINI, R., S. BIGLIANI, E. S. CURTONI and G. LEIGHEB, 1969, Transplant. Proc. *1*, 390.

CLARKE, C. A., 1967, Brit. Med. J. *4*, 7.

CLARKE, C. A., R. FINN, R. B. MCCONNELL and P. M. SHEPPARD, 1958, Int. Arch. Allergy *13*, 380.

COHEN, C., 1958, J. Immunol. *80*, 73.

COHEN, C., 1955, Genetics *40*, 770.

COHEN, B. H., 1960, Am. J. Human Genetics *12*, 180.

FLORY, L. L., 1968, Immunology *14*, 787.

FORSSMAN, J., 1911, Biochem. Z. *37*, 78.

FRANKS, D., 1962a, Ann. N.Y. Acad. Sci. *97*, 235.

FRANKS, D., 1962b, Nature *195*, 580.

HEARD, D. H., 1955, J. Hygiene *53*, 408.

HILDEMANN, W. H. and N. COHEN, 1967, Weak histoincompatibilities: emerging immuno-genetic rules and generalizations. *In:* E. S. Curtoni, P. L. Mattiuz and R. M. Tosi, eds.: Histocompatibility testing 1967. Copenhagen, Munksgaard. pp. 13–20.

HILDEMANN, W. H., 1970, Transplant. Rev. *3*, 5.

JOYSEY, V. C., 1955, J. Exptl. Biol. *32*, 440.

KAPLAN, M. H., 1967, Multiple nature of the cross-reactive relationship between antigens of group A streptococci and mammalian tissue. *In:* J. J. Trentin, ed.: Cross-reacting antigens and neoantigens. Baltimore, Williams and Wilkins. pp. 48–60.

KONUGRES, A. A., 1964, Immunological tolerance of the A and B antigens. *In:* L. Holländer, ed.: Proc. 9th Congr. Int. Soc. Blood Transf., Mexico 1962. Basel, New York, S. Karger. pp. 746–750.

LEVINE, P., 1958, Human Biol. *30*, 14.

LEVINE, P., B. S. CELANO and F. FALKOWSKI, 1963, Transfusion *3*, 278.

MARSH, W. L., 1961, Brit. J. Haematol. *7*, 200.

MAYEDA, K., 1962, Am. J. Human Genetics *14*, 281.

MYNORS, L. S., D. H. HEARD and R. R. A. COOMBS, 1950, J. Hygiene *48*, 458.

OWEN, R. D., H. R. WOOD, A. G. FOORD, P. STURGEON and L. G. BALDWIN, 1954, Proc. Natl. Acad. Sci. U.S. *40*, 420.

RACE, R. R. and R. SANGER, 1968, Blood groups in man, 5th Ed. Philadelphia, F. A. Davis Co.

REIF, A. E. and J. M. V. ALLEN, 1964, J. Exptl. Med. *120*, 413.

SCHIFF, F. and L. ADELSBERGER, 1942, Z. Immun. Forsch. *40*, 335.

SIMONSEN, M., 1970, Transplant. Rev. *3*, 22.

SPRINGER, G. F., R. E. HORTON and M. FORBES, 1959, J. Exptl. Med. *110*, 221.

UHLENBRUCK, C., G. V. F. SEAMAN and R. R. A. COOMBS, 1967, Vox Sang. *12*, 420.

WARD, A. K., R. J. WALSH and O. KOOPTZOFF, 1957, Nature *179*, 1352.

WEINER, W., A. G. GORDON and D. ROWE, 1964, Vox Sang. *9*, 684.

WIENER, A. S., L. J. UNGER, L. COHEN and J. FELDMAN, 1956, Ann. Intern. Med. *44*, 221.

WOODROW, J. C., 1970, Series Haematologica *3*, 1.

WORLLEDGE, S. M. and C. ROUSSO, 1965, Vox Sang. *10*, 293.

PART II

Function of host

CHAPTER 10

The inductive phase of antibody production*

MICHAEL FELDMAN and AMIELA GLOBERSON

Department of Cell Biology, Weizmann Institute of Science, Rehovot

10.1. Introduction

The 'decision' of lymphoid cells as to whether to respond to an antigenic stimulation with antibody production or whether to acquire a state of immunological tolerance seems to depend on the types of antigenic signal received by the cells. In stimulating antibody production, an immunogen elicits diverse cellular events. These can be classified into events which (a) determine whether or not antibody production will be initiated, (b) control the level of the immune response, and (c) are irrelevant to the production of antibodies.

In the present review, we made no attempt to cover the whole spectrum of experimental approaches to the induction of antibody response, but we tried to evaluate experimental evidence relating to the first category of cellular events, namely, to processes that might determine the initiation of the immune response.

10.2. Immunogenic function of macrophages

10.2.1. Induction of a primary response

10.2.1.1. Viral and bacterial antigens

The macrophage appears to represent the first target cell of the injected antigen. Is the interaction between an antigen and a macrophage an essential step in the primary induction of antibody production? Indications that macrophages might play a determining role in initiating an immune response were presented by Fishman (1961) who studied the *in vitro* induction of antibody to T2 phages. In this system, a primary

---

* Our studies reviewed in the present chapter were supported by Grants from the Max and Ida Hillson Foundation, New York and from D.G.R.S.T., France.

response to T2 phage was produced by rat lymph node cells only if the latter were cultured in the presence of peritoneal exudate cells (PEC).

Further analysis of the system led Fishman and Adler (1963) to conclude that the macrophage factor inducing reactivity in the lymphocytes consisted mainly of RNA. The observations regarding the immunogenic activity of RNA, whether from macrophages or from spleen cells, were confirmed by others using the T2 antigen (Friedman et al. 1965; Gottlieb et al. 1967), haemocyanin (Askonas and Rhodes 1965), or sheep red blood cells (SRBC) (Cohen and Parks 1964; Abramoff and Brien 1968). Some of these studies demonstrated that the non-RNA component of this factor contained the antigen (Fishman and Adler 1963; Friedman et al. 1965; Askonas and Rhodes 1965). Recently, Fishman and Adler (1967) and Adler et al. (1966) reported that an RNA molecule free of antigen is active in addition to the RNA-antigen complex. The level of response obtained in these experiments was relatively low. Furthermore, no attempt was made to determine which type of cell of the peritoneal exudate was responsible for the effect. Additional studies were therefore required to establish this point.

Our approach to clarifying the immunogenic function of macrophages was triggered by observations made in our laboratory on the induction of immunological tolerance to protein antigens in adult rabbits (Nachtigal and Feldman 1963, 1964). While studying the induction of tolerance to horse serum albumin (HSA) in rabbits exposed to total body x-irradiation, it was found that tolerance was induced even when the antigen was injected as late as 30 days following exposure to a sublethal dose of 550 r (Nachtigal et al. 1968). At this- stage, there was a complete regeneration of the lymphoid system, as determined by the levels of circulating lymphocytes. These experiments therefore suggested that the induction of tolerance following exposure to x-rays was not due to the state of differentiation of the lymphoid cells (Nachtigal 1967). It seemed that another cell type determines whether tolerance or immunity will be produced. The macrophage was an obvious candidate.

Experiments were therefore designed to test whether x-irradiation suppresses antibody response by inactivating the immunogenic function of macrophages (Gallily and Feldman 1966). The first series of experiments tested whether macrophages from normal mice, after interacting *in vitro* with *Shigella* antigen, would evoke antibody production in mice exposed to sublethal doses of total body x-irradiation. Peritoneal exudate cells (PEC) of normal C57Bl mice were incubated *in vitro* with *Shigella* antigen, then inoculated into mice exposed 2 days previously to 550 r total body irradiation. The inoculation of such antigen-treated PEC lead to the formation of antibody in irradiated animals whereas injection of antigen by itself did not result in a detectable response (Gallily and Feldman 1967a).

The peritoneal cell populations used in the previous experiments consisted of 80% macrophages, yet they were not free of lymphocytes. To test whether macrophages *per se* were the cells which, following interaction with the antigen, triggered the production of antibody, further experiments were carried out in which pure populations of macrophages were obtained by culturing peritoneal cells *in vitro* (Gallily and Feldman 1967a). These macrophages were exposed to *Shigella* in culture, then injected into x-irradiated mice. The results showed that lymphocyte-free macrophage populations, obtained following *in vitro* culturing of peritoneal cells, induced the production of antibody in the X-rayed recipients.

Experiments were then carried out to define the cells which produce antibody following the inoculation of antigen-treated macrophages into x-rayed animals. To test whether the recipients' lymphocytes are the cells which respond to the macrophage 'signal', different levels of lymphoid depletion were obtained by exposing mice to different doses of total body x-irradiation. Each group of mice, having been exposed to a different dose of irradiation, was then inoculated with antigen-treated macrophages. The results showed that there was an inverse relationship between the levels of total body irradiation and the levels of antibody produced following injection of the 'primed' macrophages. It was therefore inferred that normal macrophages, following interaction with *Shigella* antigen, can 'instruct' cells of the sublethally irradiated mice to produce antibodies (Feldman and Gallily 1967).

Macrophages were found to be capable of inducing antibody production across genetic barriers. Macrophages from C57Bl mice (H-2^b), which had interacted *in vitro* with *Shigella* antigen, elicited antibody production in x-irradiated Balb/c animals (H-2^d), and *vice versa* (Feldman and Gallily 1967). It appears, however, that their capacity to signal antibody production depended upon their function as intact living cells within the recipient animals. This was deduced from experiments in which normal C57Bl or Balb/c animals were immunized against the iso-antigens of the prospective macrophage donors. The iso-immunized mice were then exposed to 550 r and inoculated with 'primed' macrophages of the genotype against which they had been immunized. The results showed that the immunogenic effect of the macrophages was completely inhibited if the recipients had previously been sensitized against the prospective donors.

To further substantiate the participation of two cell types in the production of antibodies to *Shigella* and the lymphoid nature of the cells responding to the macrophage 'signal', reconstruction experiments were attempted. Mice were exposed to a lethal dose of total body x-irradiation (850 r). One group was inoculated with antigen-treated macrophages, a second with antigen-treated lymphocytes of either thoracic duct or lymph node origin, and a third group with a mixed cell population composed of antigen-treated macrophages and nontreated lymphocytes. Only animals of the third group produced a significant titre of agglutinins (Gallily and Feldman 1967b).

Experiments were then performed to test directly whether x-irradiation does in fact inactivate the immunogenic properties of macrophages. Macrophages from mice exposed to total body x-irradiation were incubated *in vitro* with antigen, then tested for their immunogenic activity in other x-irradiated recipients. The results showed that x-irradiation suppressed the capacity of the peritoneal cells to elicit agglutinin production in other sublethally irradiated mice (Feldman and Gallily 1967). To test whether the effect of x-irradiation on the immunogenic function of macrophages is direct, macrophages from normal animals were irradiated *in vitro*, then incubated with *Shigella* antigen and tested for their immunogenic effect in mice exposed to 550 r. The result was that the *in vitro* irradiation, just as the irradiation of the whole animal, abolished the capacity of macrophages to signal antibody production (Feldman and Gallily 1967). The inactivation of the immunogenic properties of macrophages by x-rays cannot be attributed to the suppression of the capacity of macrophages to take up antigenic material (Feldman and Gallily 1967a). It thus appears that x-irradiation impairs the 'processing' of antigen within the cells in a manner as yet unknown.

The studies of Gallily and Feldman suggest that impairment of response of sublethally irradiated mice is a result of inactivity of macrophages. The question was raised whether the lymphocytes interacting with the macrophages are cells which survived irradiation or whether the lymphocytes were also affected by irradiation but recovered soon after exposure. To distinguish between these two possibilities, the organ culture system for antibody response was employed (Globerson and Auerbach 1965, 1966). The idea was that if macrophages interact with cells residing in the peripheral lymphoid organs of the irradiated recipient, then spleens explanted from such mice and cultured in the presence of macrophages should respond to *Shigella* when the latter was applied *in vitro*. The results of such experiments were negative (Globerson and Feldman 1969). On the other hand, antibodies to *Shigella* were formed when thymus explants were added to the system. To test whether the thymic lymphocytes themselves participated in the production of antibodies, or whether the thymus cells induced reactivity of cells within the spleen tissue, we performed a transfilter combination experiment (Globerson and Feldman 1970a, b). The thymus was cultured across the millipore filter barrier from the spleen tissue and macrophages. The tissues were separated 4 days later and cultured individually in different dishes. Antibodies were found only in the spleen cultures and not in those of the thymus. Thus, antibodies were formed by cells of spleen origin. It may therefore be concluded that both lymphocytes and macrophages are affected by the sublethal doses of irradiation, yet reactivity of lymphocytes is regained soon after exposure.

10.2.1.2. *Sheep red blood cells (SRBC)*

How general is this phenomenon of macrophages playing a determining role in the induction of antibody formation? Do other types of antigens have to interact with macrophages in the same manner as the *Shigella* in order to initiate a response?

Experiments employing SRBC in the same system as that used for the *Shigella* experiments were conducted in our laboratory (Gershon and Feldman 1968). Mice were total-body irradiated at sublethal doses and then injected with macrophages previously incubated with SRBC. Agglutinin formation was subsequently followed. It was found that in contrast to the *Shigella* system, no response to SRBC could be detected under the same experimental conditions. Using a similar system of irradiated mice, Frisch and Wilson (1969) obtained contradictory results, showing that irradiated animals treated with macrophages and SRBC did respond at a level higher than the controls which had not been treated with macrophages. It should be noted, however, that in these studies irradiation did not completely eliminate the response to SRBC as in the experiments of Gershon and Feldman (1968).

The negative findings of Gershon and Feldman can be explained by either of the following suggestions: (a) Macrophages do not play any decisive role in the response to SRBC although they are essential for initiation of a response to *Shigella*, or (b) macrophages are required for the response to SRBC, yet an additional cell type, which is radiosensitive, must cooperate in the reaction.

The first possibility appears unlikely, since studies employing different experimental systems demonstrate participation of macrophages in antibody formation to SRBC. Thus, Argyris (1968) and Braun and Lasky (1967) have shown that PEC conferred immune reactivity on newborn mice. These observations, however, require further analysis, since in Braun's experiments the response could be attributed to lymphocytes present in a large number in the inoculum of peritoneal cells used.

Another approach was recently reported by Braun (personal communication). He found that treatment with thorotrast inhibited the response to SRBC. Since thorotrast is known to block the activity of macrophages, it was concluded that macrophages are essential for antibody production to this antigen.

The alternative hypothesis, namely that an additional cell type is involved in the reaction to SRBC, gains support from the *in vitro* studies of Mosier (1967) and Mosier and Coppleson (1968). Using the system of Mishell and Dutton (1967), Mosier found that the appearance of plaque-forming cells in culture depends on the presence of adherent and non-adherent cells (Mosier 1967). Further analysis of these observations indicated that the population of non-adherent cells may contain two cell types which are involved in the response (Mosier and Coppleson 1968). If we accept the view that the adherent cells are macrophages, then we may conclude that in addition to macrophages two other cell types participate in the reaction to SRBC. The question whether the adherent cells are identical with the macrophages in the peritoneal exudates becomes more difficult in view of the results obtained by Roseman (1969). He found that the adherent cells are resistant to irradiation of 1000 r. This is in accordance with observations of Unanue and Askonas (1968) that the enhanced immunogenicity of haemocyanin bound to macrophages is not impaired by irradiation. On the other hand, the macrophages in the peritoneal exudate participating in the response to *Shigella* and to bovine serum albumin (BSA) are radiosensitive (Feldman and Gallily 1967; Mitchison 1969). Thus, the activity of the adherent cells *in vitro* may be different from that of the macrophages in the response to *Shigella* or BSA *in vivo*.

The contradictory conclusions derived from different experimental approaches can be explained on the basis of analyses recently reported by Hoffman (1970). Using the same system as Mosier (1967), he found that one may obtain different results depending on the numerical ratios of macrophages to lymphocytes. Under certain conditions, macrophages lead to a response, whereas when the macrophages are in excess, antibody production as assayed by haemolysin plaque formation is reduced. This explains the observation of Perkins and Makinodan (1965), claiming an inhibitory effect of macrophages on anti-SRBC responses.

10.2.1.3. Protein antigens

Does the response to soluble antigens (e.g., serum proteins) depend on activity of macrophages?

Dixon and Weigle (1957) made preliminary tests of the cells which determine the immunological deficiency of newborn animals. The injection of BSA into newborn rabbits did not result in antibody production. Neither were antibodies produced when the antigen was admixed with lymphocytes from lymph nodes of an adult organism. Martin (1966) confirmed these results which seemed to suggest that it was not the lack of functional lymphocytes which prevented the newborns from making antibodies. However, when PEC which had been incubated with alum-precipitated BSA were inoculated to newborns at doses of 3×10^7 (containing 0.25–5 mg of antigen), followed by a second injection of BSA in solution, 20 animals out of 48 responded with antibody production. If the macrophages are indeed the functional cells in the peritoneal exudates employed, then these experiments represent an additional indication of the necessity of macrophages for triggering antibody production.

Further support to the idea that macrophages play a significant role in response to protein antigens was presented by Pribnow and Silverman (1967). They found that rabbits which had been total-body irradiated at sublethal doses were able to respond to BSA when inoculated with macrophages.

A detailed analysis of the immunogenic effect of macrophages in the induction of antibody formation to protein antigens was carried out by Mitchison (1969). He tested the response to BSA, human serum albumin (HSA), ovalbumin and lysozyme, fed to PEC *in vivo*. The peritoneal cells of CBA mice, treated with either BSA or HSA, were inoculated into normal adult syngeneic mice, and the immune response obtained was found to be 100–1000 times higher than that produced by the inoculation of the free antigen. With lysozyme and ovalbumin the difference was smaller than that, probably because the free form of these antigens, unlike that of HSA and BSA, is readily taken up by the recipient macrophages. As in the experiments with *Shigella* (Feldman and Gallily 1967), intact cells seemed to be the functional elements, since syngeneic combinations of PEC recipients gave a higher response than allogeneic combinations. One could argue that the active cell in the PEC is the lymphocyte and not the macrophage. If this were the case, then transfer of PEC to tolerant animals should break down the tolerant state, since normal lymphocytes have been shown to terminate tolerance. PEC-bound BSA inoculated into adult mice, tolerant to BSA, did not bring about breakdown of tolerance. Hence, the macrophage, and not the lymphocyte, is the functional cell in triggering antibody production by PEC-bound BSA. Furthermore, PEC from tolerant animals, when incubated with BSA, were as active as cells from untreated donors in eliciting antibody response to BSA following transfer to normal syngeneic recipients.

It should be noted that in Mitchison's experiments free antigen also elicited a response, although at a much lower level. This can be explained by the possibility that part of the free antigen was taken up by the recipients' macrophages and could have been involved in antibody formation. Whether antibodies to HSA and BSA can be produced by the lymphocytes of the recipient without the participation of macrophages thus requires further analysis.

10.2.2. Induction of a secondary response

In inducing a secondary response, do macrophages perform the same immunogenic function as in the primary response? Mitchison (1969) conducted experiments in which spleen cells from mice primed to BSA were inoculated into animals which had been exposed to 600 r total body irradiation. One day later the recipients received an injection of either free antigen or PEC-bound BSA, or heat-killed PEC-bound antigen. All groups manifested a secondary response of the same level. This, however, need not indicate that macrophages are not necessary for the secondary response, since the spleen cells inoculated most probably contained antibody bound to macrophages, and these could have taken up the free antigen very readily. It appears therefore that, so far, we have no definite answer to whether or not macrophages are necessary for the induction of a secondary immune response.

10.2.3. The immunogenic signal

10.2.3.1. The type of macrophages involved and localization of antigen

Which are the macrophages that function in signalling antibody production? It has been suggested that the reticular dendritic cells in the germinal centers of the lymphatic follicles are the operative macrophages, since they entrap antigen at their cell surfaces (Nossal 1967). It appears, however, that the concentration of antigen at the surface of these cells is irrelevant to the induction of a primary response, since antigen appears on the cell dendrites only *after* antibodies have been produced (Humphrey 1969). The trapping of antigen is therefore due to the localization of antibodies and thus follows rather than precedes antibody production.

In fact, antigen trapping by dendritic cells seems to be irrelevant even to the induction of a *secondary* immune response. This is deduced from the ingenious experiments carried out by Askonas (1970). Mice were primed by small doses of alum-precipitated 4-hydroxy-3-iodo-5-nitro-phenylacetyl(NIP)-bovine γ-globulin (BGG). They produced antibodies which reacted with the hapten (NIP) when the latter was attached to different carriers. For the production of a secondary response, the animals were immunized with either [121]I NIP-BGG or ^{125}I NIP-BSA, namely, with the hapten coupled to either a homologous or a heterologous carrier. As expected from previous studies (Ovary and Benacerraf 1963; Mitchison 1966; Rajewsky and Rottlander 1967), only the homologous conjugate elicited antibody production, yet both conjugates were concentrated on the follicular cell to the same degree. It thus appears that antigen trapping at the surface of the dendritic cells of the follicles is not associated with the induction of antibodies in the primary response and in the secondary response. Hence, motile macrophages rather than the sessile dendritic cells, may be the immunogenic cells.

When keyhole limpet haemocyanin (KLH) is administered to an animal, the antigen can be localized both inside the cell and at the cell surface (Askonas 1970). Seven days after antigen injection, 15–25% of the antigen is found on the surface of the macrophages. Is the surface antigen the immunogenic substance? Experiments in which the haemocyanin was coupled to SRBC or mouse red blood cells (MRBC) or to methylated BSA showed a 10- to 40-fold increase in uptake. EDTA did not remove any antigenic material, since all of it was located inside the macrophage. Yet, although these macrophages contained no surface antigen, they manifested a remarkably high immunogenic effect. On the other hand, the results of Unanue (Unanue and Cerottini 1970) indicate that the membrane-bound antigen might represent the active signal. One may suggest that the 'intracellular' antigen in Askonas' experiments could have moved to the cell surface prior to the actual immunogenic function of the macrophages. Macrophages retained their immunogenic capacity even when most of the antigen was excreted from the cells. Thus, Askonas (Askonas 1970) working with Maia squinado haemocyanin (MSH) found that 24–72 hrs following administration of the antigen, only 15% of the antigen originally taken up by the macrophages was retained by these cells. Yet, there had been no decrease in the immunogenic effect of such macrophages, i.e., they did elicit antibody production at a level which was higher by a factor of 60 than that obtained by free antigen.

10.2.3.2. Mechanism of action of the macrophages

How do the macrophages function in triggering antibody production? One possibility is that the macrophages take up the antigen and concentrate it. However, it appears unlikely that such an activity is responsible for the role of macrophages in initiation of a response, because (1) macrophages from x-rayed animals or macrophages exposed *in vitro* to x-rays lose their capacity to trigger antibody production although they show no impairment of their phagocytic properties (Feldman and Gallily 1967). Furthermore, had the function of the macrophage been to present the antigen simply in a higher concentration, the PEC-bound antigen should be at least as potent in maintaining the state of tolerance as free antigens. CBA mice tolerant to BSA were injected with either free BSA or PEC-bound BSA at a stage when signs of tolerance breakdown where observed (Mitchison 1969). The amounts of antigen presented with the PEC were similar to those injected in the free form. Yet, the free BSA prevented tolerance breakdown, whereas the cell-bound antigen facilitated it. It is therefore concluded that the immunogenic function of macrophages in inducing a primary response cannot be attributed merely to their capacity to take up and concentrate the antigen. Neither can it be attributed to the degradation of the antigen by the macrophages since the conformation of the antigenic molecule must be preserved if production of specific antibodies is to be signalled (Sela et al. 1967). Fishman's experiments (Fishman and Adler 1963, 1967; Adler et al. 1966) raised the possibility that an RNA-antigen complex is formed by the macrophage which can trigger production both *in vitro* and *in vivo*. Whether or not the macrophage acts, under *normal in vivo* conditions of immunization, by producing an antigen-RNA complex is still an open question. Mitchison (1969) claims that PEC-bound BSA loses its immunogenic properties if subjected to mild heating. From this it seemed to him improbable that the macrophage functions *via* a 'superantigen' or an RNA-antigen complex. In fact, this improbability could also derive from the experiments indicating that living cells are required to signal antibody production (Feldman and Gallily 1967; Mitchison 1969). Their destruction by graft reaction in allogeneic combinations has prevented their immunogenic function. On the other hand, it could be argued that both the heating experiment and the results of allogeneic combinations do not exclude the possibility that the macrophage effect is *via* a superantigen, if a continuous production and release of such a complex by living cells is necessary for the achievement of a measurable amount of antibodies.

10.3. *Antigen recognition by cells*

10.3.1. *Recognition of hapten*

10.3.1.1. *The secondary response*
The production of specific antibodies following antigenic stimulation should be preceded by a phase of antigen recognition by cells. Cells capable of recognizing antigenic determinants are expected to possess

receptors which should bind specifically the corresponding antigens. The existence of such receptors on cells of immunized animals could be deduced from experiments on competitive inhibition of the antigenic stimulation. Two types of specific inhibition of antibody production are relevant to the concept of antigen-binding receptors. One is the inhibition of antigenic stimulation by passively administered antibodies. Late antibodies, i.e., antibodies of higher affinity, were found to be more potent in suppressing antibody production (Finkelstein and Uhr 1964; Wigzell 1966), indicating that the passively inoculated antibodies compete with cell receptors possessing affinities of the same order of magnitude. The second is inhibition of antibody production to hapten, following immunization with hapten-protein conjugates by an excess of unconjugated hapten (Dutton and Eady 1964; Brownstone et al. 1966). These experiments were carried out *in vivo*, testing the suppression of a secondary response. Thus, following earlier observations by Dutton and Eady (1964), Mitchison (1967) used spleen cells from animals (CBA mice) pre-immunized with NIP-BGG. The cells were incubated *in vitro* either with NIP-BGG or with NIP-BGG plus unconjugated NIP, then were inoculated into syngeneic animals which had been exposed to total body x-irradiation. The result was that free NIP inhibited the production of a secondary immune response by the NIP-BGG conjugate. As expected from a competitive inhibition, it was achieved only within a certain range of concentrations, and only within a limited time interval between the application of the hapten and of the immunogen. The fact that these results measured the production of antibodies *in vivo* and were related only to a secondary reaction necessitated further studies to test whether cell receptors do exist prior to the first induced experience with the antigen, in a system amenable to cellular analysis.

10.3.1.2. Secondary and primary response in vitro

In our laboratory, we have tested the effect of free hapten on the *in vitro* induction of secondary as well as primary responses by adapting the organ culture 'millipore' filter-well method for antibody production (Globerson and Auerbach 1966) to chemically-defined antigens (Segal et al. 1970). We induced a primary immune response in spleen explants to the dinitrophenyl group (DNP), using as antigens DNP-haemocyanin (DNP-Hcy) or α-DNP-poly-L-lysine (DNP-pLL). Antibodies were detected in the culture medium by the inactivation of T4 bacteriophage coupled with DNP (Haimovich and Sela 1966). The specificity of the reaction was manifested by the lack of the capacity of the medium to inactivate the unmodified bacteriophage and by the inhibition of the inactivation of DNP-T4 with DNP-lysine. This system was then used to test whether an excess of free DNP-lysine might inhibit induction of antibody response to DNP induced by DNP-protein conjugates, when the antigen was administered in culture together with the free hapten. The results were that DNP-lysine, when applied either simultaneously with the immunogen, or up to 4 hrs prior to the application of the DNP-protein conjugate, decreased significantly the production of antibodies to the dinitrophenyl group (Segal et al. 1971a). Thus, DNP-lysine appears to compete with DNP-protein conjugates for cell receptors to DNP which exist prior to the primary stimulation with antigen. What, then, is the structure of such cell-receptors for antigens? It was suggested that the receptors are antibody-like molecules located in the membranes of the recognizing cells. That immunoglobulins do indeed exist at the cell surface was deduced from experiments demonstrating that antibodies to immunoglobulins induced lymphoblastic transformation in lymphoid cells (Sell 1967a, 1967b).

A further, more detailed, indication of the existence of immunoglobulins on the cell surface of lymphocytes was provided by the studies of Klein (1970). Cells of Burkitt lymphomas and chronic lymphatic leukaemias were found to possess IgM molecules of kappa specificity at the cell membrane. She was able to select cell lines, growing in culture, which do not secrete immunoglobulins, yet manifest IgM on their surfaces. Cytotoxic reaction was obtained with anti-IgM anti-kappa. Using the chloroform-ethanol extraction method, fractions of plasma membranes were obtained which retained the IgM marker.

If the cell receptors are in fact antibody-like entities, they should manifest the same properties as free antibodies. For example, antibodies to haptens bind covalently to affinity-labelling reagents of the corresponding haptens (Weinstein et al. 1969), so, if the cell receptors are identical with the antigen-binding sites of the antibody, affinity-labelling reagents of haptens should bind covalently to the receptor and thus block the receptors irreversibly at the recognition site. The free hapten, in contrast, should give only a reversible 'block', manifested in a temporary inhibition of the immunogenic effect of the hapten-protein conjugates.

To test this, experiments were carried out on the effect of affinity-labelling reagents of DNP on the production of antibodies in organ culture, both to a primary and a secondary stimulation with DNP-protein conjugates (Segal et al. 1971b, Segal et al. 1969).

We prepared the affinity-labelling reagents α-N-bromoacetyl-ϵ-N-(2 4-dinitrophenyl)-lysine (BADL) and N-bromoacetyl-N-(2,4-dinitrophenyl)-ethylenediamine (BADE) by introducing a reactive bromoacetyl group into homologous derivatives of the dinitrophenyl (DNP) hapten

(Weinstein et al. 1969). BADL and BADE bind covalently with rabbit anti-DNP antibodies leading to a loss in activity of the antibody site. Binding to antibodies could be inhibited by excess of DNP-lysine; no binding was observed when the reagents were tested with normal rabbit IgG (Weinstein et al. 1969).

Therefore, we tested the effect of BADL and BADE applied in culture on the production of antibodies to DNP by DNP-haemocyanin and DNP-rabbit serum albumin (DNP-RSA). Each explant was incubated for 4 hrs in phosphate buffered saline (PBS) containing 5×10^{-6} M DNP-lysine, or BADL or BADE at pH 7.3. The explants were washed twice in culture medium and incubated for either 20 or 44 hrs in culture medium. The cultures were then rinsed and supplemented with $5 \mu g$ of either DNP-RSA or DNP-Hcy, or poly-DL-ala-RSA. The antigen-containing medium was replaced 24 hrs later by fresh medium which was subsequently assayed for anti-DNP antibodies and anti-poly-DL-alanyl antibodies. Antibodies were determined by two methods: (1) the modified phage technique making use of the inactivation of DNP-T4 (Haimovich and Sela 1966) or poly-D-ala-T4 phages by anti-DNP and anti-poly-alanine antibodies, respectively; and (2) the immunoadsorbent method, based on binding of the antibodies to the hapten coupled to bromoacetyl-cellulose, then applying rabbit anti-mouse [131]IgG to determine the amount of anti-hapten antibodies bound by the immunoadsorbents (Klinman and Taylor 1969).

The results indicated that treatment with BADL and BADE had a marked inhibitory effect on the production of anti-DNP antibodies, by DNP-RSA and DNP-Hcy whereas DNP-lysine had a limited effect. Unlike DNP-lysine, BADL and BADE prevented antibody production even when the antigen was applied 44 hrs after the removal of the affinity-labelling reagents. The effect was specific, since BADL and BADE did not inhibit production of antibodies to poly-DL-alanine haptens. These experiments thus strongly suggest that the reagents become covalently bound to antibody-like molecules on the surface of cells within the spleen explants, which may represent the antigen-recognition receptors of the antigen-reactive cells.

Similar experiments were carried out by Plotz (1969), using affinity-labelling reagents of NIP. NIP-azide was mixed with a cell suspension from spleens of CBA mice pre-immunized with NIP-chicken γ-globulin (CGG). After 1 hr of incubation, the cells were washed and injected into syngeneic recipients irradiated with 600 r. Antibody response to NIP was significantly lower in such mice as compared to that of the control in which no incubation of the cells with NIP-azide had been performed. Thus, NIP-azide interfered with the induction of a secondary response to NIP-CGG. These results were attributed to the blocking of cell receptors for NIP.

Is there any correlation between the affinity of the receptor and the affinity of the antibody produced by the cell? It appears that it is easier to inhibit a cell which forms antibodies of low affinity than a cell which has been sensitized and appears at the secondary response stage. Thus, the affinity of the cell receptor to the antigen seems to have increased in parallel with the increased affinity of the antibody. The cell receptor then behaves similarly to, and is possibly identical with, the antibody produced by that cell.

One would have liked to isolate the receptor in order to characterize it in greater detail. Aiming at this, Mäkelä (personal communication) immunized rats with NIP-BSA, then drained the thoracic duct lymphocytes (TDL) from the immunized animals. These cells did not produce anti-NIP antibodies, yet they were found to possess anti-NIP antibodies on their membranes. This was evident from experiments in which the lymphocytes were disrupted in Triton X-100, and the plasma membrane fraction was obtained. This fraction showed anti-NIP activity and was found to be sensitive to 2-mercaptoethanol. The sensitivity of the assay system used was such that a minimum of 40 receptors per cell, in a population of 10^7 cells, could be detected. It seemed possible that the antibody activity of plasma membranes of TDL in these studies represented the cell receptor for the NIP hapten.

10.3.2. Recognition of the carrier molecule

10.3.2.1. Secondary and primary response

What does the receptor recognize in the antigen? Does it recognize the same molecular determinant that the antibody recognizes, or perhaps a larger (or smaller) part of the molecule? The question might not have been raised at all, had it not been for rather unexpected results obtained in experiments in which a secondary response to a hapten group was studied in animals immunized with hapten-protein conjugates. Ovary and Benacerraf (1963) found that rabbits primed with DNP-BGG produce a secondary response to DNP only if challenged with an immunogen in which the DNP is coupled to a carrier protein identical to the protein used for priming, i.e., with DNP-BGG. When the second immunization was carried out with a DNP-HSA conjugate, the response to DNP was of the primary type. Similar observations on the carrier effect were reported by Mitchison (1966) who studied the response to NIP coupled to either BSA or ovalbumin. The studies of Rajewsky and Rottländer (1967) also point to the same phenomenon. In their system the protein of porcine LDH-III was used which behaves like a hapten-carrier complex, where the A subunit acts as a carrier and the B as a hapten. These results suggested that the cell receptor for the hapten could recognize in the immunogen a part of the molecule comprising both the hapten and an adjacent sequence of amino acids of the carrier molecule. Mitchison (1967) tested this notion by assuming that if it is correct, then animals primed with NIP-BSA should behave, when challenged with NIP-BSA in which a spacer molecule has been inserted (NIP-(L-ala)-4-BSA), like animals immunized with NIP coupled to a non-cross reacting carrier. However, the result was that the NIP-(L-ala)-4-BSA elicited a secondary anti-NIP response similar to the one obtained by immunizing secondarily with NIP-BSA. Hence the phenomenon of carrier specificity cannot be ascribed to a difference in pattern of recognition of the antigen between the antibody and the cell receptor.

An alternative explanation of the carrier effect assumes the following: The induction of antibody response depends on the interaction between two cells, each of them capable of recognizing certain determinants of the antigen (Mitchison 1967). Accordingly, in the production of anti-hapten antibodies following immunization with hapten-carrier conjugate, one cell has to be capable of recognizing the hapten and of forming antibodies to it. The other cell should recognize antigenic determinants, but need not actually release antibodies. The latter could be defined as an antigen-sensitive cell (ASC). Antibody production to determinants of the carrier will thus result from an interaction between an antigen-sensitive cell and an antibody-producing cell (APC), both of which are equipped with specific receptors for carrier determinants. Antibody production to the hapten will result from an interaction between an antigen-sensitive cell specific either for the carrier or for the hapten, and an antibody-producing cell specific for the hapten. Upon priming with hapten-carrier conjugate, the antigen must first be recognized by the ASC. Theoretically, it could be recognized either by the ASC specific for the carrier or by the ASC specific for the hapten. However, because of the multiplicity of antigenic determinants of the carrier, and, possibly, the relatively higher affinity of carrier determinants for their corresponding receptors on the ASC, the latter will be stimulated during the primary response to a much greater extent than the hapten-specific ASC. Consequently, the population of cells with specific receptors for the carrier determinants will increase. Upon the secondary challenge with the hapten-carrier, the antigen will be recognized by the increased population of carrier-specific ASC, produced during the primary stimulation. The probability of interaction between ASC to the carrier determinants and APC to the hapten *via* the linking antigen is thus very much increased, leading to a higher level of antibody production. On the other hand, if the secondary stimulation is carried out by hapten coupled to a heterologous carrier, the primary stimulation would not, according to the proposed model, enhance the immunogenic effect. If this concept is correct, one would predict that spleens of animals, primed with the carrier protein alone, should respond to a secondary stimulation *in vitro* with hapten-carrier by producing anti-hapten antibodies at a level similar to that produced by spleens from animals primed with the conjugates.

To test this model as well as some other properties of the role of the carrier, we employed the *in vitro* system (Segal et al. 1970). First, we tested whether the carrier effect can be obtained in the secondary response induced in organ culture (Segal et al. 1971a). Mice were primed with DNP-Hcy, and their spleens were removed to culture 7 days, 6 months, or 12 months later. The explants were then challenged *in vitro* with DNP coupled to either Hcy or a non-cross reacting carrier, HSA. A secondary response to DNP was manifested only when the antigenic challenge was with DNP-Hcy, i.e., when the DNP was coupled to the same carrier as the one used for the production of the primary response. Thus, the carrier in this *in vitro* system plays a specific role in determining the antibody response to the hapten, similarly to its role shown previously in the *in vivo* experiments.

Experiments were then carried out in which mice were immunized with RSA and 8 months, or else 1–4 days later, the spleens were removed for culture. These, and spleen explants from non-immunized control donors, were challenged *in vitro* with DNP-RSA. The result was that priming with the carrier *alone* had sensitized the spleens to respond to a subsequent stimulation with the DNP-carrier conjugates. The enhanced response to DNP was specific with regard to the carrier, since spleens from animals immunized with RSA showed an intensified production of anti-DNP antibodies only when challenged *in vitro* with DNP-RSA, but not when challenged with DNP-Hcy. However, the response to DNP was characterized as a primary one.

The bicellular co-operation as a basis for antibody production was derived from studies of Mitchison (1967) and Rajewsky et al. (1969). Mitchison showed that when irradiated mice were injected with spleen cells of donors immunized against NIP-ovalbumin (OA) they did not respond to NIP-BSA. However, they did respond to NIP-BSA when they received cells immunized against BSA in addition to the cells immunized against NIP-OA. Similarly, Rajewsky et al. reported that a response to sulphanil-azo-HGG could be obtained following priming with sulphanil-azo-BSA, provided the animals were treated with HGG.

Thus, in these experimental systems, as well as in ours, the establishment of response to the carrier itself determines the production of antibodies to the hapten coupled to it.

A second test of the proposed model is based on the following prediction: If the production of anti-DNP antibodies involves an interaction *via* the antigen between an antigen-sensitive cell specific for the carrier determinant, and an antibody-producing cell specific for the hapten, i.e., between a cell with receptors for the carrier and a cell with receptors for the hapten, then free carrier applied with the DNP-carrier conjugate should inhibit the production of anti-DNP antibodies. Spleen cultures from mice primed with RSA and/or DNP-RSA were challenged *in vitro* with either DNP-RSA or DNP-RSA plus free RSA. Only spleens of the former group manifested antibodies. Free RSA had thus inhibited the DNP-RSA stimulated production of antibodies to DNP. Similarly, spleens immunized *in vitro* with DNP-pLL failed to produce antibodies to DNP if incubated with poly-L-lysine simultaneously with, or 3 hrs prior to the application of DNP-pLL.

10.3.2.2. Immunological tolerance

A third type of experiment testing the model stems from the following prediction: If tolerance ensues when ASC are blocked, then spleen cultures of animals tolerant to a carrier protein, e. g., RSA, should not produce anti-DNP antibodies when stimulated *in vitro* with DNP-RSA. They should, however, produce anti-DNP antibodies when challenged with DNP coupled to a non-cross-reacting carrier. Experiments were conducted in our Laboratory and the results confirmed this prediction (Segal et al. 1971b). It should be noted here that in other systems of tolerance to a carrier protein, immunization with the hapten-carrier conjugate does result in the production of antibodies to the hapten (Nachtigal and Feldman 1964). Thus, rabbits made tolerant to HSA then immunized with arsanil-azo-HSA or sulphanil-azo-HSA, or normal rabbits immunized with arsanil- or sulphanil-azo-RSA, produced anti-sulphanilic antibodies. In these cases, however, the coupling of the antigen results in the production of a new antigenic determinant, comprising part of the carrier protein (Nachtigal and Feldman 1964, Nachtigal et al. 1968). In our system only 5 molecules of DNP are attached to each carrier molecule. We suggest that whenever the coupling of a hapten does not modify the antigenic properties of the carrier, anti-hapten antibodies will not be produced in an animal tolerant to the carrier protein. This is in accordance with the model of bicellular interaction, suggesting that tolerance is determined at the level of the antigen-sensitive cells.

All these experiments are compatible with and in fact can best be explained by·assuming that each cell, whether it is an antigen-sensitive cell or an antibody-producing cell, can recognize one or possibly just a few determinants. This notion has recently been supported experimentally by observations of Wigzell and Andersson (1969) who developed a method for the removal, from a lymphoid cell population, of cells with receptors to a specific antigen. When a lymphoid cell population from a nonimmunized animal was passed through a column of plastic beads covered with an antigen, the cells which came through the column were found incapable of responding with antibody production to that particular antigen, while retaining their reactivity to other antigens. A similar approach was adopted by others (Abdou and Richter 1969; Truffa-Bachi and Wofsy 1970) leading to similar results.

10.4. *Origin and properties of interacting lymphocytes*

The production of antibodies to haptenic determinants, as analysed in the previous section, were interpreted on the basis of a bicellular interaction. Each of the co-operating cells is capable to recognize specific antigenic determinants of the immunogenic (hapten-carrier) molecule. Yet, only one of them produces the antibodies to the hapten.

Is this cell co-operation based on the existence of two cell populations, with distinct properties and of distinct origin? The analysis of this question is based on studies in which the immunogens used were foreign red blood cells, mostly SRBC. In fact, these studies had preceded the deductions made from the response to hapten determinants.

10.4.1. *Co-operation between cells of thymus and of bone marrow origin*

Studies of Davies et al. (1966) employing mouse radiation-chimeras which had been thymectomized before irradiation and re-grafted with thymus tissue have demonstrated that the thymus cells were triggered to replicate when antigenic stimulation was applied. Yet these were not the cells which actually produced antibodies. Antibodies were produced by bone marrow-derived cells (BDC) and not by thymus-derived cells (TDC) (Davies et al. 1967). It raised the question of whether the proliferation of thymus-derived cells is at all relevant to the process of antibody response. Involvement of bone marrow-derived and thymus-derived cells in antibody formation to SRBC was also shown in the experiments of Claman et al. (1966). They found that irradiated mice injected with bone marrow and thymus cells produce antibodies to SRBC at a level higher than mice injected with either bone marrow or thymus cells only. The synergistic result observed could not be attributed to an additive effect. These observations were confirmed by Miller and Mitchell (1969). Although originally these authors tended to believe that thymus-derived cells are the precursors of antibody-forming cells (Miller and Mitchell 1967), they very soon discovered that the antibody-forming cells were not of the same origin as the inoculated thymus cells (Mitchell and Miller 1968). Thus, neonatally thymectomized mice inoculated with either thymus cells or thoracic duct cells responded to SRBC applied simultaneously with the cells. Since in this system semi-allogeneic cells were also effective, the workers were able to identify the origin of the antibody-forming cells by using anti-H-2 sera, and they found that the cells were of host origin. Further studies were performed on adult thymectomized irradiated mice repopulated with bone marrow. Such mice responded to SRBC when inoculated with thymus cells (Mitchell and Miller 1968). In this case, as in the neonatally thymectomized mice, the use of semi-allogeneic combinations and applications of anti-H-2 sera demonstrated that the antibody-forming cells were derived from the bone marrow.

In most of the studies discussed above, co-operation of cells of thymus and of bone marrow origin was shown in a system using radiation-chimeras. The final tests for responses were performed on the spleens of these animals. We have raised the question as to whether thymus and bone marrow cells can interact directly in the presence of irradiated spleen tissue, or whether the cells have to reside within the spleen tissue *in vivo* in order to be able to effect a response.

Spleens from total body irradiated mice were cultured in millipore-filter-wells in the presence of thymus explants with or without bone marrow tissue (Globerson 1966). SRBC were added to the cultures and the response was followed. The result was (Globerson and Feldman 1970a, b) that no antibodies to SRBC could be detected in any of these combination cultures. In contrast to this, spleens explanted from lethally irradiated mice that had been treated with bone marrow and thymus cells, did respond to SRBC under such experimental conditions. Thus, the response is probably carried out by cells of the bone marrow and thymus which underwent a certain phase of differentiation within the spleen of the irradiated host. This may explain the failure of Bussard et al. (1970) to obtain a response by cells of different tissue origins admixed *in vitro* with peritoneal cells. However, it should be noted that Doria et al. (1970) did obtain a response *in vitro* by bone marrow-derived cells maintained in the system of Mishell and Dutton (1967) when mixed with cells of thymus tissue.

According to these results, one should distinguish between two separate events: (1) the development of thymus-derived cells (TDC) and of bone marrow-derived cells (BDC) within the spleen of the irradiated mouse, and (2) immunological interaction of these cell populations in response to antigenic stimulation. That the micro-environment within the spleen tissue may have an effect on development of cells lodged in the spleen has been demonstrated for various systems, e.g., haemopoietic cells (Till and McCulloch 1961), leukaemic cells (Feldman et al. 1964), and lymphoid cells (Globerson 1966; Auerbach 1966). If these two events are indeed distinct it may be predicted that immunological interactions of TDC and BDC could be carried out *in vitro* in the presence of antigenic stimulation. Thus, lethally irradiated mice (900 r) were injected with either bone marrow or thymus cells. Spleens were removed 24 hrs later and paired *in vitro*. SRBC were added to the cultures and the response was followed. It was found that cultures composed of spleens with TDC and spleens with BDC produced antibodies, whereas controls consisting of pairs of fragments from either bone marrow- or thymus-treated mice failed to respond (Globerson and Feldman 1970b). It may therefore be concluded that the immunological interaction can take place *in vitro*.

In view of these results, and in view of the studies reported on the role of macrophages in the response to SRBC, one may raise the question whether bone marrow-derived cells or thymus-derived cells contain the precursors of the adherent cells involved in the response *in vitro* (Mosier 1967). To answer this question, Mosier et al. (1970) cultured spleen cells from thymectomized irradiated mice treated with either bone marrow or thymus cells. Adherent and non-adherent cells were prepared from each of these spleens, and mixtures were cultured in various combinations. Active adherent cells were found in the spleens containing bone marrow-derived cells, whereas the non-adherent population participating in the response was composed of cells from spleens of donors treated with thymus as well as bone marrow. It thus appears as if the bone marrow contributes two cell types participating in the response, one of which acts as adherent cell population.

10.4.2. *The role of thymus-derived cells*

The role of the thymus-derived cells could be explained by either of the following hypotheses:

(a) Cells of bone marrow origin are induced by the thymus cells to become immunocompetent (Globerson and Auerbach 1967), possibly by a humoral factor (Trainin et al. 1969).

(b) Cells of thymus origin interact with the antigen and trigger the response in bone marrow-derived cells.

The distinction between these two possibilities was based on the notion that if the second hypothesis is correct, then tolerance could block the activity of thymus cells towards the tolerogen, but will have no effect on the response to other non-cross reacting antigens. Thus, Miller and Mitchell (1969) tested the ability of thymus cells from mice made tolerant to SRBC to lead to antibody formation in neonatally thymectomized mice. It was found that such thymus cells failed to enhance the response to SRBC whereas they did affect the response to horse red blood cells. It was thus suggested that the thymus cells recognize the antigen and interact with it specifically in inducing anti-SRBC response. They can thus be considered to be antigen-sensitive cells.

These results cannot be regarded as conclusive, since this system involved neonatally thymectomized mice which could be restored to activity by thymus cells alone, without addition of bone marrow cells. When the response was tested in thymectomized, irradiated mice, thymus cells from tolerant mice were as effective in leading to a response in the presence of bone marrow cells as thymus cells from normal mice (Miller and Mitchell 1970). Specific blocking of activity of thymus cells by paralyzing against SRBC was also reported by Gershon et al. (1968). In contrast to this, Playfair (1969) has demonstrated that cells from bone marrow, and not from the thymus, were responsible for unresponsiveness in tolerance to SRBC. On the other hand, Chiller et al. (1970) concluded that both bone marrow and thymus cells are defective during immunological unresponsiveness to HGG, whereas Taylor (1969), also using soluble antigens (BSA), demonstrated that the thymus cells are specifically unresponsive. These contradictory conclusions may be attributed to differences in the experimental conditions employed (i.e., low zone and high zone tolerance). Yet, if we consider the idea that TDC and BDC probably represent antigen-sensitive and antibody-producing cells, and hence both cell populations may be equipped with specific cell receptors, it would appear quite possible that under appropriate conditions each of these cells may be blocked. In any case, the experimental evidence presented shows that interaction of TDC and BDC depends on antigen.

Does the carrier effect described in the previous chapter involve the thymus-derived cells? To analyse this question we studied the response to DNP in spleens of radiation chimeras (Kunin et al. 1971). (Balb × BL)F_1 mice were total body irradiated at a dose of 750 r and injected i.v. with 10^8 thymus cells from untreated syngeneic donors. One day later they were injected i.p. with RSA in complete Freund's adjuvant. On day 6–8 they were further injected with 3–4×10^7 bone marrow cells, and 2–4 days later the animals were sacrificed and the spleens were cultured and stimulated with DNP-RSA under conditions enabling a response to the hapten (Segal et al. 1970). It was found that such spleens produced antibodies to DNP. No response was detected in any of the control groups which had been treated with either thymus or bone marrow cells only, or when treatment with bone marrow cells preceded injection of the thymus cells. Thus, the carrier effect in antibody response to DNP (Segal et al. 1971a) involves TDC which act as antigen-sensitive cells. Further studies are now being conducted in our Laboratory to find out whether thymus-derived cells from mice tolerant to RSA will show a specific failure to participate in the response to DNP-RSA.

Since both TDC and BDC are essential for the initiation of a response, which of these cells determine the class of immunoglobulin produced? Cudkowicz et al. (1969) and Shearer et al. (1969) have approached this question by employing limiting dilutions of either thymus cells or bone marrow cells in treatment of irradiated recipients. They found that when bone marrow cells were applied in limiting dilutions in mixtures with an excess number of thymus cells, the antigen-sensitive unit obtained produced either IgM or IgG. The number of antigen-sensitive units was proportional to the number of bone marrow cells injected (Cudkowicz et al. 1969). On the other hand, when thymus cells were given in limiting dilutions with bone marrow cells in excess, the results suggested that one TDC can interact with more than one BDC (P-PFC) regardless of the type of antibodies produced (Shearer et al. 1969). Thus, the class of antibodies is determined by the BDC in the antigen-sensitive unit.

10.5.   *The open questions*

The experiments discussed in this review deal with events involved in initiation of antibody response. We have raised the following questions: Is the macrophage-antigen interaction an essential step for inducing antibody production? If it is, what is the nature of the signal emitted by the macrophage-antigen complex? How is the immunogenic signal recognized by the lymphoid cells? Does the bicellular lymphocyte co-operation represent a general principle in the process of triggering antibody production? Finally, what are the basic intracellular events which 'translate' the recognition processes to the induction of antibody synthesis?

Macrophage-antigen complexes were found to increase dramatically the immunogenic capacity of quite a number of antigens. T2 bacterio-phages, *Shigella*, SRBC, and certain protein antigens such as BSA, HSA, and haemocyanin, after incubation with macrophages, elicited an immune response which was significantly higher than that produced following the inoculation of the free antigen. This was observed in experiments in which macrophages took up antigen either *in vivo* or *in vitro*, and in which macrophages were inoculated into normal recipients (Mitchison 1969; Unanue and Askonas 1968), into x-irradiated recipients (Gallily and Feldman 1967a, b; Mitchison 1969; Pribnow and Silverman 1967), or into newborn recipients (Argyris 1968; Braun and Lasky 1967). Although in some experiments PEC were used at doses in which the non-macrophage cell types reached an absolute high number (Braun and Lasky 1967), in others, evidence was brought to indicate that the active cell in PEC was not the lymphocyte but rather the macrophage (Mitchison 1969; Gallily and Feldman 1967b). In experiments in which the macrophages were used following elimination of lymphocytes and granulocytes, no diminution of the immunogenic effect was observed (Gallily and Feldman 1967b).

It should, however, be noted that the reports on positive participation of macrophages apply, so far, to a limited number of antigens tested and may not apply to others. Furthermore, even with regard to the 'macrophage-dependent' antigens, one faces the question of whether antigen-macrophage interaction is essential for inducing initiation of antibody production, or whether such an interaction only amplifies the response which would be initiated by an antigen even without being taken up by macrophages. At the present stage, it is impossible to answer this question in a final way, since in those cases where the free antigen does elicit an immune response, although of a significantly lower level than that elicited by an antigen-macrophage complex, it could be argued that the inoculated free antigen *was* taken up by recipient macrophages, though to a limited degree. This might apply both to *Shigella* inoculated into X-rayed animals, and to free BSA and HSA. This is in accordance with the observations that the large molecular weight haemocyanin was immunogenic in its free form, most probably because it was taken up readily by the recipient macrophages (Askonas 1970). Macrophages, therefore, might play a determining role in inducing antibody production, yet a final proof of this notion must await more rigorous experiments.

The nature of the immunogenic signal exerted by the macrophage is still a controversial matter. Mitchison's experiments indicate that it is not just a quantitative concentration of antigen, although tests of the effects of macrophages in the initiation of the response to SRBC suggest that quantitative parameters might determine whether the macrophages will inhibit or induce antibody production (Hoffman 1970). It is therefore conceivable that the macrophage might alter the antigen in an as yet unknown manner. Whether or not we define this notion of molecular alteration as the 'processing' of antigen by macrophages, it should be stated that, at least with regard to protein antigens, this is *not* a process of degradation (Sela et al. 1967). Whether the process consists in coupling the antigen to macrophage-originated molecular components such as an RNA, remains an open question. Fishman's experiments (Fishman 1961; Fishman and Adler 1963; Fishman and Adler 1967; Adler et al. 1966) are suggestive in this respect, at least with regard to T2 phage, yet even in this system it is not clear whether the normal *in vivo* participation of macrophages in the induction of anti-T2 antibodies involves an RNA-antigen complex. So far, the activity of RNA-antigen was demonstrated in a very limited number of cases, let alone the 'template' activity or RNA, eliciting antibody of the macrophage allotype specificity (Adler et al. 1966).

The observations regarding the function of the membrane-bound antigen tend to suggest that under normal conditions, the macrophage might exert its immunogenic effect *via* contact interaction with other cells, the obvious candidate being the antigen-sensitive lymphocyte. Indeed, morphological evidence that surface contacts between macrophages and lymphocytes are formed coincidentally with the application of an immunogen have been presented (Schoenberg et al. 1964). Whether these manifest the immunogenic signal of macrophages to lymphocytes requires further tests. Fischer's recent cinematographic analysis indicates that the contact between macrophages and lymphocytes of the omentum is associated with the replication of the lymphocytes (Fischer, personal communication). Using a different morphological approach, Sulitzeanu arrived at similar observations (Sulitzeanu et al. 1969). This obviously suggests a possible immunogenic significance to the contact interaction.

One possible explanation of the increase in the final manifestation of antibody production is to assume that lymphocytes interacting with macrophages undergo replication.

A *simple* explanation of the carrier effect can be based on a signal for replication of carrier ASC. This could be elicited by a macrophage-carrier complex. Yet, it is obvious that theoretically the carrier effect could be obtained not only by increasing the population of antigen-sensitive cells, but also by increasing the number of specific receptors per cell. To test whether the increase in the population of carrier antigen-sensitive cells is the process operating in the system, we carried out experiments in which we blocked cell replication with vinblastine at different time intervals following the *in vivo* immunization with the carrier. The result was that the application of vinblastine simultaneously with the carrier prevented the subsequent *in vitro* response to the hapten-carrier conjugate. Yet, if the vinblastine was given just 24 hrs following the immunization with the carrier, a significant carrier effect was obtained. We interpret these results as an indication that in order to confer a carrier effect cell replication is essential; but in fact, the minimal requirement may be just one cycle of replication. If gene de-repression can take place here, as in other systems, only on a newly synthesized DNA strand, then it seems conceivable that the single cycle of antigen-sensitive cell replication is required for the production of more receptor molecules per cell. Accordingly, the carrier effect is based primarily on the increase in number of carrier cell receptors which will take place only when DNA replication is initiated.

The co-operation between antigen-sensitive cell and antibody-producing cell as a basic mechanism in inducing antibody production was either shown or inferred for quite a number of different antigens (Davies 1969; Miller and Mitchell 1969; Claman and Chaperon 1969; Taylor 1969). Whether the antigen, in all these cases is a 'macrophage-processed' molecule remains an open question. Whether the co-operation is indeed based on *contact via* the antigen bridging between the antigen-sensitive cell and the antibody-producing cell is generally assumed but still requires further evidence. Alternatively, one could explain the co-operative effect on the basis of an antigen signal emitted by the antigen-sensitive cell, and received by a circulating antibody-producing cell. Be the nature of the interaction *via* the antigen as it may, the *main* question which remains unsolved and which has as yet hardly been touched upon experimentally is: How does the cell-cooperation switch on the production of antibodies in the antibody-producing cells?

Theoretically, at least three alternative mechanisms can be envisaged: (1) The co-operation leads just to the initiation of an exponential pattern of replication of antibody-producing cells which, to begin with, were producing antibodies. That clones of antibody-producing cells appear following immunization has been assumed (Burnet 1959) long ago. (2) The function of the antigen interacting with the antibody-receptor of the antibody-producing cell is to elicit the shedding-off of this receptor in the form of free antibody – after which a new 'receptor' will be synthesized homeostatically. (3) The antigen-receptor complex formed on the surface of the antibody-producing cell elicits an intracellular signal to the genome, resulting in a continuous synthesis of antibodies.

To test the first possibility, we asked the following question: Is antibody production following antigenic stimulation causally related to an exponential replication of antibody-producing cells? To test this, we applied cytosine-arabinoside in spleen organ cultures at different time intervals following *in vitro* immunization with DNP-Hcy (Segal et al. 1969). The result was that the application of cytosine-arabinoside simultaneously with the antigen prevented the production of anti-DNP antibodies. Yet, when the cytosine-arabinoside was applied just 24 hrs after the immunogen, a significant anti-DNP response was obtained. Thus, the minimal requirement in terms of cell proliferation is one cycle of replication – similar to the requirement for the antigen-sensitive cell in eliciting the carrier effect. This, therefore, makes the first possible mechanism very unlikely.

The second possible mechanism, based on the shedding-off of the receptor by the antigen seems improbable for the simple reason that it requires the persistence of antigen on the antibody-producing cell. No experimental evidence so far supports this requirement.

We are, therefore, left with the third rather 'conventional' mechanism of the antigen functioning as an inducer of a state of protein biosynthesis, similarly to inducers of cell differentiation in other developmental systems. This is also in accordance with the necessity for one cycle of cell replication, since gene derepression might require a new, yet unrepressed DNA. The great questions then are – what is the precise molecular signal which is conveyed from the cell receptor to the genome of the antibody-producing cell, how does that signal cause specific gene derepression, and what is the precise function of co-operation between antigen-sensitive cell and antibody-producing cell in eliciting the functional intracellular signal from the antibody-producing cell receptor to its genome?

It should be noted that in many developmental systems, particularly in the embryo, differentiation is triggered by contact interaction between cells (Grobstein 1955). From this point of view the induction of antibody formation represents a model for the induction of cell differentiation. The attractiveness of this model stems from the fact that the inducer, in our case the antigen, is chemically defined, and the end result of the differentiating event is characterized by a specific molecular marker – the antibody. Yet, the main question of how the signal of the defined inducer triggers the formation of the antibody remains open.

References

ABDOU, N. I. and M. RICHTER, 1969, J. Exptl. Med. *130*, 141.

ABRAMOFF, P. and N. B. BRIEN, 1968, J. Immunol. *10*, 1210.

ADLER, F. L., M. FISHMAN and S. DRAY, 1966, J. Immunol. *97*, 554.

ARGYRIS, B. F., 1968, J. Exptl. Med. *128*, 459.

ASKONAS, B. A. and L. JAROŠKOVÁ, 1970, Antigen in macrophages and antibody induction. *In*: R. van Furth, ed.: Mononuclear phagocytes. Blackwell Scientific Publications. pp. 595–610.

ASKONAS, B. A. and J. M. RHODES, 1965, Nature *205*, 470.

AUERBACH, R., 1966, Embryogenesis of Immune Systems. *In*: G. E. W. Wolestenholme and R. Porter, eds.: CIBA Foundation Symp. on the Thymus. London, Churchill. pp. 39–49.

BRAUN, W. and L. J. LASKY, 1967, Federation Proc. *26*, 642.

BROWNSTONE, A., N. A. MITCHISON and R. PITT-RIVERS, 1966, Immunology *10*, 481.

BURNET, M., 1959, The clonal selection theory of acquired immunity. London, Cambridge University Press.

BUSSARD, A. E., G. J. V. NOSSAL, J. C. MAZIE and H. LEWIS, 1970, J. Exptl. Med. *131*, 917.

CHILLER, J. M., G. S. HABICHT and W. O. WEIGLE, 1970, Proc. Natl. Acad. Sci. U.S. *65*, 551.

CLAMAN, H. N., E. A. CHAPERON and R. F. TRIPLETT, 1966, J. Immunol. *97*, 828.

CLAMAN, H. N. and E. A. CHAPERON, 1969, Transplant. Rev. *1*, 92.

COHEN, E. P. and J. J. PARKS, 1964, Science *144*, 1012.

CUDKOWICZ, G., G. M. SHEARER and R. L. PRIORE, 1969, J. Exptl. Med. *130*, 481.

DAVIES, A. J. S., 1969, Transplant. Rev. *1*, 43.

DAVIES, A. J. S., E. LEUCHARS, V. WALLIS, R. MARCHANT and E. V. ELLIOT, 1967, Transplantation *5*, 222.

DAVIES, A. J. S., E. LEUCHARS, V. WALLIS and P. C. KOLLER, 1966, Transplantation *4*, 438.

DIXON, F. J. and W. O. WEIGLE, 1957, J. Exptl. Med. *105*, 75.

DORIA, G., M. MARTINOZZI, G. AGAROSSI and S. DI PIETRO, 1970, Experientia *26*, 410.

DUTTON, R. W. and J. D. EADY, 1964, Immunology *7*, 40.

FELDMAN, M. and R. GALLILY, 1967, Cold Spring Harbor Symp. Quant. Biol. *32*, 415.

FELDMAN, M., D. YAFFE and A. GLOBERSON, 1964, Some cellular and molecular aspects of cytodifferentiation. *In*: P. Emmelot and O. Mühlbock, eds.: Cellular control mechanisms and cancer. London, Elsevier. pp. 60–79.

FINKELSTEIN, M. S. and J. W. UHR, 1964, Science *146*, 67.

FISHMAN, M. and F. L. ADLER, 1963, J. Exptl. Med. *117*, 595.

FISHMAN, M., 1961, J. Exptl. Med. *114*, 837.

FISHMAN, M. and F. L. ADLER, 1967, Cold Spring Harbor Symp. Quant. Biol. *32*, 343.

FRIEDMAN, H. P., A. B. STAVITSKY and J. M. SOLOMON, 1965, Science *149*, 1106.

FRISCH, A. W. and B. J. WILSON, 1969, Proc. Soc. Exptl. Biol. Med. *132*, 42.

GALLILY, R. and M. FELDMAN, 1966, Israel J. Med. Sci. *2*, 358.

GALLILY, R. and M. FELDMAN, 1967a, Immunology *12*, 197.

GALLILY, R. and M. FELDMAN, 1967b, The cellular components in the induction of antibody by x-irradiated animals. *In*: Germinal centers in immune responses, Symp. Proc. Berlin, Springer-Verlag. pp. 333–336.

GERSHON, H. and M. FELDMAN, 1968, Immunology *15*, 827.

GERSHON, R. K., V. WALLIS, A. J. S. DAVIES and E. LEUCHARS, 1968, Nature *218*, 380.

GLOBERSON, A., 1966, J. Exptl. Med. *123*, 25.

GLOBERSON, A. and R. AUERBACH, 1965, Science *149*, 991.

GLOBERSON, A. and R. AUERBACH, 1966, J. Exptl. Med. *124*, 1001.

GLOBERSON, A. and R. AUERBACH, 1967, J. Exptl. Med. *126*, 223.

GLOBERSON, A. and M. FELDMAN, 1969, In vitro reactivation of antibody response in explants of irradiated spleens. *In*: L. Fiore-Donati and M. G. Hanna, eds.: Lymphatic tissue and germinal centers in immune response. New York, Plenum Press. pp. 407–414.

GLOBERSON, A. and M. FELDMAN, 1970a, Macrophages and the bicellular mechanism of antibody response. *In*: R. van Furth, ed.: Mononuclear phagocytes. Blackwell Scientific Publications. pp. 613–624.

GLOBERSON, A. and M. FELDMAN, 1970b, In vitro reactivation of immunocompetence following X-irradiation. In: L. Severi, ed.: Immunity and tolerance in oncogenesis. Division of Cancer Research, Perugia. pp. 989–1000.

GOTTLIEB, A. A., V. R. GLISIN and P. DOTY, 1967, Proc. Natl. Acad. Sci. U.S. *57*, 1849.

GROBSTEIN, C., 1955, Tissue interaction in the morphogenesis of mouse embryonic rudiments in vitro. *In*: D. Rudnick, ed.: Aspects of synthesis and order in growth. Princeton, Princeton University Press. pp. 233–256.

HAIMOWICH, J. and M. SELA, 1966, J. Immunol. *97*, 338.

HOFFMANN, M., 1970, Immunology *18*, 791.

HUMPHREY, J. H., 1969, Antibiot. et Chemotherap. *15*, 7.

KLINMAN, N. R. and R. B. TAYLOR, 1969, Clin. Exptl. Immunol. *4*, 473.

KUNIN, S., G. M. SHEARER, S. SEGAL., A. GLOBERSON and M. FELDMAN, 1971, Cell Immunol. *2*, 229.

MARTIN, M. J., 1966, Aust. J. Exptl. Biol. Med. Sci. *44*, 605.

MILLER, J. F. A. P. and G. F. MITCHELL, 1970, J. Exptl. Med. *131*, 675.

MILLER, J. F. A. P. and G. F. MITCHELL, 1969, Transplant. Rev. *1*, 3.

MILLER, J. F. A. P. and G. F. MITCHELL, 1967, Nature *216*, 659.

MILLER, J. F. A. P. and G. F. MITCHELL, 1969, Transplant. Proc. *1*(1), 535.

MISHELL, R. I. and R. W. DUTTON, 1967, J. Exptl. Med. *126*, 423.

MITCHELL, G. F. and J. F. A. P. MILLER, 1968, Proc. Natl. Acad. Sci. U.S. *59*, 296.

MITCHELL, G. F. and J. F. A. P. MILLER, 1968, J. Exptl. Med. *128*, 821.

MITCHISON, N. A., 1969, Immunology *16*, 1.

MITCHISON, N. A., 1966, Proc. Biophys. and Mol. Biol. *16*, 3.

MITCHISON, N. A., 1967, Cold Spring Harbor Symp. Quant. Biol. *32*, 431.

MOSIER, D. E., 1967, Science *158*, 1573.

MOSIER, D. E. and L. W. COPPELSON, 1968, Proc. Natl. Acad. Sci. U.S. *61*, 542.

MOSIER, D. E., F. W. FITCH, D. A. ROWLEY and A. J. S. DAVIES, Nature (London) *225*, 276.

NACHTIGAL, D., 1967, Lymphoid regeneration following X-ray treatment and the susceptibility to the induction of immune tolerance. *In*: Germinal centers in immune responses, Symp. Proc. Berlin, Springer-Verlag. pp. 329–332.

NACHTIGAL, D. and M. FELDMAN, 1963, Immunology *5*, 356.

NACHTIGAL, D. and M. FELDMAN, 1964, Immunology *7*, 616.

NACHTIGAL, D., E. GREENBERG and M. FELDMAN, 1968, Immunology *15*, 343.

NOSSAL, G. J. V., 1967, Inductive steps in antibody formation and tolerance. *In:* J. Killander, ed.: Gamma globulins, Proc. 3rd Nobel Symp. Stockholm, Almqvist and Wiksell. pp. 428–442.

OVARY, Z. and B. BENACERRAF, 1963, Proc. Soc. Exptl. Biol. Med. *114*, 72.

PERKINS, E. H. and T. MAKINODAN, 1965, J. Immunol. *94*, 765.

PLAYFAIR, J. H. L., 1969, Nature *222*, 882.

PLOTZ, P. H., 1969, Nature *223*, 1373.

PRIBNOW, J. F. and M. S. SILVERMAN, 1967, J. Immunol. *98*, 225.

RAJEWSKY, K., V. SCHIRRMACHER, S. NASE and N. K. JERNE, 1969, J. Exptl. Med. *129*, 1131.

RAJEWSKY, K. and E. ROTTLÄNDER, 1967, Cold Spring Harbor Symp. Quant. Biol. *32*, 547.

ROSEMAN, J., 1969, Science *165*, 1125.

SCHOENBERG, M. D., V. R. MUMAW, R. D. MOORE and A. S. WEISBERGER, 1964, Science *143*, 964.

SEGAL, S., A. GLOBERSON and M. FELDMAN, 1969, Israel J. Med. Sci. *5*, 444.

SEGAL, S., A. GLOBERSON, M. FELDMAN, J. HAIMOVICH and D. GIVOL, 1969, Nature *223*, 1374.

SEGAL, S., A. GLOBERSON, M. FELDMAN, J. HAIMOVICH and M. SELA, 1970, J. Exptl. Med. *131*, 93.

SEGAL, S., A. GLOBERSON and M. FELDMAN, 1971a, Cell. Immunol. *2*, 205.

SEGAL, S., A. GLOBERSON and M. FELDMAN, 1971b, Cell. Immunol. *2*, 222.

SELA, M., B. SCHECHTER, I. SCHECHTER and F. BOREK, 1967, Cold Spring Harbor Symp. Quant. Biol. *32*, 537.

SELL, S., 1967a, J. Exptl. Med. *125*, 289.

SELL, S., 1967b, J. Exptl. Med. *125*, 393.

SHEARER, G. M., G. CUDKOWICZ and R. L. PRIORE, 1969, J. Exptl. Med. *130*, 467.

SULITZEANU, D., G. RASOOLY, D. BENEZRA and I. GERY, 1969, Israel J. Med. Sci. *5*, 443.

TAYLOR, R. B., 1969, Transplant. Rev. *1*, 14.

TILL, J. E. and E. A. MCCULLOCH, 1961, Radiation. Res. *14*, 213.

TRAININ, N., M. SMALL and A. GLOBERSON, 1969, J. Exptl. Med. *130*, 765.

TRUFFA-BACHI. P. and L. WOFSY. 1970, Proc. Natl. Acad. Sci. U.S. *66*, 685.

UNANUE, E. R. and B. A. ASKONAS, 1968, Immunology *15*, 287.

UNANUE, E. R. and J. C. CEROTTINI, 1970, J. Exptl. Med. *131*, 711.

WEINSTEIN, Y., M. WILCHEK and D. GIVOL, 1969, Biochem. Biophys. Res. Commun. *35*, 694.

WIGZELL, H. and B. ANDERSSON, 1969, J. Exptl. Med. *129*, 23.

WIGZELL, H., 1967, Cold Spring Harbor Symp. Quant. Biol. *32*, 507.

CHAPTER 11

Heriditary aspects of
the capacity to respond immunologically

JACK R. BATTISTO and FRANK LILLY

*Department of Microbiology and Immunology and Department of Genetics, Albert
Einstein College of Medicine, Bronx, N.Y.*

11.1. Introduction

One of the several variables that determines whether an immune response will be made to an introduced antigen, has long been suspected
to be the host's genetic composition. Attempts to solve the question of
whether heredity controls the ability to respond immunologically to
antigens have taken several avenues over the years.

Perhaps the earliest information in this area derives from observations
on allergic diseases of humans. Many investigators involved in the study
of allergies have noted the peculiar distribution of allergic disorders in
some families (see review by Schwartz 1952). Most of the reports in
this area comprise family pedigrees and mathematical treatments of
large clinical analyses. Data from neither of these sources, coming as
they do from interrogation of or tests upon humans, have been definitive
enough to reveal precise hereditary control of immunological responsiveness.

In some of the earliest experimental trials random-bred animals were
immunized to determine which were responding and which non-responding. Usually these were subsequently mated to yield families of high- and
low-responding individuals and speculations on the genetic control of
the response were made. As will be shown these were followed by
assessments of the data that developed counter-claims and much
confusion.

Investigators in the next wave were led to the use of highly inbred
animals in attempts to get an answer concerning genetic influences. Unfortunately a large number of workers used complex antigens such as
microorganisms or xenogeneic erythrocytes and these have tended to
obscure results. This was especially true when tests for antibody did
not differentiate sufficiently between multiple antigens on a cell's surface.
A host incapable of responding to a major antigen of a mosaic might well

respond to a minor one and be recorded phenotypically as a responding animal.

More recently immunization of highly inbred animals with single antigenic determinants, some synthetic and others naturally occurring, has led to results that are more easily interpreted. In addition, information on methods for inducing immunological tolerance has promoted use of immunization techniques that avoid this source of confusion.

As far as practicable, then, presentation of the information on this particular subject will be made in an historical manner. Attempts have been made to group studies in a particular species of animals since there is some evidence that genetic control of immune response for certain antigens may be unigenic in one species whereas in other species it may be polygenic. In addition, where possible, every attempt has been made to keep separate the responses of the humoral antibody type and of the delayed hypersensitivity variety, in the event that separate genetic paths control initiation of each. Finally, a separate section is devoted to a description of the mechanisms used to explain genetic influence upon the heritability of immune responses.

11.2. Early experimental attempts to determine whether initiation of the immune response is under genetic control

One of the earliest experimental attempts to determine whether initiation of the immune response is under genetic control was by Gorer and Schultze (1938). These workers tested four lines of mice for ability to produce antibodies to 'H' and 'O' antigens of bacteria *Salmonella typhimurium* and *Salmonella enteritidis*. Two of the mouse lines were not inbred and two others had been brother-sister inbred for over 30 generations. After immunization with *S. typhimurium*, female mice of all four lines were found to give higher 'H' and 'O' titres of circulating antibody than did the males. After immunizing with *S. enteritidis*, antibody production showed no correlation along sexual lines. However, the mice of the inbred pure lines gave better antibody responses than did the non-inbred, selected lines. This evidence was suggestive that initiation of antibody synthesis is under genetic control.

The first attempts to purposely breed animals with reference to susceptibility to skin sensitization with simple chemical compounds (delayed hypersensitivity) were undertaken by Landsteiner and Chase (1940) and by Chase (1941). They proved it possible to derive two colonies of guinea-pigs with significantly different susceptibilities towards a compound 2,4-dinitrochlorobenzene (DNCB). One strain gave uniformly intense cutaneous reactions in the great majority of cases while the other responded with low-grade sensitivity but was not entirely refractory. These investigations thus provided direct evidence that contact sensitization is influenced by heredity. Chase put forward the view that, because the sensitivities showed continuous transitions and did not fall into sharply discrete grades, a single pair of genetic factors could hardly control reactivity.

In addition to using DNCB, these investigators (Landsteiner and Chase 1939) used another sensitizer, poison ivy extract, to develop guinea-pig lines that were high and low in responsiveness. To learn whether susceptibility to sensitization is general or varies with the substances employed, both DNCB and poison ivy extract were applied to offspring from the four developed families. The degrees of sensitivity engendered to each of the two sensitizers were in 93 instances closely parallel. Nevertheless, 35 animals were noted where sensitivity to DNCB was high while that to poison ivy was low. In addition, cases of the reverse were seen. Thus, inheritance of immunological responsivity to one antigen does not carry over to a second, unrelated antigen. The authors emphasized the complexity of the hereditary basis for contactant-type allergy.

The hereditary predisposition to dermal sensitization in guinea-pigs was confirmed by Jacobs et al. (1941), who used allyl isothiocyanate as hapten. Although only a small percentage of unselected guinea-pigs was sensitizable, by selective breeding a strain was obtained in which practically all the members could be strongly sensitized. A non-sensitizable strain wâs also bred.

In a provocative report Landsteiner et al. (1939) analysed the data from an experiment on humans by Sulzberger and Rostenberg (1939). They suggested that individual differences exist among humans as regards susceptibility to eczematous sensitization with simple chemical substances. Among 82 persons in whom experimental sensitization was attempted with p-nitrosodimethylaniline (A) and with 2,4 dinitrochlorobenzene (B), 36.6% became sensitized to A and 40% to B. Of the 50 individuals who became sensitive, 21 were sensitive to approximately the same degree to both substances. However, a group of 20 became sensitized chiefly to B and another group of 9 sensitized mainly to A. A distinct direction of susceptibility to sensitization was thus shown to exist in certain individuals. These investigators called attention to the fact that studies among races, families and of identical twins would help to define the cause of the selective direction in susceptibility to eczematous sensitization in humans.

Although the use of simple chemical haptens might be thought to be useful for genetic studies of immunological capacity to respond, they possess a serious drawback if used in the nascent condition in the animal. Virtually all of the chemicals that are sensitizers couple chemically with various body components. In this condition they may present more than a single antigenic determinant to the immunological apparatus and thus become similar to more complex natural antigens.

Chase (1953, 1961) investigated still another instance of heritability to sensitization. In this case the conjugated antigen, picrylated homologous erythrocyte ghosts, was incorporated into an adjuvant mixture consisting of killed mycobacteria in paraffin oil (referred to hereafter as Freund's adjuvant). He noted that although guinea-pigs of the susceptible and resistant responding families reacted well to the constituents of mycobacteria that induced tuberculin hypersensitivity, members of the resistant colony remained deficient in acquiring cutaneous hypersensitivity to the picryl moiety of the conjugated antigen. In addition, they were unable to synthesize circulating antibody to the conjugated antigen. Thus, two independently variable sensitizing properties of the dead tubercle bacilli became apparent, one for developing sensitivity to tuberculin and the other an adjuvant effect for directing immune responses to the incorporated conjugated antigen. It is obvious that sensitizability for both are separately inherited.

Stone (1962) made studies on the inducibility of tuberculin delayed-type sensitivity in guinea-pigs of the Hartley strain and Wright strains 2 and 13. He found that there were differences in the amount of killed dried *Mycobacterium tuberculosis* necessary to sensitize them well. For instance, 1 microgram was sufficient for Hartley guinea-pigs but 5 micrograms were needed for strain 2 animals. Differences were also noted between sexes, e.g., 1–5 μg sensitized strain 13 males but 5 μg were needed for strain 13 females. Stone also showed that a genetic effect was operative in the ease with which autoimmune diseases could be initiated. When an excess of all sensitizing materials was used for inducing allergic encephalomyelitis including 2.5 mg of mycobacteria, strain 13 males were much more susceptible to the disease than were strain 2 males (10 out of 10 deaths in strain 13 vs. 2 out of 10 deaths in strain 2).

A genetic influence was also observed in another autoimmune disease, experimental allergic thyroiditis of guinea-pigs (McMaster et al. 1965). The incidence of thyroiditis was seen to be greater in the Hartley strain of guinea-pigs than in strain 13 animals after immunization with Freund's complete adjuvant containing low doses of homologous thyroid extract.

A similar type observation was made in mice. Gorstein and Lerner found greater susceptibility among animals of the Swiss strain than among those of the C57BL strain (quoted as personal reference in McMaster et al. 1965).

It has long been known that guinea-pigs varied in their ability to synthesize circulating antibody capable of neutralizing the effects of diphtheria toxin. Prigge (1937) called attention to the fact that inbred strains of guinea-pigs should be used in experiments involving immunization against diphtheria since they show a smaller range of variation in the amount of antigen necessary to develop a given resistance to the toxin. Scheibel (1943) using the diphtheria antitoxin response of guinea-pigs was first to suggest that antitoxin-producing faculties might be controlled by dominant hereditary factors. By selection and inbreeding Scheibel was able to separate a guinea-pig population into 2 strains, one consisting of good and another made up of poor producers of antitoxin. Isozygosity in either strain was not achieved because the animals were bred for only a few generations. Nevertheless, the number of antitoxin producers rose in one generation to over 90% in the good strain while 5 generations were required to obtain an equivalent percentage of nonproducers among the poor strain. The ability to respond was not a sex-linked property. Although the results of these experiments were not decisive as to whether one or several genes were responsible, the strong influence of a few generations suggested an uncomplicated dominant gene type of inheritance.

Carlinfanti (1948) took issue with Scheibel's interpretation that the mode of inheritance of antitoxin production was by dominance. He insisted that control of antibody synthesis is accomplished by heredity in the absence of dominance. He analysed the genetic capacity for producing iso-antibodies to blood group antigens A_1 and B by means of correlation tables between the haemagglutinin titres of the parents and those of the children. Carlinfanti felt that a coefficient of 0.3 would imply the existence of dominant and recessive alleles in the determination of these antibody levels, whereas a coefficient of 0.5 would imply no dominance, or codominance. His findings were all coefficients between these two values, and he interpreted them as being closer approximations of 0.5 than 0.3. Since codominance has been observed in most of the recent experimental systems, this interpretation was probably well founded.

11.3. Newer attempts to uncover the hereditary control of immune responses

11.3.1. Use of sheep erythrocytes and bovine serum albumin

A number of laboratories have contributed to the study of the immune response of mice to sheep erythrocytes. Stern et al. (1956) studied the occurrence of natural sheep erythrocyte agglutinins among various inbred strains of mice. They found high levels of agglutinins in the normal sera of C57BL mice; C3H mice showed much lower levels of the agglutinins; and C3H X C57BL F_1 hybrids showed levels of activity only slightly higher than the parental C3H mice. Studies in segregating generations were compatible with determination of the trait by one or a small number of genes.

Claringbold et al. (1957) studied the heritability of the response to immunization with sheep erythrocytes in mother-daughter combinations in a line of random-bred mice and found a heritability factor of 42% in the primary response. This was surprisingly high considering the complexity of the antigen and the absense of information about the fathers' responses. Dineen (1964) determined the response to sheep erythrocytes of individual mice of several inbred strains and found the interstrain differences to be 4.7 times as large as the intrastrain differences. Playfair (1968) studied the development of immunologic responsiveness to sheep erythrocytes and showed that NZB mice responded significantly at 5 days of age, whereas Balb mice did not do so until 14 days and C57BL mice did not attain the same level of reactivity until 28 days or longer. Studies in crosses of NZB and Balb suggested that about three genes influenced the difference in responsiveness between the two strains.

Sobey and his colleagues (1966) also studied the phenomenon of immunological unresponsiveness to bovine serum albumin in random-bred mice. Breeding experiments showed that selection for non-responders led within five generations to a line of mice which consistently showed about a 90% level of unresponsiveness to this antigen. Later, Hardy and Rowley (1968) showed that the non-responder phenomenon in this case was due to a susceptibility to the induction of immunological paralysis by the antigen, since a lower dose of the substance readily induced an antibody response in other mice of the same 'non-responder' line.

11.3.2. Use of synthetic antigens

The production of synthetic polypeptide molecules and their use in immunological studies was a prime element in the current renaissance of interest in genetic factors which control the specificity of the immune response. These molecules comprise, by comparison with even the simplest of natural proteins, a very restricted range of structural and therefore of antigenic complexity. They are either homopolymers (polymers of a single α-amino acid residue) or random copolymers of two or more amino acids.

In the studies of Pinchuck and Maurer (1965) homopolymers tended to be non-antigenic (e.g., polyalanine, glutamic acid, tyrosine or lysine), but the property of antigenicity was acquired as the degree of complexity of the polymers increased. Copolymers of glutamic acid with either lysine, alanine or tyrosine elicited specific antibody formation in some animals of some species but in none of the mice tested. However, terpolymers of glutamic acid, lysine and alanine (GLA) were antigenic in random-bred Swiss mice. The percentage of mice able to make antibodies to GLA increased as the percentage of alanine incorporated in the polymer increased. When only 5% alanine – the lowest percentage studied – was present in the polymer (GLA_5), 47% of Swiss mice responded to the antigen; when 10% or more alanine was present (GLA_{10}, GLA_{20}, etc.), virtually all the mice responded.

Breeding experiments with Swiss mice indicated that the pattern of response or non-response to GLA_5 was inherited as a single-gene trait, with the ability to respond dominant over non-response. The published data were inadequate to indicate whether heterozygous responders made the same or reduced amounts of antibody by comparison with homozygous responders.

Studies of mice of inbred strains immunized with GLA_5 appeared consistent with the finding in random-bred mice of single-gene determination of the antibody response: animals of a given strain were either all responders (C3H/He, BALB/c and 129) or all non-responders (C57BL, A and CBA). The F_1 progeny of two different crosses, each involving a responder and a non-responder strain (C3H $\times$ C57BL and BALB/c $\times$ A), were all responders. No attempts to localize this as yet unnamed gene on the linkage map of the mouse genome have been reported.

There may be a gene, separate from the locus determining responsiveness to GLA_5, which governs the ability of mice to respond to a terpolymer of glutamic acid, alanine and tyrosine ($G_{60}A_{30}T_{10}$); both C57BL and CBA mice were responders to GLA_5, whereas C57BL were non-responders and CBA were responders to $G_{60}A_{30}T_{10}$ (Pinchuck and Maurer 1968).

When Swiss mice were immunized with DNP-conjugated polymers, anti-hapten (DNP) antibodies were elicited in all cases except that of DNP-polylysine, the only homopolymer conjugate used in the study.

However, when the same antisera were examined for anti-carrier (polymer) specificity, activity was found only in cases in which the non-conjugated polymer alone was known to be antigenic. Thus immunization with DNP-conjugated $G_{60}L_{40}$ elicited a response specific for DNP in all of 33 mice, but none of these mice appeared to have responded to the copolymer determinants. Immunization with DNP-GLA$_5$ conjugate elicited a hapten-specific response in all of 18 mice tested, but a polymer-specific response was detected in only 8 of them (44%).

Later studies of Pinchuck et al. (1968) indicated that normally non-responding C57BL mice could be made to produce antibodies specific for the terpolymer $G_{60}A_{30}T_{10}$. Peritoneal macrophages from responder mouse strains, rats or rabbits were exposed briefly *in vitro* to the terpolymer, and RNA extracted from the cells then elicited the appearance of the antibodies upon inoculation into C57BL mice. The RNA so obtained contained about 0.02% by weight of the specific antigen. RNA from cells exposed *in vitro* to a different polymer, $G_{36}L_{24}A_{40}$, also initiated a response specific for the homologous antigen, but a mixture of this RNA with the antigen $G_{60}A_{30}T_{10}$ failed to initiate a response to the admixed antigen. Treatment of the extracted RNA with a high concentration of RNase destroyed its ability to initiate the *in vivo* antibody response. The authors concluded that the specificity of the response resided in the RNA transferred and not in the antigen associated with it. If this be the case, it would seem to follow that the non-responder state was due to the absence of a species of RNA.

11.3.3. Ir-1 gene

Another type of synthetic polypeptide antigen (Sela 1969) which has received some careful attention is that involving complex molecules consisting of a backbone of polylysine (pL) bearing long side-chains of poly-DL-alanine (pA–pL). This portion alone of the synthetic substances was non-antigenic in mice. However, the further attachment at the free ends of the polyalanine side-chains of short, random copolymers of either tyrosine and glutamic acid, p(T, G)-pA–pL, histidine and glutamic acid, p(H, G)-pA–pL, or phenylalanine and glutamic acid, p(Phe, G)-pA–pL, rendered the molecules antigenic.

Studies of McDevitt and Sela (1965, 1967) showed that immunization of mice of various inbred strains with any one of these antigens resulted in an antibody response* which was readily classifiable as high or low

---

* The level of antibody response of individual mice was determined by incubating their sera with radioactive antigen (^{125}I or ^{131}I label) followed by precipitation of the mouse antibodies with rabbit anti-mouse γ-globulin anti-serum; the results were then expressed as 'per cent antigen bound'.

response. In general, the response of low responder mice was near the threshold of detectability. F_1 hybrids of a cross involving a high and a low responder strain produced somewhat reduced amounts of antibody by comparison with the high responder parents (i.e., the response was codominant), and in segregating generations of such a cross the distribution of antibody levels produced by the segregants was compatible with single-gene determination of the trait.

The fact that mice of a given strain were high responders to one of these antigens did not necessarily indicate that animals of the same strain would be high responders to another of the antigens. C57BL mice showed a high level of response to $p(T, G)$-pA–pL and a low level to $p(H, G)$-pA–pL; the reverse was true of CBA mice, which showed a low level of response to $p(T, G)$-pA–pL and a high level to $p(H, G)$-pA–pL. In the ·case of each antigen, backcross populations appeared to indicate segregation at 1:1 ratios of the appropriate response levels, suggesting single-gene determination. These experiments did not, however, indicate if the same gene or two different genes governed the responses to the two related antigens.

The single-gene hypothesis for major control of this antibody response received unexpected confirmation in the finding that the histocompatibility-2 locus (*H-2*) was closely associated with this character (McDevitt and Tyan 1968). Studies involving the *H-2*-congenic mouse strains* developed by Snell (1958) showed that mice differing essentially only with respect to the chromosomal region bearing the *H-2* locus might also differ strongly in their level of response to these synthetic antigens. Thus, whereas the A/J (*H-2^a*) and C3H (*H-2^k*) mouse strains were both low responders to $p(T, G)$-pA–pL, the congenic A . BY and C3H . SW (both *H-2^b*) strains were both high responders to the same antigen. Each of these same four strains showed exactly the opposite response to the antigen $p(H, G)$-pA–pL.

The close linkage of *H-2* with the *Ir-1* gene, the name given to the locus governing the response to both $p(T, G)$-pA–pL and $p(H, G)$-pA–pL, was confirmed by examining appropriate backcross populations, in which there was a nearly complete correlation in the segregation patterns of these traits. Subsequent studies (see McDevitt and Benacerraf 1969) of mouse strains bearing internally recombinant *H-2* alleles** revealed

---

* Ideally, two strains are congenic when their genetic make-up differs only with respect to a single locus. In practice, even the best methods of creating such a pair of strains will result only in a relatively close approximation of this condition.

** The *H-2* locus includes the determinants of the presence or absence on the cell surface of a large number of isoantigens. These isoantigen determinants have in many cases been

that *Ir-1* was within the *H-2* region itself, located to the right of the *Ss* sublocus and within or extremely near the *K* sub-locus of the complex *H-2* region.

In further studies of McDevitt and Chinitz (1969) *Ir-1* also governed the level of response to p(Phe, G)-pA–pL, as demonstrated by studies in the DBA/1 × SJL cross. DBA/1 mice responded well to p(Phe, G)-pA–pL and poorly to p(T, G)-pA–pL, whereas the opposite was true of SJL mice, which responded poorly to p(Phe, G)-pA–pL and well to p(T, G)-pA–pL. Studies in backcross populations from this cross showed that in each case the level of antibody response segregated in a manner closely correlated with the segregation of *H-2* antigens.

There is no answer as yet to the question of whether or not the determinants of antibody response levels to each of the three substances, p(T, G)-pA–pL, p(H, G)-pA–pL and p(Phe, G)-pA–pL, are separate subloci within the *Ir-1* locus. If they are separable subloci, then each *Ir-1* allele includes a sublocus determining either high or low response to a single one of the antigens. If they are not separable regions, then *Ir-1* is a polyallelic gene with at least 5 different alleles of a possible 8 already identified: those associated with $H\text{-}2^a$ (and $H\text{-}2^k$), $H\text{-}2^b$, $H\text{-}2^d$, $H\text{-}2^q$, and $H\text{-}2^s$. It will be very difficult or impossible to distinguish between these two possibilities by classical genetic techniques; although the three antigens are quite different in their abilities to elicit antibody production on the various *Ir-1* backgrounds, the antibodies, once obtained with any one antigen, cross-react extensively with the other two antigens, so that simultaneous immunization with two or more of them appears to be meaningless.

An aspect of the association between *Ir-1* and *H-2* which merits discussion is the possible relationship of *Ir-1* with *Rgv-1*, a gene which governs the host susceptibility to leukaemia induction by Gross virus (Lilly 1966). *Rgv-1*, like *Ir-1*, has also been localized to the *K* subregion of *H-2*. It is conceivable (Lilly 1970a) that *Rgv-1* exerts its influence on viral leukaemogenesis by influencing the host's reactivity to antigens associated with either the leukaemogenic virus or with cells infected by the virus, and thus the further possibility exists that *Rgv-1* and *Ir-1* are identical.

A further degree of subtlety in the determination of immune responsiveness to this type of synthetic, branched polypeptide antigen was

---

mapped in one of several subloci. Recombination occurring within the *H-2* locus and between two subloci has been demonstrated at very low frequencies, and the resulting recombinant alleles have proven extremely useful in studies of the fine structure of the *H-2* region.

revealed by Mozes et al. (1969) in studies of two related antigen molecules: p(T, G)-pPro–pL and p(Phe, G)-pPro–pL, in which poly-L-proline side chains replaced the poly-DL-alanine side-chains of the previously discussed antigens.

SJL mice were high responders and DBA/1 mice low responders to p(T, G)-pPro–pL. Genetic analysis of this difference gave somewhat equivocal information concerning single *vs.* multiple gene determination of the trait, but in any case there was no indication of linkage, as there had been with p(T, G)-pA–pL, between the level of antibody response and *H-2* type, implying that *Ir-1* was irrelevant in the determination of the response to p(T, G)-pPro–pL.

However, studies of the p(Phe, G)-pPro–pL antigen in this same strain combination produced results which, to a first approximation, helped to clarify the situation. Mice of both parental strains, the F_1 and the two backcross generations showed nearly equally high responses to p(Phe, G)-pPro–pL when their sera were assayed with the homologous antigen. When these same sera were assayed for their ability to bind p(T, G)-pPro–pL, the results revealed a parental strain difference and segregation data consistent with single-gene determination and *no* linkage with *H-2*. Similar antisera to p(Phe, G)-pPro–pL were then assayed for reactivity with the p(Phe, G)-pA–pL antigen, and this time the parental strain difference and backcross segregation pattern indicated single-gene determination and *close* linkage with *H-2*.

From these findings it appears that DBA/1 mice immunized with p(Phe, G)-pPro–pL made antibody largely specific for the (Phe, G) terminal sequences of the polypeptide molecule, whereas SJL mice responded largely to the poly-L-proline side-chain portions of the same molecule. In each case the ability to respond immunologically appeared to be determined by a different gene: *Ir-1* governed the response to the chain terminal segments, and an independently segregating locus named *Ir-3* governed the response to poly-*l*-proline specificities.

In an attempt to clarify the mechanism of the genetic determination of these antibody responses, a number of cell transfer studies were carried out by McDevitt and Tyan (1968). The ability to mount a primary response to p(T, G)-pA–pL could be transferred from hybrid responder mice to homozygous non-responder mice. Inoculation of 100–150 million spleen cells for normal (C3H × C57BL) F_1 donors to lethally irradiated C3H mice was successful in 19/28 attempts to establish a responder phenotype in these hosts. The success of these transfers was independent of whether or not the C3H hosts had been thymectomized or whether the immunization of the recipients was begun immediately after irradiation or three weeks later.

The adoptive transfer of a secondary response to this same antigen was accomplished in a similar manner. Irradiated C3H non-responders received 125–150 million spleen cells from (C3H × C57BL) F_1 responders previously immunized with p(T, G)-pA–pL. Thereafter the C3H hosts showed a level of antibodies similar to that in the immunized donor mice, whether or not the hosts received a secondary antigenic stimulus following the cell transfer.

Another cell transfer study (Tyan et al. 1969) showed that mice which normally respond well to one antigen and poorly to another could be converted to the opposite phenotype. Thymectomized and lethally irradiated (C57BL × DBA/2) F_1 mice, which are normally good responders to p(T, G)-pA–pL and poor responders to p(H, G)-pA–pL, received a thymus implant and foetal liver cells from CBA mice, which are poor responders to p(T, G)-pA–pL and good responders to p(H, G)-pA–pL. A first course of immunization of these chimeras with p(T, G)-pA–pL failed to elicit an antibody response to this antigen. However, a further course of immunization, this time with p(H, G)-pA–pL, elicited a good response in 12/13 mice. Thus, in the opinion of the authors, this conversion of the recipients from one phenotype to its opposite (i.e., the transfer both of responsiveness to one antigen and of unresponsiveness to another antigen) showed that the *Ir-1* locus does not govern some phase of metabolizing or processing of antigen, but rather that it exerts its control directly upon the process of antibody formation.

Vaz and Levine (1970) studied the immune response in inbred mice to four protein-hapten conjugates: benzylpenicilloyl and dinitrophenyl conjugates of bovine gamma-globulin and benzylpenicilloyl conjugates of hen's ovomucoid and bovine pancreatic ribonuclease. Following a single, large dose immunization (100 μg), all strains tested showed a low to moderate antibody response. However, following two low dose immunizations (1 μg each), there was a marked strain specificity in the levels of antibody response observed. Among twenty inbred strains tested, the incidence of a consistently high level of response was closely correlated with the occurrence among the mouse strains of the $H\text{-}2^a$ and $H\text{-}2^k$ alleles. These two alleles differ in their D and Ss subregions, but they share the same K subregions. Since it is the K subregion of $H\text{-}2$ with which the *Ir-1* gene is associated, it appears likely that the ability to respond to these antigens is also a function of *Ir-1*.

With respect to the finding of no strain specificity in the immune response to a single, high dose of antigen, the authors speculate that high antigen doses might (a) stimulate a response in more cells which produce antibodies with low antigen binding affinity, or (b) increase the level of response to minor antigenic determinants of the conjugate.

11.3.4. *Immune response to isoantigens*

Gasser (1969) has shown that a single-gene polymorphism exists among mice in the ability to make antibodies specific for antigens governed by the *Ea-1* locus. *Ea-1ᵃ* and *Ea-1ᵇ* are allelic erythrocyte antigens absent from all tested inbred mouse strains (which possess the allele *Ea-1ᵒ*) but present in wild populations. Immunization with a mixture of cells bearing the *Ea-1ᵃ* and *Ea-1ᵇ* antigens elicited haemagglutinating antibody production in 70% of strain YBR mice, but no mice of the BALB/c or CBA strains produced detectable levels of antibody. F_1 crosses of YBR and either BALB/c or CBA mice were all non-responders. *In vivo* absorption studies confirmed that non-responsiveness was not due to possession of either the homologous or a crossreacting antigen. This ability to react to the *Ea-1* antigens segregated in about a 1 : 1 ratio in appropriate backcross populations, and the gene governing the trait was named *Ir-2*.

A potentially interesting aspect of these findings was the linkage of *Ir-2* and *agouti* with a recombination frequency of about 20%. Three different histocompatibility genes are also linked to *agouti: H-13, H-3* and *H-6*, all on the same side of the *agouti* marker, with recombination frequencies of 2, 17 and 25%, respectively. It is thus possible that *Ir-2* is closely associated with *H-3* or *H-6*, just as *Ir-1* is closely associated with *H-2*. If this is true, it may indicate that *Ir* genes are regularly associated with histocompatibility antigen loci, and the implications of this hypothesis are immense.

Another gene which appears to fall into the category of immune response genes was recently discovered by Cudkowicz (1969) in his studies of the ability of lethally irradiated (700–900 r) mice to reject allogeneic bone marrow cells. The antigens primarily responsible for this rejection were associated with the *D* subregion of the *H-2* locus – specificities H-2.2 and H-2.4 (and perhaps H-2.7) in particular. The presence of any one of these specificities on bone marrow cells led to graft rejection by hosts lacking it. Lethally irradiated *H-2ᵈ* homozygotes rejected bone marrow cells from both *H-2ᵇ* homozygotes and *H-2ᵇ/H-2ᵈ* heterozygotes, although the rejection was stronger against fully allogeneic than against semi-allogeneic cells.

However, an *Ir* gene (not yet named) which segregated independently of *H-2* strongly influenced the host's reactivity to the isoantigens. Some inbred mouse strains possessed the dominant allele for strong reactivity to these antigens (C57BL, DBA/2Cum), whereas other mouse strains possessed the recessive allele for weak reactivity (BALB/C, DBA/2J, A). The gene has not been mapped in the mouse genome.

The mechanism of this gene is entirely unstudied at present. It is not known if the reactivity governed is specific for all antigens involved in this relatively radiation-resistant type of rejection phenomenon or for just the antigen specificities of the *D* sublocus of *H-2*. Furthermore, unirradiated DBA/2J mice are fully capable of making cytotoxic anti-H-2.2 antibodies, although they possess the weak response allele with respect to this H-2.2-associated bone marrow rejection system. Thus this weak response allele appears to be specific for a particular type of immune response. However, it may be relatively non-specific in the sense that it affects the level of responsiveness to both the H-2.2 and H-2.4 specificities in the bone marrow system, whereas cytotoxic antibodies to these two antigens do not cross-react.

It is well known that the delayed hypersensitivity type of immune response is much more radiation-resistant than is the humoral-type (Uhr and Scharff 1960). Should rejection of bone marrow cells in this instance be found to be mediated by delayed hypersensitivity, then the responsible gene would be the first in this species shown to control a non-humoral type of immune response. Furthermore, the delayed hypersensitivity to the H-2.2 and H-2.4 specificities would have had to be spontaneously engendered in the recipient mice prior to irradiation and cell transfer. A condition such as this, i.e., spontaneously existing delayed-type iso-hypersensitivity to a heritable serum factor antigen, has been reported to exist in another species, the guinea-pig (Battisto 1960, 1968).

Recent studies of Lilly (1970) have demonstrated the existence of another genetically controlled immune unresponsiveness specific for the H-2.2 isoantigen of the *D* sublocus. Immunization with cells of a C57BL strain (*H-2^b*) leukaemia induced both cytotoxic and haemagglutinating antibodies to H-2.2 in BALB/c, A and (BALB/c × HTI)F₁ mice but failed to elicit a detectable level of antibodies in HTI, B10.A and (B10.BR × B10.D2)F₁ mice. In mice of the (BALB/c × HTI) × B10.D2 backcross generation, the inability to make anti-H-2.2 antibodies segregated in ratios compatible with determination by a single gene independent of *H-2* itself and of the *agouti* locus. Thus the immune response gene was not related to *Ir-1* or to *Ir-2*. It did not appear to influence the ability to make antibodies to several other antigens of the *H-2* complex, including H-2.4, H-2.11, H-2.31 and H-2.33. It is not yet known if this genetically determined inability to make anti-H-2.2 antibodies is accompanied by an inability to respond to the same antigen in cell-mediated immunologic systems, such as skin graft rejection.

11.4. Attempts to reveal hereditary control of immune responses in guinea-pigs

11.4.1. Insulin as antigen

Genetic control of the combining sites of insulin antibodies produced by guinea-pigs was studied by Arquilla and Finn (1963, 1965). They found that highly inbred Wright strain 2 guinea-pigs produced antibody to portions of the insulin molecule to which Wright strain 13 guinea-pigs could not. The system for revealing this difference is quite novel and merits description. An insoluble insulin complex was first saturated with anti-insulin antibody synthesized by partially inbred strain III rabbits. Thereafter insulin-specific antisera from guinea-pigs of strains 2 and 13 were incubated with aliquots of the saturated complex. All of the strain 2 antisera contained significant amounts of antibodies which bound at sites on the insulin molecule to which the rabbit antibody could not bind. None of the strain 13 antisera contained significant amounts of antibody capable of binding to the insulin aggregate saturated with antibodies from the rabbits. Thus, certain sections of the insulin molecule caused strain 2 guinea-pigs, but not strain 13 animals, to produce antibodies.

When antibodies from strain 13 animals were used to saturate the insulin aggregate, no binding of antibodies from strain 2 guinea-pigs occurred. Similarly, when antibodies from strain 2 guinea-pigs were used to saturate the insulin aggregate, no binding of antibodies from strain 13 animals was observed. In like manner it was not possible to demonstrate antibody differences among individual animals of the same strain.

To explain these results the authors hypothesized that binding sites of the antibodies from strain 2 guinea-pigs are near the binding sites of the antibodies from strain 13 guinea-pigs. Thus, by steric hindrance, each type of guinea-pig antibody prevented the other from binding. The site of the insulin molecule to which the rabbit antibodies are directed is close to that for which strain 13 antibodies are specific but more distant from the site to which strain 2 antibodies are directed. In this way rabbit antibody bound to insulin aggregates does not interfere with the binding of strain 2 antibodies but prevents binding of strain 13 antibodies.

When antisera from $(2 \times 13)F_1$ hybrids were tested, the antibody combining sites of all but one were similar to the combining sites of both parents. The authors view the exception as possibly due to an unrecognized error in breeding.

When antisera from F_2 animals were tested, segregation of the differences in antibody-combining site configuration was noted. Of 7 F_2 antisera, 4 had antibodies that overlapped the determinants to which the insulin antibodies in both strain 2 and 13 were directed, 1 had antibody combining site configurations different from strain 2 antibodies but similar to those of strain 13, and 2 had antibodies with combining site configurations different from the antibodies in strain 2 and strain 13 antisera. Thus, F_2 offspring produce antibodies directed to portions of the insulin molecule to which neither of the inbred grandparents do. These data suggest that the configuration of the antibody-combining site in guinea-pigs is controlled by more than one gene and not by different alleles at a given gene locus.

11.4.2. Use of synthetic antigens

As has been indicated, the advent of synthetic antigens offers certain advantages which are particularly useful in elucidating the heritable nature of the immune response. Theoretically it should be possible to synthesize antigens for which an animal presumably has not had prior exposure and to make molecules with a single antigenic determinant.

In one of the earliest applications of synthetic molecules to a study of the heritable nature of immune responses, Kantor et al. (1963) used hapten-conjugated and unconjugated poly-α-amino acids to study circulating antibody and delayed hypersensitivity responses of guinea-pigs. The haptenic 2,4-dinitrophenyl group was coupled with poly-L-lysine and with a copolymer of lysine and glutamic acid to yield DNP-PLL and DNP-poly-Glu-Lys, respectively. The haptenic group was attached to enhance immunogenicity, since Gill and Doty (1961) and Maurer and associates (1963) had already shown that polymers of single amino acids such as poly-L-lysine or poly-L-glutamic acid lacked antigenicity in guinea-pigs. Maurer (1963) had also shown that copolymers of glutamic acid and lysine having ratios of 6:4, 7:3 or 5:5 are antigenic in 20 to 50% of Hartley strain guinea-pigs. He had noted both delayed and immediate-type hypersensitivity among the animals responding.

When DNP-PLL was incorporated into complete Freund's adjuvant and administered to randomly bred Hartley guinea-pigs, Kantor et al. (1963) observed 30 to 40% of the animals developed delayed and immediate skin reactivity as well as precipitating antibody to DNP-PLL. The authors interpreted this to mean that constitutional differences existed among the animals assayed. They also observed that the percentage of animals responding to DNP-PLL decreased as the degree of DNP conjugation increased. The greatest number of animals responded with 1 to 2% conjugation of DNP to PLL and half this number responded to PLL that was 10% conjugated with DNP. In addition they found that only animals responding to DNP-PLL responded to the immunologically distinct DNP-poly-Glu-Lys.

In order to determine whether the ability of an individual guinea-pig to respond immunologically to a given hapten-PLL conjugate is dependent on the structure of the haptenic group, Levine et al. (1963a) immunized random-bred Hartley strain guinea-pigs with PLL conjugated separately with different haptens. They injected DNP-PLL, dimethylaminonaphthalenesulphonyl-PLL, *o*-toluenesulphonyl-PLL and benzylpenicilloyl-PLL either consecutively or simultaneously. They found essentially an all or none response, i.e., individual animals of the Hartley strain were either capable of developing an immune response to all four hapten-PLL conjugates or the individual was unable to develop an immune response to any of these conjugates. Thus, the haptenic groups did not exercise primary control upon the initiation of the immune response whereas the PLL backbone of the conjugate did.

At this point, Levine et al. (1963b) presented the first evidence for the genetic transmission of the ability of guinea-pigs to respond immunologically to synthetic antigens. They immunized offspring of Hartley parents that had responded to DNP-PLL and found 82% capable of response. All of the offspring of non-responding parents were unable to respond to DNP-PLL. Further, they found none of strain 13 guinea-pigs and all of strain 2 guinea-pigs were responders.

11.4.3. PLL-gene

To help determine how the ability to respond immunologically to hapten-PLL is transmitted, heterozygous Hartley strain responders were mated with Hartley non-responders and their offspring were immunized (Levine and Benacerraf 1965). If transmission were through a Mendelian dominant gene, 50% of the offspring of these matings would be expected to be responders. Since responders are phenotypically alike, animals were considered to be heterozygous when they produced at least one non-responder offspring. Non-responders were looked upon as homozygous, since mated pairs of non-responders produced only non-responder offspring. When 31 offspring of these matings were immunized with DNP-PLL in complete adjuvant, 14 were seen to be responders (45.3%). No unusual distribution along sex lines was noted. Since the actual observation was not significantly different from the theoretically expected result, the capacity to respond immunologically to PLL conjugates was considered genetically transmitted as a unigenic Mendelian dominant trait.

In contrast to PLL conjugates that are immunogenic in certain guinea-pigs, benzylpenicilloyl conjugate of poly-D-lysine (BPO-PDL) was found to be non-antigenic in 35 randomly bred guinea-pigs (Parker and Thiel 1963). These results were confirmed by Levine (1964a) who immunized two groups of strain 2 guinea-pigs with different doses of BPO_{20}-PDL_{144}, in Freund's complete adjuvant. Animals of both groups were unable to exhibit Arthus or delayed skin reactions to the conjugate and their sera contained no antibodies directed to the BPO group. The very same animals were next injected with BPO_{40}-PLL_{286} in adjuvants and after a 14 day interval all showed strong Arthus and delayed skin reactions to BPO-PLL and their sera contained anti-BPO antibodies. Thus, guinea-pigs of strain 2 that are genetically endowed to respond immunologically to a hapten conjugate of PLL, failed to make responses to the same hapten coupled to PDL.

Strain 2 guinea-pigs injected with maximally coupled conjugate BPO_{265}-PLL_{525} were unable to recognize it as antigenic. In some way the excessive number of BPO groups interfered with the processing of the molecule. When few BPO groups were conjugated to PLL and the remaining epsilon-amino groups were succinylated, the resulting conjugate, although taken up by macrophages, was also non-antigenic (Levine 1964b).

As these findings suggested that the difference between responder and non-responder guinea-pigs may reside in their abilities to metabolize the PLL carrier, Levine and Benacerraf (1964) investigated the enzymatic degradation of haptenic conjugates of PLL by tissues of the two types of animals. Fluorescein conjugates of PLL, PDL and exhaustively succinylated PLL were introduced into aqueous extracts of spleens from responder and non-responder guinea-pigs. Succinylated and un-succinylated PLL conjugates were enzymatically degraded by tissue extracts from either type of animal. Since both responder and non-responder guinea-pigs degraded PLL conjugates, responders were thought to process the degradation products by certain additional specific metabolic steps that are as yet unidentified. Presumably, these steps are absent in non-responder guinea-pigs.

As regards the minimum size of DNP-PLL that is immunogenic in guinea-pigs possessing the PLL gene, Schlossmann et al. (1965) have shown that α-DNP-oligo-L-lysine compounds containing 7 to 9 lysine residues or more possessed antigenicity. In view of this finding it would be of interest to know whether non-responders are unable to form an immune response because they degrade PLL conjugates into units containing less than 7 lysines.

Confirmation of the genetic control of immunogenic responses of guinea-pigs to synthetic polymers came from Ben-Efraim and Maurer (1966). They studied the antigenicity of random copolymers of amino acids and aggregates of polymers with methylated plasma albumin in inbred guinea-pig strains 2 and 13 and (2×13) F_1 hybrids. Oligolysine coupled with copolymers glutamic acid-alanine and glutamic acid plus methylated guinea-pig plasma albumin aggregate were found to be immunogenic for inbred strain 2 and non-immunogenic for inbred strain 13 animals. When 100% of the F_1 hybrids of these strains responded immunologically, strong evidence was provided for inheritance on a dominant Mendelian gene basis.

Additional information on the manner in which the two inbred strains of guinea-pigs respond immunologically to lysine-containing synthetic antigens was provided by Ben-Efraim and Leskowitz (1966). Upon immunization with arsanilic acid conjugates of poly-L-lysine (ars-L) and poly-L-glutamic acid-L-lysine-L-tyrosine (ars-GLT), they observed positive delayed skin responses in guinea-pigs of inbred strain 2, immediate and delayed skin reactions in random-bred Hartley animals but no responses in guinea-pigs of strain 13.

To test the idea that the mere presence of sequences of lysine molecules in an otherwise antigenic substance would convert the latter into a non-antigen for strain 13 guinea-pigs, animals of strains 2 and 13 were immunized with polylysyl rabbit serum albumin (Ben-Efraim et al. 1966). Whereas rabbit serum albumin alone provoked immune responses in animals of both strains, attachment of lysine peptides to the albumin resulted in a substance that was immunogenic in strain 2 but not in strain 13.

Several other linear and multi-chain synthetic polypeptides were studied for immunogenicity in strains 2 and 13 guinea-pigs (Ben-Efraim et al. 1966). As before, linear and branched copolymers containing lysine were found to be immunogenic in strain 2 and negative in strain 13. A linear copolymer of tyrosine, glutamic acid and alanine was found to be immunogenic in both strains but a linear copolymer of tyrosine and glutamic acid had a behaviour diametrically opposite to that of the lysine-containing polymer. Still, the authors did not claim that control of the immune response to this antigen is genetically determined. If it should prove to be so, then this would be an instance where recessiveness controls an immune response. This would be true in view of the fact that (2×13) F_1 animals acquire the non-responsiveness of strain 2 parents which would make lack of response to this antigen dominant.

Immune responses to hapten-coupled PLL and to copolymers of glutamic acid with L-lysine were thought to occur in PLL-gene-possessing guinea-pigs primarily because of specific recognition of PLL sequences (Benacerraf et al. 1967). In actuality, Green et al. (1969) have found that the PLL gene controls immune responses to a wide variety of positively charged substances. All strain 2 and PLL-gene-positive Hartley strain guinea-pigs were found to respond immunologically to poly-L-arginine (PLA), protamine, DNP-PLA, DNP-protamine and DNP-poly-L-ornithine. The animals for some reason were unable to make responses to poly-L-ornithine (PLO) alone. Non-responder strain 13 guinea-pigs on the other hand did not respond to any of these polymers under regular immunizing procedures. Thus, the PLL gene controls immune responses to a wide variety of antigenic substances that are like PLL-containing antigens only because of their highly charged nature.

11.4.4. Localization of site of action of PLL gene

In efforts to pinpoint the site in the immunological apparatus where the PLL gene exerts its control, two types of studies involving transfers of lymphoid tissues were undertaken. The first involved attempts to transfer passively pre-formed DNP-PLL or DNP-GL delayed hypersensitivity to guinea-pigs possessing or lacking the PLL gene (Green et al. 1967). Lymph node cells from 3 highly sensitive donors were injected into individual Hartley strain guinea-pigs without knowledge of their PLL gene status. Each recipient was tested within 2 hours of transfer with 10 μg of DNP-PLL and dermal reactions observed at 24 hours. With this knowledge in hand the animals were thereafter actively immunized with DNP-PLL in Freund's adjuvant to ascertain their responsiveness. For DNP-PLL, positive passive transfers were accomplished in 12 of 12 responder animals but in only 2 of 25 non-responder guinea-pigs. As regards sensitivity for DNP-GL, 6 of 7 transfers into responder type animals were positive whereas 1 of 14 transfers into non-responder type animals were successful. The inability to transfer to PLL-gene negative animals could not be attributed to destruction of transferred cells since delayed hypersensitivity to ovalbumin was readily transferred from PLL gene (+) to PLL gene (−) animals. Of course attempts to transfer 'reactivity' from non-responder guinea pigs that had been 'immunized' were not successful no matter whether the recipients were responders (0/6) or non-responders (0/15).

So it may be seen that, animals without the PLL gene could not be induced to give a delayed dermal response to DNP-PLL or DNP-GL even when they were made recipients of pre-developed reactivity in the form of highly sensitized lymph node cells. Thus, the host of passively conferred immunity takes an active part in displaying a visible dermal manifestation of the reactivity transferred, and in this special instance this activity is linked to possession of the PLL gene.

The second type of study involves transfer of lymphoid cells from normal responder animals into genetically non-responder guinea-pigs followed by attempts to actively sensitize the latter (Foerster et al. 1969). Two attempts were made; one with Hartley strain animals as donors and recipients and the other with strain 13 guinea-pigs as recipients of $(2 \times 13)F_1$ donor tissue. Hartley animals were first screened for responder status to DNP-PLL by active immunization in one pair of paws. Non-responders were lethally irradiated and given bone marrow cells from the responder animals. Those animals that survived graft-*versus*-host reactions were again immunized in the other pair of paws. When assayed for anti-DNP antibodies, delayed dermal hypersensitivity to DNP-PLL, and DNP-PLL-stimulated lymph node cell uptake of tritiated thymidine, 12 of 14 animals were seen to have responded.

To eliminate the disease seen in the Hartley recipients of allogeneic bone marrow cells, strain 13 non-responder guinea-pigs were lethally irradiated and given either bone marrow from (2×13) F_1 responder animals or strain 13 bone marrow and (2×13) F_1 lymph node and spleen cells. Approximately 15 days after cell transfer the animals were actively immunized with hapten-PLL in adjuvant. Animals given strain 13 bone marrow and (2×13) F_1 lymph node and spleen cells made immune responses to DNP-PLL (3 of 3) and to DNP-GL (7 of 10). The majority of animals given (2×13) F_1 bone marrow alone did *not* respond to DNP-GL (only 1 of 6 responded).

To determine whether non-responder strain 13 animals were involved in the response following reconstitution with (2×13) F_1 cells, anti-strain 2 histocompatibility antisera (cytotoxic for F_1 cells) were incubated with lymph node cells from immunized animals prior to testing *in vitro*. Such antibody destroyed the blastogenic stimulation of lymph node cells *in vitro* by antigen and eliminated anti-DNP antibody-producing cells. This information supports the idea that strain 13 cells apparently take no part in the response of F_1 cells to hapten-PLL conjugates (Ellman et al. 1970). Thus, although bone marrow contains all the cells required for the expression of the PLL gene, lymphocytes rather than monocytes and macrophages may be the cells through which the PLL-gene exerts its control over immune responses to these synthetic antigens.

11.4.5. *Instances of abrogation of PLL gene control*

Certain conditions exist under which PLL gene control of the initiation of immune responses apparently can be abrogated (Green et al. 1966; Benecerraf et al. 1967; Green et al. 1969a; Stone and Goode 1970). When complexed to foreign antigenic albumins such as bovine serum albumin or ovalbumin, DNP-PLL will cause non-responder guinea-pigs to synthesize about 1 mg/ml of anti-DNP-PLL antibodies. However, when homologous albumin is used as carrier, the animals act as true non-responders (Green et al. 1966). In addition, immune responses to DNP-PLL and to BSA were considerably reduced when tolerance to BSA was induced prior to attempted immunization with DNP-PLL-BSA (Green et al. 1966). This information can be explained on the basis that the albumin serves as carrier or 'Schlepper' for DNP-PLL which in this case is considered a hapten. Thus, recognition of the PLL backbone of the antigen would not appear to be essential when a different carrier, i.e., foreign albumin, is used in immunization to get the PLL beyond a certain processing step.

Yet even in this instance genetic control in non-responders is retained for the development of delayed-type hypersensitivity to DNP-PLL. For despite the fact that non-responders formed anti-DNP-PLL antibodies when injected with DNP-PLL-BSA, they were unable to develop delayed cutaneous reactions and their lymph node cells exposed *in vitro* to DNP-PLL were unable to show increased DNA synthesis. In contrast, responder guinea-pigs immunized with DNP-PLL without albumin demonstrated antigen-specific humoral antibodies, delayed dermal responses and *in vitro* uptake of tritiated thymidine into lymph node cells.

Another condition that apparently alters full genetic control over the immune response is the quantity and strain of mycobacteria incorporated into the adjuvant required for immunization (Green et al. 1969a). Thus, PLL-gene negative animals produced anti-DNP antibodies when immunized with DNP-protamine in adjuvant containing 10 mg/ml of *Mycobacterium tuberculosis*. They did so, also, when immunized with DNP-poly-L-ornithine in adjuvant having 0.5 mg/ml of mycobacteria.

This observation was extended using DNP-PLL and DNP-GL as antigens (Green et al. 1969a). Non-responder strain 13 and Hartley animals produced anti-DNP antibodies following immunization with DNP-PLL and 0.5 mg/ml of *Mycobacterium butyricum*. When the same amount of this mycobacterium was injected with DNP-GL, the animals reflected their actual non-responder status. All PLL-gene negative animals synthesized anti-DNP antibodies to DNP-PLL mixed with *M. tuberculosis* at 10 mg/ml. The levels of antibodies obtained were lower than those seen in PLL-gene positive guinea-pigs. Despite the fact that they synthesized anti-DNP antibody, all PLL-gene-negative guinea-pigs, immunized with DNP-PLL or DNP-GL in adjuvants containing either small or large amounts of mycobacteria, failed to develop antigen-specific delayed hypersensitivity. This apparent breakdown in the gene control of the initiation of the immune response could be attributed to the fact that mycobacteria can act equally effectively as carriers for the highly positively charged antigens as do the foreign albumins. Thus, genetic control of immunologic responses to antigens containing PLL appears more perfectly directed to delayed hypersensitivity than to circulating antibody synthesis.

If the highly charged synthetic antigens adsorb so readily to components of either adjuvants or of the body then their great advantage in the study of genetic factors would appear to be impaired. Indeed, use of molecules that are not highly charged would appear to be indicated.

A third condition under which strict genetic control of the immune response is apparently relaxed has to do with the observation of Stone and Goode (1970). They have shown that stimulation of non-responder-type strain 13 guinea-pigs with DNP-PLL in *incomplete* Freund's adjuvant followed by intradermal injections of DNP-PLL results in Arthus type skin reactions. Whether dermal responses attributable to delayed hypersensitivity developed in the animals could not be ascertained since Arthus responses ordinarily obscure delayed reactions. As no mycobacteria were present in the Freund's adjuvant, synthesis of antibody by PLL-gene negative guinea-pigs under these conditions would appear to weaken the "Schlepper hypothesis".

Stone and Goode further showed that initiation of immune responses to bovine serum albumin would simulate PLL-gene control, if a tiny dose of BSA were used in immunization. When given 10 μg of BSA in complete Freund's adjuvant (2.5 mg of *M. tuberculosis*), strain 2 guinea-pigs responded with both delayed hypersensitivity and circulating antibody whereas strain 13 guinea-pigs did not. Increasing the dose of BSA to 100 μg caused animals of both strains to respond identically (Stone, personal communication). (See note added in proof on page 332.) Thus, antigen dose-dependence would appear to be a complicating factor in unravelling hereditary aspects of immune responses.

More recent data have shown that linkage exists between the major histocompatibility locus of inbred strain 2 guinea-pigs and the PLL-gene (Ellman et al. 1970). The correlation was demonstrated by ascertaining which offspring of (2 × 13) F_1 backcrosses to non-responding 13 parents were capable of response to antigen PLL. These offspring were also assayed for possession of strain 2 histocompatibility antigens by two methods. One procedure was by the mixed leucocyte interaction test in which cells from strain 13 animals immunized to strain 2 antigens demonstrated blastogenic transformation in the presence of the latter. The other test was to measure release of chromium-51 from labelled lymph node cells coming from the backcross guinea-pigs upon exposing them to anti-strain 2 isoantiserum and complement. When all of the responder backcross guinea-pigs showed the presence of strain 2 isoantigen by the two tests, linkage between the histocompatibility locus and the PLL-gene was established.

The linkage observed in mice between the *H-2* locus and the *Ir-1* locus has thus been extended to another species and to a different immunological system.

11.5. Genetic control of immune responses in rats

Using a multi-determinant antigen, bovine serum albumin, the primary humoral response of a number of inbred and random-bred strains of rats was studied (James et al. 1969). In addition, the effect of anti-lymphocytic antibody on this process was investigated. Marked differences in the primary responses between hooded inbred rats, hooded random bred rats, Wistar random-bred and Sprague-Dawley random-bred rats were noted as was considerable variation within each of the groups.

In addition to these differences considerable variation in the immuno-suppressive effect of anti-lymphocytic antibody upon the primary immune response to BSA was observed. Although the anti-lymphocytic antibody readily suppressed the primary immune response to BSA in hyper-responsive rats it was seen to be relatively ineffective in rats exhibiting a smaller responsiveness to the antigen.

Genetic control of the immune response in rats to a synthetic antigen poly $Glu^{52}Lys^{33}Tyr^{15}$ has been systematically studied. Simonian et al. (1968) immunized 6 inbred (BN, BUF, F344, WF, LEW and ACI) and one random-bred (WIST) strain of rats. They observed a highly variable antibody response which they attributed to random genetic fluctuations in the population. They concluded that the ability to make antibody was transmitted as a complex genetically controlled mechanism involving several genes.

In follow-up studies (Gill et al. 1970a; Gill et al. 1970b) attention was concentrated upon the high and low responding strains of rats (ACI and F344 respectively) as well as their F_1 and backcross offspring. Poly $Glu^{52}Lys^{33}Tyr^{15}$ elicited large amounts of antibody formation in ACI strain animals (ave. 775 $\mu g/ml$) but small amounts in F344 rats (ave. 420 $\mu g/ml$). Backcrosses of F_1 animals with parental strains showed segregation of the response into 3 separate populations.

Their results are compatible with the view that genetic control of the antibody response is by 2 independently segregating genes. One is thought to operate at the level of recognizing antigen (R-gene) while the other controls the quantity of antibody formed (Q-gene). In addition, as the females of the ACI strain made a higher and more heterogeneous antibody response than did males, there is sex influence which may also be genetically controlled.

Antigen dosage emphasized the differences between the two strains of rats. ACI rats made more antibody as the dose of antigen increased up to 1.5 mg; then the amount of antibody leveled off. On the other hand F344 rats made low, erratic responses to antigen doses up to 1.5 μg and thereafter antibody concentrations slowly increased until all

the animals responded. A curious finding is that ACI made IgM predominantly at low antigen doses but with increased antigen dose antibody was found in all immunoglobulin classes. In contrast F344 rats
always made IgG and little if any IgM. The authors suggested that the
inability of F344 rats to make IgM to poly Glu Lys Tyr may account for
their generally poor immunological response to this antigen.

11.6. Hereditary control of immune responsiveness in rabbits

Rabbits have not been used extensively in the study of genetic control
of immune responsiveness. Nevertheless, a few investigations have been
made using synthetic antigens. Humphrey (1965) has immunized rabbits
with multi-chain polymers of tyrosine, glutamic acid, alanine and lysine,
$p(TG)$-pA-pL, incorporated in Freund's complete adjuvant. He found
that Himalayan rabbits responded well, Sandylops rabbits responded
badly and Dutch rabbits responded in an intermediate manner between
the other two. Animals of each of the strains are known to respond well
to naturally occurring antigens. The question of whether the response
to $p(TG)$-pA-pL is under genetic control is being pursued.

Another investigation was made using synthetic polypeptide Glu^{56}-
$Lys^{38}Tyr^6$ in 8 strains of rabbits of varying degrees of inbreeding and
in genetically heterogenous New Zealand white rabbits (Gill 1965).
Significant differences among the amounts of antibody produced in the
different strains was taken as evidence for genetic control of the ability
of the various strains to respond to the antigen. The animals of C strain
produced the greatest amount of antibody (347 μg antibody N per ml)
and those of OS strain produced least (87 μg antibody N per ml). No
report was made on either F_1 or backcross progeny in either of these
studies on rabbits.

11.7. Genetic control of immunological tolerance induction

Closely associated with the induction of immunological responses is
the phenomenon of immunologic unresponsiveness (tolerance). The first
to suggest that specific immunological unresponsiveness may be genetically controlled were Sobey and Magrath (1965). They studied immunological unresponsiveness in mice injected neonatally with bovine plasma
albumin and indicated that the degree of inhibition of the immune
response is dependent in part upon the genetic constitution of the

animals. Confirmation for the suggested heritable control of immuno-logical tolerance was provided by data from rabbits and mice (Sobey et al. 1966). During the routine production of antibody to bovine serum albumin (BSA) in rabbits, a buck was found incapable of synthesizing anti-BSA. It was mated to 2 normal does which produced 8 offspring all capable of anti-BSA synthesis. Intercrosses between the F_1 animals and backcrosses with the negative buck produced results suggestive of genetic control of the negative phenomenon. As the backcrosses produced 10 negative offspring and 55 positive young, two or three genes rather than a single gene would appear to control the inheritance of the negative phenomenon.

Essentially the same sort of information was gathered by the above-mentioned authors from their studies of unresponsiveness to BSA in mice. Again the data presented did not fit a single gene model but rather suggested that two or three genes were involved.

Confirmation of the genetic control for immunologic unresponsiveness came from Golub and Weigle (1969). Using human gamma-globulin as antigen they were able to show variation in the dose of ultracentrifuged HGG required for induction of specific unresponsiveness in different strains of inbred mice. Trace amounts of aggregated HGG remaining in preparations of unaggregated HGG were processed efficiently by BALB/cJ mice, thus resulting in an immune response. In contrast C57BL/6J mice developed unresponsiveness to the same HGG preparation doses. When cross-matings were made between C57BL/6J and other strains, the F_1 mice were rendered unresponsive by the same dose effective in the C57BL/6J parent. A study of F_2 mice and backcrosses ruled out single gene control of the phenomenon.

11.8. Use of polysaccharides as antigens in studies on hereditary control of immune responses

Two requirements for studying the genetic control of immune responsive-ness are to use antigenic determinants that are well characterized and secondly to have them limited in number. The fewer the antigenic determinants offered, the less complicated is assessment of the immune response. While synthetic antigens have shown promise with regards these criteria some have disadvantages such as possessing structural vagaries as well as coupling spontaneously to adjuvant or bodily com-ponents. Another group of antigenic substances that may fulfil the requirements under discussion are microbial carbohydrates. Some of these have structures that are well characterized and certain of them are known not to adsorb to carrier substances in adjuvant or in the host. An additional advantage that this group of antigens possesses is that in some animals they cause production of homogeneous populations of antibodies (cf. Kunkel, H. G., Symposium on homogeneous antibody populations, Federation Proc. *29, 55,* 1970).

Immunization of over 100 rabbits with streptococcal vaccines caused the majority to produce precipitins to the group-specific carbohydrates (A, A-variant and C) in concentrations between 1 to 10 mg/ml of anti-serum and the minority to make 11 to 32 mg/ml (Braun et al. 1969). In addition the offspring of rabbits with high concentrations of antibody produced significantly higher concentrations of antibody than did offspring of low concentration producing parents. Thus, it would appear that the magnitude of the immune response to these carbohydrates is controlled genetically.

Pneumococcal vaccines of Types III and VIII were used in another extensive study in rabbits (Pincus et al. 1970). Whereas all 232 rabbits immunized demonstrated anti-pneumococcal polysaccharide antibodies in their sera, only a minority of the animals possessed antibody restricted electrophoretically to the gamma globulin region, i.e., 7% of those immunized with III and 9% of those given VIII. These data suggest some sort of genetic control is operative in the immune response of rabbits to these antigens.

The immune responses to still another carbohydrate, dextran, have been suggested to be under genetic control (Battisto et al. 1968). A highly purified dextran of large molecular weight induced delayed dermal reactions and circulating antibody formation in approximately 50% of guinea-pigs of the Abyssinian strain. The vast majority of Pirbright, Hartley and all Wright 13 guinea-pigs did not develop immune responses to dextran.

Furthermore, the dextran-specific circulating antibody elicited in guinea-pigs was found to be of the homocytotropic variety that mediates passive cutaneous anaphylaxis reactions. Despite repeated attempts to develop precipitating antibody none has so far been produced. Thus, guinea-pig anti-dextran antibody may represent a source of homogeneous immunoglobulin.

Adoptive transfer of delayed dermal reactivity for dextran was accomplished with lymphoid cells from sensitive Abyssinian animals to normal, responding type, Abyssinian animals but not to Pirbright, non-responding type, animals. It should be recalled that a parallel situation exists with regard to positive adoptive transfers of passive immunity for DNP-PLL from responder to responder guinea-pigs, and negative transfers from responder to non-responder guinea-pigs (Green et al. 1967).

The fact that a large majority of Hartley guinea-pigs do not recognize dextran as antigenic indicates that genetic control of immunological responses to this antigen is separate from the PLL-gene and from the genes controlling responses to insulin.

Another interesting aspect of the response of guinea-pigs to polysaccharides has to do with the observation by Gerety et al. (1970) that pneumococcal polysaccharide Type II (Pn IIS) induces delayed dermal reactivity in virtually all random-bred guinea-pigs. Pn IIS is composed of L-rhamnose, D-glucose and D-glucuronic acid in the ratio of $3:1:2$. In spite of the fact that rhamnose accounts for about 50% of the molecule, antisera to Pn IIS cross reacts with dextran. The latter is composed entirely of D-glucose predominantly coupled by $1:6$ linkages. It is interesting to note that the restricted and homogeneous composition of dextran in contrast to the varied composition of Pn IIS causes dextran's immunogenicity, but not that of Pn IIS, to be limited to only certain guinea-pigs.

11.9. Discussion and summary

From the data collected in four species of animals immunized with synthetic and natural antigens of known composition, some clear-cut information and some inconsistencies are emerging concerning genetic control of the capacity to respond immunologically. Little doubt now remains that heredity influences the kind of antigens to which an individual will respond immunologically. Genes have been described that perform this function in three species of animals, namely: mice, guinea-pigs and rats.

The levels at which these genes exert their influence vary. For instance, the genes of guinea-pigs that affect the immunological response to insulin apparently control the specificity of the immunoglobulin combining sites. In addition, the *Ir-1* locus in mice is thought to control the synthesis of antibody and not the processing of antigen. In contrast, the PLL-gene of guinea-pigs is operative at an earlier stage of the immune response that has to do with recognition and/or processing of highly charged molecules such as PLL and protamine. It is possible that the gene determining the response to GLA_5 antigen in mice is homologous to the PLL-gene of guinea-pigs. The fact that separate genes may eventually be found that control the synthesis of a specific immunoglobulin to a particular antigen, has already been alluded to for rats (Gill et al. 1970) and for guinea-pigs (Battisto 1968).

By passive transfer studies the genetic control appears to be operative through lymphocytes. With them the phenotype of irradiated non-responding animals was changed to responder-type. This has shown to be true for mice where spleen cells were used and for guinea-pigs where bone marrow cells alone as well as spleen and lymph node cells were found to be effective.

There is considerable variation in the number of genes that have been claimed to control immune responses in guinea-pigs. Using haptens that couple spontaneously to body components and Freund's adjuvant containing mycobacteria, Chase concluded that at least three genes, two dominant and one recessive, are involved. With insulin as antigen, Arquilla and Finn arrived at two genes for control. In contradistinction, using synthetic antigens containing PLL as backbone, Benacerraf and co-workers have observed a single dominant gene that controls initiation of the immune responses. This seeming inconsistency in the number of genes controlling immunological responses in guinea-pigs may be explainable on the basis of the varied antigenic determinants used by the different investigators. Haptens such as those used by Chase couple to body constituents and alter the latter sufficiently so that complex antigenic determinants could result. From the work of Arquilla and Finn, insulin is known to possess at least two and perhaps more antigenic moieties. In contrast, DNP-PLL presumably presents the animal with a single antigenic determinant. Thus, the fewer determinants offered, and ideally only one should be introduced, the easier is assessment of hereditary influences upon immunological responses. An alternative explanation for the varied number of genes involved may have to do with the stage of the immune response at which they are operative. Clear-cut differences in this respect have already been described.

A discrepancy that is more apparent than real has to do with passive transfer of *preformed* immunity from responder-type to non-responder-type animals. It has been claimed, for instance, that this type of transfer is accomplished readily in mice (McDevitt and Tyan 1968) but has not succeeded in guinea-pigs (Green et al. 1967). In actuality these investigators examined quite separate immunological responses. McDevitt and Tyan were successful at transferring circulating antibody responses while Green et al. were unsuccessful at transferring delayed hypersensitivity reactions. In the dextran system both of these conditions have been seen in the passive transfers accomplished in guinea-pigs. Battisto et al. (1968) have shown, for instance, that passive transfer from responder to non-responder type guinea-pigs is successful for circulating antibody response but is not successful for delayed-type dermal hypersensitivity. The latter authors have viewed the inability of non-responder type animals to demonstrate delayed dermal responses to dextran following adoptive transfer of competent lymphoid cells as a defect that has been termed an inability of 'translation'.

Another peculiarity is the vital part that L-lysine plays in the genetic response of guinea-pigs to antigens containing this amino acid. Its presence in antigens given to mice has little relevance in determining the immune response in this species. This must reflect a basic species difference in the manner in which this chemical substance is processed.

Some genes controlling immune responses have been shown to be linked to histocompatibility antigens: the *Ir-1* gene in mice and the PLL gene in guinea-pigs. The fact that this has been seen in separate species and to separate antigenic moieties may perhaps point to a relatively important principle, namely, that histocompatibility antigens in some way control immunological responsiveness (Lilly 1970a). Whether the other genes that have been described in these species as well as those that have been described for other species, e.g., the rat, will be shown to be so linked, remains to be determined.

11.9.1. Hypotheses for genic control of immune responses

Several hypotheses to explain the manner in which gene control of the immune response is operative have been put forward. Cinader (1960) has suggested, for instance, that antigens controlled by genes within an individual would be expected to cause tolerance for similar or cross-reacting antigens found in nature. This would insure a non-responsiveness. Lack of such antigens (or recessiveness) would control the responsive state. This situation may be operative in the instance of blood group antigens in humans but it would not be possible in situations that equate dominant genes with responsiveness.

As Pinchuck et al. (1968) have suggested, genes involved in the initiation of immune responses may control productivity of varieties of RNA effective to couple to certain antigens only. For a particular antigen possession of the proper RNA results in a responsive individual and lack of such RNA would result in a non-responder.

Alternatively, genes may control catabolic processing or entry of antigen into critical sites and in this way contribute to responsivity (Levine and Benacerraf 1964). Compatible with this view is the thought that the genes control histocompatibility antigens and perhaps the latter are responsible for receptivity or entry of the immunizing antigens (Lilly 1970a).

Much work remains to be done in this highly important area that has recently witnessed several dramatic breakthroughs. Indeed, the overall view one gains from the literature collected thus far is that the subject is still in its infancy.

Added in proof. Green et al. (1970) have shown the response of strain 2 guinea-pigs to limiting doses of BSA is under dominant genetic control linked with the PLL-gene. While strain 13 animals were found to make no antibody to 0.1 μg HBSA, Hartley responders made antibody as well as strain 2. With the same antigen dose Hartley non-responders were divisible into two types: (I) those making a response significantly smaller than responders, and (II) those making little or no detectable response.

References

ARQUILLA, E. R. and J. FINN, 1963, Science *142*, 400.

ARQUILLA, E. R. and J. FINN, 1965, J. Exptl. Med. *122*, 771.

BATTISTO, J. R., 1960, Nature *187*, 1969.

BATTISTO, J. R., 1968 J. Immunol. *101*, 743.

BATTISTO, J. R., G. CHIAPPETTA and R. HIXON, 1968, J. Immunol. *101*, 203.

BENACERRAF, B., I. GREEN and W. E. PAUL, 1967, Cold Spring Harbor Symp. Quant. Biol. *32*, 567..

BEN-EFRAIM, S., R. ARNON and M. SELA, 1966, Immunochemistry *3*, 491.

BEN-EFRAIM, S. and S. LESKOWITZ, 1966, Nature *210*, 1068.

BEN-EFRAIM, S. and P. H. MAURER, 1966, J. Immunol. *97*, 577.

BRAUN, D. G., K. EICHMANN and R. M. KRAUSE, 1969, J. Exptl. Med. *129*, 809.

CARLINFANTI, E., 1948, J. Immunol. *59*, 1.

CHASE, M. W., 1953, Trans. N. Y. Acad. Sci. *15*, 79.

CHASE, M. W., 1941, J. Exptl. Med. *73*, 711.

CHASE, M. W., 1961, Symposium on the genetic aspects of the experimental animal. *In*: Carworth Quarterly Letter, no. 62.

CINADER, B., 1960, Nature *188*, 619.

CLARINGBOLD, P. J., W. R. SOBEY and K. M. ADAMS, 1957, Austral. J. Biol. Sci. *10*, 367.

CUDKOWICZ, G., 1968, Int. Convoc. on Immunol., Buffalo, N.Y. Basel and New York, Karger, 1969. p. 193.

DINEEN, J. K., 1964, Nature *202*, 101.

ELLMAN, L., I. GREEN and B. BENACERRAF, 1970, Federation Proc. *29*, 769.

FOERSTER, J., I. GREEN, J. P. LAMELIN and B. BENACERRAF, 1969, J. Exptl. Med. *130*, 1107.

GASSER, D. L., 1969, J. Immunol. *103*, 66.

GERETY, R. J., R. W. FERRARESI and S. RAFFEL, 1970, J. Exptl. Med. *131*, 189.

GILL, T. J., III, 1965, J. Immunol. *95*, 542.

GILL, T. J., III and P. DOTY, 1961, J. Biol. Chem. *236*, 2677.

GILL, T. J., III, H. W. KUNZ and K. F. AUSTEN, 1970a, Federation Proc. *29* (2), 825.

GILL, T. J., III, H. W. KUNZ, D. J. STECHSCHULTE and K. F. AUSTEN, 1970b, J. Immunol. *105*, 14.

GORER, P. A. and H. SCHÜTZE, 1938, J. Hyg. *38*, 647.

GREEN, I., B. BENACERRAF and S. H. STONE, 1969a, J. Immunol. *103*, 403.

GREEN, I., J. K. INMAN and B. BENACERRAF, 1970, Proc. Natl. Acad. Sci. U.S. *66*, 1267.

GREEN, I., W. E. PAUL and B. BENACERRAF, 1966, J. Exptl. Med. *123*, 859.

GREEN, I., W. E. PAUL and B. BENACERRAF, 1967, J. Exptl. Med. *126*, 959.

GREEN, I., W. E. PAUL and B. BENACERRAF, 1969b, Proc. Natl. Acad. Sci. U.S. *64*, 1095.

HARDY, D. and D. ROWLEY, Immunology, 1968, *14*, 401.

HUMPHREY, J. H., 1965, *in*: J. Šterzl, ed.: Molecular and cellular basis of antibody formation. Prague, Publishing House of the Czechoslovak Acad. of Sci. p. 85.

JACOBS, J. L., J. J. KELLEY and S. C. SOMMERS, 1941, Proc. Soc. Exptl. Biol. Med. *48*, 639.

JAMES, K., D. M. PULLAR and V. S. JAMES, 1969, Nature *222*, 886.

KANTOR, F. S., A. OJEDA and B. BENACERRAF, 1963, J. Exptl. Med. *117*, 55.

KUNKEL, H. G., 1970, Federation Proc. *29*, 55.

LANDSTEINER, K. and M. W. CHASE, 1940, Breeding experiments in reference to drug allergy in animals. *In*: 3rd International Congress for Microbiology, Abst. of Commun. p. 772.

LANDSTEINER, K., A. ROSTENBERG, JR. and M. B. SULZBERGER, 1939, J. Invest. Dermatol. *2*, 25.

LEVINE, B. B., 1964a, Nature *202*, 1008.

LEVINE, B. B., 1964b, Proc. Soc. Exptl. Biol. Med. *116*, 1127.

LEVINE, B. B. and B. BENACERRAF, 1964, J. Exptl. Med. *120*, 955.

LEVINE, B. B. and B. BENACERRAF, 1965, Science *147*, 517.

LEVINE, B. B., A. OJEDA and B. BENACERRAF, 1963a, Nature *200*, 544.

LEVINE, B. B., A. OJEDA and B. BENACERRAF, 1963b, J. Exptl. Med. *118*, 953.

LILLY, F., 1966, Genetics *53*, 529.

LILLY, F., 1970a, 2nd Int. Convoc. on Immunol., Buffalo, N.Y. Basel and New York, Karger (in press).

LILLY, F., 1970b, Immunogenetics of the *H-2* System, Prague. Basel and New York, Karger (in press).

MCMASTER, P. R. B., E. M. LERNER and P. S. MUELLER, 1965, Science *147*, 157.

MCDEVITT, H. O. and B. BENACERRAF, 1969, Adv. Immunol. *11*, 31.

MCDEVITT, H. O. and A. CHINITZ, 1969, Science *163*, 1207.

MCDEVITT, H. O. and M. SELA, 1965, J. Exp. Med. *122*, 517.

MCDEVITT, H. O. and M. SELA, 1967, J. Exp. Med. *126*, 969.

MCDEVITT, H. O. and M. L. TYAN, 1968, J. Exp. Med. *128*, 1.

MAURER, P. H., 1963, J. Immunol. *90*, 493.

MOZES, E., H. O. MCDEVITT, J. C. JATON and M. SELA, 1969, J. Exp. Med. *130*, 1273.

PARKER, C. W. and J. A. THIEL, 1963, J. Lab. Clin. Med. *62*, 988 (Abstract).

PINCHUCK, P., M. FISHMAN, F. L. ADLER and P. H. MAURER, 1968, Science *160*, 194–195.

PINCHUCK, P. and P. H. MAURER, 1965, J. Exp. Med. *122*, 673–679.

PINCHUCK, P. and P. H. MAURER, 1968, *in*: B. Cinader, ed.: Regulation of the Antibody Response. Springfield, C. C. Thomas. pp. 97–113.

PINCUS, J. H., J. C. JATON, K. J. BLOCH and E. HABER, 1970, J. Immunol. *104*, 1143.

PLAYFAIR, J. H. L., 1968, Immunology *15*, 35–50.

PRIGGE, R., 1937, Ztschr. f. Hyg. u. Infectionskr. *119*, 186.

SCHEIBEL, I. F., 1943, Acta Pathol. et Microbiol. Scand. *20*, 464.

SCHLOSSMAN, S. F., A. YARON, S. BEN-EFRAIM and H. A. SOBER, 1965, Biochemistry *4*, 1638.

SCHWARTZ, M., 1952, Heredity in brochial asthma. Copenhagen, Munksgaard.

SELA, M., 1969, Science *166*, 1365–1374.

SIMONIAN, S. J., T. J. GILL and S. N. GERSHOFF, 1968, J. Immunol. *101*, 730.

STONE, S. H. and J. H. GOODE, JR., 1970, Federation Proc. *29*, 769 (Abstract).

SNELL, G. D., 1958, J. Nat. Cancer Inst. *21*, 843–877.

SOBEY, W. R. and J. M. MAGRATH, 1965, Aust. J. Biol. Sci. *18*, 947.

SOBEY, W. R., J. M. MAGRATH and A. H. REISNER, 1966, Immunology *11*, 511.

STERN, K., K. S. BROWN and I. DAVIDSOHN, 1956, Genetics *41*, 517–527.

STONE, H. S., 1962, Int. Arch. Allergy *20*, 193.

STONE, S. H. and GOODE J. H., 1970, Federation Proc. *29*, 769 (Abstract).

SULZBERGER, M. B. and A. ROSTENBERG, JR., 1939, J. Immunol. *36*, 17.

TYAN, M. L., H. O. MCDEVITT and L. A. HERZENBERG, 1969, Transpl. Proc. *1*, 548–550.

UHR, J. W. and M. SCHARFF, 1960, J. Exp. Med. *112*, 65.

VAZ, N. M. and B. B. LEVINE, 1970, Science *168*, 852–854.

CHAPTER 12

Hormonal regulation of host immunity

ABRAHAM WHITE and ALLAN L. GOLDSTEIN

Department of Biochemistry, Albert Einstein College of Medicine, Bronx, N.Y.

12.1. Introduction

The regulatory influences of hormones on immunogenic responses in the mammalian organism may be divided, for purposes of discussion and indeed classification, into two categories. The first includes actions resulting in alterations in the rates of synthesis of humoral antibody, and the second, effects contributing to changes in host immunological competence other than those primarily dependent upon humoral antibody. The second category has, in general, been termed cell-mediated immunological competence and this designation will, for convenience, be used in this chapter. However, it is recognized that the term, cell-mediated immune responses, is not adequately descriptive of all manifestations of host immunological resistance other than those based upon the production of humoral antibody alone.

Host immunogenic responses may be examined in the light of the cells known to contribute to the synthesis of humoral antibody and to cell-mediated immunological competence, and with the background of knowledge of the actions of hormones on the functioning of these cells. Considerations of the chemistry of the major classes of humoral antibodies are not discussed in this chapter but have been reviewed adequately elsewhere (cf. Burnet 1969). Also, such phenomena as the mechanism of antibody synthesis and its related aspects, e.g., immunological tolerance, autoimmune reactions, cell-cell interaction, lymphocyte properties, etc., will not be discussed here but aspects of these topics are presented elsewhere in this volume as well as in recently published monographs (Elves 1966; Ling 1968; Burnet 1969) and symposia (Wolstenholme and O'Connor 1960; Cinader 1968; Landy and Braun 1969; Lawrence and Landy 1969; Sorkin 1969). Rather, our attention in this chapter will be directed to hormonal influences on the rate or extent of antibody formation and on selected cell-mediated immune phenomena.

12.2. Synthesis of humoral antibody

12.2.1. Cell types involved in immune globulin synthesis

Two types of cell populations have been implicated in antibody synthesis, namely, the macrophage and the lymphocyte. The involvement of the former was recognized in the latter part of the nineteenth century, when Metchnikoff initiated his classical and monumental researches leading to the establishment in 1884 of the doctrine of phagocytosis (cf. Metchnikoff 1905). Although more recent investigations permit the conclusion that phagocytosis of antigens by macrophages is not an absolute prerequisite for the subsequent synthesis of all antibodies (cf. Mitchison 1969; Sela et al. 1967; Sela 1969) or for cell-mediated immune phenomena (Burnet 1969), it is clear that prior engulfment and processing of antigenic materials allows for a maximum antibody response. Indeed, the immunogenic capacity of a protein can be related to its susceptibility to phagocytosis (Biozzi et al. 1957; Frei et al. 1965). Thus, the functioning of the phagocytic cells of the reticuloendothelial system, and the hormonal regulation of this function, are of prime importance in affecting the rates of production of humoral antibody.

Considerations of the second type of cell populations involved in antibody synthesis focuses attention on the prime role of lymphoid tissue in antibody formation (cf. McMaster 1953). The demonstration that lymphocytes from normal animals have protein components with an electrophoretic mobility identical with that of serum β- and γ-globulins (White 1948) and that lymphocytes from immunized animals contain antibody globulin (Dougherty et al. 1944) provided evidence that these cells contain and/or synthesize immunoglobulins. From these studies and in view of the continuing synthesis of antibody globulin by transplanted proliferating malignant lymphocytes from immunized animals without further antigenic challenge (Dougherty et al. 1945b), it was established that lymphocytes are the major site of antibody synthesis. Moreover, the latter data indicate that the prerequisite information (or residual antigen?) for continuation of antibody production can be transmitted to daughter cells for a period of several generations.

It may also be pointed out that what is of additional significance for a discussion of the roles of lymphocytes in immune phenomena is the fact that these cells infiltrate readily into all the tissues and organs of the body, resulting in their ubiquitous distribution throughout the organism. In view of the presence in lymphocytes of specific antigenic determinants, and of antibody in the lymphocytes of immunized animals, it is apparent that lymphocytes may function as conveyors of immunologically potent and reactive components to distant tissues and organs.

This aspect of lymphoid cell biology could provide a basis for the cell-mediated immunological competence which is of prime significance in host resistance to a variety of noxious assaults, e.g., autoimmune phenomena (cf. Good and Gabrielson 1964; Metcalf 1966; Miller and Osoba 1967; Burnet 1969).

12.2.2. Hormonal effects on structure and functions of phagocytic cells

Investigations of the influence of hormones on phagocytosis have generally been based upon a technique utilizing intravenous administration of either finely divided carbon particles or chromium phosphate, or cells, generally erythrocytes, labelled with a radioactive marker. In addition, the rate of uptake by macrophages of intraveneously administered trypan blue has been utilized to contribute data on the influence of hormones on phagocytosis. The assembled data in Table 12.1 are, for the most part, derived from studies utilizing one of these procedures, with measurements made of the rate of disappearance from the circulation of the injected particulate material. In some instances, these data have been supplemented by accompanying measurements of the rate of appearance of the detectable administered substance in cells of the reticuloendothelial system.

TABLE 12.1

Influence of hormones on the phagocytic activity of the reticuloendothelial system.

Hormone or gland	Direction of effect	Reference*
Somatotropin	None	Snell and Nicol (1957)
Thyrotropin		
Thyroxine, triiodothyronine	Increase	Lurie (1960)
Corticotropin		
Cortisol, corticosterone	Increase (small doses)	Nicol and Bilbey (1960); Snell (1960)
	Decrease (large doses)	DiCarlo et al. (1963)
Gonadotropins		
Oestrogens	Increase	Nicol and Bilbey (1960)
Androgens	None	Nicol and Bilbey (1960)
Progesterone	None	Nicol and Bilbey (1960)
Thymus**	None	Miller and Howard (1964); Morrow and DiLuzio (1965); Schooley et al. (1965)

* Wherever possible references have been selected to review articles. For additional references see text and bibliography.

** Cell-free thymic fractions have not as yet been examined for possible phagocytic activity; these references are to results in animals post-thymectomy.

While it is true that the above mentioned techniques probably provide an index of the rates of phagocytosis, it must be emphasized that these experimental approaches do not necessarily reveal the *direct* effects of hormones on the structure and functions of phagocytic cells. Although indices are utilized which *reflect* phagocytic activity, hormonal actions can be exerted on parameters other than the phagocytic cell itself. Thus, relatively little attention has been directed toward hormonal actions on the production of factors which influence phagocytosis, e.g., opsonins and complement, as well as on processes providing the energy requirements for phagocytosis, e.g., rates of glycolysis in macrophages.

As indicated in Table 12.1, only three classes of hormones, namely those of the thyroid, the adrenal cortex, and the ovary have been reported to alter the phagocytic rates of reticuloendothelial cells. In general, the most potent stimulants of phagocytosis, as established experimentally, are the oestrogenic hormones. The influence of the latter group of hormones on the phagocytic activity of the reticuloendothelial system appears to bear a direct relationship to their known oestrogenic activity (cf. Nicol and Bilbey 1960). It may be noted that although the androgen testosterone has little or no effect on the rate of phagocytosis, it, as well as thyroxine, will potentiate the activity of the oestrogens when administered together with the latter. This particular property of testosterone is unexpected since, in general, the actions of this steroid generally are antagonistic to the biological responses to the oestrogens. The data may reflect the possibility that the oestrogen molecule has two biological activities, one acting on the reticuloendothelial system and the other on the reproductive tract, and that these actions may be manifested independently (Nichol and Vernon-Roberts 1965b).

A detailed study was described by Nicol and Vernon-Roberts (1965a) of the influence of the oestrus cycle, pregnancy and ovariectomy on reticuloendothelial activity. This was based on previous observations by Nicol (1935) that the administration of oestrogenic hormones stimulated the appearance and activity of phagocytic cells in the endometrium of the uterine horns of the guinea-pig. Other studies from the same laboratory had indicated that substances possessing oestrogenic activity were among the most potent stimulators of reticuloendothelial cell activity (cf. Nicol and Bilby 1960). Utilizing a standard carbon clearance technique, Nicol and Vernon-Roberts (1965a) observed two peaks of reticuloendothelial activity in the rat and mouse during the oestrus cycle, one during the follicular phase and the other during the luteal phase at the time of endometrial degeneration. Two peaks of activity were also noted during pregnancy, one at the time of implantation and the other approaching the end of pregnancy prior to parturition. After ovariectomy, reticuloendothelial activity declined. The results are in accord with knowledge regarding variations in blood levels of oestrogens in the human during the phases of the oestrus cycle as well as during pregnancy. The data also indicate a role for oestrogens as a stimulant of body defenses based upon immunogenic responses and dependent upon an early phagocytic augmentation.

Although as pointed out previously, the processing of antigen prior to the latter's contact with antibody-producing cells may not always be a prerequisite for antibody synthesis, nonetheless in the majority of instances phagocytosis of both soluble and particulate antigens is an initial step in the sequence of events leading to the synthesis of humoral antibody. Thus a causal relationship obtains between reticuloendothelial structure and function and antibody formation (cf. LaVia et al. 1960; Thorbecke and Benacerraf 1962; Rowley 1966).

12.2.3. Hormonal effects on structure and functions of lymphoid cells

Although the preceding comments have been devoted primarily to the phagocytic activity of the major loci of *reticuloendothelial* cells in the mammalian organism, attention should be directed to the important role of lymphoid tissue in phagocytosis. While the number of fixed histiocytes or macrophages found in normal lymphoid tissue is small, they do appear in increased numbers with the entry of soluble or particulate foreign material into the nodes *via* the circulation, as well as in the circumstances of lymphocyte destruction by specific hormones. These phagocytic cells play an initial prime role in the sequence of events leading to the synthesis of immunoglobulins by lymphoid cells. This role is based to a significant degree on the arterial blood supply of a lymph node. Histologically, the arterial supply of a lymph node branches upon entering the structure. While one branch passes to the capsule, the other ends in a germinal center. This is an *end* artery and is the first place in the lymph node at which blood-borne agents, such as antigens, hormones, *etc.*, would leave the capillary. This locus is also the site of initial and maximal effects of these blood-borne agents. Indeed, the nuclear material from destroyed lymphocytes at the termini of such capillaries in lymph nodes was described by Flemming (1885) in the latter part of the 19th century and these aggregates of nuclear debris have been referred to as 'Flemming's tingible bodies.' Flemming also recognized the increased numbers of these bodies in lymph nodes following challenge of an animal by a foreign protein as well as by what today would be termed 'stressful stimuli'. The effect of a wide variety of the latter on the release of adrenocorticotropin from the adenohypophysis and the consequent lymphoid cell dissolution have been reviewed by Dougherty and White (1947) and will be considered further below.

The above apparent generalization of the initial point of entry and localization of blood-borne agents must, however, be considered with caution if extended to all antigens, particularly in view of the large number of materials classified as antigens. Extensive studies of the localization in lymph nodes of a wide variety of antigens indicates that the latter may show an affinity for either the germinal center reticular macrophages or the medullary macrophages, or both (cf. Humphrey 1969).

Although the role of lymphoid tissue in antibody formation and release is well established, some confusion may exist with regard to the specific cell type of the lymphoid system which can be described as *the* antibody-forming cell. Part of the difficulty arises from the rather unrestricted designation of all lymphocytes with basophilic staining cytoplasm as plasma cells. The nomenclature of lymphocytes suggested by Fagraeus (1960) for immunologically competent cells has clarified some of the ambiguity of terms in the literature. Distinction was made between *large* and *medium lymphocytes* on the one hand and *small lymphocytes* on the other. Among the former two types of cells it was suggested that there are lymphocytes which are active mitotically and metabolically and have typical block-structure chromatin and a richer basophilic cytoplasm. The term, plasma cells, was assigned to cells with an extensive, strongly basophilic cytoplasm and a juxta-nuclear clear area.

It is not completely clear whether the types of cells and their designations listed by Fagraeus are considered as separated developmentally from one another or whether consideration is given to interconversions of diverse cell types. This point is made here because of two possible points of view: (1) the background of knowledge relating initial phagocytosis of antigenic material by the macrophage to possible subsequent interactions of these and/or the phagocytosed material with lymphoid cells (plasma cells) in which antibody synthesis occurs; *versus* (2) a possible macrophage-lymphocyte interconversion and the question of a common stem cell origin, e.g., the reticular lymphocyte from which develops the potential antibody-forming cell (cf. White 1958; McMillan and Engelbert 1963).

For the present discussion it may suffice to consider that the non-thymic lymphoid tissues contain plasma cells and their precursor cells, in addition to lymphocytes and reticular cells. It may be noted that there are data supporting the existence of lymphocytes with differing potentiality and function (Gowans et al. 1962). This evidence may be related to the fact that since the distinction proposed by Fagraeus (1960) in the lymphocyte series between *large* and *medium* lymphocytes on the one hand and *small* lymphocytes on the other, recognition must now be given to two classes of small lymphocytes. These two have been termed the *short-lived* and the *long-lived small lymphocytes* (cf. Gatti et al. 1970). This distinction is of significance for our subsequent considerations of cell-mediated immune phenomena. For the latter, perhaps another useful classification of lymphocytes in the peripheral structures would be into thymus-dependent and thymus-independent populations (see below). Indeed, on the basis of recent studies in our laboratory (cf. Goldstein and White 1970, 1971a, b; White and Goldstein 1970b) as well as the rapidly expanding interest in the origin, distribution and fate of lymphoid cell populations, we wish in this presentation to postulate three possible classes of lymphocytes, two thymus-dependent populations and one thymus-independent population. This will be considered later in this chapter.

For our present discussion of hormones influencing humoral antibody synthesis, let us examine briefly what is known of hormonal actions on lymphoid tissue structure and function. Several reviews of this topic are available (White 1948, 1949a, 1963; Dougherty 1952; Dougherty et al. 1964; Ernström 1965).

The constancy in the size of the lymphoid tissue and in the numbers of circulating lymphocytes suggest that the rate of growth of lymphocytes, their entry into the circulation, and their peripheral disposal are regulated by physiological mechanisms which control body homeostasis. The latter is subject to the influence of the two major control mechanisms available to mammals, i.e., the nervous system and the endocrine system. It is significant that the major endocrine gland regulating the constancy of the structure and function of lymphoid tissue is the adenohypophysis. The importance of this endocrine gland stems from two considerations:

(1) The hormonal secretions of the adenohypophysis are controlled in their rates by factors, termed releasing factors, which are synthesized and secreted by the hypothalamus. Thus, this hypothalamic-adenohypophyseal interdependence represents the confluence of the two major pathways in the mammalian organism for maintaining homeostasis by disseminating information throughout the body, namely, transmission *via* the nervous system and transmission *via* the blood.

(2) The hormones of the adenohypophysis, multiple in number, comprise the controlling mechanisms for regulating the rates of secretion of the diverse hormones which act upon lymphoid tissue.

Table 12.2 lists the endocrine glands affecting lymphoid tissue structure and functions. As indicated above and will be discussed below, the influential role of the adenohypophysis on lymphoid tissue is established

TABLE 12.2

Influence of hormones on lymphoid tissue structure and functions.

Homone	*Direction of effect*	*Reference**
Somatotropin	Increase	Dougherty (1952); Pierpaoli and Sorkin (1969)
Thyrotropin		
Thyroxine, triiodothyronine	Increase	Dougherty (1952); Sorkin (1969)
Corticotropin	Decrease	White (1948);
Cortisol, corticosterone		Dougherty (1952)
Gonadotropins		
Oestrogens	Increase	Dougherty (1952)
Androgens	Decrease	Dougherty (1952)
Thymosin	Increase	White and Goldstein (1968, 1970a); Goldstein et al. (1970); Goldstein and White (1970; 1971a, b)

* See footnote Table 12.1.

for all of its hormones. Less clear at present is whether the production
and release of thymic hormone(s), including thymosin, is dependent upon
a trophic influence of the adenohypophysis. As will be discussed later,
Pierpaoli and Sorkin (1968, 1969) and Pierpaoli et al. (1969) have
provided evidence in support of the concept that somatotropin, of the
adenohypophysis, may function as a thymotropic hormone.

It might also be pointed out that the diversity of humoral agents
affecting lymphoid tissue structure and function, and the control of
their rates of secretion by higher centers of the nervous system, are
factors in the wide variety of derangements, encountered as a reflection
of alterations in the contribution of lymphoid cells to host humoral and
cell-mediated immunity.

Of the hormones listed in Table 12.2 which affect lymphoid tissue
structure and function, those of the adenohypophyseal-adrenal cortical
secretory axis may receive special emphasis. This is due in large measure
to (1) the extreme sensitivity and augmentation of this secretory response
to a wide variety of unrelated stimuli (Dougherty and White 1947), and
(2) the profound and acute morphological effects of adrenal cortical
steroids, whether released endogenously or administered, on the
structure of lymphoid tissue (Dougherty and White 1945). Inasmuch as
the latter changes are characterized by a pyknosis and karyorrhexis of
lymphocyte nuclei, with a subsequent dissolution of lymphocytes in
the thymus and lymph nodes, and an acute inhibition of mitosis of

lymphocytes, it is apparent that any stimulus causing elevated blood levels of adrenal cortical steroids will have serious deleterious consequences on immunological phenomena which are based on normal numbers and functions of lymphoid cells. Thus, exposure of the organism to environmental influences such as cold, heat, or anoxia, to traumatic conditions such as tissue injury, fractures or hemorrhage, to bacterial toxins, to toxic chemicals, e.g., arsenic or benzene, to anesthetics, e.g., nembutal, to foreign proteins, or to minute amounts of a variety of compounds normally produced in the organism, such as histamine, insulin, epinephrine and thyroxine, will produce an increased rate of secretion of adenohypophyseal corticotropin. The resulting accelerated release of adrenal cortical hormones caused by any one of these stimuli does not occur in the absence of the hypophysis.

These observations serve to explain why the various physiological alterations which are affected by pituitary-adrenal cortical secretion may be seen to a qualitatively similar extent in response to a wide variety of agents and in diverse circumstances. This endocrine mechanism is undoubtedly the physiological basis for the so-called 'accidental involution' of lymphoid tissue, and for the decrease in lymphoid tissue size seen in the 'alarm reaction' of Selye (1946) inasmuch as stress, whether physical or chemical, is one of the potent activators of pituitary-adrenal cortical secretion. Thus, the fact that the histological and physiological responses of lymphoid tissue are so greatly influenced by a particular endocrine mechanism, the hypophyseal-adrenal cortical relationship, which in turn may be augmented by many stimuli, suggests a reason for the difficulty in finding uniformly, at biopsy or autopsy, a normal appearance of lymphoid structures. It would appear that the latter are, literally, in a state of perpetual histological and physiological flux in response to continual variations in the secretory rate of the pituitary-adrenal cortical mechanism. This rate is, in turn, influenced markedly by a variety of diverse stimuli which may have their origin either within the organism or in its environment.

It should be emphasized that stimuli operating independently of the pituitary-adrenal cortical mechanism may also influence profoundly the size and structure of lymphoid tissue. This is evident from experience which shows that certain agents may cause lymphoid tissue involution in the absence of the hypophysis or the adrenals. For example, exposure to x-irradiation, or injection of toxic chemicals such as nitrogen mustard, urethane, or deoxypyridoxine, results in lymphoid tissue involution in the hypophysectomized or the adrenalectomized animal. Thus, a direct effect of any one of these agents on lymphoid tissue without endocrine mediation is well established. It may be pointed out, however, that in the intact animal, a portion of these effects may be endocrine-mediated, since these toxic agents do augment pituitary-adrenal cortical secretion (White 1948, 1949a). It is not unlikely that this is also the case for other commonly used immunosuppressive agents.

It is apparent from the foregoing that the steroids of the adrenal cortex are particularly potent agents in suppressing lymphoid tissue structure and function, including those reflected in immune phenomena. This earlier evidence for the action of these hormones on lymphoid tissue has provided the logical basis for their use clinically as immunosuppressive agents. However, the relatively lesser degree of effectiveness of the adrenal steroids in comparison with other approaches, may now find explanation in recent studies. Although the earlier observations of the action of adrenal cortical steroids on lymphoid cells had clearly established that the target cell most affected was the small and the medium-sized lymphocytes (Dougherty and White 1945; Dougherty 1952, 1960), subsequent histological and immunological data have revealed the existence of two distinct populations of small lymphocytes, namely, the short-lived and the long-lived, with the latter being of greater importance in immunological phenomena (cf. Gatti et al. 1970). Recently, Esteban (1968) has demonstrated that when rats are injected intra-peritoneally with a lymphocytolytic steroid (cortisol), at four-hour intervals, the short-lived lymphocytes are significantly more susceptible to the destructive effects of the steroid than are the long-lived lymphocytes. These observations are in accord with observations of Warner (1964), Craddock et al. (1967), J. J. Miller and Cole (1967), Blomgren and Andersson (1969), and Levine and Claman (1970). However, it may be noted that Lance and co-workers (1970) have recently reported that the type of lymphocyte affected by cortisol is related to the dose of steroid administered. Thus, in studies in rabbits of the distribution and recirculation of lymphocytes labeled with radioactive chromium, these investigators found that, in small doses, cortisol acts upon immature thymocytes. In contrast, the action of larger doses of the steroid was upon peripheral lymphocytes.

A second secretory axis with profound influence on lymphoid tissue structure and function is the adenohypophyseal-thyroid axis. The stimulatory action of thyrotropin releases two hormones, thyroxine and triiodothyronine, each of which exerts a proliferative influence on lymphoid tissue. The role of the thyroid in the regulation of lymphoid tissue structure and function has been reviewed (Dougherty 1952; Ernström 1965). The lymphocytosis and lymphoid hyperplasia of hyperthyroidism have been well documented. Although the thyroid hormones may also act as non-specific agents in causing augmented release of adrenocorticotropic hormone, it is clear that the proliferative action of thyroxine on lymphoid tissue is seen in adrenalectomized, gonadectomized, adrenalectomized-gonadectomized and hypophysectomized animals (cf. Ernström 1965). Thus this action of thyroxine is not dependent upon mediation by other endocrine glands. It is also of interest for the present discussion that clinical coexisting thyrotoxicosis and myasthenia gravis have been recorded, accompanied occasionally by thymomas.

In considering thyroid-lymphoid tissue relationships, mention should also be made of the investigations of Comsa. This investigator has stressed an older point of view attributing a role for the thymus in mediating the action of the trophic hormones of the adenohypophysis (cf. White and Goldstein 1968; Goldstein and White 1970). Comsa (1966) reported the isolation of an electrophoretically homogeneous glycopeptide from thymic tissue. The product was described as effective in preventing the creatinuria seen in the castrated, thymectomized, thyroidectomized guinea-pig following endogeneous or exogeneous elevation of circulating thyroid hormone. This reported hypophyseal-thymic-thyroidal relationship remains to be explored further, particularly with respect to its possible significance for considerations of the immunogenic roles ascribed to the thymus (see below).

The actions of the gonads on the structure and function of lymphoid tissue appear to be unidirectional only in the case of the male secretion. Administration of testosterone results in involution of lymphoid tissue (Dougherty 1952). A dramatic example of this action of androgens was described by Szenberg and co-workers (cf. Warner and Szenberg 1964). Thus, injection of androgenic steroids into chick embryos caused marked involution of bursal lymphoid cells, as well as a decrease in the epitheleal elements of the bursa. Castration has been reported to cause a significant enlargement of lymphoid structures (cf. Pierpaoli and Sorkin 1968a). A striking demonstration of the influence of the male gonad on lymphoid tissue is seen in the differences in the size of lymphoid tissue occurring in fasting, intact male mice as compared to fasting, castrate mice (Szego and White 1951). Indeed, the marked involution of lymphoid tissue resulting from fasting in adult mice was reduced markedly in severity by prior gonadectomy in either male or female mice, illustrating the suppressive action of either androgens or oestrogens on lymphoid tissue size. Nonetheless, in the case of oestrogens, small doses of these hormones may augment the secretion of adrenocorticotropin, thus leading to thymic involution. However, prolonged administration of the female sex hormones leads to lymphoid tissue hypertrophy, characterized initially by active epithelial cell proliferation of the thymus.

Prolonged exposure of mice of a specific strain to oestrogens can lead to lymphoid tumours (Gardner et al. 1944). It is interesting in connection with the present discussion that the total amount of lymph nodes and splenic lymphatic tissue is generally greater in female than in male experimental animals. This may be of significance for the greater degree of immune responsiveness frequently exhibited by the female.

The influence of somatotropin (growth hormone) on lymphoid tissue structure and function is of particular interest because it appears to be directed more specifically to the thymus as a target lymphatic tissue (cf. Dougherty 1952; Pierpaoli and Sorkin 1969). Administration of somatotropin increased the size of the thymus of intact and hypophysectomized animals. Moreover, it has been suggested that growth hormone might have a specific thymotropic action since hypophysectomized animals treated with hypophyseal growth hormone-containing extracts had larger thymi but not lymph nodes and spleens than operated control animals given the same quantity of food. However, administration of a somatotropin preparation to fasted, intact or fasted adrenalectomized mice did not affect the composition or weight of lymphatic tissue, or the size of lymphatic tissue of hormone-treated, fasted mice (Szego and White 1949).

In addition to the evidence mentioned above as well as that reviewed by Dougherty (1952) regarding the effects of somatotropin on the structure and functions of lymphoid tissue, other publications have supported and extended a role for this hormone in influencing lymphoid tissue size and, as will be considered later, its contributions to immunological phenomena. In earlier studies, Moon et al. (1950) described the effects of prolonged injection into rats of growth-hormone containing extracts. At autopsy, a number of the animals had lymphoid hyperplasia and lymphosarcomas localized in the lung tissue. Apparently, this proliferation of lymphoid tissue was a consequence of the stimulation by growth hormone of areas of peribronchial lymphoid tissue. All extra-thoracic lymph nodes were normal.

Stimulatory effects of growth hormone on lymphoid organs such as spleen, thymus and lymph nodes have also been reported (Moon et al. 1952; Dougherty 1955a; Shrewsbury and Reinhardt 1959). Growth hormone administration accelerated plasma cell development in mice treated with mineral oil as a tumorigenic stimulus, as well as the production of lymphosarcomas in mice given growth hormone either with or without mineral oil (Takakura et al. 1967). Tumour masses were found in the thymus, lung, peritoneal cavity, spleen and liver, with infiltration of lymphocytes into the spleen and distinct enlargement of spleen and lymphoid tissue surrounding the thymus. Other investigators (Hayashida and Li 1957; Lundin 1958; Gyllensten 1962; Ernström 1965; Pierpaoli et al. 1969) have reported that somatotropic hormone and thyroxine might act either alone or synergistically in the maturation and differentiation of the lymphoid organs.

Of particular interest to these considerations of the role of somatotropin in influencing lymphoid tissue structure and function are the recent reports (Pierpaoli and Sorkin 1968b, 1969) that the administration to young mice of rabbit immune globulins isolated from an antiserum to purified bovine somatotropic hormone caused inhibition of growth, thymic atrophy, involution of splenic lymphoid tissue, and a wasting syndrome. The simultaneous administration of somatotropin together with the immune globulins completely prevented the effects of the latter.

A rather dramatic reflection of the role of somatotropin in the regulation of lymphoid tissue structure and function is seen in the failure of the development of the thymo-lymphatic tissue in mice (Snell-Bagg dw) with hereditary hypopituitary dwarfism (Baroni 1967a, b). In these animals the hypophysis is characterized by a lack or absence of somatotropic and thyrotropic hormone-producing cells. These hormonal deficiencies are accompanied by hypoplasia of central and peripheral lymphoid tissues. Treatment of the mice with somatotropin and thyroxine, in combination, prevented the thymus involution and the cellular depletion in the peripheral lymphoid tissue (Baroni et al. 1969). The combination of both hormones was more effective in restoration of normal lymphoid tissue structure than was the case with either hormone alone.

One of the oldest of the indicated and at the same time the most recent of the accepted members of the list of endocrine glands suggested as influencing lymphoid tissue structure and function is the thymus (cf. White and Goldstein 1968, 1970a; Goldstein et al. 1970b; Goldstein and White 1970; 1971a, b). A cell-free, partially purified thymic factor, which has been termed thymosin, will, when administered to either normal adult mice, neonatally thymectomized mice, adult lethally X-irradiated mice, germ-free mice, adrenalectomized mice or normal guinea-pigs, produce a marked proliferation of peripheral lymphoid tissue. This is reflected in both an increase in lymphoid tissue weight, a stimulation of mitotic activity of lymphoid cells, and an increased degree of incorporation of radioactive labeled precursors into the total DNA, RNA and protein of peripheral lymphoid structures. Histological and radioautographic studies (Goldstein et al. 1970c) indicate that thymosin has a stimulatory effect particularly on the more primitive immature cells of proliferating lymph nodes. This may be of significance for later discussions of humoral and cell-mediated immune responses.

12.2.4. Hormonal influences on the rate of humoral antibody formation

In view of the above-described and established role of lymphoid tissue in antibody production, it may be expected that hormonal influences on the rate of formation of circulating antibody should bear some relationships to the actions of each hormone on lymphoid tissue structure and function. This is the case for most of the previously discussed hormones. Thus, prolonged administration of adrenocorticotropic hormone or of adrenal cortical steroids inhibits antibody formation (cf. Batchelor 1968). It has been pointed out above that the marked ability of these secretions to produce involution of lymphoid tissue has provided a basis for their use as immunosuppressive agents. In general, any agent that has a lymphocytotoxic effect will suppress or inhibit trends toward increased titres of circulating antibody.

In view of the dramatic lymphocytokaryorrhectic effects of adrenal cortical steroids, it is abundantly clear that these hormones, particularly when administered in large pharmacological doses, are potent immunosuppressive agents as a result of their destructive actions on antibody-producing cells. However, *augmented* antibody synthesis and release may also occur under the influence of these hormones, particularly if they are not administered for prolonged periods of time and are given in small, physiological amounts to actively immunized, or previously immunized, animals. In view of the continuing turnover of lymphoid cellular components even in the absence of the adrenals or hypophysis, the data available clearly establish that these hormones, as in the case of other endocrine secretions, merely influence *rates* of reactions which do not cease completely in the absence of the endocrine controlling factor.

In experiments following the demonstration by Dougherty et al. (1944) of the presence of antibody globulin in lymphoid cells of immunized mice, these same investigators reported that adrenal cortical extract, given either in conjunction with antigens (Chase et al. 1946) or post immunization (Dougherty et al. 1945b) would augment circulating antibody titres. At a later time, Roberts et al. (1948, 1949) examined the extent of production and release of antibody *in vitro* by tissues obtained from immunized rats and mice. The data demonstrated that the relative degree of antibody production among various tissues, notably spleen, thymus and peripheral lymph nodes, was related to the schedule and route of administration of antigen. Adrenalectomy prior to immunization delayed and depressed the production and release of immune globulins by lymphoid tissues.

These initial reports of the ability of adrenal cortical hormones to augment antibody production have been confirmed in some laboratories (Fox and Whitehead 1936; Hammond and Novack 1950; Halpern et al.

1951, 1952; Ambrose 1964) but not in others (Eisen et al. 1947; cf. also reviews by McMaster 1953; Dougherty 1955b; Gabrielsen and Good 1967). In addition, recent studies *in vitro* have demonstrated that small physiological concentrations of cortisol must be present in the medium for expression of the secondary immune response (Ambrose 1964).

Perhaps one of the more significant contributions to possible explanation of these discrepant results are the studies of Halpern et al. (1951, 1952). These investigators were able to demonstrate both effects of cortisone, i.e., an augmentation and a depression of circulating antibody titres in rabbits. The animals were immunized to egg albumin; when significant quantities of antibody were present in the serum, the rabbits received another injection of the antigen in an amount adequate to reduce almost to zero the antibody titres. The animals were then divided into two groups; one received a single injection of cortisone and the other served as controls. Within 24 to 48 hrs, the cortisone-injected animals exhibited a highly significant level of serum antibody, while antibody titres in the control rabbits were negligible. However, after the third day, the antibody levels in the steroid-treated rabbits began to drop to levels below that of the control group. When the latter had recovered completely their original level of antibody, generally after the fifth day following antigen administration, the animals treated with steroid had a lower precipitin level than the control rabbits. The remarkable increase in the serum antibody levels observed in the first 48 hrs in the cortisone injected animals was attributed to the lysis of lymphocytes which contained antibody, as suggested by Dougherty et al. (1945), since the rise in antibody titres in the serum and the decrease in the numbers of lymphocytes in the blood and tissues paralleled one another.

Experiments of the type just described emphasize the importance of the relationships of the schedules of administration of adrenal steroid and antigen in influencing the rate of antibody production. These variables may afford a possible explanation for the conflicting findings of authors who have observed an early acute increase in antibodies in the blood as a result of adrenal steroid treatment of previously immunized animals and, on the other hand, of those investigators who have reported a depressing effect of the steroid hormone on the production of antibody when administered during the sensitization period. There seems little doubt that potent adrenal cortical steroids do reduce the concentration of circulating antibody in immunized animals (Bjöerneboe et al. 1951) and decrease the number of lymphoid cells as a consequence of their lymphocytokaryorrhectic and antimitotic actions (Dougherty and White 1945).

It may be of experimental significance in resolving certain of these discrepancies of the immunogenic influence of adrenal steroids to give consideration not only to schedule of administration and dose of antigen and of steroid, but also to the ratio of these two agents. Perhaps yet another factor may be the evidence that the ratio of lymphoid cells that proliferate to those that undergo differentiation to antibody-producing cells may be influenced not only by the dose of antigen but also by its properties (Benacerraf 1969). In any event, the possibility that adrenal cortical hormones may, under specific conditions, enhance immunogenicity has been over-shadowed by the more dramatic consequences of severe immunosuppression following use of pharmacological doses of lymphocytokaryorrhectic adrenal steroids. Nonetheless, it may be noted that the secondary response, which can readily be elicited in cultures of lymph node fragments prepared from previously immunized rabbits, is dependent upon the presence in the medium of a lymphocytolytic adrenal cortical steroid, e.g., cortisol (Ambrose 1964).

In contrast to the adrenal cortical steroids, any hormone which has a proliferative action on lymphoid tissue might be expected to augment formation of humoral antibody. Mention has been made previously of the proliferative effects of oestrogens on lymphoid tissue, contrasted with the regressive influence of testosterone. Thus, in general, the immunological responsiveness of the female seems to be more pronounced than that of the male of the same species and strain.

The earlier literature on the effects of sex hormones on circulating antibody titres has been reviewed by Perla and Marmorston (1941). Since the appearance of that scholarly volume, a number of laboratories have described data for the influence of the androgens and oestrogens on antibody production (cf. Batchelor 1968). In general, the data are in accord with the earlier considerations (see page 335ff, page 339ff; Tables 12.1 and 12.2) of the influence of sex hormones on the rate of phagocytosis by the reticuloendothelial system and on lymphoid tissue proliferation. Oestrogen administration during the period of immunization will increase the rate of humoral antibody production, whereas in male animals the response to antigen is diminished in magnitude and can be maintained at higher levels by prior castration. This has been examined recently in some detail by Batchelor (1968). Indeed, it is possible to increase the levels of γ-globulin in male guinea-pigs by the injection of stilbestrol (Charles and Nicol 1961).

As might be anticipated, reports of the influence of thyroid hormones on the synthesis of humoral antibody are conflicting. The level of circulating proteins is the net result of the rate of their addition to the blood and the rate of their removal. It appears obvious that inasmuch as thyroid hormones influence the rates of cellular reactions, the balance between antibody synthesis and secretion, on the one hand, and antibody removal by the tissues, on the other may be altered by a large variety of non-thyroidal factors. For example, the production of immunity to bacterial antigens is enhanced by hyperthyroidism in guinea-pigs, monkeys and man (Long and Shewell 1955; Shewell and Long 1957), but appears to be reduced in rats, rabbits and mice (Shewell and Long 1957). Hypothyroidism has the opposite effect. Also hypothyroidism has been reported to decrease the antibody response in rabbits (Johnstone et al. 1962) as well as in guinea-pigs and primates (Nilsen 1957; Shewell and Long 1957). By way of emphasizing the above point regarding the balance determining levels of circulating protein, it may be pointed out that passive immunity is prolonged by hypothyroidism due to a slower rate of disappearance of γ-globulin from the blood (Farthing et al. 1960a, b; Trapani et al. 1959).

As indicated previously, one of the hormones exerting a significant influence on lymphoid tissue structure and functions is adenohypophyseal somatotropin. However, until recently, there has been surprisingly little interest in the possible influence of somatotropin on the regulation of the circulating antibody response. One recent and striking demonstration of an adenohypophyseal-lymphoid system interrelationship is that of the effects of somatotropin and anti-somatotropin serum on lymphatic tissue, and on the immune response. Indeed, additional evidence has accumulated to support the hypothesis that somatotropin may exert a trophic influence on the thymus (cf. also Dougherty 1952), thus influencing the rate of cellular turnover in this gland and thereby affecting the magnitude of thymic contributions to immune phenomena. This area of research has also suggested interesting relationships between somatotropin and thyrotropin, another adenohypophyseal hormone known to accelerate the proliferation of lymphoid tissue (see page 343ff. and Table 12.2).

These recent studies of hypophyseal-thymus relationships have provided added interest and significance to the role of somatotropin in the regulation of lymphoid tissue structure and function particularly as the latter relate to immunological phenomena. The background for this recent work on the relationship of somatotropin to lymphoid tissue structure and function derives from the initial observations of Baroni (1967a, b) that genetic hypopituitary dwarf mice (Snell-Bagg dw) are immunologically deficient and have lymphoid tissue abnormalities characteristic of the neonatally thymectomized mouse. Of significance for our present discussion of hormonal influences on humoral antibody synthesis are the demonstrations in three laboratories (Baroni et al. 1969; Pierpaoli et al. 1969; Pierpaoli and Sorkin 1969; Duquesnoy et al. 1969,

1970) of a diminished capacity for antibody synthesis in the Snell-Bagg dwarf mice in response to injected antigens. Moreover, the first two groups of investigators were able to reconstitute 19 S antibody production in these hormonally deficient mice by administration of somatotropic hormone together with thyroxine. Antibody globulin synthesis could be augmented by administration of somatotropin alone but complete reconstitution of the immune capacity required the injection of both somatotropin and thyroxine. These last observations recall the previously cited reports (see page 344) that somatotropin and thyroxine might influence lymphoid tissue maturation and differentiation either acting alone or synergistically.

Further interesting evidence of the important role of somatotropin in antibody production was provided by the demonstration (Pierpaoli et al. 1969b) that complete suppression of antibody formation in normal mice could be achieved by administration of a globulin fraction obtained from an anti-somatotropin serum. Surprisingly, it was also reported that somatotropin could also restore significantly the antibody forming capacity in normal mice whose immune response had been completely inhibited by treatment with globulin fractions from an antiserum against bovine thyrotropic hormone. These data with normal mice are of added significance since it might be suggested that in the dwarf mice it is somewhat more difficult to dissect the effects of an individual trophic hormone in animals with general multi-hormonal deficiencies.

An exception to the direct relationship between the capacity of a hormone to stimulate proliferation of lymphoid tissue and its effect on the rate of antibody production may be thymosin, the thymic humoral principle. Although this hormonal factor does influence cell-mediated immune responses (see below), its administration to either normal adult mice, or adult mice thymectomized at birth, or adult thymectomized lethally x-irradiated bone-marrow maintained mice, all challenged with sheep erythrocytes as antigen did not yield significant evidence of augmented 19 S or 7 S antibody production (Goldstein et al. 1970a). These studies require repetition with other antigens prior to concluding that thymosin does not play a role in humoral antibody production.

It may be noted that the secondary antibody response in lymph nodes cultured *in vitro* was stimulated by the presence of normal thymic tissue or of thymosin (Wolf and Erb 1971). Moreover, although the results from our laboratory (Goldstein et al. 1970a) indicate the inability of administered thymosin, a cell-free thymic extract, to alter antibody production in mice to sheep erythrocytes, the only antigen studied, it is clear that, from both experimental and clinical studies, the thymus has a role in humoral antibody synthesis (cf. Bruton, 1952, 1968; Gatti et al.

1970; Goldstein and White 1970, 1971a, b; Good and Gabrielson 1964; Miller and Osoba 1967; Peterson and Good 1968).

One laboratory, that of Trainin and his colleagues (Trainin and Linker-Israeli 1967; Trainin et al. 1968), has described restoration in thymectomized animals of immunological capacity with cell-free thymic extracts as reflected in 19 S antibody formation. These investigators administered a partially purified thymic extract to either neonatally thymectomized mice or to adult, thymectomized mice exposed to sublethal radiation (550 R). Challenge of the animals with sheep erythrocytes suggested that mice treated with the thymic extract had a slightly greater number of plaque-forming cells in their spleens than were seen in control animals. However, the differences between the treated and the control animals were only slight. A demonstrated role for cell-free thymic humoral factors in the regulation of 19 S antibody synthesis awaits further studies with other antigens as well as perhaps with more potent thymic fractions.

12.3. Cell-mediated immunological competence

In this section we shall not discuss the mechanism of cell-mediated immunity, but will restrict our major considerations to hormones influencing the role of lymphoid cells in cell-mediated immune phenomena. Several monographs, symposia and reviews have recently appeared concerned with the manifold aspects of the processes and reactions which form the basis of cellular immunity (cf. Good and Gabrielson 1964; Metcalf 1966; Miller and Osoba 1967; Hess 1968; Burnet 1969; Lawrence and Landy 1969; Goldstein and White 1970, 1971a, b; White and Goldstein, 1970b). In addition, this topic receives attention elsewhere in the present volume (cf. Chapters 9, 15, 16, 17). Perhaps it is necessary only to emphasize that cell-mediated immune phenomena have been given increasing emphasis during the past decade concomittant with the initial observations of the deleterious consequences of neonatal thymectomy (cf. Good and Gabrielsen 1964; Metcalf 1966; Miller and Osoba 1967; Hess 1968; Sorkin 1969; White and Goldstein 1968, 1970a, b; Goldstein and White 1970, 1971a, b). Indeed, had the discovery by Bordet of humoral immune lysis not followed within four years the classical observations of Metchnikoff on cellular phenomena involved in response to foreign materials, it may not have been necessary to look anew at the cellular basis for delayed hypersensitivity reactions, allograft rejection, many types of autoimmune diseases and resistance to malignant growths and to a variety of infectious diseases. The current emphasis in immunobiology has clearly shifted from an earlier greater concern with levels of circulating antibodies to an emphasis on immune phenomena mediated by lymphoid cells.

12.3.1. Cell types involved in cell-mediated immunity

From the initial studies of thymectomized animals mentioned above, the important conclusion evident was that the thymus gland controls the development and expression of those functions of the immunological system reflected in cell-mediated immunity and also has a role in certain aspects of the development of humoral immunity.

The contributions of the thymus gland to cell-mediated immunity are of two types, namely, endocrine and cellular. The endocrine contribution is dependent upon the production and secretion by the thymus of one or more factors, including thymosin. The role of the latter in cell-mediated immunity will be discussed below. The cellular contributions of the thymus may be two-fold in nature. One is the production and export by the thymus to the organs and tissues of the body of cellular elements destined in the appropriate environment and in the presence of specific stimuli to become immunologically competent cells. Of the latter, a proportion can function in cell-mediated immune phenomena. A second cellular contribution of the thymus may be localized within the gland itself. Multipotential, undifferentiated stem cells, from sources such as foetal liver or bone marrow, are induced to differentiate and to proliferate by passing through specific microenvironments. The thymus provides one of these important microenvironments.

Of the various lymphoid cells influenced by thymectomy, the small lymphocyte is the most susceptible. Some of these cells are thymus dependent (Parrott et al. 1966) and can be obtained in large numbers from the thoracic duct lymph (Gowans 1965). This class of small lymphocytes has been shown to be responsible for the surveillance role of lymphoid tissue in the body and for many of the typical cell-mediated responses. The small lymphocyte, or more specifically a class of small lymphocytes within this category, has been designated collectively as 'immunologically competent cells' or alternatively as 'antigen-reactive cells' and has been demonstrated to have an extremely long life span. Studies utilizing chromosomal markers have revealed that the immunologically competent cell in rats has a life span of over 100 days (Little et al. 1962) and in man of several years (Buckton and Pike 1964). This long life span probably explains the lack of immediate multiple immunological defects in adult animals following thymectomy. The number of immunologically competent cells in the circulation at the time of thymectomy would, under normal circumstances, be more than that required to parry normal pathogenic challenges. Thus, the numerous older reports of the lack of effect of thymectomy in the adult animal can now be reconciled with present immunological understanding. A decrease in lymphocyte numbers and in immunological competence is seen in adult thymectomized animals examined at a time significantly beyond operation (Metcalf 1965; Miller 1965; Taylor 1965). This slow rate of decline in the numbers of immunologically competent cells in the adult, thymectomized animal can be accelerated by destruction of the existing lymphoid cell populations by use of lymphocytolytic agents such as x-irradiation (Miller et al. 1964), anti-lymphocyte serum (Monaco et al. 1965) or cyclophosphamide (Dukor and Dietrich 1967). Adult, thymectomized animals treated in this manner cannot restore normal numbers of small lymphocytes and, histologically and immunologically, resemble the neonatally thymectomized animal in their immunological incompetence.

A striking clinical manifestation of the role of the thymus in the production of cells which are basic to cell-mediated immune responses is the DiGeorge syndrome (DiGeorge 1968). This disease is characterized by the presence at birth of either an aplastic thymus or the latter fails to develop normally. Although the antibody-producing mechanisms are intact, with normal levels of all the immunoglobulins and a normal response to many antigens, infants with the DiGeorge syndrome exhibit a total failure to elicit typical delayed hypersensitivity and homograft reactions. Hence, these infants are extremely susceptible to a wide range of infectious agents, particularly those which are viral or fungal, and survival for more than one year is rare.

12.3.2. *Hormonal effects on cells providing cell-mediated immunity*

As indicated above, the slow rate of decline in the numbers of immunologically competent cells in the adult, thymectomized animal can be accelerated by use of a variety of lymphocytotoxic agents. However, in the present discussion limited to hormonal agents altering the numbers of small lymphocytes providing cell-mediated immunity, we need focus solely again, as in previous sections of this review, on hormones which influence lymphoid tissue structure and functions. Here, however, we cannot speak of lymphoid tissue size as a whole, but are rather limited in our discussion to that population of lymphoid cells in which resides cell-mediated immunological functions, namely, the small lymphocyte. Even in the latter class we must recognize, as mentioned above, two populations of cells of differing life spans, the so-called short- and long-lived small lymphocyte. In this last group of cells, we shall propose a possible further subdivision (see below), thus distinguishing three classes of small lymphocytes.

The initial observations of Dougherty and White (1945) (see also, White 1949b, Dougherty 1952, 1960) stressed the selectivity of the lymphocytokaryorrhectic adrenal cortical steroids on the lymphoid cell population. The smaller lymphocytes of the lymphoid organs were the most sensitive to the destructive influence of these steroid hormones, while the medium-sized lymphocyte was much less attacked and the large cells were unaltered. The destruction of the smaller lymphocytes was accompanied by an inhibition of mitotic activity so that continuing differentiation of more primitive stem cells into small lymphocytes was held in abeyance. Of the lymphoid organs studied, the thymus was most sensitive to the lytic action of the adrenal steroids. These observations formed a logical basis for the subsequent practical application of adrenal cortical steroids in the treatment of certain lymphoid malignancies and the more recent use of these compounds as immunosuppressive agents (cf. Gabrielson and Good 1967).

Although the potent adrenal cortical steroids are of some value as immunosuppressive agents as a result of their deleterious effects on the small lymphocyte population, the studies of Warner (1964), Esteban (1968), Blomgren and Andersson (1969), and Levine and Claman (1970) may provide explanation, at least in part, for the lack of complete success with the use of these steroids along prior to tissue or organ transplantation. The data reveal that the short-lived cells are more susceptible to the destructive actions of the steroid than are the long-lived lymphocytes. As indicated above, it is this latter class of small lymphocytes that is responsible for the typical cell-mediated immune responses. These data must be interpreted in relation to the dose of adrenal steroid used, since, as indicated previously, the type of lymphocyte acted upon by this hormone may be influenced by the quantity of steroid administered (Lance and Cooper 1970).

The role of the somatotropic hormone of the adenohypophysis and of thyroxine in the proliferation of lymphoid tissue and the influence of these hormones on the rate of humoral antibody formation have been discussed in previous pages. It is not yet clear whether these hormones, through their influence on lymphoid tissues, may also augment significantly cell-mediated immune phenomena. That this is likely is suggested from the striking 'naturally occurring' example mentioned previously, namely, the Snell-Bragg dwarf mouse. Duquesnoy et al. (1969, 1970) have reported a decreased reactivity of the spleen cells of these dwarf mice when tested for graft-*versus*-host reactivity. Also, Pierpaoli and his colleagues (Pierpaoli et al. 1969, Pierpaoli and Sorkin 1969) have found that adult mice treated with anti-somatotropic hormone serum showed, on histological examination, a complete lack of lymphoid cells in the thymus-dependent areas (Parrott et al. 1966) of the lymphoid organs. Moreover, untreated Snell-Bragg dwarf mice develop an appearance reminiscent of the wasting disease of neonatally thymectomized mice, and usually die between 45 and 65 days after birth, presumably of infection. In contrast, treatment of the dwarf mice with somatotropin and thyroxine extended their life span to a year or more (Pierpaoli et al. 1969). These findings point to a possible role of somatotropin and thyroxine not only in the production of immunoglobulins but also in cell-mediated immune phenomena. It may be noted that hypothyroidism has been reported to prolong the survival of skin homografts in rats (Schatten et al. 1958).

The role of the thymus in the development and maturation of lymphoid tissue has been referred to in earlier pages and has also been considered in more detail in recent reviews (Miller and Osoba 1967; Gatti et al. 1970; Goldstein and White 1970; 1971a, b). We have also discussed in preceding pages the possible role of cell-free thymic fractions in regulating the rate of immunoglobulin production. The importance of the thymus in cell-mediated immune phenomena is now clearly established; support for this conclusion has been summarized recently (Good and Gabrielson 1964; Metcalf 1966; Miller and Osoba 1967; Hess 1968; Sorkin 1969; Goldstein and White 1970; 1971a, b; White and Goldstein 1970a, b). The possible role of a thymic hormonal factor as a basis for regulating aspects of cell-mediated reactions known to be thymus dependent has been stimulated by reports from several laboratories of the biological activity of cell-free thymic extracts in experimental models designed to assess cellular immunological competence (DeSomer et al. 1963; Jankovic et al. 1965; Law and Agnew 1968; Law et al. 1968; Trainin et al. 1968; Asanuma et al. 1970; Goldstein et al. 1970a, b, c; Goldstein and White 1970; 1971a, b; White and Goldstein 1970a, b).

Studies from our own laboratory have utilized primarily a partially purified cell-free preparation from calf thymic tissue, which has been designated as thymosin (Goldstein et al. 1966). The further purification of this thymic humoral factor has been described elsewhere (Goldstein et al. 1970b). Thymosin is lymphocytopoietic when injected in mice which are either normal, adrenalectomized, germ-free or lethally irradiated. To the present, as indicated previously in this review, administration of thymosin to mice in several types of experimental designs did not influence their immunological response to a challenge of sheep erythrocytes (Goldstein et al. 1970a). In contrast, thymosin administration did have a positive influence on cell-mediated immunological competence of lymphoid cells as reflected in the graft *vs.* host reaction

(Law et al. 1968; Goldstein et al. 1970a), in the rate of allograft rejection in both immunologically competent (Hardy et al. 1968) and incompetent (Quint et al. 1969a, b; Goldstein et al. 1970a) mice, and in the acceleration of development of resistance to a murine sarcoma virus-induced tumour in mice (Zisblatt et al. 1970). It may be noted that over 20 years ago, Kidd and his associates (cf. Kidd, 1950, 1970) provided evidence for the relation of lymphocytes to the necrobiosis of regressing cancer cells and to the role played by lymphocytes in host resistance to the proliferation of malignant cells.

The above described experiments indicating a positive influence of thymosin on cell-mediated immunological phenomena are supported by studies with an anti-thymosin serum prepared in rabbits (Hardy et al. 1968). In contrast to the acceleration of graft rejection in normal mice treated with thymosin, treatment with anti-thymosin serum delayed significantly first- and second-set allograft rejection (Hardy et al. 1968). This antiserum appears to be unique in that it crosses species lines and is cytotoxic to and agglutinates thymocytes of several species *in vitro* but not lymphocytes or spleen cells (Hardy et al. 1969). The potential uses of thymosin and anti-thymosin serum in conjunction with anti-lymphocyte serum to suppress the allograft response have been examined by Quint and his colleagues (1969a, b). These investigators observed that thymosin can either reduce or potentiate the immunosuppressive effects of mouse anti-lymphocyte serum (ALS) on cell-mediated immune processes depending upon the schedule of treatment. Thymosin, given 6 hours before ALS, prolonged allograft survival from 22 days with ALS alone, to more than 50 days. In contrast, thymosin given following ALS, partially reversed the severe immunosuppressive action of ALS. Control calf tissue extracts prepared from brain, liver and spleen were inactive under these experimental conditions (Quint et al. 1970). The mechanism underlying the action of thymosin in this system with ALS is not completely understood. It has been suggested (Quint et al. 1969b) that thymosin administration at a time prior to ALS increases the number, rate of development and/or maturation of immunologically competent cells present in the circulation and thus enables ALS to come into contact with and inactivate a large number of thymus-dependent cells.

In concluding this chapter, we wish to present an hypothesis which evolves from the newly defined roles of the thymus as an endocrine gland. This hypothesis is based upon our experimental findings in mice that thymosin, probably secreted by the reticuloepithelial cells of the thymus, can act in lieu of the thymus to restore cell-mediated immuno-logical competence in a number of experimental systems but is without action on humoral antibody synthesis (Goldstein and White 1970, 1971a, b; White and Goldstein 1970a, b). These findings suggest that there are at least two populations of thymus-dependent immunologically competent cells, in addition to at least one large class of thymus-independent cells, namely, potential antibody producing cells. The latter class includes the cells that act in cooperation with a thymus-dependent cell in the production of humoral antibody (Claman et al. 1966; Mitchell and Miller 1968).

Figure 12.1 diagrams our present concept of the maturation of the two classes of thymus-dependent, immunologically competent cells.

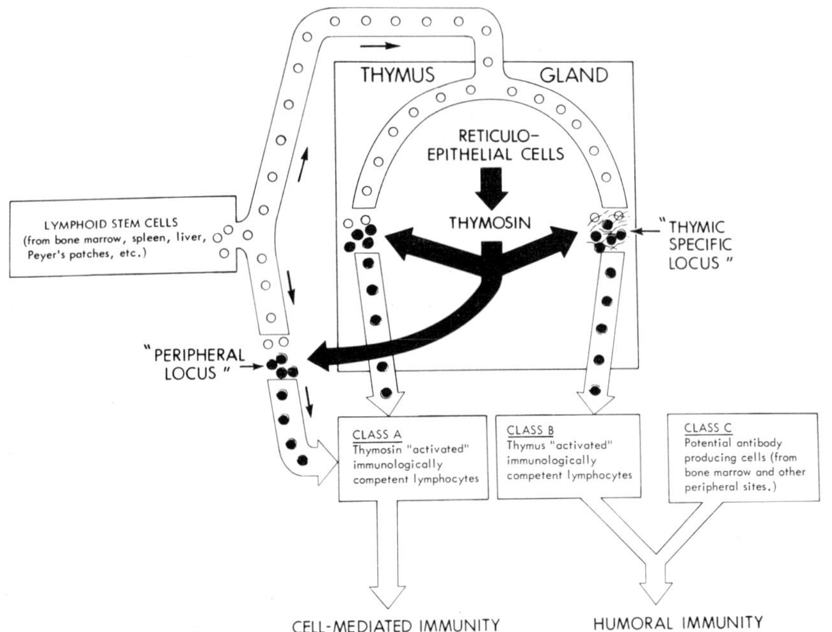

Fig. 12.1. Schematic representation of the role of thymosin in the development of immunologically competent cells. See text for details.

One type, termed *Class A cells*, can mature under the influence solely of thymosin acting upon stem cell precursors (pre- or post-thymic cell populations) from bone marrow, spleen, liver, Peyer's patches or other peripheral sites and not requiring an *in situ* thymic locus. Recent experimental findings (White and Goldstein 1970b; Bach et al. 1971; Goldstein et al. 1971) suggest that the maturation of this type of immunologically competent cell occurs rapidly and might involve derepression or activation of an incompetent cell at a specific stage in its differentiation. The development of *Class A cells* could occur either within or outside of the thymic environment. The second type of lymphocyte, which we have termed *Class B cells*, are the thymus-dependent cells involved in humoral immunity. This type of cell, once mature can recognize either soluble antigens or antigens which have been solubilized by macrophages and is capable of acting in cooperation with a population of thymus-independent cells (*Class C cells*) which contain the antibody producing mechanism and thus are necessary to elicit a humoral response. Our experimental findings indicate that the maturation of *Class B* lymphocytes requires specifically, in contrast to *Class A* lymphocytes, an intact thymic locus for proper development, as well as thymosin and/or other thymic factors. Thus, the stem cell from which *Class B* cells arise must, at some time in its development, reside within the thymus proper. The distinction between the two classes of thymus-dependent cells appears to be based upon whether or not maturation must occur within the thymic environment.

Numerous studies in the literature indicate that cells involved in cell-mediated responses are present within the thymus. It thus appears that in a normal animal the development of *Class A* cells can occur within the thymic environment, as well as peripherally. Our recent studies of the reconstitution of neonatally thymectomized mice by ad-ministration of thymosin (Law et al. 1968; Asanuma et al. 1970; Gold-stein et al. 1970a) indicate that a thymic locus is not, however, an ab-solute requirement for the maturation of these cells. It is possible that the extremely high mitotic index within the thymus is a reflection of the influence of thymic humoral factors on the maturation and/or expansion of both *Class A* and *Class B* cells that are either indigenous to the thymus or have entered the gland from the periphery.

The availability of new methods to separate distinct populations of viable lymphoid cells and the isolation and purification of thymosin offers the possibility of dissecting the intricate processes by which lymphoid cells mature and perhaps clarifying the contribution of the thymus to the normal functioning of cells of the lymphoid system.

Acknowledgements

Miss Norma Robert, Mrs. Rashalee Levine and Mr. James Oliver provided valuable technical assistance in obtaining the data referred to in this paper from our own laboratory. These data have been obtained in studies supported by grants from the Damon Runyon Fund for Cancer Research (DRG-920), the National Cancer Institute, Public Health

Service Research Grant No. CA-07470 from the American Cancer Society (P-68 and E-613), and the National Science Foundation (GB-6616X).

Allan L. Goldstein is a recipient of a Career Scientist Award of the Health Research Council of the City of New York under contract I-519.

References

AMBROSE, C. T., 1964, J. Exptl. Med. *119*, 1027.

ASANUMA, Y., A. L. GOLDSTEIN and A. WHITE, 1970, Endocrinol. *86*, 800.

BACH, J.-F., M. DARDENNE, A. L. GOLDSTEIN, A. GUHA and A. WHITE, 1971, Proc. Natl. Acad. Sci. U.S. In press.

BARONI, C., 1967a, Acta Anatomica *68*, 361.

BARONI, C., 1967b, Experientia *23*, 282.

BARONI, C. D., N. FABRIS and G. BERTOLI, 1969, Immunology *17*, 303.

BATCHELOR, J. R., 1968, Hormonal control of antibody formation. *In*: B. Cinader, ed.: Regulation of the antibody response. Springfield, Thomas. pp. 276–295.

BENACERRAF, B., 1969, Properties of antigens in relation to responsiveness and non-responsiveness. *In*: M. Landy and W. Braun, eds.: Immunological tolerance. New York, Academic Press. pp. 3–11.

BIOZZI, G., B. N. HALPERN, D. BILBERG, C. STIFFEL, B. BENACERRAF and D. MOULTON, 1957, Comp. rend. Soc. biol. *151*, 1326.

BJÖRNEBOE, M., E. E. FISCHEL and H. C. STOERK, 1951, J. Exptl. Med. *93*, 37.

BLOMGREN, H. and B. ANDERSSON, 1969, Exptl. Cell Res. *57*, 185.

BRUTON, O. C., 1952, Pediatrics *9*, 722.

BRUTON, O. C., 1968, The discovery of agammaglobulinemia. *In*: D. Bergsma, ed.: Immunological deficiency diseases in man. New York, The National Foundation. pp. 2–6.

BUCKTON, K. E. and M. C. PIKE, 1964, Nature *202*, 714.

BURNET, F. M., 1969, Cellular Immunology. London, Cambridge University Press.

CHARLES, L. M. and T. NICOL, 1961, Nature *192*, 565.

CHASE, J. H., A. WHITE and T. F. DOUGHERTY, 1946, J. Immunol. *52*, 101.

CINADER, B., ed., 1968, Regulation of the antibody response. Springfield, Thomas.

CLAMAN, H. N., E. A. CHAPERON and R. F. TRIPLETT, 1966, Proc. Soc. Exptl. Biol. Med. *122*, 1167.

COMSA, J., 1966, Arzneimittel-Forsch. *16*, 18.

CRADDOCK, C. G., A. WINKELSTEIN, Y. MATSUYUKI and J. S. LAWRENCE, 1967, J. Exptl. Med. *125*, 1149.

DESOMER, P., P. DENYS and R. LEYTEN, 1963, Life Sci. *11*, 810.

DICARLO, F. J., V. L. BEACH, L. J. HAYNES, N. J. SILVER and B. G. STANETZ, 1963, Endocrinology *73*, 170.

DIGEORGE, A. M., 1968, Congenital absence of the thymus and its immunologic consequences: concurrence with congenital hypoparathyroidism. *In*: D. Bergsma, ed.: Immunological deficiency diseases in man. New York, The National Foundation. pp. 116–123.

DOUGHERTY, T. F., 1952, Physiol. Rev. *32*, 379.

DOUGHERTY, T. F., 1955a, Effects of growth hormone on certain structures. *In*: R. W. Smith, Jr., O. H. Gaebler and C. N. H. Long, eds.: The hypophyseal growth hormone, nature and actions. New York, Blakiston. pp. 148–152.

DOUGHERTY, T. F., 1955b, Progr. Allergy *4*, 319.

DOUGHERTY, T. F., 1960, Lymphocytokaryorrhectic effects of adrenocortical steroids. *In*: J. W. Rebuck, ed.: The lymphocyte and lymphocytic tissue. New York, Hoeber. pp. 112–124.

DOUGHERTY, T. F., M. L. BERLINER, G. SCHNEEBELI and D. L. BERLINER, 1964, Ann. N.Y. Acad. Sci. *113*, 825.

DOUGHERTY, T. F., J. H. CHASE and A. WHITE, 1944, Proc. Soc. Exptl. Biol. Med. *57*, 295.

DOUGHERTY, T. F., J. H. CHASE and A. WHITE, 1945a, Proc. Soc. Exptl. Biol. Med., *58*, 135.

DOUGHERTY, T. F. and A. WHITE, 1945, Am. J. Anat. *77*, 81.

DOUGHERTY, T. F. and A. WHITE, 1947, J. Lab. Clin. Med. *32*, 584.

DOUGHERTY, T. F., A. WHITE and J. H. CHASE, 1945b, Proc. Soc. Exptl. Biol. Med. *59*, 172.

DUKOR, P. and F. M. DIETRICH, 1967, Int. Arch. Allergy *32*, 131.

DUQUESNOY, R. J., P. K. KALPAKTSOGLOU and R. A. GOOD, 1970, Proc. Soc. Exptl. Biol. Med., *133*, 201.

DUQUESNOY, R. J., G. E. RODEY, B. HOLMES and R. A. GOOD, 1969, Federation Proc. *28*, 376.

EISEN, H. N., M. M. MAYER, D. H. MOORE, R. TARR and H. C. STOERK, 1947, Proc. Soc. Exptl. Biol. Med. *65*, 301.

ELVES, M. W., 1966, The Lymphocytes. London, Lloyd-Luke.

ERNSTRÖM, U., 1965, Acta Pathol. et Microbiol. Scand. *63*, Suppl. 178.

ESTEBAN, J. N., 1968, Anat. Rec., *162*, 349.

FAGRAEUS, A., 1960, Nomenclature of immunological competent cells. *In*: G. E. W. Wolstenholme and C. M. O'Connor, eds.: Cellular aspects of immunity, Ciba Foundation Symp. Boston, Little, Brown and Co. pp. 3–4.

FARTHING, C. P., J. GERWING and J. SHEWELL, 1960a, J. Endocrinol. *21*, 83.

FARTHING, C. P., J. GERWING and J. SHEWELL, 1960b, J. Endocrinol. *21*, 91.

FISCHEL, E. E., M. LEMAY and E. A. KABAT, 1949, J. Immunol. *44*, 259.

FLEMMING, W., 1885, Arch. Mikr. Anat. *24*, 50.

FOX, C. A. and R. W. WHITEHEAD, 1936, J. Immunol. *30*, 51.

FREI, P. C., B. BENACERRAF and G. J. THORBECKE, 1965, Proc. Natl. Acad. Sci. U.S. *53*, 20.

GABRIELSEN, A. E. and R. A. GOOD, 1967, Advan. Immunol. *6*, 91.

GARDNER, W. U., T. F. DOUGHERTY and W. T. WILLIAMS, 1944, Cancer Res. *4*, 73.

GATTI, R. A., O. STUTMAN and R. A. GOOD, 1970, Ann. Rev. Physiol. *32*, 529.

GOLDSTEIN, A. L., Y. ASANUMA, J. R. BATTISTO, M. A. HARDY, J. QUINT and A. WHITE, 1970a, J. Immunol. *104*, 359.

GOLDSTEIN, A. L., Y. ASANUMA and A. WHITE, 1970b, Recent Progr. Hormone Research *26*, 505.

GOLDSTEIN, A. L., S. BANERJEE, G. L. SCHNEEBELI, T. F. DOUGHERTY and A. WHITE, 1970c, Rad. Research *41*, 579.

GOLDSTEIN, A. L., A. GUHA, M. L. HOWE and A. WHITE, 1971, J. Immunol. *106*, 713.

GOLDSTEIN, A. L., F. D. SLATER and A. WHITE, 1966, Proc. Natl. Acad. Sci. U.S. *56*, 1010.

GOLDSTEIN, A. L. and A. WHITE, 1970, The thymus as an endocrine gland: hormones and their actions. *In*: G. Litwack, ed., Biochemical actions of hormones, Vol. 1. New York, Academic Press. pp. 465–502.

GOLDSTEIN, A. L. and A. WHITE, 1971a, Advan. Metabolic Disorders *5*, 149.

GOLDSTEIN, A. L. and A. WHITE, 1971b, Role of thymosin and other thymic factors in the development, maturation and functions of lymphoid tissue. *In*: V. H. T. James and L. Martini, eds., Current topics in experimental endocrinology, Vol. 1. New York, Academic Press. In Press.

GOOD, R. A. and A. E. GABRIELSON, eds., 1964, The thymus in immunobiology. Structure, function and role in disease. New York, Hoeber-Harper.

GOWANS, J. L., 1965, Brit. Med. Bull. *21*, 106.

GOWANS, J. L., D. D. MCGREGOR, D. M. COWAN and C. E. FORD, 1962, Nature *196*, 651.

GYLLENSTEN, L., 1962, Acta Pathol. Microbiol. Scand. *56*, 29.

HALPERN, B., G. MAURIC, A. HOLTZER and M. BRIOT, 1951, Acta Allergol. *4*, 207.

HALPERN, B., G. MAURIC, A. HOLTZER and M. BRIOT, 1952, J. Allergy *23*, 303.

HAMMOND, C. W. and M. NOVAK, 1950, Proc. Soc. Exptl. Biol. Med. *74*, 155.

HARDY, M. A., J. QUINT, A. L. GOLDSTEIN, D. STATE and A. WHITE, 1968, Proc. Natl. Acad. Sci. U.S. *61*, 875.

HARDY, M. A., J. QUINT, A. L. GOLDSTEIN, A. WHITE, D. STATE and J. R. BATTISTO, 1969, Proc. Soc. Exptl. Biol. Med. *130*, 214.

HARRIS, T. N., E. GRIMM, E. MERTENS and W. E. EHRICH, 1945, J. Exptl. Med. *81*, 73.

HAYASHIDA, T. and C. H. LI, 1957, J. Exptl. Med. *105*, 93.

HESS, M. W., 1968, Experimental thymectomy. Possibilities and limitations. Berlin, Springer.

HUMPHREY, J. F., 1969, The fate of antigens and its relationship to the immune response. The complexity of antigens. *In*: E. Sorkin, ed.: The immune response and its suppression. New York, Karger. pp. 7–23.

JANKOVIC, B. D., K. ISAKOVIC and J. HORVAT, 1965, Nature *208*, 356.

JOHNSTONE, D. E., J. W. HOWLAND and S. MICHAELSON, 1962, J. Allergy *33*, 6.

KIDD, J. G., 1950, Proc. Inst. Med. Chicago *18*, 50.

KIDD, J. G., 1970, Morphological findings in relation to immune reactions against cancer with special reference to the part played by lymphocytes in overcoming transplanted cancer cells as they grow in alien hosts. *In*: L. Severi, ed.: Immunity and tolerance in oncogenesis. Univ. of Perugia, pp. 63–88.

LANCE, E. M. and S. COOPER, 1970, Part II effects of cortisol and antilymphocyte serum on lymphoid populations. *In*: G. E. W. Wolstenholme and J. Knight, eds.: Hormones and the immune response. London, Churchill. pp. 13–99.

LANDY, M. and W. BRAUN, eds., 1969, Immunological tolerance. New York, Academic Press.

LA VIA, M. F., F. W. FITCH, C. H. GUNDERSON and R. H. WISSLER, 1960, The relation of antibody formation to reticuloendothelial structure and function. *In*: J. H. Heller, ed.: Reticuloendothelial structure and function. New York, Ronald Press. pp. 45–63.

LAW, L. W. and H. D. AGNEW, 1968, Proc. Soc. Exptl. Biol. and Med. *127*, 953.

LAW, L. W., A. L. GOLDSTEIN and A. WHITE, 1968, Nature, *219*, 1391.

LAWRENCE, H. W. and M. LANDY, eds., 1969, Mediators of cellular immunity. New York, Academic Press.

LEVINE, M. A. and H. N. CLAMAN, 1970, Science *167*, 1515.

LING, N. R., 1968, Lymphocyte stimulation. Amsterdam, North-Holland.

LITTLE, J. R., G. BRECHER, T. R. BRADLEY and S. ROSE, 1962, Blood *19*, 236.

LONG, D. A. and J. SHEWELL, 1955, Brit. J. Exptl. Pathol. *36*, 351.

LUNDIN, P. M., 1958, Acta Endocrinologia *28*, Suppl. 40.

LURIE, M. B., 1960, Ann. N.Y. Acad Sci. *88*, 83.

MCMASTER, P. D., 1953, Sites of antibody formation, *In*: A. M. Pappenheimer, Jr., ed.: The significance of the antibody response. New York, Columbia University Press. pp. 13–45.

MCMILLAN, D. B. and V. E. ENGELBERT, 1963, Am. J. Pathol., *42*, 315.

METCALF, D., 1965, Nature, *208*, 1336.

METCALF, D., 1966, The thymus. Its role in immune responses, leukaemia development and carcinogenesis. New York, Springer-Verlag.

METCHNIKOFF, E., 1905, Immunity in infective diseases (transl. from the French by F. G. Binnie). Cambridge University Press.

MILLER, J. F. A. P., 1965, Nature *208*, 1337.

MILLER, J. F. A. P. and J. G. HOWARD, 1964, J. Reticuloendothelial Soc. *1*, 369.

MILLER, J. F. A. P., E. LEUCHARS, A. M. CROSS and P. DUKOR, 1964, Ann. N.Y. Acad. Sci. *120*, 205.

MILLER, J. F. A. P. and D. OSOBA, 1967, Physiol. Rev. *47*, 437.

MILLER, J. J., III and L. J. COLE, 1967, J. Exptl. Med., *126*, 109.

MITCHELL, G. F. and MILLER, J. F. A. P., 1968, J. Exptl. Med., *128*, 821.

MITCHISON, N. A., 1969, Cell populations involved in immune responses. *In*: M. Landy and W. Braun, eds.: Immunological tolerance. New York, Academic Press. pp. 115–116, 178–179.

MONACO, A. P., M. L. WOOD and P. S. RUSSELL, 1965, Science *149*, 432.

MOON, H. D., M. E. SIMPSON, C. H. LI and H. M. EVANS, 1950, Cancer Res. *10*, 297.

MOOD, H. D., M. E. SIMPSON, C. H. LI and H. M. EVANS, 1952, Cancer Res. *12*, 448.

MORROW, S. H. and N. R. DILUZIO, 1965, Nature, *205*, 193.

NICOL, T., 1935, Trans. Roy. Soc. Edinburgh *58*, 449.

NICOL, T. and D. L. J. BILBEY, 1960, The effects of various steroids on the phagocytic activity of the reticuloendothelial system. *In*: J. H. Heller, ed.: Reticuloendothelial structure and function (Ronald Press, New York) pp. 301–320.

NICOL, T. and I. D. HELMY, 1951, Nature *167*, 199.

NICOL, T. and B. VERNON-ROBERTS, 1965a, J. Reticuloendothelial Soc. *2*, 15.

NICOL, T. and B. VERNON-ROBERTS, 1965b, J. Reticuloendothelial Soc. *2*, 351.

NILSEN, Å., 1957, Acta Allergol. *11*, 45.

PARROTT, D. M. V., M. A. B. DESOUSSA and J. EAST, 1966, J. Exptl. Med. *123*, 191.

PERLA, D. and MARMORSTON, J., 1941, Natural resistance and clinical medicine. Boston, Little, Brown and Co.

PETERSON, R. D. A. and R. A. GOOD, 1968, Ataxia-Telangiectasia, *In*: D. Bergsma, ed: Immunological deficiency diseases in man. New York, The National Foundation. pp. 370–377.

PIERPAOLI, W., C. BARONI, N. FABRUS and E. SORKIN, 1969, Immunology *16*, 217.

PIERPAOLI, W. and E. SORKIN, 1968a, Brit. J. Exptl. Pathol. *49*, 288.

PIERPAOLI, W. and E. SORKIN, 1968b, J. Immunol. *101*, 1036.

PIERPAOLI, W. and E. SORKIN, 1969, Effect of growth hormone and anti-growth hormone serum on the lymphatic tissue and the immune response. *In*: E. Sorkin, ed.: The immune response and its suppression. New York, Karger. pp. 122–134.

QUINT, J., M. A. HARDY and A. P. MONACO, 1969a, Federation Proc. *28*, 694.

QUINT, J., M. A. HARDY and A. P. MONACO, 1969b, Surg. Forum *20*, 252.

QUINT, J., M. A. HARDY and A. P. MONACO, 1970, private communication.

ROBERTS, S., E. ADAMS and A. WHITE, 1948, J. Biol. Chem. *174*, 379.

ROBERTS, S., E. ADAMS and A. WHITE, 1949, J. Immunol. *62*, 155.

ROWLEY, D., 1966, Experientia *22*, 1.

SCHATTEN, W. E., D. M. BERGENSTAL, W. M. KARMER and H. WEXLER, 1958, Plastic Reconstruc. Surg. *21*, 20.

SCHOOLEY, J. C., L. S. KELLY, E. L. DOBSON, C. R. FINNEY, V. W. HAVENS and L. N. CANTOR, 1965, J. Reticuloendothelial Soc. *2*, 396.

SELA, M., 1969, Effects of antigen dosage, *In*: M. Landy and W. Braun, eds.: Immunological tolerance. New York, Academic Press. pp. 99–101.

SELA, M., B. SCHECHTER, I. SCHECHTER and F. BOREK, 1967, Antibodies to sequential and conformational determinants. *In*: L. Frisch, ed.: Cold Spring Harbor Symposia on Quantitative Biology, Vol. XXXII. New York. pp. 537–545.

SELYE, H., 1946, J. Clin Endocrinol. *6*, 117.

SHEWELL, J. and D. A. LONG, 1957, J. Hyg. *57*, 202.

SHREWSBURY, M. M. and W. O. REINHARDT, 1959, Endocrinology *65*, 858.

SNELL, J. F., 1960, Relationship of chromium phosphate clearance rates to resistance: 1. The effects of some corticosteroids on blood clearance rates in mice, *In*: J. H. Heller, ed.: Reticuloendothelial structure and function. New York, Ronald Press. pp. 321–322.

SNELL, R. S. and T. NICOL, 1957, Nature *179*, 473.

SORKIN, E., ed., 1969, The immune response and its suppression. New York, Karger.

SZEGO, C. M. and A. WHITE, 1949, Endocrinology *44*, 150.

SZEGO, C. M. and A. WHITE, 1951, Endocrinology *48*, 576.

TAKAKURA, K., H. YAMADA and V. P. HOLLANDER, 1967, Cancer Res. *27*, 2034.

TAYLOR, R. B., 1965, Nature *208*, 1334.

THORBECKE, G. J. and B. BENACERRAF, 1962, Progr. Allergy *6*, 559.

TRAININ, N., M. BURGER and M. LINKER-ISRAELI, 1968, Restoration of homograft response in neonatally thymectomized mice by a thymic humoral factor (THF). *In*: J. Dausset, J. Hamburger and E. Mathé, eds.: Advance in transplantation. Baltimore, Williams and Wilkins. pp. 91–95.

TRAININ, N. and M. LINKER-ISRAELI, 1967, Cancer Res. *27*, 309.

TRAPANI, I. L., A. LEIN and D. H. CAMPBELL, 1959, Nature *183*, 982.

WARNER, N. L. 1964, Australian J. Exptl. Biol. Med. Sci. *42*, 401.

WARNER, N. L. and A. SZENBERG, Ann. Rev. Microbiol. *18*, 253.

WHITE, A., 1948, Harvey Lectures *43*, 43.

WHITE, A., 1949a, Ann. Rev. Physiol. *11*, 355.

WHITE, A., 1949b, Annals Otology, Rhinology and Laryngology *58*, 523.

WHITE, A., 1958, Ann. N.Y. Acad. Sci. *73*, 79.

WHITE, A., 1963, Ann. Allergy *21*, 417.

WHITE, A. and A. L. GOLDSTEIN, 1968, Perspectives Biol. Med. *11*, 475.

WHITE, A. and A. L. GOLDSTEIN, 1970a, The role of the thymus gland in the hormonal regulation of host resistance, *In*: G. E. W. Wolstenholme and J. Knight, eds.: Control processes in multicellular organisms, Ciba Foundation Symp. London, Churchill. pp. 210–237.

WHITE, A. and A. L. GOLDSTEIN, 1970b, Thymosin, a thymic hormone influencing lymphoid cell immunological competence. *In*: G. E. W. Wolstenholme and J. Knight, eds.: Hormones and the immune response, Ciba Foundation Symp. London, Churchill. pp. 3–23.

WOLF, B. and S. D. ERB, 1971, Proc. 4th Leukocyte Culture Conf. Philadelphia, Appleton, Century, Croft. pp. 207–217.

WOLSTENHOLME, G. E. W. and C. M. O'CONNOR, eds., 1960, Cellular aspects of immunity, Ciba Foundation Symp. Boston, Little, Brown and Co.

ZISBLATT, M., A. L. GOLDSTEIN, F. LILLY and A. WHITE, 1970, Proc. Natl. Acad. Sci. U.S. *66*, 1170.

CHAPTER 13

Effects of antimetabolites and other pharmacological agents

M. EARL BALIS

Division of Cell Metabolism, Sloan-Kettering Institute for Cancer Research, New York, N.Y.

13.1. Introduction

Potential sites of immunosuppression are:
  (1) activation and recognition of antigen
  (2) preparation for antibody synthesis
  (3) synthesis and release of antibody.
The first and second involve synthesis and function of nucleic acids and proteins in specialized ways. The third in this context can be viewed as a special case of protein synthesis, with the usual needs for messenger, transfer, and ribosomal nucleic acids, and the enzymes and structural entities of protein synthesis. It is obvious that interference with the activation and synthesis of any substance pecularily required for processes one and two might specifically prevent the immunological reaction without necessarily producing other direct effects. On the other hand, inhibition of protein synthesis might well be generally toxic. Thus, it is not possible to design an antimetabolite which can specifically inhibit immune response until the molecular mechanisms of the process are understood. Most of the metabolite antagonists which have been shown to be active inhibitors of the immune process are substances known to inhibit protein and nucleic acid synthesis in general. This empirical knowledge that certain substances can block antibody production can be enlightening indicators of the biochemistry of immunological reactions.

No matter how immunosuppression is achieved on the empirical basis of the active compounds known, it would appear that it is a special manifestation of inhibition of the synthesis and function of nucleic acids and/or proteins. Thus, the effective inhibitors can be classified and studied as inhibitors of the metabolism of nucleic acid intermediates, inhibitors of nucleic acid *per se*, and inhibitors of protein synthesis.

13.2. Inhibition of nucleic acid intermediates

Control of nucleic acid synthesis and function can be exerted by antimetabolites which interfere with syntheses and transformations of the purine and pyrimidine nucleotides. Many substances have been found which function in this way and several have powerful immunosuppressive potential.

13.2.1. Purine metabolism

Presumably all anabolic transformations of purines occur at the nucleotide levels. In most systems there are two enzymes which convert purines to nucleotides (pyrophosphorylases), one acts on adenine, adenosine 5'-monophosphate (AMP): pyrophosphate phosphoribosyltransferase, the other on hypoxanthine and guanine, inosine 5'-monophosphate (IMP): pyrophosphate phosphoribosyltransferase (Kornberg et al. 1955; Korn et al. 1955). The adenylate pyrophosphorylase also uses 2,6-diaminopurine as a substrate (Fig. 13.1) (Remy and Smith

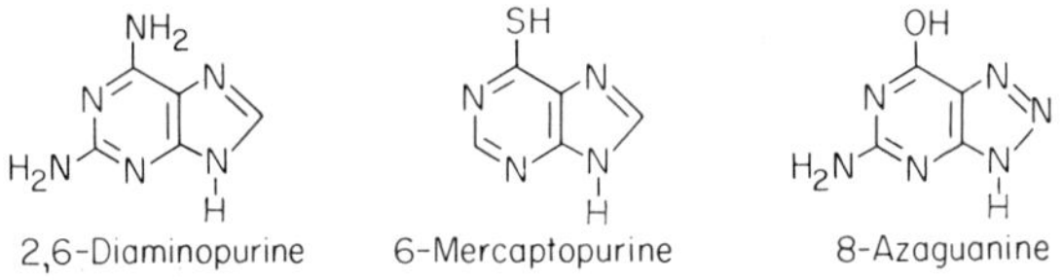

2,6-Diaminopurine   6-Mercaptopurine   8-Azaguanine

Fig. 13.1.

1957); that for inosinate and guanylate also converts 6-mercaptopurine (Fig. 13.1) (Lukens and Herrington 1957), and 8-azaguanine (Fig. 13.1) (Way and Parks 1958) to ribonucleotides.

The first step of purine synthesis is considered to be the reaction between phosphoribosylpyrophosphate and glutamine because this reaction is the point at which feedback inhibition is exerted (Caskey et al. 1964; Nierlich and Magasanik 1965). That analogues of naturally occurring purines might interfere with the normal synthesis *de novo* of purines and also possibly with their interconversion has been recognized for some time. For example, 2,6-diaminopurine, an analogue of a naturally occurring purine, was shown to be a precursor of polynucleotide guanine in the rat (Bendich and Brown 1948; Bendich et al. 1950). No evidence of incorporation of unchanged diaminopurine into polynucleotides has been detected, and very little conversion into nucleic acid adenine is found. In a similar way, 6-mercaptopurine (6-MP) can serve as a substrate, be converted into the normal nucleic acid purines, and reduce normal purine synthesis in several strains of *Streptococcus faecalis* (Balis et al. 1958). Unlike diaminopurine, small amounts of 6-MP and thioguanine are incorporated as the unnatural purine, thioguanine (Scannell and Hitchings 1966).

In 1959, Gots and Gollub postulated that purine analogues could, as their nucleotides, prevent synthesis *de novo* of purines by a type of pseudo feedback inhibition. They further suggested that the three most potent analogs, 2,6-diaminopurine, 6-MP, and 6-thioguanine, may owe some of their inhibitory activity to this feedback mechanism. Substance was lent to this concept by the demonstration of McCollister et al. (1964) that thioinosinate could serve as a feedback inhibitor of amidotransferase, and there is no question that *in vitro* this nucleotide does act as an analogue of the natural ribonucleotides in inhibiting the first step of purine synthesis. The possibility that the mechanism found *in vitro* is operative *in vivo* was investigated extensively by Bennett et al. (1963) who studied the utilization of various purine precursors in animals treated with 6-MP. The expected blockade by 6-MP of the utilization of small precursors was extensive, while the uptake of purines *per se* was not reduced, so the contention that 6-MP acts *in vivo* by feedback inhibition of purine synthesis has experimental support. The biologic significance of analogue feedback is not easily evaluated, however.

The inhibition of purine synthesis produced by 6-MP usually has been determined shortly after the administration of the inhibitor. Since the better-seen biological effects are often the result of a sequence of metabolic events, this short-term inhibition of purine synthesis doubtless triggers a chain of subsequent events. A series of studies on formate incorporation, made one and eight days after administration of 6-MP, predictably produced a somewhat different pattern (Salser et al. 1967). Extensive inhibition of purine synthesis in some tissues was seen eight days after administration of a single dose of 6-MP, and both kidney and liver synthesized more soluble nucleotide when the animals had received 6-MP twenty-four hours vs. eight days prior to the incorporation study, i.e., the total effect of 6-MP may differ from tissue to tissue. That these effects last so long after the administration of the inhibitor indicates that none of the proposed explanations is complete.

Azathioprine (6[(1-methyl-4-nitroimidazole-5-yl)thio]purine) is a derivative of 6-MP that acts by similar or identical biochemical mechanisms (Elion et al. 1963). This compound has assumed a role of major significance as an immunosuppressant. The biochemical basis for its unique value relative to 6-MP is not completely apparent.

Thioguanylic acid as a purine nucleotide analog inhibits a number of steps in purine metabolism. Like 6-thio IMP, 6-thio GMP is an inhibitor of the amidotransferase (Wyngaarden and Ashton 1955), and this probably plays some role in its activity (Sartorelli and Lepage 1958). It has been shown that 6-thio GMP inhibits IMP dehydrogenase (Miech et al. 1967), thus leading to a decrease in available supplies of guanine nucleotides. On the other hand, 6-thio GMP does not necessarily produce inhibition per se, since as was shown with the Mecca lymphosarcoma, the accumulation of 6-thio GMP does not necessarily lead to inhibition of growth (Lepage et al. 1964). Thus, it appears that there may be two general metabolic areas which are sensitive to 6-thioguanylate: (1) incorporation into DNA and (2) an analogue inhibition resembling that seen with 6-MP.

The first purine derivative synthesized *de novo* is inosinic acid. This compound is converted enzymatically in two steps to adenylic acid and guanylic acid (Fig. 13.2). Not surprisingly, analogue nucleotides

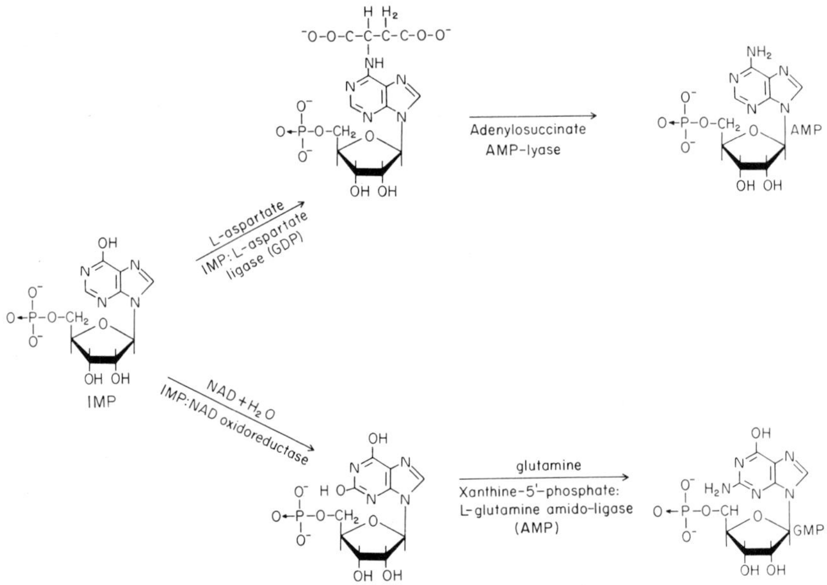

Fig. 13.2.

can inhibit these reactions and much of the antimetabolic activity of 6-MP is attributable to such a blockade by its nucleotide, 6-thioinosinate. This analogue nucleotide is formed by the action of the same enzyme that converts hypoxanthine to inosinate. Studies of cell-free preparations (Salser et al. 1969) showed that the first reaction of the sequence which leads to AMP is inhibited by thioinosinate. Studies with crude extracts containing inosinate dehydrogenase activity indicated in a similar manner, that inhibition of xanthylate synthesis can be brought about by thio-inosinate. It is, of course, difficult to be sure what the concentrations of particular precursors are at critical sites within the cell, but certainly the concentration of thioinosinate decreases extremely rapidly, shortly after administration of 6-MP (Salser and Balis 1965).

The antibiotic, mycophenolic acid, inhibits the conversion of inosinic acid to xanthylic acid and of xanthylic acid to guanylic acid (Franklin and Cook 1969).

Mitchell et al. (1950) showed that 8-azaguanine-^{14}C is incorporated into the nucleic acids of tumour-bearing mice. Up to 40% of the RNA guanine of *Bacillus cereus* may be replaced by 8-azaguanine (Smith and Matthews 1957). Even though extensive substitution of 8-azaguanine for guanine can occur in RNA, very little, if any, of the analogue is found in DNA (Mandel et al. 1954).

A major amount of azaguanine is incorporated into the transfer RNA (Levin 1963). Analysis of 8-azaguanine-containing transfer RNA revealed that only guanine residues are replaced by the analogue, and that the nucleotide sequence is not otherwise altered. However, the analogue-containing RNA has less secondary structure, as evidenced by a diminution in the temperature-dependent hyperchromicity (Levin and Litt 1965). This analogue-containing transfer RNA does, however, appear to function normally despite the fact that one might predict *a priori* that slight alterations in the structure of tRNA might so alter the specificity that miscoding would result (Weinstein and Grunberger 1965; Levin 1965).

The suggestion has been made that 6-thioguanine exerts its inhibitory action by virtue of its incorporation into nucleic acid (Lepage 1960). More specifically, it was found that the incorporation is primarily into DNA in susceptible tumours, and largely into RNA in resistant lines (Lepage and Jones 1961). Both ring-labelled and sulphur-labelled mercaptopurines have also been shown to be incorporated into DNA. Surprisingly the bulk of the material in the DNA was found to be in the form of 6-thioguanine deoxyribonucleoside derivatives (Scannell and Hitchings 1966). Since exogenous 6-MP yields as much DNA-linked deoxythioguanosine as does exogenous 6-thioguanine itself, it would seem most unlikely that the incorporation of this amount of thioguanine into DNA is the cause of the inhibition exerted by 6-thioguanine.

13.2.2. *Pyrimidine metabolism*

The regulation of pyrimidine synthesis apparently takes place at the point of carbamoyl aspartate synthesis (Yates and Pardee 1956). Despite the well-defined feedback system, and although pyrimidine analogues (or their derivatives) do act as inhibitors *in vitro*, there has been little or no evidence that their analogues exert their *in vivo* activity primarily by mimicking feedback inhibition, as has been suggested for several purine derivatives. There are, however, examples where such behaviour is at least partially responsible for the activity of analogues, e.g., 5-fluoro-cytosine, 6-azauracil and 6-azauridine, inhibit aspartate carbamoyl-transferase (Smith and Sullivan 1960; Bresnick and Hitchings 1961).

13.2.3. Pyrimidine interconversion

The action primarily responsible for the major inhibitory effects of most of the antifolates is the inhibition of folic reductase, the enzyme that catalyses the reduction of both folic acid and dihydrofolic acid (DHF) to tetrahydrofolic acids (THF).

Studies of the fate of injected methotrexate in experimental animals have revealed that some of the material remains in host tissues for many months although most of the compound is rapidly eliminated (Fountain et al. 1953). Similar observations have been made in man (Condit 1960). As only a small amount can be bound at any one time, administration of larger amounts is not much more effective because the excess is rapidly eliminated.

Non-dividing tissues, such as liver and kidney, have large stores of tetrahydrofolate. However, many rapidly dividing tissues contain much smaller amounts of this cofactor (Nichol 1953). The more rapidly growing tissues are constantly oxidizing the tetrahydrofolate derivatives into di-hydrofolate in the process of synthesizing thymidylate. Not surprising-ly, the tissues which normally contain higher amounts of folate are the tissues which bind the largest amount of methotrexate (Fountain et al. 1952); these are also the tissues with the largest amount of dihydrofolate reductase (Bertino et al. 1964; Werkheiser 1961), so that the cells which concentrate the largest amount of inhibitor are not necessarily the ones most affected by the compound.

Evans et al. (1961) showed that arabinosyl cytosine (Ara-C) is inhibitory to a number of transplanted tumours in mice, but ineffective against rat tumour cultures (Chu and Fischer 1962). The incorporation of tritiated uridine into RNA of these cells is not suppressed by Ara-C but the synthesis of DNA is. The inhibition of DNA formation could be reversed by the addition of deoxycytidine. These findings led to the proposal that Ara-C acts by interfering with the conversion of cytosine nucleotides to corresponding deoxycytidine derivatives.

Regardless of the specific mechanism of inhibition, phosphorylation is probably a necessary step in the inactivation of Ara-C. This is sup-ported by the fact that a variety of resistant cells lack the Ara-C kinase and these cells are deficient in their ability to transport the inhibitor into the cells. The activity of Ara-C depends to a large extent not only on its conversion to the nucleotide but also inversely on the activity of the degradation enzyme. That the deamination of Ara-U can be of significance in living cells is shown by the fact that addition of Ara-U to cells growing in tissue culture tends to minimize the deamination of Ara-C (Smith et al. 1965). It is also quite possible that Ara-C is a substrate for deoxycytidine 5′-monophosphate deaminase.

13.3. Inhibitors of nucleic acid intermediates as immunosuppressants

A variety of analogues of the naturally occurring purines have been studied, and many shown to have immunosuppressant properties. Malmgren et al. (1952) demonstrated that 2,6-diaminopurine can block the production of antibodies against sheep red cells in mice. Much of the current interest in the action of metabolic antagonists against immunization resulted from the demonstration by Schwartz et al. (1958) that 6-MP would completely suppress antibody response in rabbits. Azathioprine, Imuran, a derivative of 6-mercaptopurine, which is used extensively in clinical immunosuppressive regimens probably acts by virtue of the fact that it is cleaved to 6-mercaptopurine *in vivo* (Elion et al. 1963). It has an advantage over 6-MP clinically, in that it appears to be less toxic to the epithelium of the gut, which reduces the toxicity normally associated with 6-mercaptopurine. 6-Thioguanine, which in many ways behaves similarly to 6-mercaptopurine, but whose mechanism of action is probably not identical also inhibits antibody production in mice (Nathan et al. 1961). 6-Thioguanine has been used rather little clinically as an immunosuppressant. However, in view of the fact that in some patients it has been a valuable substitute for 6-mercaptopurine in the therapy of leukaemia because of rare idiosyncrasies it is possible that it may have some value clinically as an immunosuppressant (I. H. Krakoff, personal communication).

Alanosine, though an analog not of a purine, but apparently of aspartate, a compound important in purine intermediary metabolism, has also been shown to be effective as an immunosuppressant (Gale et al. 1968; Fumarola 1969). Mycophenolic acid which blocks the other interconversion of inosinic acid, that leading to guanylic acid, has also been found to be active (Mitsui et al. 1969).

8-Azaguanine is one of the first purine analogues to be shown by Malmgren et al. (1952) to have some immunosuppressive activity. This compound has not received any great clinical trial possibly because of the high toxicity noted when it was given as a possible antitumour agent, and possibly because of the inconsistent results observed by Šterzl (1961). Some of the lack of reproducibility found in the earlier tests of this analogue may be attributed to the fact that early samples were quite impure, and often may not have been purified prior to administration to the experimental animals. Recently Uteshev et al. (1969) reported immunological response in mice was completely inhibited by azaguanine, administered subcutaneously, 10 mg/kg/daily × 4, beginning at the time of immunization. They suggested that azaguanine works in mice immunized with soluble antigen, but not in rabbits with corpuscular antigen and that the effect is selective, working on some antibodies, not others.

The results of attempts to inhibit the immune process with pyrimidine analogues have been relatively unsuccessful. The activity of arabinosylcytosine is mentioned below as an inhibitor of DNA. Somewhat better effects have been claimed for a derivative of Ara-C (adamantoyl arabinosylcytosine) (Gray and Mickelson 1970).

Uphoff and Pitkin (1962) and Thomas et al. (1962) demonstrated that it is possible to induce tolerance through the use of methotrexate, a compound which has a variety of inhibitory effects, but probably is most effective by virtue of its inhibition of DNA formation through blockade of thymidine phosphate synthesis. The possibility that even more useful immunosuppressive effects can be achieved with drugs currently available by altered therapeutic regimens is demonstrated by dosage-related protection seen with methotrexate (Storb et al. 1970). These workers were able to obtain long term survival of marrow grafts with long-term therapy even in mismatched dogs while other regimens were far less effective.

Several workers have examined the possible mechanism of action of antifolates on the immune response. Turk and his associates (Turk 1964; Diengdoh and Turk 1966; Turk and Stone 1963) in a series of studies, showed that the uptake of thymidine was not reduced by treatment with methotrexate, but that the uptake of uridine and leucine was reduced. This was interpreted as suggesting that interference with RNA rather than DNA metabolism was at the basis of the immunosuppressive action. They had shown that methotrexate prevented the development of immunoblasts in the lymph nodes and that furthermore, increases in glucose-6-phosphate dehydrogenase and alkaline phosphatase that followed antigenic stimulation were blocked by methotrexate. Though one cannot question their observations, their interpretation of them is in doubt, since the action of methotrexate is on the synthesis of thymidylic acid from deoxyuridylic acid, the administration of tracer doses of thymidine should actually show an increased uptake, since there would be less dilution with endogenous thymidylate. The fortuitous observation that there was no major change in uptake therefore sheds little light on the biochemical action. On the other hand, if cell division is decreased, and if the conversion of deoxyuridine and thymidylate is inhibited, there should be a reduced uptake of uridine, and inhibited cells would be expected to synthesize less protein. Thus, their interpretation of the mechanism of action as independent of the usual blockade of dihydrofolate reductase has probably not been established.

Berenbaum and Brown (1965) have noted that despite the fact that the toxicity of folic acid can sometimes be reversed by later administration of folinic acid, a similar reversal of the immunological inhibition is not seen. Berenbaum and Brown suggested the explanation that the stimulated immunological cells are unable to withstand folic acid deficiency for as long a period of time as gut and bone marrow. One reason might be that all the stimulated cells enter into S phase at the same time, while in the intestine and the marrow, many of the cells which are potentially inhibited by the binding of antifolate to folate reductase would suffer no ill effects until they enter into S phase. Those cells which are either in G_0 or those which have just come out of S phase would be safe for a long time. This observation, if it can be extended, might serve as a basis for a very useful protocol in the clinical use of immunosuppressant agents. If it is generally true, toxic doses of inhibitors could be given followed shortly thereafter, as was done in this case, by agents which would reverse the toxicity in host cells, but be unable to reverse the immunosuppressant action.

The recent demonstration of inhibitory effects of cyclic AMP on antibody synthesis by spleen cells *in vitro* (Gericke et al. 1970) suggests a new approach to the problem. Since endogenous cyclic AMP levels are subject to regulation by a variety of drugs as well as hormones, it might be possible to effect secondary immunosuppression with them. Cyclic AMP has been shown to change the rate of mitosis of thymine lymphocytes (MacManus and Whitfield 1969), and some tumour lines in culture (Heidrick and Ryan 1970). It thus may be that it can act also by blocking proliferation of competent cells.

13.4. Nucleic acid synthesis and function

Several functional roles in the immunologic process have been ascribed to DNA and the various RNA's. Thus, some drugs which affect these macromolecules might be expected to be immunosuppressive. The syntheses of these complex polynucleotides are subject to many kinds of inhibitors.

13.4.1. Compounds binding DNA

A large number of antibiotics and synthetic polycyclic molecules have the requisite properties to bind nucleic acids and, as a consequence, prevent transcription and duplication of the polymer. Some of the most potent members of this class of compounds are the actinomycins, the most active of which is actinomycin D (Fig. 13.3). In extremely small

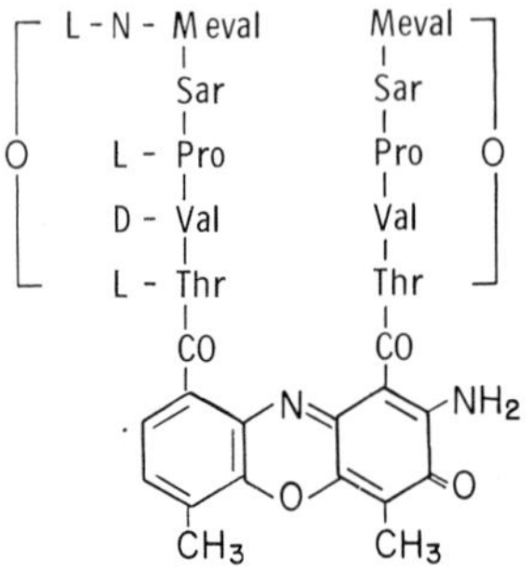

Fig. 13.3.

concentrations actinomycin D is toxic to both mammalian cells (Reich et al. 1961) and microorganisms (Kirk 1960). Actinomycin D is toxic by virtue of its inhibitory effect on RNA synthesis (Kirk 1960; Reich et al. 1961; Harbers and Muller 1962), and it does not normally inhibit DNA synthesis.

With concentrations of actinomycin that produce partial inhibition of growth, there is differential inhibition of the synthesis of various classes of RNA (Perry 1962; Georgiev et al. 1963; Franklin 1963; Revel and Hiatt 1964), while with higher concentrations, all RNA synthesis is blocked (Reich et al. 1962b). Additional insight into the mechanism by which the inhibition is exerted is gained from the fact that the antibiotic also inhibits the action of RNA polymerase *in vitro* (Goldberg and Rabinowitz 1962; Reich et al. 1962a). Just as DNA synthesis is less sensitive than is RNA synthesis *in vivo*, DNA polymerase is much less sensitive to the antibiotic than is RNA polymerase *in vitro* (Kirk 1960; Hurwitz et al. 1962). In studies of a variety of different actinomycins, it was found that the extent of the inhibition of polymerase is proportional to the ability of the antibiotic to complex with DNA (Reich et al. 1962a; Hartmann et al. 1962).

The DNA-actinomycin complexes are relatively stable, as is demonstrated by their resistance to dissociation by electrophoresis (Kawamata and Imanishi 1961), dialysis (Kirk 1960), ultracentrifugation (Rauen et al. 1960), or passage through molecular exclusion gels (Hartmann et al. 1962).

Actinomycin binds very poorly to crab DNA, which is low in guanine and cytosine, and not at all to synthetic poly deoxyadenylatethymidylate mixtures; furthermore, it is inhibitory only when bound. These facts led to the suggestion that guanine in the helical configuration is necessary for that binding of actinomycin to DNA which leads to its activity. Furthermore, the amount of actinomycin bound parallels the guanine content of the DNA but is not directly proportional to it (Goldberg et al. 1962). The need for the double stranded structure is shown by the fact that maximal binding by single stranded DNA is far less than that with the equivalent amount of native DNA. That the binding sites on DNA surface may be related spatially to the sites of attachment of RNA polymerase is suggested by the finding that DNA bound to RNA polymerase is displaced by actinomycin. Actinomycin may, in binding to DNA, block the sites normally occupied by the enzyme (Reich and Goldberg 1964; Goldberg et al. 1963).

X-ray diffraction studies of DNA containing one molecule of actinomycin for every eighteen nucleotides led to the proposal of a model for the actinomycin-DNA complex (Hamilton et al. 1963), in which the actinomycin is attached directly to the guanine 7-nitrogen and its deoxyribose moiety, and is bound in the minor groove of the helical DNA by 7 hydrogen bonds. This model accounts for the role of the functional groups of actinomycin which are essential and for the observed biological and biochemical activity of the antibiotic.

Though a variety of effects have been attributed to actinomycin, its principal action at lower concentrations is undoubtedly due to specific binding to DNA guanine which prevents normal transcription.

The binding of proflavine to nucleic acid has been well established (Peacocke and Skerrett 1956; Freifelder et al. 1961; Lerman 1961; Kleinwachter and Koudelka 1964). In the presence of proflavine, the *in vitro* synthesis of DNA and RNA is blocked (Hurwitz et al. 1962). The complex formed by proflavine and DNA is more stable than any enzyme-DNA complex. Also, acridine orange and acriflavine each protect DNA from hydrolysis by DNase (Leith 1963). That this may also be the basis of the *in vivo* activity follows from the fact that the synthesis of DNA in cells treated with acriflavine is greatly inhibited while protein and RNA synthesis are less so (Pecora and Balis 1964). The 'messenger' fraction from cells exposed to proflavine has significantly less capacity to stimulate amino acid incorporation *in vitro*, and such RNA prevents stimulation by RNA from normal cells (Scholtissek 1965).

Following Hurwitz's demonstration that proflavine inhibits synthesis of DNA-primed RNA *in vitro*, Woese et al. (1963) demonstrated that proflavine blocks transcription and the synthesis of labile RNA in growing bacteria. In general, nevertheless, the inhibition by proflavine of RNA and of protein is best interpreted by assuming as a primary attack, a DNA-dependent step (Soffer and Gros 1964).

Lerman (1964) studied the reactivity of amino groups of DNA: amino-acridine complexes, and showed that diazotization by nitrite is strongly inhibited. Those amino groups which would be expected to fall inside the van der Waal's contour figure are greatly protected, while those lying outside the contour are relatively unguarded.

These findings support an intercalated model, which explains the action of proflavine and congeners as mutagens and the inhibition by these compounds of DNA-primed RNA and DNA synthesis. The acridines force the bases twice as far apart, which could result in insertion or deletion of base pairs in transcription leading to grossly altered or missing proteins (Brenner et al. 1961).

A large number of biologically active, synthetic compounds, have been shown to interact with DNA, and there has been a tendency to attribute their biological activity to this. For example, chloroquine and quinacrine (atebrin) form complexes with DNA (Kurnick and Radcliffe 1962; Allison et al. 1965), presumably by ionic attraction, and quinine forms a urea sensitive complex which has been attributed to hydrogen bond formation. As a result the double helix is apparently stabilized. DNA bound to these antimalarials is less active biologically (Stollar and Levine 1963), and in their presence the synthesis of nucleic acid is inhibited both *in vivo* and *in vitro* (Cohen and Yielding 1965; Ciak and Hahn 1966). Because of the chemical similarity to the acridine dyes, it appears reasonable to attribute the interaction to similar molecular mechanisms.

13.4.2. *Alkylating agents*

Despite the fact that current thinking usually first attributes their activity to reaction with nucleic acid, nevertheless, there have been well documented examples of alkylating agents interfering at the enzyme level: nitrogen mustard caused an increase in adenosinetriphosphatase and $5'$-nucleotidase in spleen and thymus of treated mice and rats (Dubois et al. 1956) and in nicotinamide adenine dinucleotide glyco-hydrolase of tumours (Green and Bodansky 1962).

The most active alkylating agents, those which are bifunctional, can theoretically cross-link by reacting with different substrate molecules (Goldacre et al. 1949). However, monofunctional alkylating agents are also active in this way, so that their biological effects do not depend solely upon cross-linking.

Examination of the *in vitro* reaction between DNA and alkylating agents led to the conclusion that the most active site is the N-7 position on the guanine moieties (Lawley and Wallick 1957; Reiner and Zamenhof 1957; Brookes and Lawley 1960). Watson and Crick (1953) had proposed that mutations would arise if a base in the DNA was in its less common tautomeric form, thereby causing it to pair with a 'wrong' base in the other strand. The observation of Lawley and Brookes (1961) that 7-alkyl deoxyguanosine has a much more acidic character than does deoxyguanosine, suggested that this could cause anomalous base pairing by such a mechanism. The nitrogen atom in position one of N-7 alkyl-guanylic acid would tend to lose a proton and this ionized guanine would preferentially pair with a thymine rather than a cytosine in replication. Alkylation with mustard was shown by Brookes and Lawley (1961) to lead to a product which was unstable to mild hydrolytic conditions.

As these authors point out, the early loss of 7-alkylguanine from the DNA would be expected and the resultant apurinic acid would be less stable than native DNA.

Mustard treated DNA reaggregates at a lower salt concentration than control DNA, as measured by the return of the optical density to the initial value (Lawley and Brookes 1963). In studies of the thermal properties of DNA treated with nitrogen mustard, Wheeler and Stevens (1965) obtained evidence which was consistent with the postulate that there is, in fact, cross-linking.

An interesting compound which may act pharmacologically by virtue of its ability to alkylate is 1-methyl-2-para-(isopropylcarbamoyl)-benzyl-hydrazine hydrochloride (MBH) (procarbazine) (Fig. 13.4). It has been

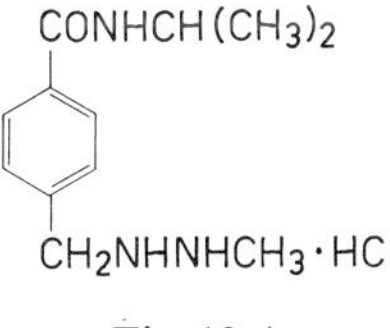

Fig. 13.4.

reported both to inhibit experimental tumours (Bollag and Grunberg 1963) and to induce tumours (Kelly et al. 1964). Two close analogues of MBH, one which lacks the N-terminal methyl group and the N-ethyl analog are not carcinostatic (Bollag and Grunberg 1963), which suggests a functional role for that methyl group. Studies with labeled material demonstrated that this is a source of labile methyl groups (Kreis and Yen

1965) and the compound is capable of ultimately transmethylating purine bases. Kreis has recently demonstrated that the action involves direct alkylation of RNA, especially transfer RNA (Kreis 1970).

There have been reports of the isolation of *E. coli* resistance to alkylating agents and cross-resistance to mitomycin C (Kontani et al. 1959; Greenberg et al. 1961; Mandel et al. 1961). This cross-resistance suggests a similarity of action of alkylating agents and mitomycin C. Schwartz et al. (1963) suggested that mitomycin C is reduced *in vivo* and this reduction unmasks the potential alkylating capacity of the aziridine ring. The link of mitomycin with DNA was demonstrated directly by Iyer and Szybalski (1963), who showed that exposure of bacterial cells to inhibitory concentrations of mitomycin C resulted in covalent linkage of the complementary DNA strands.

Mitomycin C treatment results in changes in DNA quite similar to those described for the other alkylating agents and support the contention that this is a major action of the antibiotic.

Busch et al. (1962) concluded that the action of mustard involves RNA as well as DNA and suggested that the primary action might be a suppression of the biosynthesis of acid-insoluble nuclear proteins due to the binding of RNA by these alkylating agents.

There is no question that alkylation of the bases of both RNA and DNA can occur *in vitro* and *in vivo* and that excision of some altered bases can occur chemically and enzymatically. In terms of current molecular biology these lead to satisfying explanations of mutations and changes in metabolic patterns. However, no direct correlations of such substitutions and biological activities have been conclusively demonstrated.

13.5. Nucleic acid synthesis and immunosuppression

13.5.1. RNA synthesis

There is an increase in RNA synthesis after stimulation with antigen (Ortiz-Ortiz and Jaroslow 1969; Church et al. 1968; Vasil'chenko et al. 1969). In rabbits immunized with typhoid vaccine incorporation of ^{32}P into the RNA and DNA was increased two to four hours after the antigen administration (Grutman 1968). This initial synthesis is sensitive to RNase (Adler et al. 1966). Similarly, a role of specific RNA in transferring immunologic information has been demonstrated (Cohen and Parks 1964; Michelazzi et al. 1964; Friedman 1965; Sato and Mitsuhashi 1965). Heightened immunity can be brought about by inoculation of cells previously incubated with RNA extracted from sensitized nodes (Mannick and Egdahl 1964; Sabbadini and Sehon 1968). The immunosuppressive action of ribonucleases is also a well confirmed observation (Mowbray et al. 1969; Mowbray 1967). The early action of inhibitors of RNA synthesis may be directed against this function of RNA, however, treatment of animals with at least one inhibitor (6-mercaptopurine) results in inhibitions of nucleic acid synthesis, which persisted for such a period of time that it is difficult to attribute immunosuppressive action to this early RNA synthesis (Salser et al. 1967).

Two species of rapidly labelled RNA were detected in rabbits which had been immunized with bovine serum albumin (Kuechler and Rich 1969a). The properties, including molecular weight of these RNAs suggest that they represent messengers with the property of coding for the two antibody chains, one consisting of approximately 215 and the other 430 amino acids. These latter, specific RNAs were not found in non-immunized animals (Kuechler and Rich 1969b). Thus, it is possible that specific inhibition could be achieved, though not by any of the agents presently known. The possibility has been suggested that there is a deficit of the monomolecular precursors of nucleic acid (Johnson and Hoekstra 1966), and as a consequence inhibitors of purine and pyrimidine synthesis should be especially effective in blocking immune response; however, rapidly dividing tissues in general have this same deficit and this may not provide a site of specificity.

13.5.2. DNA synthesis

Rapid proliferation of cells requires synthesis of new DNA and there is no reason to assume any distinction in susceptibility to inhibitors between this DNA and the DNA of other rapidly dividing cells. The uptake of labeled thymidine by spleen cells from previously immunized rabbits is stimulated by the addition of antigen *in vitro* (Dutton and Eady 1964). The stimulation is apparently specific and dose-dependent. This was seen as a counterpart of cellular proliferation which is seen in whole animals. The possible role of DNA replication was also indicated by the observations that nitrogen mustard could act as an immunosuppressant in rabbits, preventing serum sickness in the majority of animals who received large doses of horse serum (Bukantz et al. 1948). Arabinosylcytosine, a metabolic inhibitor whose mode of action consists primarily of interferring with DNA synthesis (Balis 1968) has also been shown to be an inhibitor of the immune process (Evans et al. 1964; Buskirk et al. 1965). Thus, it appears quite definite that DNA production is involved (cf. 13.5.3).

Mitomycin C, which blocks functions and/or synthesis of DNA, probably by alkylation (cf. 13.4.2), is also immunosuppressive (Lemmel and Good 1969). Other compounds which bind DNA, such as acriflavine, are immunosuppressive (Samuelson et al. 1965). Zeleznick et al. (1969) compared the potency of a number of compounds which had previously been demonstrated to bind DNA. They were struck by the surprising degree of correlation between the immunosuppressive potency and the ability to bind DNA as measured by the displacement of associated methyl green. Two compounds, 6-chloro-9-amino-2-methoxyacridine and chlorocrine were exceptions to the generalization that the more firmly a compound bound the more potent it should be as an inhibitor. Chlorocrine had activity which exceeded its ability to bind and it was suggested that it may act in other ways, not simply by binding; the chloroaminomethoxyacridine bound firmly, but was not active. This may be due to a difference between comparing *in vivo* and *in vitro* conditions. On the other hand, Yamaki et al. (1969) examined a number of compounds, some of which bound, some of which didn't, and found that puromycin was effective, while bleomycin, phenomycin and angustmycin were ineffective. Puromycin certainly binds firmly to DNA, on the other hand, bleomycin, under the proper conditions also binds (Nagai et al. 1969), but is not effective as an immunosuppressant in their system.

13.5.3. Inhibitors of DNA synthesis

Just as many compounds are effective in treatment of transplanted tumours in one species and not another, so there have been numerous reports of compounds being active in one species as immunosuppressants and inactive in others. Many investigators, of course, have referred to the similarity between the groups of compounds which act on these two systems and have observed a similarity between drugs which are effective as immunosuppressants and those which are tumour inhibitors. At first glance it would appear to be due to the fact that in both cases one wishes to destroy rapidly dividing tissue and, in fact, effective compounds can be quite toxic. However, the specificity of compounds is often striking. Some substances which are very effective in one system are not effective in another and some agents which are known to inhibit particular biochemical steps are effective immunosuppressants or tumour inhibitors and others which are equally active at the same metabolic site do not have biological specificity. Perhaps related to this is the observation recorded by several investigators, that compounds which are moderately effective, individually, seem to have synergistic interactions. Griswold and Uyeki (1969) reported such behavior for salicylate and quinine against suspensions of sensitized mouse spleen cells. Similarly, Jennings (1969) reported mutual stimulation of this nature between actinomycin D and radiation (Grozdanovic et al. 1969).

The timing of the administration of the antigen and the immunosuppressant obviously are of great importance. Several investigators have suggested that disagreements in the literature can be attributed to such differences in protocol. Amiel (1969), for example, suggested that agents which interfere with DNA synthesis are active when given before the antigen while cyclophosphamide and methylhydrazine compounds which react with DNA *per se*, are most active when given afterward. Contradictory results have been attributed to different therapeutic schedules (Mackiewicz et al. 1969; Gisler and Bell 1969).

Methylhydrazines as a group, have been shown to have antitumour activity and to be immunosuppressant. Perhaps the most active and useful is procarbazine (1-methyl-2-*p*-isopropylcarbamoylbenzohydrazine hydrochloride) (MBH). The compound is effective in preventing transplantation of tumours in mice (Bollag 1963), and rejection of skin homografts in mice (Floersheim 1966). Procarbazine has been considered by some investigators as one of the most useful and potentially valuable immunosuppressants currently available on the basis of the results in these systems and also in its effectiveness in blocking haemoglobin synthesis in rabbits (Stewart and Cohen 1969).

Silagi (1965) has shown that with mouse fibroblast cultures tritiated arabinosylcytosine (Ara-C) is found to be firmly associated with DNA and to a lesser extent with RNA. She suggested that perhaps the inhibition of synthesis of functional DNA and the lethality of Ara-C could be attributed to this.

13.5.4. Alkylating agents

One of the more commonly used alkylating agents in immunosuppression has been cytoxan (2[bis(2-chloroethyl)amino]2H-tetrahydro-1,3,2-oxaza-phosphorine, 2-oxide) (also known as cyclophosphamide). This compound has been designed to require activation *in vivo* and preliminary partial hydrolysis is, in fact, required (Foley et al. 1961). Once activated it presumably behaves as a 'traditional' alkylating agent. It was first reported as an immunosuppressant by Stender et al. in 1959 and its activity was more extensively examined by Maguire and Maibach (1961a. b) in guinea-pigs. It has been shown to be effective in various rat (Santos and Owens 1962) and mouse systems (Berenbaum 1962a) and it protected skin grafts in rabbits (Jones et al. 1963). Frisch and Davies (1965) felt that the primary benefit of cytoxan is its ability to inhibit the evolution of potential antibody-producing cells into more mature cells.

Attempts to correlate time of inhibition with function of immunocytes and with their relative differentiation with known pharmacological activity of immunosuppressants have not been, as yet, successful. Berenbaum (1962b) has divided the inhibitors into classes and attempted to correlate their pharmacological activity with the time of the greatest efficiency. Unfortunately, he has been forced to separate compounds which have very similar biochemical activities; probably because though gross effects of all these inhibitors are known, it is not possible in many cases to define a specific cytologic site in terms of cellular function. Most of these compounds have multiple actions and the relative significance of each is not established.

One of the more intriguing aspects of the action of immunosuppressant drugs is the antigenic specificity of unresponsiveness that may be shown by adjusting the timing of drug administration in relation to that of antigen. In one of their early studies Schwartz and Dameshek (1959) showed that rabbits made immunologically tolerant to human serum albumin remained unresponsive to this foreign protein on repeated challenges, even though administration of the immunosuppressive agent (6-mercaptopurine) had been discontinued. At the same time the animals responded normally to bovine γ-globulin. Thus, the retained capacity for antibody production in general showed that a 'gross dysfunction of the information-storing device had occurred.' This type of specific unresponsiveness is not peculiar to the antigen, the host, or the inhibitor employed. For example, the administration of cyclophosphamide and sheep red blood cells induced immunological tolerance to the latter in mice (Aisenberg and Wilkes 1967). A similar antigenic specificity to that observed by Schwartz was seen and interpreted as evidence of the high specificity of immunocompetent cells and as support of the clonal selection theory of antibody formation. An interesting synergism in this regard was seen between 6-MP and chloramphenicol by Cruchaud (1966). In view of the lack of precision in our knowledge of the action of chloramphenicol in mammalian systems (cf. 13.7) it is difficult to understand the biochemical basis for this interaction. Cruchaud (1966) suggested that perhaps both compounds acted, though somewhat indirectly, on DNA synthesis. Santos (1967) reviewing a similar series of experiments with methotrexate, suggested in the same vein that all cells capable of response to a given antigen are sent into mitosis and are then killed. The implications seem to be that no reserve of competent cells exist and that specialized division is a highly synchronous activity.

13.6. Protein synthesis

The mechanism of protein synthesis as it is now generally understood can be summarized as follows: the activating enzyme (aminoacyl-RNA-synthetase), specific for a given amino acid, catalyzes the reversible production of an enzyme-aminoacyl-adenylate complex which in turn reacts with one of the proper transfer RNAs (tRNA) to form a 2' (3') aminoacyl-tRNA. The terminal nucleoside of active tRNA is adenosine. The aminoacyl-tRNA reacts with a messenger RNA (mRNA)-ribosome complex (a polysome). Then in a series of as not completely understood steps, polymerization and release of the complete polypeptide occurs. The intricacies of the activation and elongation of the growing peptide chain are probably not relevant to this subject.

Many inhibitors block protein synthesis by interference with the nucleic acids. This role is exemplified by the inhibitor, puromycin, a structural analogue of the natural purine ribonucleosides. Though puromycin blocks protein synthesis it does so without interfering with RNA or DNA production in bacterial or mammalian tissues (Takeda et al. 1960; Gorski et al. 1961). Fortunately, the initial observations of Creaser (1955) were concerned with the formation of β-galactosidase, since Sells (1965) has recently shown that the induction of β-galactosidase by thiomethyl-galactosidase is inhibited to a greater extent than is protein synthesis in general.

Puromycin inhibits the incorporation of leucine into protein by crude extracts of rat liver, and it does this neither by interfering with ATP generation, nor by blockade of the activating enzyme. Similarly, puromycin does not prevent the synthesis of leucinyl-tRNA, but does block the incorporation of leucinyl-RNA into protein (Yarmolinsky and De la Haba 1959). Nathans and Lipmann (1961) confirmed the findings of Yarmolinsky and De La Haba and postulated that puromycin specifically prevents the ultimate polymerization, but leaves intact a 'partial reaction' in amino acid transfer.

Chloramphenicol (Fig. 13.5) is an antibiotic with a broad specificity, whose isolation was reported independently by Ehrlich et al. (1947) and Carter et al. (1948). It has been known for some time that addition of relatively small amounts of chloramphenicol to growing bacteria results in extensive and even complete inhibition of protein synthesis (Gale

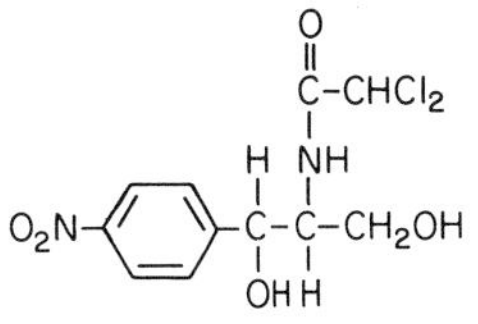

Chloramphenicol

Fig. 13.5.

and Folks 1953; Wissman et al. 1954). As a result of studies of the relationships between structure and activity of various derivatives Shemyakin et al. (1955) concluded that there is interaction with protein.

There has not been, however, any unequivocal demonstration of specific inhibition of protein synthesis in mammalian systems or yeast by chloramphenicol, perhaps due to failure of the compound to be bound intracellularly (Vazquez 1964). Examination of the protein synthesizing complex from rabbit reticulocytes and an analogous one from *E. coli* suggested complete resistance of the rabbit system to chloramphenicol (Von Ehrenstein and Lipmann 1961).

In contrast is the report of Nirenberg and Matthaei (1961) who were able to obtain almost complete inhibition of protein synthesis in a mammalian system with 0.15 mM chloramphenicol as well as the observation of Weisberger et al. (1964) that the antibiotic is active against a cell-free protein-synthesizing system obtained from maturing rabbit erythrocytes.

Though Von Ehrenstein and Lipmann found no inhibition of ^{14}C leucine incorporation with 1 mM chloramphenicol and endogenous messenger, in other experiments Weisberger et al. (1964) using a similar system confirmed this but also reported 50% inhibition of the attachment of template RNA to ribosomes by the same amount of chloramphenicol. Others have attempted unsuccessfully to confirm these findings (Zelkowitz et al. 1968).

The concept that the mechanism (of action of the drug) involves a ribosomal site is supported by the observation of Rendi and Ochoa (1962) that a messenger-like RNA accumulates in chloramphenicol-inhibited bacterial systems. At the present time it is not clear how chloramphenicol acts and very little is known about the basis for the difference between the response of mammalian and bacterial systems.

Though it has not been shown conclusively, the data in general support the suggestion that cycloheximide is effective in preventing assemblage of peptides by a reversible interaction with ribosomes, which is also manifested by interference with aggregation of ribosomes into polysomes. Isolation of a yeast resistant to cycloheximide permitted analysis of the function of various cell components, and as a result it could be shown that resistance and susceptibility depend upon the ribosomes, not on the supernatant enzymes (Siegel and Sisler 1965). Apparently resistance is attributable to a function of the 60S ribosomal subunit.

Cycloheximide, like several other inhibitors of protein formation also blocks DNA synthesis. However, it is not active against DNA polymerases and necessary kinases in cell-free systems and no binding of the inhibitor to DNA is demonstrable. The inhibitions are so rapid that it is not possible to develop a temporal relationship; at the present time we cannot say that inhibition of protein synthesis must precede that of DNA (Bennett et al. 1964).

The tetracyclines inhibit protein synthesis in microorganisms without blocking nucleic acid production (Gale and Folkes 1953; Hash et al. 1964) but possibly affect nitrogen balance in man (Bateman et al. 1954). They also block the synthesis of protein in the rat (Yeh and Shils 1966).

Bacterial RNA synthesized during chlorotetracycline inhibition is contained in ribosome-like particles which sediment more slowly than do normal ribosomes (Holmes and Wild 1965). These particles are more sensitive to ultrasonic and RNase degradation than are normal ribosomes, and they differ also in their behaviour on DEAE cellulose.

Ultracentrifugal studies have shown that tetracycline is bound by ribosomal subunits and the chelating properties of tetracycline are of such a magnitude as to cause dissociation of 100S polyribosomes into constituent 70S monomers. Day (1966) found no dissociation of the 70S into 30S and 50S subunits which is in contrast to the report by Yokota and Akiba (1962) that tetracycline brings about a complete breakdown of 70S ribosomes. It is quite possible that the two groups were working with different sublines with differing sensitivities.

Chlorotetracycline reduces the incorporation of ^{14}C leucine *in vitro* with rat liver and *E. coli* preparations. The drug prevents transfer of the amino acid from the tRNA to the ribosome-protein complex, but does not interfere with the attachment of the amino acid to the tRNA.

Cell-free systems from sensitive and resistant bacteria in general have the same sensitivity to inhibition by tetracycline (Okamoto and Mizuno 1964; Laskin and Chan 1964). On the other hand, Yokota and Akiba (1962) have reported the isolation of a cell free system from a mutant of *E. coli* in which resistance is located in the ribosomes. The fact that cell-free preparations from resistant strains are just as sensitive to inhibition as are those from sensitive strains may suggest that inhibitory action *in vivo* is not directed against protein synthesis *per se*.

13.7. Inhibition of protein and antibody synthesis

As has been mentioned above, a specific messenger RNA is apparently necessary for the synthesis of the immunologically active proteins, and thus inhibitors which prevent protein synthesis should prevent the synthesis of antibodies. On the other hand, protein synthesis may also be involved in the early stages of recognition and preparation for multiplication of active cells. Thus, it is not surprising that a variety of responses to the inhibitor, actinomycin D, have been reported. Inhibition has been seen if the antibiotic was given early, but no effect if it was given late (Brown 1964; Wust et al. 1964). Smiley et al. (1964) reported that at low concentrations (1 mg/ml) there was inhibition of RNA synthesis, while at the same time there was uneffected or even increased antibody synthesis when actinomycin D was administered to an assay system of responsive anamnestic lymphoid cells. In the same assay, puromycin, which inhibits protein synthesis *per se*, was effective in reducing antibody synthesis. This led Smiley to suggest that the messenger RNA which regulates antibody production, was long-lived. Similar experiments reported by Speirs (1965) led to the suggestion that messenger RNA synthesized during primary response may be utilized as a template for antibody synthesis during the anamnestic response (Speirs 1965). Similarly, Lazda and Starr (1965) found with rabbit spleen cells that RNA synthesis could be reduced by approximately 75%, while in cells which had been obtained from hyperimmune rabbits, antibody synthesis continued for at least 18 hours. Differential stability of mammalian messenger RNAs is not unique to these systems, of course (Scott and Bell 1964; Imondi et al. 1970). That the effect of actinomycin D is not simply on transcription of DNA for production of antibody-specific messenger comes from the observations that the *in vivo* differentiation of spleen cells following administration of antigen is also inhibited (Abramoff et al. 1968; Geller and Speirs 1968). Studies, on the other hand, by Ivanyi et al. (1968) would seem to indicate that it might be possible to separate multiplication and immunocyte maturation from specific messenger RNA synthesis.

The action of actinomycin D on acquisition of immune tolerance to bovine globulin (a phenomenon in itself little understood), reported by Claman and Bronsky (1965), may be related to the drug's immuno-suppressive action. However, the failure of 6-MP on cyclophosphamide to behave similarly suggests a more unique explanation. The assumption that one can stop production of a protein of interest with actinomycin and have no other profound effect on living cells has been shown to be naive. For example, one often finds that the resultant inhibition of degradation of a given protein is as significant as the prevention of synthesis. (Kenney 1967; Auricchio et al. 1969). Thus, though these observations are stimulating, their true import is not as yet discernible.

Inhibition of protein synthesis *per se* at the level of translation or beyond, obviously could also prevent production of antibodies. Speirs (1965) showed that puromycin, streptomycin and erythromycin, inhibitors of protein synthesis, did not prevent the primary immune response while actinomycin did, but it has been demonstrated that puromycin blocks antibody synthesis *in vitro* (Smiley et al. 1964).

Ambrose and Coons (1963) were also able to demonstrate inhibition *in vitro* with lymph nodes from stimulated rabbits. Chlorotetracycline caused a dose-related depression of agglutinin titres in vaccinated chickens (Prochazka et al. 1968). Cycloheximide, a well known, well established inhibitor of protein synthesis, is also effective (Sutton et al. 1963).

L-asparaginase presumably has as one of its primary sites of action, destruction of exogenous levels of asparagine. Not only is it effective in the inhibition of acute lymphoblastic leukaemia, but has been shown to be immunosuppressive in experimental animals. It prevented sloughing of skin grafts in mice (Bertelli et al. 1968) and caused at the same time a pronounced drop in leucocytes and involution of lymph nodes and spleen. It inhibited the tuberculin reaction in guinea-pigs (Madaus 1969). It was also shown to be immunosuppressive in other murine systems by Hobik (1969) and Schwartz (1969).

Chloramphenicol has been reported to be effective in blocking antibody production in mammals. Ambrose, in 1962, demonstrated it to be effective *in vitro*, and several investigators have shown it to be effective *in vivo* (Weisberger et al. 1964; Cruchaud and Coons 1964). Weisberger and his associates have been responsible for much of this work. Recently they demonstrated that chloramphenicol interfered with antibody synthesis, but not to nearly the same extent with general protein synthesis (Schoenberg et al. 1967). The nature of the inhibition by chloramphenicol is not clear; the bulk of the evidence from laboratories other than Weisberger's suggests that chloramphenicol is not inhibitory to protein synthesis in mammalian cells; certainly it is not inhibitory in the same way as it is in bacteria.

Many workers have suggested that the mechanism of chloramphenicol activity might involve interaction with RNA. Michelazzi et al. (1968) proposed that immunosuppression by chloramphenicol is due to this mechanism. What is more interesting, they found that RNA from rabbits treated with both antigen and chloramphenicol was less effective in transferring sensitivity than was the RNA from animals which had received the antigen alone.

Cycloleucine (1-amino-cyclopentylcarboxylic acid), while not an inhibitor of protein synthesis *per se*, does block the uptake of methionine and glycine (Ahmed and Schoenfield 1962), and as such, is presumably active at blocking protein synthesis indirectly; it too inhibits antibody production (Frisch 1969).

It is quite well established that a variety of substances capable of blocking cell division by virtue of their inhibition of nucleic acid or protein synthesis or function, can act as immunosuppressants. No specific aspect of the action of these macromolecules can be indicated as critical. In view of the ability of these compounds in general to inhibit cellular proliferation of normal and neoplastic tissues, and the role of cell multiplication in the immunologic process, nothing more specific can be said than to state the evidence and coincidence. At present, the knowledge of actions of these inhibitors and of development of anti-bodies is not sufficiently advanced to do more than indicate the mechanisms of immune suppression; however, the rate of progress in both areas of research is such as to promise rapid advances in the design and use of active compounds.

References

ABRAMOFF, P., C. HINTZKE and N. BRIEN, 1968, Res., J. Reticuloendothelial Soc. *5*, 498.

ADLER, F. L., M. FISHMAN and S. DRAY, 1966, J. Immunol. *97*, 554.

AHMED, K. and P. G. SCHOENFIELD, 1962, Can. J. Biochem. Physiol. *40*, 1101.

AISENBERG, A. C. and B. WILKES, 1967, Nature *213*, 498.

ALLISON, J. L., R. L. O'BRIEN and F. E. HAHN, 1965, Science *149*, 1111.

AMBROSE, C. T., 1962, Federation Proc. *21*, 30.

AMBROSE, C. T. and A. H. COONS, 1963, J. Exptl. Med. *117*, 1074.

AMIEL, L., 1969, Recent Results in Cancer Research *21*, 41.

AURICCHIO, F., D. MARTIN, JR. and G. TOMKINS, 1969, Nature *224*, 806.

BALIS, M. E., 1968, Antagonists and nucleic acids. Amsterdam, North-Holland.

BALIS, M. E., V. HYLIN, M. K. COULTAS and D. J. HUTCHISON, 1958, Cancer Res. *18*, 440.

BATEMAN, J. C., C. T. KLOPP and R. SAMSON, 1953–4, Antibiotics Ann. 531.

BENDICH, A. and G. B. BROWN, 1948, J. Biol. Chem. *176*, 1471.

BENDICH, A., S. S. FURST and G. B. BROWN, 1950, J. Biol. Chem. *185*, 423.

BENNETT, L. L., JR., L. SIMPSON, J. GOLDEN and T. L. BARKER, 1963, Cancer Res. *23*, 1574.

BENNETT, L. L., JR., D. SMITHERS and C. T. WARD, 1964, Biochim. Biophys. Acta *87*, 60.

BERENBAUM, M. C., 1962a, Nature *196*, 384.

BERENBAUM, M. C., 1962b, Biochem. Pharmacol. *11*, 29.

BERENBAUM, M. C. and I. N. BROWN, 1965, Immunology *8*, 251.

BERTELLI, A., L. DONATI and E. TRABUCCHI, JR., 1968, Arch. Ital. Patol. Clin. Tumori *11*, 475.

BERTINO, J. R., B. SIMMONS and D. M. DONOHUE, 1964, Biochem. Pharmacol. *13*, 225.

BOLLAG, W., 1963, Experientia *19*, 304.

BOLLAG, W. and E. GRUNBERG, 1963, Experientia *19*, 130.

BRENNER, S., L. BARNETT, F. H. C. CRICK and A. ORGEL, 1961, J. Mol. Biol. *3*, 121.

BRESNICK, E. and G. H. HITCHINGS, 1961, Cancer Res. *21*, 105.

BROOKES, P. and P. D. LAWLEY, 1960, Biochem. J. *77*, 478.

BROWN, I. N., 1964, Nature *204*, 487.

BUKANTZ, S. C., G. J. DAMMIN, K. S. WILSON and M. C. JOHNSON, 1948 J. Lab. Clin. Med. *33*, 1463.

BUSCH, H., H. ADAMS and M. MURAMATSU, 1962, Federation Proc. *21*, 1093.

BUSKIRK, H. H., J. A. CRIM, H. G. PETERING, K. MERRITT and A. G. JOHNSON, 1965, J. Natl. Cancer Inst. *34*, 747.

CARTER, H. D., D. GOTTLIEB and H. W. ANDERSON, 1948, Science *107*, 113.

CASKEY, C. T., D. M. ASHTON and J. B. WYNGAARDEN, 1964, J. Biol. Chem. *239*, 2570.

CHU, M. Y. and G. A. FISCHER, 1962, Biochem. Pharmacol. *11*, 423.

CHURCH, R. B., U. STORB, B. J. MCCARTHY and R. S. WEISER, 1968, J. Immunol. *101*, 399.

CIAK, J. and F. E. HAHN, 1966, Science *151*, 237.

CLAMAN, H. N. and E. A. BRONSKY, 1965, J. Immunol. *95*, 718.

COHEN, E. P. and J. J. PARKS, 1964, Science *144*, 1012.

COHEN, S. M. and K. L. YIELDING, 1965, Proc. Natl. Acad. Sci. U.S. *54*, 521.

CONDIT, P. T., 1960, Cancer *13*, 229.

CREASER, E. H., 1955, J. Gen. Microbiol. *12*, 288.

CRUCHAUD, A., 1966, J. Immunol. *96*, 832.

CRUCHAUD, A. and A. H. COONS, 1964, J. Exptl. Med. *120*, 1061.

DAY, L. E., 1966, J. Bacteriol. *92*, 197.

DIENGDOH, J. V. and J. L. TURK, 1966, Int. Arch. Allergy *29*, 224.

DUBOIS, K. P., D. F. PETERSEN and G. R. ZINS, 1956, Proc. Soc. Exptl. Biol. Med. *91*, 244.

DUTTON, R. W. and J. D. EADY, 1964, Immunology *7*, 40.

EHRLICH, J., Q. R. BARTZ, R. M. SMITH, D. A. JOSLYN and P. R. BURKHOLDER, 1964, Science *106*, 417.

ELION, G. B., S. CALLAHAN, R. W. RUNDLES and G. H. HITCHINGS, 1963, Cancer Res. *23*, 1207.

ELLIOTT, W. H., 1963, Biochem. J. *86*, 562.

EVANS, J. S., E. A. MUSSER, G. D. MENGEL, K. R. FORSBLAD and J. H. HUNTER, 1961, Proc. Soc. Exptl. Biol. Med. *106*, 350.

EVANS, J. S., E. A. MUSSER, L. BOSTWICK and G. D. MENGEL, 1964, Cancer Res. *24*, 1285.

FLOERSHEIM, G. L., 1966, Nature *211*, 638.

FOLEY, G. E., O. M. FRIEDMAN and B. P. DROLET, 1961, Cancer Res. *21*, 57.

FOUNTAIN, J. R., D. J. HUTCHISON, G. B. WARING and J. H. BURCHENAL, 1952, Proc. Soc. Exptl. Biol. Med. *81*, 193.

FOUNTAIN, J. R., D. J. HUTCHISON, G. B. WARING and J. H. BURCHENAL, 1953, Proc. Soc. Exptl. Biol. Med. *83*, 369.

FRANKLIN, T. J. and J. M. COOK, 1969, Biochem. J. *113*, 515.

FREIFELDER, D., P. F. DAVISON and E. P. GEIDUSCHEK, 1961, Biophys. J. *1*, 389.

FRIEDMAN, H., 1965, Nature *207*, 1315.

FRISCH, A. W., 1969, Biochem. Pharmacol. *18*, 256.

FRISCH, A. W. and G. H. DAVIES, 1965, Cancer Res. *25*, 745.

FULLER, W. and M. J. WARING, 1964, Ber. Bunsenges. Physik. Chem. *68*, 805.

FUMAROLA, D., 1969, Boll. Ist. Sieroter. *48*, 184.

GALE, E. F. and J. P. FOLKES, 1953, Biochem. J. *53*, 493.

GALE, G. R., W. E. OSTRANDER and L. M. ATKINS, 1968, Biochem. Pharmacol. *17*, 1823.

GELLER, B. D. and R. S. SPEIRS, 1968, Immunology *15*, 707.

GEORGIEV, G. P., O. P. SAMARINA, M. I. LERMAN, M. N. SMIRNOV and A. N. SEVERTZOV, 1963, Nature *200*, 1291.

GERICKE, D., P. CHANDRA, I. HAENZEL and A. WACKER, 1970, Z. Physiol. Chem. *351*, 305.

GISLER, R. H. and J. P. BELL, 1969, Biochem. Pharmacol. *18*, 2115.

GOLDACRE, R. J., A. LOVELESS and W. C. J. ROSS, 1949, Nature *163*, 667.

GOLDBERG, I. H. and M. RABINOWITZ, 1962, Science *136*, 315.

GOLDBERG, I. H., M. RABINOWITZ and E. REICH, 1962, Proc. Natl. Acad. Sci. U.S. *48*, 2094.

GOLDBERG, I. H., E. REICH and M. RABINOWITZ, 1963, Nature *199*, 44.

GORSKI, J., Y. AIZAWA and G. C. MUELLER, 1961, Arch. Biochem. *95*, 508.

GOTS, J. S. and E. G. GOLLUB, 1959, Proc. Soc. Exptl. Biol. Med. *101*, 641.

GRAY, G. D. and M. M. MICKELSON, 1970, Transplantation *9*, 176.

GREEN, S. and O. BODANSKY, 1962, J. Biol. Chem. *237*, 1752.

GREENBERG, J., J. D. MANDEL and P. L. WOODY, 1961, Cancer Chemother. Rept. *11*, 51.

GRISWOLD, D. E. and E. M. UYEKI, 1969, Eur. J. Pharmacol. *6*, 56.

GRUTMAN, M. I., 1968, Byull. Eksp. Biol. Med. *65*, 70.

HAMILTON, L. D., W. FULLER and E. REICH, 1963, Nature *198*, 538.

HARBERS, E. and W. MULLER, 1962, Biochem. Biophys. Res. Comm. *7*, 107.

HARTMANN, G., U. COY, and G. KNIESE, 1962, Z. Physiol. Chem. *330*, 227.

HASH, J. H., M. WISHNICK and P. A. MILLER, 1964, J. Biol. Chem. *239*, 2070.

HEIDRICK, M. L. and W. L. RYAN, 1970, Cancer Res. *30*, 376.

HOBIK, H. P., 1969, Naturwissenschaften *56*, 217.

HOLMES, I. A. and D. G. WILD, 1965, Biochem. J. *97*, 277.

HURWITZ, J., J. J. FURTH, M. MALAMY and M. ALEXANDER, 1962, Proc. Natl. Acad. Sci. U.S. *48*, 1222.

IMONDI, A. R., M. LIPKIN and M. E. BALIS, 1970, J. Biol. Chem. *245*, 2194.

IVANYI, J., M. MALER, L. WUDL and E. SERCARZ, 1968, J. Exptl. Med. *127*, 1149.

IYER, V. N. and W. SZYBALSKI, 1963, Proc. Natl. Acad. Sci. U.S. *50*, 355.

IYER, V. N. and W. SZYBALSKI, 1964, Science *145*, 55.

JENNINGS, B. R., 1969, J. Reticuloendothelial Soc. *6*, 50.

JOHNSON, A. G. and G. HOEKSTRA, 1967, Acceleration of the primary antibody response. *In*: R. T. Smith, R. A. Good and P. A. Miescher, eds.: Ontogeny of immunity. Gainesville, Fla., Univ. of Florida Press. pp. 187–190.

JONES, J. W., G. L. BRODY, R. M. ONEAL and R. F. HAINES, 1963, J. Surg. Res. *3*, 189.

KELLY, M. G., R. W. O'GARA, K. GADEKAR, S. T. YANCEY and V. T. OLIVERIO, 1964, Cancer Chemother. Rept. *39*, 77.

KENNEY, F. T., 1967, Science *156*, 525.

KIRK, J. M., 1960, Biochim. Biophys. Acta *42*, 167.

KLEINWACHTER, V. and J. KOUDELKA, 1964, Biochim. Biophys. Acta *91*, 539.

KONTANI, H., S. SHIBA, T. TAGUCHI and A. TERAWAKI, 1959, Gann *50*, 30.

KORN, E. D., C. N. REMY, H. C. WASILEJKO and J. M. BUCHANAN, 1955, J. Biol. Chem. *217*, 875.

KORNBERG, A., I. LIEBERMAN and E. S. SIMMS, 1955, J. Biol. Chem. *215*, 417.

KREIS, W., 1970, Cancer Res. *30*, 82.

KREIS, W. and W. YEN, 1965, Experientia *21*, 284.

KUECHLER, E. and A. RICH, 1969a, Proc. Natl. Acad. Sci. U.S. *63*, 520.

KUECHLER, E. and A. RICH, 1969b, Nature *222*, 544.

KURNICK, N. B. and I. E. RADCLIFFE, 1962, J. Lab. Clin. Med. *60*, 669.

LASKIN, A. E. and W. M. CHAN, 1964, Biochem. Biophys. Res. Comm. *14*, 137.

LAWLEY, P. D. and P. BROOKES, 1961, Nature *192*, 1081.

LAWLEY, P. D. and P. BROOKES, 1963, Exptl. Cell Res. (Suppl.) *9*, 512.

LAWLEY, P. D. and C. A. WALLICK, 1957, Chem. and Industry 633.

LEITH, J. D., JR., 1963, Biochim. Biophys. Acta, *72*, 643.

LEMMEL, E. M. and R. A. GOOD, 1969, Int. Arch. Allergy *36*, 554.

LEPAGE, G. A., 1960, Cancer Res. *20*, 403.

LEPAGE, G. A. and M. JONES, 1961, Cancer Res. *21*, 1590.

LEPAGE, G. A., I. G. JUNGA and B. BOWMAN, 1964, Cancer Res. *24*, 835.

LEPECQ, J., P. YOT and C. PAOLETTI, 1964, Compt. rend. Acad. Sci. *259*, 1786.

LERMAN, L. S., 1961, J. Mol. Biol. *3*, 18.

LERMAN, L. S., 1964, J. Mol. Biol. *10*, 367.

LEVIN, D. H., 1963, J. Biol. Chem. *238*, 1098.

LEVIN, D. H., 1965, Biochem. Biophys. Res. Comm. *19*, 654.

LEVIN, D. H. and M. LITT, 1965, J. Mol. Biol. *14*, 506.

LUKENS, L. N. and K. A. HERRINGTON, 1957, Biochim. Biophys. Acta *24*, 432.

MACKIEWICZ, U., S. MACKIEWICZ and J. KONYS, 1969, Ann. Immunol. *1*, 59.

MACMANUS, J. P. and J. F. WHITFIELD, 1969, Exptl. Cell Res. *58*, 188.

MADAUS, W. P., 1969, Klin. Wschr. *47*, 1237.

MAGUIRE, H. C. and H. I. MAIBACH, 1961a, J. Allergy *32*, 406.

MAGUIRE, H. C. and H. I. MAIBACH, 1961b, J. Invest. Dermatol. *37*, 427.

MALMGREN, R. A., B. E. BENNISON and T. W. MCKINLEY, JR., 1952, Proc. Soc. Exptl. Biol. Med. *79*, 484.

MANNICK, J. A. and R. H. EGDAHL, 1964, J. Clin. Invest. *43*, 2166.

MANDEL, J. D., P. L. WOODY and J. GREENBERG, 1961, J. Bacteriol. *81*, 419.

MATSUMOTO, I. and K. G. LARK, 1963, Exptl. Cell Res. *32*, 192.

MCCOLLISTER, R. J., W. R. GILBERT, JR., D. M. ASHTON and J. B. WYNGAARDEN, 1964, J. Biol. Chem. *239*, 1560.

MICHELAZZI, L., G. NANNI, I. BALDINI and A. NOVELLI, 1964, Experientia *20*, 447.

MICHELAZZI, L., U. M. MARINARI and I. BALDINI, 1968, Experientia *24*, 1268.

MIECH, R. P., R. E. PARKS, JR., J. H. ANDERSON, JR., and A. C. SARTORELLI, 1967, Biochem. Pharmacol. *16*, 2222.

MITCHELL, J. H., JR., H. E. SKIPPER and L. L. BENNETT, JR., 1950, Cancer Res. *10*, 647.

MITSUI, A. and S. SUZUKI, 1969, J. Antibiot. *22*, 358.

MOWBRAY, J. F., 1967, J. Clin. Pathol. (Suppl.) *20*, 499.

MOWBRAY, J. F., A. W. BOYLSTON, J. D. MILTON and M. WEKSLER, 1969, Antibiot. Chemother. *15*, 384.

MURAKAMI, H., 1966, J. Theoret. Biol. *10*, 236.

NAGAI, K., H. YAMAKI, H. SUZUKI, N. GANAKA and H. UMEZAWA, 1969, Biochim. Biophys. Acta *179*, 165.

NATHAN, H. C., S. BIEBER, G. B. ELION, and G. H. HITCHINGS, 1961, Proc. Soc. Exptl. Biol. Med. *107*, 796.

NATHANS, D., 1961, Proc. Natl. Acad. Sci. U.S. *51*, 585.

NICHOL, C. A., 1953, Proc. Soc. Exptl. Biol. Med. *83*, 167.

NIERLICH, D. P. and B. MAGASANIK, 1965, J. Biol. Chem. *240*, 358.

NIRENBERG, M. S. and J. H. MATTHAEI, 1961, Proc. Natl. Acad. Sci. U.S. *47*, 1588.

OKAMOTO, S. and D. MIZUNO, 1964, J. Gen. Microbiol. *35*, 125.

ORTIZ-ORTIZ, L. and B. N. JAROSLOW, 1969, Nature *211*, 1153.

PEACOCKE, A. R. and J. N. H. SKERRETT, 1956, Trans. Faraday Soc. *52*, 261.

PECORA, P. F. and M. E. BALIS, 1964, Biochem. Pharmacol. *13*, 1071.

PERRY, R. P., 1962, Proc. Natl. Acad. Sci. U.S. *48*, 2179.

PROCHAZKA, Z., L. RODAK and J. KREJČI, 1968, Folia Microbiologica *13*, 490.

RAUEN, H. M., H. KERSTEN and W. KERSTEN, 1960, Z. Physiol. Chem. *321*, 139.

REICH, E., and I. H. GOLDBERG, 1964, Progr. Nucleic Acid Res. and Mol. Biol. *3*, 183.

REICH, E., R. M. FRANKLIN, A. J. SHATKIN and E. L. TATUM, 1961, Science *134*, 556.

REICH, E., I. H. GOLDBERG and M. RABINOWITZ, 1962, Nature *196*, 743.

REICH, E., R. M. FRANKLIN, A. J. SHATKIN and E. L. TATUM, 1962b, Proc. Natl. Acad. Sci. U.S. *48*, 1238.

REINER, B. and S. ZAMENHOF, 1957, J. Biol. Chem. *228*, 475.

REMY, C. N. and M. S. SMITH, 1957, J. Biol. Chem. *228*, 325.

RENDI, R. and S. OCHOA, 1962, J. Biol. Chem. *237*, 3711.

REVEL, M. and H. H. HIATT, 1964, Biochem. Biophys. Res. Comm. *17*, 730.

SABBADINI, E. and A. H. SEHON, 1968, Induction of accelerated graft rejection and enhanced graft-versus-host reaction with RNA from lymphoid organs of animals immunized with allogeneic tissues. *In*: O. J. Plescia and W. Braun, eds.: Nucleic acids in immunology. New York, Springer-Verlag. pp. 560–572.

SALSER, J. S. and BALIS, M. E., 1965, Cancer Res. *25*, 539.

SALSER, J. S., D. J. HUTCHISON and M. E. BALIS, 1960, J. Biol. Chem. *234*, 429.

SALSER, J. S., D. G. MILLER and M. E. BALIS, 1967, Exptl. Mol. Pathol. *6*, 199.

SAMUELSON, J. S., P. B. STEWART, S. C. KRAFT and R. S. FARR, 1965, J. Immunol. *95*, 314.

SANTOS, G. W., 1967, Federation Proc. *26*, 907.

SANTOS, G. W. and A. H. OWENS, JR., 1962, Blood *20*, 111.

SARTORELLI, A. C. and G. A. LEPAGE, 1958, Cancer Res. *18*, 1329.

SATO, I. and S. MITSUHASHI, 1965, J. Bacteriol. *90*, 1194.

SCANNELL, J. P. and G. H. HITCHINGS, 1966, Proc. Soc. Exptl. Biol. Med. *122*, 627.

SCHOENBERG, M. D., R. D. MOORE and A. S. WEISBERGER, 1967, Advan. Exptl. Med. Biol., 345.

SCHOLTISSEK, C., 1965, Biochim. Biophys. Acta *103*, 146.

SCHWARTZ, H. S., J. E. SODERGREN and F. S. PHILIPS, 1963, Science *142*, 1181.

SCHWARTZ, R. S., 1969, Nature *224*, 275.

SCHWARTZ, R. S. and W. DAMESHEK, 1959, Nature *183*, 1682.

SCHWARTZ, R. S., J. STACK and W. DAMESHEK, 1958, Proc. Soc. Exptl. Biol. Med. *99*, 164.

SCOTT, R. B. and E. BELL, 1964, Science *145*, 711.

SELLS, B. H., 1965, Science *148*, 371.

SHEMYAKIN, M. M., M. N. KOLOSOV, M. M. LEVITOV, K. I. GERMANOVA, M. G. KARAPETYAN, Y. B. SHVETSOV and E. M. BAMDAS, 1955, Dokl. Akad. Nauk S.S.S.R. *102*, 953.

SIEGEL, M. R. and H. D. SISLER, 1965, Biochim. Biophys. Acta *103*, 558.

SILAGI, S., 1965, Cancer Res. *25*, 1446.

SMILEY, J. D., J. G. HEARD and M. ZIFF, 1964, J. Exptl. Med. *119*, 881.

SMITH, C. G., H. H. BUSKIRK and W. L. LUMMINS, 1965, Proc. Am. Assoc. Cancer Res. *6*, 60.

SMITH, J. D. and R. E. F. MATTHEWS, 1957 Biochem. J. *66*, 323.

SMITH, L. H. and M. SULLIVAN, 1960, Biochim. Biophys. Acta *39*, 554.

SOFFER, R. L. and F. GROS, 1964, Biochim. Biophys. Acta *87*, 423.

SPEIRS, R. S., 1965, Nature *207*, 371.

STENDER, H. S., D. RINGLEB, D. STRAUCH and H. WINTER, 1959, Strahlentherapie (Suppl.) *43*, 392.

ŠTERZL, J., 1961, Nature *189*, 1022.

STEWART, P. B. and V. COHEN, 1969, Science, *164*, 1082.

STOLLAR, D. and L. LEVINE, 1963, Arch. Biochem. Biophys. *101*, 335.

SUTTON, W. R., F. VAN HAGEN, H. B. GRIFFITH and F. W. PRESTON, 1963, Arch. Surg. *87*, 840.

TAKEDA, Y., S. HAYASHI, H. NAKAGAWA and F. SUZUKI, 1960, J. Biochem. *48*, 169.

THOMAS, E. D., J. A. BAKER, E. A. BLUMENSTOCK, H. HECHTMAN and J. W. FERREBEE, 1962, Blood *20*, 112.

TRUXOVA, G. and Z. VICH, 1969, Neoplasma *16*, 225.

TURK, J. L., 1964, Int. Arch. Allergy *24*, 191.

TURK, J. G. and S. H. STONE, 1963, Implications of the cellular changes in lymph nodes during the development and inhibition of delayed type hypersensitivity. *In*: B. Amos, and H. Koprowski, eds.: Cell-bound antibodies. Philadelphia, Wistar Institute Press. pp. 51–59.

UPHOFF, D. E. and L. PITKIN, 1962, Blood *20*, 113.

VASIL'CHENKO, V. N., A. G. D'YACHENKO, E. S. VASI'EVA and I. N. TODOROV, 1969, Biokhimiya *34*, 170.

VAZQUEZ, D., 1964, Nature *203*, 257.

VON EHRENSTEIN, G. and F. LIPMANN, 1961, Proc. Natl. Acad. Sci. U.S. *47*, 941.

WARING, M. J. 1966, Biochim. Biophys. Acta *14*, 234.

WARING, M. J., 1965, J. Mol. Biol. *13*, 269.

WATSON, J. D. and F. H. C. CRICK, 1953, Nature *171*, 964.

WAY, J. L. and R. E. PARKS, JR., 1958, J. Biol. Chem. *231*, 467.

WEINSTEIN, I. B. and D. GRÜNBERGER, 1965, Biochem. Biophys. Res. Comm. *19*, 647.

WEISBERGER, A. S., T. M. DANIEL and A. HOFFMAN, 1964, J. Exptl. Med. *120*, 183.

WEISBERGER, A. S., S. WOLFE and S. ARMENTROUT, 1964, J. Exptl. Med. *120*, 161.

WERKHEISER, W. C., 1961, J. Biol. Chem. *236*, 888.

WHEELER, G. P. and Z. H. STEPHENS, 1965, Cancer Res. *25*, 410.

WISSEMAN, C. L., JR., J. E. SMADEL, F. E. HAHN and H. E. HOPPS, 1954, J. Bacteriol. *67*, 662.

WOESE, C., S. NAONO, R. SOFFER and F. GROS, 1963, Biochem. Biophys. Res. Comm. *11*, 435.

WUST, C. J., C. L. GALL and G. D. NOVELLI, 1964, Science *143*, 1041.

WYNGAARDEN, J. G. and D. M. ASHTON, 1959 Nature *183*, 747.

YAMAKI, H., N. TANAKA and H. UMEZAWA, 1969, J. Antibiot. *22*, 315.

YARMOLINSKY, M. D. and G. L. DE LA HABA, 1959, Proc. Natl. Acad. Sci. U.S., *45*, 1721.

YATES, R. A. and A. B. PARDEE, 1956, J. Biol. Chem. *221*, 757.

YEH, S. D. J. and M. E. SHILS, 1966, Proc. Soc. Exptl. Biol. Med. *121*, 729.

YOKOTA, T. and T. AKIBA, 1962, Med. Biol. (Tokyo) *64*, 39.

ZELEZNICK, L. D., J. A. CRIM and G. D. GRAY, 1969, Biochem. Pharmacol. *18*, 1823.

ZELKOWITZ, L., G. K. ARIMURA and A. A. YUNIS, 1968, J. Lab. Clin. Med. *71*, 596.

Effects of vitamins and dietary factors

J. M. STARK

Department of Bacteriology and Immunology, University of Glasgow

14.1. Introduction

A major deficiency of an important nutrient may lead to a major cellular deficiency. It is therefore not surprising that a natural or induced lack of a dietary constituent should have its effect on the immunological reponse where cells must differentiate efficiently and speedily to fulfil their function. The effect of some deficiencies on the response is barely detectable whereas others cause profound alterations on the mode of its expression. The studies outlined below show that by dietary changes the reception or recognition of antigen may be altered, the ability to proliferate or differentiate in the potentially responding cell may be impaired, or the balance between humoral antibody and the cellular delayed-type response may be modified. Most often only the end result is known; the intimate mechanism remains to be elucidated.

14.2. The vitamins

Although refinement in nutritional and immunological technique has allowed the influence of vitamins on the immunological response to be examined in greater depth, the order of immunological impairment brought about by most deficiencies had been recognized by 1951 (Ludovici and Axelrod). Since that time, attention has been paid to those deficiencies most actively affecting the response, whereas others such as vitamin D and K deficiencies have been relatively neglected.

14.2.1. Vitamin A
The role of vitamin A has not been regarded as major in the immune response. Nevertheless there are continued reports to show that lack of the vitamin leads to a less than optimal response to an antigen. Harmon and his colleagues (1963) have demonstrated in pigs that dietary

deficiency of the vitamin leads to a poorer response to *Salmonella pullorum* phenolized antigen. Panda and Combs (1963) also have shown a poor response to *Salmonella pullorum* in chicks on a similarly deficient diet. The older literature, although containing much that is contradictory, provides some evidence that a sufficiency of the vitamin aided the immune response of the human species where, for example, antibody titres to prophylactic agents such as triple typhoid vaccine (TAB) and diphtheria toxoid have been improved by an increased intake of vitamin (Scaglione 1938; Schmeckebier 1945).

The mechanism of action has not been elucidated in such observations and a relationship to the known physiological action of the vitamin in vision has not been established. The action of the vitamin in high pharmacological doses has proved of immunological interest. Its use in immunological systems has stemmed from the knowledge of the lysosome derived from the work of de Duve (1959) and also the observations of the action of vitamin A in organ culture made by Dingle et al. (1961); proteolytic enzymes were released from the lysosomal vesicles within the cells and were allowed to spread throughout the cell and also into the tissue culture fluid.

Uhr and Weissman had shown (1965) that vitamin A did affect the response against phage ϕX 174 so that the 19S response was prolonged although without any increase in antibody titre. These authors also demonstrated the digestion of phage antigen within the large granule fraction of the guinea-pig liver by the loss of ability of the phage particles to form plaques on a lawn of susceptible bacteria. They found that the number of plaque-forming units fell, but that the immunogenicity of the digested material increased. How vitamin A affected this digestive process, was not defined.

Adjuvant activity of vitamin A has been found with other antigens. Bovine gamma globulin (BGG) given intravenously in mice induces tolerance unless an adjuvant stimulus is also given (Dresser 1960). The vitamin has adjuvant activity in this model, when given subcutaneously in high dosage without local antigen at the site of adjuvant injection (Dresser 1968). To act as adjuvant the vitamin need not be given parenterally. Oral vitamin A has an adjuvant action in CBA mice with BGG (Stark 1970a) and HSA (human serum albumin) as antigens. Fig. 14.1 shows the response to 1 mg. HSA given intravenously to mice treated with 30,000 i.u. vitamin A orally (Stark, unpublished work); a primary response could not be detected in the untreated control group; a brisk secondary response is found in each of the treated mice, only one untreated mouse showing a secondary response and that a later one. Spitznagel and Allison (1970) examined the adjuvant effect of several

                    J. M. Stark

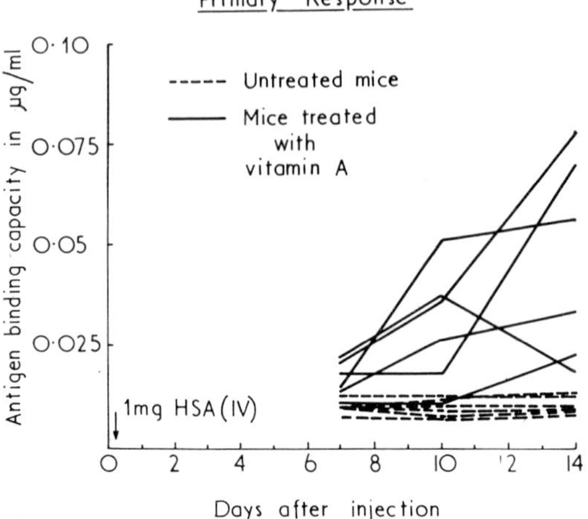

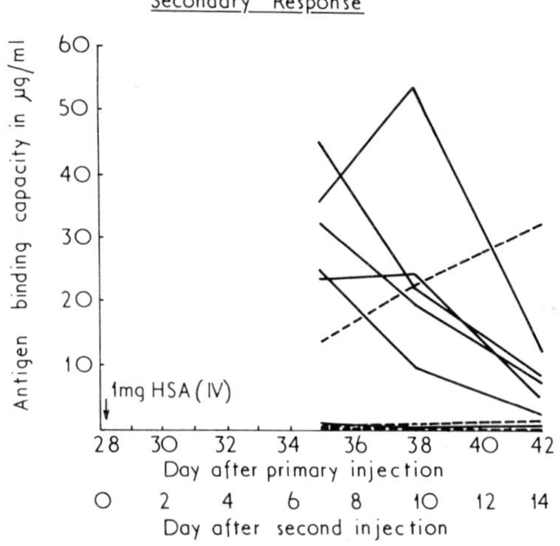

Fig. 14.1. Influence of oral vitamin A on the response to human serum albumin (HSA) in CBA mice. The primary and secondary antibody responses to 1 mg HSA of control (— — — —) and test mice (————) are shown, measured as antigen binding capacity in µg/ml. Samples were taken on the 7th, 10th, and 14th day of the response. The test mice received 10,000 i.u. vitamin A on the three days before the primary antigen injection only.

agents known to labilize lysosomes including vitamin A alcohol. They found a correlation between this ability and ability to stimulate an immune response to bovine serum albumin in CBA mice, this antigen being ordinarily poorly immunogenic.

The adjuvant activity of vitamin A resembles endotoxin in that delayed-type hypersensitivity is not produced and also in that a local granuloma is not required. The vitamin will not stimulate delayed-type hypersensitivity in guinea-pigs (White 1968) and indeed there is evidence that acute hypervitaminosis will depress previously induced delayed hypersensitivity (Uhr et al. 1963); this has been related to the reduced inflammatory response of animals whose lysosomes have been depleted of many enzymes by the hypervitaminosis (Weissman et al. 1963). Also hypervitaminosis A has depressed in guinea-pigs the production by Freund-type adjuvants of experimental thyroiditis and antibodies against thyroid (Jansz et al. 1967). (Paradoxically in this experiment the thyroid glands of animals receiving only the vitamin did show lymphoid infiltration.)

The impaired antigen catabolism, implied although not proved in the report of Uhr and Weissman (1965), compares with slowed catabolism of antigen (BGG) in the period before antibody is produced in mice treated with vitamin A (Stark 1970). In this respect vitamin A is unlike other adjuvant substances which accelerate the elimination of antigen in the preimmune phase of elimination.

The exact explanation of the adjuvant action of vitamin A is by no means elucidated. The polar conjugated molecule has surface activity. Gall (1966) has asked whether more antigen might not enter the immuno-competent cell, through alterations in cell permeability brought about by surface active agents. This would allow passage of information regarding the shape of antigen to some effector site. Dresser (1968) has based another interpretation of the mode of vitamin action on observations of lysosomal behaviour before cell division or lymphocyte transformation (Allison and Mallucci 1964; Hirschhorn et al. 1962). One cycle of division in the presence of antigen, set off by leakage of ribonuclease from unduly permeable lymphoid lysosomes, is suggested as sufficient to initiate the immune response.

The intimate action of the vitamin on the membranes of lysosomes or other cellular structures is not known, but Dingle (1968) has suggested that a reversible *cis-trans* transformation of the vitamin molecule may be related to the altered permeability found with high concentrations.

The integrity of the beta-ionone ring is important for some of the biological activities of vitamin A. The opening of the ring as in lycopene destroys for example the ability of the compound to stimulate in rats the formation of properdin (Isliker et al. 1960).

14.2.2. *The vitamin B group*

Deficiencies of vitamins of this group have long been associated with reduction in antibody production to antigenic stimuli. The more recent experience has been in keeping with this. Harmon et al. (1964) describe a typical experiment where diets deficient in pantothenic acid, pyridoxine, or riboflavine were tested in four-week old pigs. The test pigs with any of the diets produced significantly lower titres than did the control pigs against *Salmonella pullorum* or sheep red cells. In an accompanying paired feeding experiment the control pigs gained weight significantly faster, more efficiently and produced higher titres. On their return to a normal diet the formerly deficient pigs regained the ability to produce antibody, but gained weight more slowly. The response to live infective agents is similarly affected. Muranyi et al. (1964) have shown in albino rats that a riboflavine-deficient diet for 24 days reduced the antibody response to *Leptospira icterohaemorrhagiae* 32 days later. Thiamine deficiency in the mouse increases its susceptibility to *Cryptococcus neoformans*. Gadesbusch and Gikas (1963) relate this to a defect in the alveolar macrophages which allows greatly increased invasion of brain and heart. The organism itself requires thiamine for growth so that relative deficiency has biased the outcome in favour of the organism.

Vitamin B6 (pyridoxine, deficiency produces a much more complete inhibition of the immune response and has therefore been more fully investigated. These researches, particularly by Axelrod and his colleagues (reviewed by Axelrod and Pruzansky 1955, and Axelrod and Trakatellis 1964) are the logical extension of the observations of Stoerk and Eisen (1946) that in pyridoxine deficient rats there was a poor production of antibody to sheep red cells and that this was associated with a reduction of lymphoid tissue mass. In later studies the pyridoxine-deficient animals were shown to have impaired responses to antigenic stimuli such as human red cells, diphtheria toxoid and influenza virus. Hypersensitivity reactions were also altered by the deficiency. The Arthus reaction in guinea-pigs against diphtheria toxoid was reduced. A reduction was also found in the reaction to purified protein derivative (PPD) in guinea pigs sensitized by injections of either live or killed BCG 20 days previously. The giving of pyridoxine to the previously sensitized animals restored the response.

Delayed type hypersensitivity in vitamin B6 deficiency was also shown to be depressed in experiments with skin grafts; vitamin-deficient mice did not reject grafts as readily as control mice on a normal diet. Better results could be obtained if the vitamin deficients were first made tolerant by injections of cells or cellular fractions (splenic cells, ribosomes, or RNA extracts) from animals syngeneic with the skin donors (Axelrod and Trakatellis 1964). The mice were grafted after return to a normal balanced diet, yet the grafts remained unrejected. This experience contrasts with tuberculin hypersensitivity, where the ability to react to tuberculoprotein was restored with the giving of pyridoxine. The deficiency could be further accentuated by giving the competitive antagonist deoxypyridoxine as well. This regime has allowed skin grafts to be made from CBA males to C3HHeJ male mice and also across the histocompatibility barrier between male and female C57B1J mice (Trakatellis and Axelrod 1969).

Three groups of observations have also been made on cellular metabolism during pyridoxine deficiency which were thought to be related to this response. First there was a reduction in the synthesis of nucleic acid (DNA and RNA) in liver and spleen (Trakatellis and Axelrod 1965). There was also a decreased protein synthesis in the polysomes of these organs (Trakatellis and Axelrod 1964). More recently Kumar and Axelrod (1968) have shown by the Jerne plaque technique that there was a severe reduction in the number of antibody forming cells. This was unrelated to inanition and was abolished by giving pyridoxine before immunization.

The poor antibody response may indeed be part of the generalized depression of protein metabolism in liver and spleen, yet an inability to recognize antigen could also be partially responsible. Phagocytosis itself as tested by carbon clearance in rats is depressed in vitamin B6 deficiency (Fisher et al. 1964). This persists for some time on return to a normal diet and could also be brought about by administration of the specific vitamin B6 antagonist, deoxypyridoxine. The application of a skin homograft however overcomes the depression of the RES, so that it does not necessarily explain the prolonged graft survival in this deficiency. The vitamin acts as an apoenzyme and affects many enzyme systems in protein and amino acid metabolism. Its absence seems to allow the more ready development of tolerance which suggests that this must be a relatively passive phenomenon, not requiring the vitamin-dependent enzymes. The research emphasis has been on protein metabolism, but it may be mistaken to neglect its effect on the metabolism of fatty acids and cholesterol (Mueller 1964), particularly in view of the depression of the reticulo-endothelial system noted by Fisher et al. (1964).

Mihich (1962) and Mihich and Nichol (1965) have also shown the effects of vitamin B6 deficiency on tumour suppression. The regression of Sarcoma 180 (S180) in pyridoxine-deficient mice appears to depend on an immunological response of the host, because when irradiation was added to the deficient state either before or within three days of implantation, the mice could no longer rid themselves of the tumour so successfully. The vitamin B content of the tumour itself was not altered by irradiation. The process of regression was not susceptible at a later stage to either irradiation or the reintroduction of vitamin B6. Further evidence of an underlying immunological mechanism was found when a subline of the tumour (S180/B6), capable of growing in a pyridoxine-deficient mouse, was implanted in deficient mice into which the parent tumour strain had previously been introduced. The subline regressed only when implanted at least 8–14 days after the parent strain.

The pyridoxine antagonist, 4-deoxypyridoxine, is itself unable to bring about regression and for it to be effective, the animals have to be put on a deficient diet when drug treatment begins. The inhibition of the tumour which results is not so great as that produced by the deficient diet given for 14 days before implantation, and is not followed by complete tumour regression. However the antagonist is able to bring about regression of the pyridoxine-resistant subline. Not all vitamin B6 antagonists act identically on the immunological system (Mihich and Nichol 1965). Unlike deoxypyridoxine, thiosemicarbazide was effective against S180 whether or not there was any dietary deficiency and could bring about complete tumour regression. Isonicotinic acid hydrazide, itself relatively ineffective in preventing tumour regression, greatly enhanced the effect of deoxypyridoxine.

Neonatal thymectomy, but not splenectomy, reduced the tumour regression obtained by the vitamin-deficient state. A possible interpretation is that the dietary deficiency impairs to a lesser degree the cell-mediated delayed-type reaction (Ferrer and Mihich 1968). The different results obtained with the vitamin antagonists would then imply different effects on the balance between the antibody and cell-mediated response.

Folic acid deficiency had been shown to reduce antibody production in various animals to a number of stimuli (Axelrod and Pruzansky 1955). Further evidence of its importance in the immune response has been demonstrated indirectly in the use of folic acid antagonists. Berenbaum and Brown (1965) have shown that the immune response of mice to TAB vaccine is susceptible to the action of methotrexate, that the drug requires only 6–8 hours to have its effect, and that this can be partially or completely prevented by the early administration of folinic acid. The clearance of carbon by the reticulo-endothelial system (RES) is also depressed by methotrexate (Megirian and Leonardi 1966). The effect can again be reversed by administration of folinic acid, but also by exposure of the carbon to normal serum suggesting a depression of the production of an opsonin in the methotrexate-treated animal.

Vitamin B12 has been variously reported as affecting the immune response (Ludovici and Axelrod 1951; Wertman and Sarandria 1952) but there are few recent reports on this topic. Tashmukhamedov (1966) has shown an increased response to tetanus toxoid in rabbits receiving vitamin B12 (10 μg/μg). In untreated animals there was a correlation between the serum concentration of vitamin B12 and the antibody concentration, whereas the treated animals saturated with the vitamin did not show this.

Although in autoimmune states associated with chronic gastritis (Schwartz 1960; Jeffries et al. 1962) antibodies are found against the intrinsic factor which effects the absorption of the vitamin, there is nothing at present to suggest that the physiological link with the vitamin molecule brings about sensitization to the protein entity.

14.2.3. Vitamin C

Recent work has not revealed the lowered antibody production associated with this deficiency in the past (Hartley 1942; 1948; Long 1950) but has indicated that there may be accessory defects in the tissue reactions in the hypersensitivity states. In severely scorbutic guinea-pigs Kumar and Axelrod (1968) failed to show a reduction in antibody in the primary and secondary responses to diphtheria toxoid. On skin testing these animals responded with a reduced early Arthus-type hypersensitivity. A similar reduction was also detectable in their reaction to the non-specific irritant histamine which suggested that the defect in the response was not in the antibody-forming system. A peripheral defect has also been suggested as existing in the tuberculin sensitivity of guinea-pigs sensitized while on a scorbutic diet (Zweiman et al. 1966). The *in vitro* mitotic response of their lymphocytes to phytohaemagglutinin and Old Tuberculin was no less than those of normal guinea-pigs. These cells could also transfer the specific sensitivity to unimmunized control animals.

A scorbutic diet does not abolish immunological memory of the previously established skin response to purified protein derivative (PPD) (Kies et al. 1964). The response returns with the restoration of the vitamin to the diet. Further studies were made by the same authors in the induction of experimental allergic encephalitis (EAE). This process is set up by injection of encephalitogen together with mycobacterial adjuvant, but can be prevented by injection beforehand of either encephalitogen or adjuvant alone. The separate injection of either agent does not however protect scorbutic guinea-pigs; EAE will develop in such animals if vitamin C is restored to the diet when the encephalitogenic challenge is made. Thus lack of vitamin C has had an effect on the reception of the encephalitogen as well as on the reaction to adjuvant.

14.2.4. Vitamins E and K

Vitamin E deficiency has seldom been examined for its effect on antibody production and vitamin K seems to have escaped attention in this respect. Stowe and Whitehair (1964) have found that antibody production is not reduced in vitamin E-deficient mink.

The addition of these vitamins (and also of the other fat-soluble vitamins, A, D, or A and D together) to the diet of normal mice does not alter the phagocytic activity of the RES (Cordingley and Nichol 1961). These authors point out that this might be expected under conditions of normal metabolism; the hyperactivity of infection may however increase vitamin requirements. Vitamin E will counteract the RES depression caused by oxidized cod liver oil (McKay et al. 1964).

Vitamin K deficiency does lead to a reduced level of serum complement in chickens (Weber et al. 1963). There is a slow resynthesis when vitamin K is restored to the diet, normal complement activity returning more slowly than prothrombin activity.

14.3. Lipids

Lipids, not contributing to the formation of protein antibody and only rarely regarded as antigenic, have been neglected in the immunological context. A few observations have been made of the effects of dietary lipids on the reticulo-endothelial system. Trioleate has a depressant effect when given orally in the diet (Berken and Benacerraf 1966) despite its known stimulating effect when given intravenously (Stuart et al. 1960). Cod liver oil, both oxidized and fresh, in the diets of Columbia-Sherman female rats was found by Mckay et al. (1964) to depress reticulo-endothelial function.

14.4. Proteins

14.4.1. Effects on the resistance to infection

At least since the time of Cannon (1942) an adequate protein intake and amino-acid metabolism have been thought of as important in allowing an effective immune response and indeed there has been much to substantiate this. Bertok and Kemenes (1962), for example, have shown in rats infected with leptospires that reduction in the protein content of the diet reduced the ability to respond with antibody formation. Kenney et al. (1968) examined the primary response to sheep red cells in protein-deficient rats. At six days the spleens of the protein-deficient animals were smaller, with fewer cells, less RNA, and more DNA per cell than those of the control group. The lowering of the antibody titre was associated with a reduction in the antibody forming cells in the spleen, the numbers being reduced by two thirds.

Increased susceptibility to infection in protein-deficient animals is not always explained by a reduction in antibody production. Katz and Plotkin (1967) have demonstrated the increased susceptibility of weanling mice to *Herpes simplex* after one week on a protein-free diet; the virus spreads more readily within the body, a smaller dose is required to initiate infection, a higher mortality and a heightened viraemia are found. Encephalitis, rare in the control group, was consistently found in the protein-deficient group. Within the time of observation both groups produced an interferon-like substance in like amount but neither produced antibody. The breach in the defences lay elsewhere. Chickens on two protein diets (15 and 30% protein) behaved differently when infected with viral and bacterial agents (Boyd and Edwards 1963). Animals on the lower protein diet were more susceptible to inoculation with *Escherichia coli* than when on the higher protein diet. Those animals on the higher protein diet were more susceptible to Newcastle disease.

Diets sufficient for weight gain are not necessarily those which best allow resistance to infection to develop. This finding in mice (Howie and Porter 1950) has been confirmed in chicks (Fisher et al. 1964). Birds, initially given a high protein (28% protein) or control (22% protein) diet, were subsequently fed a diet lacking an essential aminoacid and were then challenged with Newcastle disease virus. Those birds fed the high protein diet before the deficient diet had been fortified in some way, since weight gain, resistance, and humoral antibody levels were greater.

In many dietary studies including those concerned with protein requirements, the effects of the dietary changes are tested by the infectivity, morbidity, or mortality after exposure to an infective agent. This has provided useful information in studies of population nutrition or animal husbandry, but does not define the specific effect on the immunological response. Dubos and Schaedler (1959) have emphasized that the effectiveness of the immune response in such models could only be one of several influences determining the outcome of the encounter with the pathogen; the rate of its multiplication and elimination, the effects of toxin, and the susceptibility to toxaemia all play their part.

14.4.2. Delayed-type hypersensitivity

The ability to react with delayed-type hypersensitivity is affected by the protein calorie malnutrition of Kwashiorkor in African children. It has been possible, however, to restore tuberculin sensitivity to such children by passive transfer of sensitized lymphocytes (Brown and Katz 1964). There is therefore only a difficulty in initiating the response and not in producing the accessory cellular and humoral factors for the hypersensitive reaction. Further evidence of difficulty in cellular proliferation is seen during infections in such children when they are unable to mount a leucocyte response. Their leucocytes at such times contain more alkaline phosphatase (Tejada et al. 1964).

14.4.3. Effects on leucocytes

From observations made in normal and thymectomized rats, Aschkenazy (1965, 1966) has deduced that atrophy of the thymus accounts for a large part of the fall in the number of the larger and medium-sized lymphocytes which follows protein deficiency. Restoration of protein to the diet results in a rapid increase in their number but the omission of an essential amino acid is sufficient to prevent the recrudescence of the lymphocyte population.

Protein also influences leucocyte mobilization. Gray (1964) extending his experiments on lysine deficiency (*v. infra*) in rats on a gluten diet found that the deficient animals do not sustain a leucocyte response and that the relative number of monocytes is reduced by more than 50%. The less resistant animals also mobilized more slowly fewer intraperitoneal leucocytes after injection of an intraperitoneal irritant. In man a reduction in the polymorphonuclear leucocytes and lymphocytes was found in prolonged total starvation (Shapiro 1964).

14.4.4. Induction of tolerance

The inability of protein-deficient hosts to mount an effective immune response may be related in part to their rate of protein clearance or catabolism. Where protein intakes are low, the specific dynamic action of protein is lost and the metabolic rate falls. Not only host but also foreign proteins are removed from the circulation more slowly. This in experimental systems has been associated with poorer responses to antigen, possibly because unprocessed antigen has persisted and has remained to inhibit the appropriate clones. For example in Sobey mice with bovine serum albumin as antigen, those individuals eliminating the antigen slowly do not respond by producing antibody (Hardy and Rowley 1968). Also in CBA mice a high carbohydrate diet led to slowed excretion of the protein antigen, bovine gamma globulin; such animals gave a poorer antibody response to bovine gamma globulin after stimulation with a mycobacterial adjuvant than did animals on a balanced diet (Stark 1970b).

14.4.5. Protein antigens by the oral route

The oral route of antigen administration has been avoided in experimental work because of the possibility of the antigen being digested in the gastrointestinal tract before absorption, yet observations have been made to show that the arrival of antigen or hapten by the oral route is part of the host's immunological experience. The oral introduction of hapten may inhibit the response to the complete antigen as is seen in guinea pigs with dinitrochlorobenzene (the Sulzberger-Chase phenomenon). In man an antibody response may be stimulated by the oral route. When bovine serum albumin (BSA) was given either orally or subcutaneously to human adults an increase in antibodies to BSA could be detected in the serum of those individuals who had retained from childhood the ability to respond (Korenblat et al. 1968). About 80% of the adults have lost this childhood ability but why this should be so is not known.

14.5. Amino acid deficiencies

In rats antibodies against the synthetic antigen poly-Glu^{52}Lys^{33}Tyr^{15} (no. 3) or sheep red cells were decreased on a diet with tryptophan or phenylalanine deficiency (Gershoff et al. 1968). Methionine did not alter the response; the methionine antagonist, ethionine, decreased the antibody response, an effect which could not be reversed by adenine or methionine. Gill and Gershoff (1967) in a primate (*Cebus albifron*) found that methionine deficiency or excess or ethionine did not alter the primary response. Ethionine had some depressive effect on the early secondary phase. Several amino acid deficiencies decreased the antibody response of rats to *Leptospira icterohaemorrhagiae*; methionine, glycine, isoleucine, or tryptophan (the last three in increasing order of effectiveness) had this action. The addition of ethionine to a concentration of 0.36% in a normal diet resulted in such a reduced response that a large number of the animals died (Bertok et al. 1962; Bertok and Kemenes 1963).

Gray (1963) has demonstrated the increased susceptibility of rats on a lysine-deficient diet to several concentrations of *Bacillus anthracis* spores given subcutaneously. Lysine, added to the gluten diet producing the deficiency, restored resistance only partially. Gray demonstrated by the carbon clearance technique a decreased clearing ability in the RES during lysine deficiency and postulated an increased retention of spores within the body. In contrast, Dubos and Schaedler (1959) in similar experiments with different bacterial species found the same content of organisms in the organs of normal and deficient animals. In

                    J. M. Stark

lysine-deficiency oxygen utilization is increased but is not increased further during phagocytosis. This has been taken to mean that there is lessened ability to destroy organisms once they are engulfed (Wojcik and Gray 1966). Basically charged polypeptides from polymorphs are lethal for anthrax and other organisms (Skarnes and Watson 1956; Spitznagel 1961). A deficiency in the basic amino-acid lysine might result in deficiencies in these polypeptides.

14.6. Starvation

During food restriction the serum components taking part in natural or acquired resistance are conserved, the other proteins providing a labile reserve for tissue utilization and maintenance. This was the conclusion of Weimer et al. (1963, 1964) who had examined the effect of food restriction in rats at three levels of weight loss. Complement levels were down at 12% weight loss and increased at 26% and 33% but as depletion continued there was a gradual return to normal. Alpha-2 and gamma-globulin were either normal or increased although other protein concentrations had fallen. Kenney et al. (1965) have also shown that although antibody levels fell in the first six weeks of protein depletion in rats, complement and properdin levels did not do so.

A 28 day period of dietary restriction in rabbits suppressed the early stages of the immune response to bovine serum albumin, but did not induce an extended paralysis (Samuelson et al. 1965). This suppression was unrelated to depletion of serum protein and was not abolished by daily vitamin supplement.

Lowered opsonic activity may be the cause of the poorer resistance found in profound malnutrition (Saba and di Luzio 1968). RES activity was observed by the clearance of a gelatinized lipid emulsion and was found to be decreased. Exposure of the test emulsion to normal serum beforehand abolished the RES depression brought on by the starvation, but serum from starved rats did not have this opsonic activity.

Megirian (1964) also observed the behaviour of the RES in the rat by carbon clearance and clearance of ^{32}P chromium phosphate, and noted a reduced performance after a five day period of reduced food intake. A reduced blood flow as well as a reduced phagocytic activity was postulated to explain this finding.

References

ALLISON, A. C. and L. MALLUCCI, 1964, Lancet *2*, 1371.
ASCHKENAZY, A., 1965, Experientia *21*, 225.

ASCHKENAZY, A., 1966, Compt. Rend. Soc. Biol. *160*, 1787.

AXELROD, A. E. and J. PRUZANSKY, 1955, Vitamins Hormones *13*, 1.

AXELROD, A. E. and A. C. TRAKATELLIS, 1964, Vitamins Hormones *22*, 591.

BERENBAUM, M. C. and I. N. BROWN, 1965, Immunology *8*, 251.

BERKEN, A. and B. BENACERRAF, 1966, Proc. Soc. Exptl. Biol. Med. *128*, 793.

BERTOK, L. and F. KEMENES, 1962, Z. Immun.-Forsch. *124*, 270.

BERTOK, L. and F. KEMENES, 1963, Z. Immun.-Forsch. *125*, 438.

BERTOK, L., F. KEMENES and G. SIMON, 1962, Z. Immun.-Forsch. *124*, 280.

BOYD, F. M. and H. M. EDWARDS, 1963, J. Infect. Diseases *112*, 53.

BROWN, R. E. and M. KATZ, 1967, J. Pediatr. *70*, 126.

CANNON, P. R., 1942, J. Immunol. *44*, 107.

CHASE, M. W. 1946, Proc. Soc. Exptl. Med. Biol. *61*, 257.

CORDINGLEY, J. and T. NICHOL, 1961, Nature *191*, 82.

DE DUVE, C., 1959, Lysosomes, a new group of subcellular particles. *In*: T. Hayashi, ed.: Subcellular particles. New York, Ronald Press.

DINGLE, J. T., 1968, Brit. Med. Bull. *24*, 141.

DINGLE, J. T., J. A. LUCY and H. B. FELL, 1961, Biochem. J. *79*, 497.

DRESSER, D. W., 1960, Immunology *3*, 289.

DRESSER, D. W., 1968, Nature *217*, 527.

DUBOS, R. J. and R. W. SCHAEDLER, 1959, J. Pediatr. *55*, 1.

FERRER, J. F. and E. MIHICH, 1968, *28*, 1116.

FISHER, B., E. R. FISHER and E. SAFFER, 1964, Transplantation *2*, 235.

FISHER, H., J. GRUN, R. SHAPIRO and J. ASHLEY, 1964, J. Nutr. *83*, 165.

GADESBUSCH, H. H. and P. W. GIKAS, 1963, J. Infect. Diseases *112*, 125.

GALL, D., 1966, Immunology *11*, 369.

GERSHOFF, S. N., T. J. GILL, III, S. J. SIMONIAN and A. I. STEINBERG, 1968, J. Nutr. *95*, 184.

GILL, T. J., III and S. N. GERSHOFF, 1967, J. Immunol. *99*, 883.

GRAY, I., 1963, J. Exptl. Med. *117*, 497.

GRAY, I., 1964, Proc. Soc. Exptl. Biol. Med. *116*, 414.

HARDY, D. and D. ROWLEY, 1968, Immunology *14*, 401.

HARMON, B. G., E. R. MILLER, J. A. HOEFER, D. E. ULLREY and R. W. LUECKE, 1963, J. Nutr. *79*, 263.

HARTLEY, P., 1942, Proc. Roy. Soc. Med. *36*, 147.

HARTLEY, P., 1948, Proc. Roy. Soc. Med. *41*, 328.

HIRSCHHORN, R., J. M. KAPLAN, A. F. GOLDBERG, K. HIRSCHHORN and G. WEISSMAN, 1965, Science *147*, 55.

HOWIE, J. W. and G. PORTER, 1950, J. Nutr. *4*, 175.

ISLIKER, H., F. WEBER and O. WISS, 1960, Z. Physiol. Chem. *320*, 126.

JANSZ, A., H.-D. FLAD, D. KOFFLER and P. MIESCHER, 1967, Int. Arch. Allergy *31*, 69.

JEFFRIES, G. H., D. W. HOSKINS and M. H. SLEISENGER, 1962, J. Clin. Invest. *41*, 1106.

KATZ, M. and S. A. PLOTKIN, 1967, J. Nutr. *93*, 555.

KENNEY, M. A., L. ARNRICH, E. MAR and C. E. RODERUCK, 1965, J. Nutr. *85*, 213.

KENNEY, M. A., C. E. RODERUCK, L. ARNRICH and F. PIEDAD, 1968, J. Nutr. *95*, 173.

KIES, M. W., S. MUELLER and E. C. ALVORD, 1964, Z. Immun.-Forsch. *126*, 228.

KORENBLAT, P. E., R. M. ROTHBERG, P. MINDEN and R. S. FARR, 1968, J. Allergy *41*, 226.

KUMAR, M. and A. E. AXELROD, 1968, J. Nutr. *96*, 53.

KUMAR, M. and A. E. AXELROD, 1969, J. Nutr. *98*, 41.

LONG, D. A., 1950, Brit. J. Exptl. Path. *31*, 183.

LUDOVICI, P. P. and A. E. AXELROD, 1951, Proc. Soc. Exptl. Biol. Med. *77*, 526.

MCKAY, D. G., W. MARGARETTEN and J. ROTHERBERG, 1964, Lab. Invest. *13*, 54.

MEGIRIAN, R., 1964, J. Reticuloendothelial Soc. *1*, 333.

MEGIRIAN, R. and D. LEONARDI, 1966, J. Reticuloendothelial Soc. *3*, 295.

MIHICH, E., 1962, Cancer Research *22*, 218.

MIHICH, E. and C. A. NICHOL, 1965, Cancer Research *25*, 153.

MUELLER, J. F., 1964, Vitamins Hormones *22*, 787.

MURANYI, F., L. BERTOK and F. KEMENES, 1964, Z. Immun.-Forsch. *127*, 1.

PANDA, B. and G. F. COMBS, 1963, Proc. Soc. Exptl. Biol. Med. *113*, 530.

SABA, T. M. and N. R. DI LUZIO, 1968, Proc. Soc. Exptl. Biol. Med. *128*, 869.

SAMUELSON, J. S., S. C. KRAFT and R. S. FARR, 1965, J. Immun. *95*, 1013.

SCAGLIONE, G., 1938, Boll. 1st. Sieroter. *17*, 408.

SCHMECKEBIER, M., 1945, Amer. J. Dis. Child. *66*, 25.

SCHWARTZ, M., 1960, Lancet *2*, 1263.

SHAPIRO, Y. L., 1964, Federation Proc. Trans. Suppl. *23*, 447.

SKARNES, R. C. and D. S. WATSON, 1956, Proc. Soc. Exptl. Biol. Med. *93*, 267.

SPITZNAGEL, J. K., 1961, J. Exptl. Med. *114*, 1063.

SPITZNAGEL, J. K. and A. C. ALLISON, 1970, J. Immunol. *119*, 104.

STARK, J. M., 1970a, Immunology *19*, 457.

STARK, J. M., 1970b, Immunology *19*, 449.

STOERK, H. C. and H. N. EISEN, 1946, Proc. Soc. Exptl. Biol. Med. *89*, 323.

STOWE, H. D. and C. K. WHITEHAIR, 1964, Amer. J. Vet. Res. *25*, 1542.

STUART, A. E., G. BIOZZI, C. STIFFEL, B. N. HALPERN and D. MOUTON, 1960, Brit. J. Exptl. path. *41*, 599.

SULZBERGER, M. B., 1930, Arch. Derm. Syph. *22*, 839.

TASHMUKHAMEDOV, F. R., 1966, Federation Proc. Trans. Suppl. *25*, 143.

TEJADA, C., V. ARGUETA, M. SANDREZ and C. ALBERTAZZI, 1964, J. Pediatr. *64*, 753.

TRAKATELLIS, A. C. and A. E. AXELROD, 1969, Proc. Soc. Exptl. Biol. Med. *132*, 46.

UHR, J. W. and G. WEISSMAN, 1965, J. Immunol. *94*, 544.

UHR, J. W., G. WEISSMAN and L. THOMAS, 1963, Proc. Soc. Exptl. Biol. Med. *112*, 287.

WEBER, F., O. WISS and H. ISLIKER, 1963, Experientia *19*, 142.

WEIMER, H. E., J. F. GODFREY, R. E. MEYERS and J. N. MILLER, 1963, J. Nutr. *81*, 405.

WEIMER, H. E., J. N. MILLER, R. L. MEYERS, D. BAXTER, D. M. ROBERTS, J. F. GODFREY and C. M. CARPENTER, 1964, Cancer Research, *24*, 847.

WEISSMAN, G., J. W. UHR and L. THOMAS, 1963, Proc. Soc. Exptl. Biol. Med. *112*, 284.

WERTMAN, K. and J. L. SARANDRIA, 1952, Proc. Soc. Exptl. Biol. Med. *81*, 395.

WHITE, R. G., 1968, Proc. Roy. Soc. Med. *61*, 1.

WOJCIK, J. D. and I. GRAY, 1966, Proc. Soc. Exptl. Med. Biol. *123*, 435.

ZWEIMAN, B., R. W. BESDINE and E. A. HILDRETH, 1966, J. Immunol. *96*, 672.

CHAPTER 15

Histocompatibility in transplantation immunity

J. R. BATCHELOR

McIndoe Memorial Research Unit, Queen Victoria Hospital, East Grinstead, Sussex

and

L. BRENT

Department of Immunology, St. Mary's Hospital Medical School, London W.2

15.1. Introduction

We now have a fair understanding of the genetic basis of tissue transplantation in several species, and recent years have seen a steady unravelling of the chemistry of histocompatibility antigens; yet we remain very uncertain as to the precise meaning and the biological causes of immunogenicity in this field. That skin allografts transplanted between certain mouse strains incite a violent response leading to rapid rejection, whilst in other strain combinations the response is weaker in varying degrees, has been known for at least 10 years. Furthermore, we now realize that the 'strength' of an antigenic disparity provides us with one of the most important variables in the formation of serum antibodies and the induction of immunological tolerance. Although we can define the genetic conditions that make some strain combinations 'strong' and others 'weak' (for recent reviews see Lengerová 1969; Hildemann 1970a, b; Simonsen 1970) we remain at a loss to explain these concepts in molecular terms. It is true that the immunogenicity of histocompatibility antigens can be increased by the use of adjuvants, as for other kinds of antigens. This does not, however, answer the central question concerning the nature of 'the built-in adjuvanticity' that dictates whether a response is strong or weak. Perhaps the definitive answer will have to await the outcome of attempts now being made to supplement the genetic information by dissecting the complex of antigenic determinants present on the cell surface of any one individual or strain by the chemical and physical isolation of single, soluble antigens, so that their biological properties may be studied separately.

Before discussing the immunogenic properties of histocompatibility

409

antigens it is necessary to survey present-day knowledge of their genetics, distribution and chemistry (Sections 15.2 and 15.3). This is followed by a consideration of their biological properties with special reference to the fields of immunity (Section 15.4.1), tolerance (Section 15.4.2) and enhancement (Section 15.4.3). The concept of antigenic strength and its possible mechanisms are discussed in Section 15.5.

We have confined ourselves to a consideration of antigens playing a role in the rejection of tissues and organs transplanted to recipients belonging to the same species as the donor. Such grafts are known as allografts or allogeneic grafts (homografts or homologous grafts according to the old terminology; see Gorer et al. 1961). Grafts transplanted from one member of a homogeneous inbred strain to another belonging to that strain will be referred to as syngeneic grafts.

15.2. *Genetics of histocompatibility antigens*

Virtually all the initial studies on the immunogenetics of transplantation antigens have been conducted using mice, and there is a comprehensive body of information for this species which is lacking for others. However, what is known about other species indicates close similarity to the mouse. We shall therefore describe here the transplantation antigens of the mouse, with special reference to the problems of immunogenicity. In addition, because current ideas on the genetic structure of the most potent human transplantation antigen system (HL-A) are beginning to influence our concepts of the analogous mouse H-2 system, we shall also describe the current state of knowledge of human transplantation antigen systems.

15.2.1. *Mouse transplantation (histocompatibility or H) antigen systems*
Although it had been previously known that genetic factors influenced the growth of transplantable mouse tumours, C. C. Little (1914) was the first to postulate the existence of multiple, independent genetic systems controlling the growth of transplanted tissue. In order to test Little's hypothesis rigorously it was necessary to have available genetically homogeneous mice, and therefore large-scale inbreeding of mice was undertaken. By the fourth decade of this century several well-inbred mouse strains had been developed, and they were used to establish both Little's hypothesis and its various corollaries, which are usually referred to as the genetic laws of transplantation (Snell 1958a).

During the work which led to the establishment of the laws of transplantation, estimates of the precise number of independent genetic systems which influenced graft survival were made. These estimates, which were based on a formula derived by Little, varied considerably depending upon the particular pair of inbred strains of mice tested and the tumour selected for grafting (Bittner 1935). It was obvious that graft survival was determined by several independent genetic systems, but at the time it was puzzling that there should apparently be so much variation in the number estimated to be involved. Now that the immunological basis of transplantation is understood (Gorer 1937, 1938; Medawar 1944, 1945) we know that the variation in estimates of the number of genetically independent transplantation antigen systems was partially due to variations in immunogenicity of the products of the different systems. Only very approximate estimates of the total number of transplantation antigen systems can be made, most previous ones having been underestimates (Barnes and Krohn 1957; Prehn and Main 1958; Bailey and Mobraaten 1964). Nevertheless it is useful to have an indication, and Hildemann and Cohen (1967) suggest as many as 30–100 loci in mice.

Thanks largely to the studies of G. D. Snell and his co-workers, thirteen autosomal H antigen loci have been individually identified (Snell and Stevens 1961; Snell and Bunker 1965). Snell (1958b) has also developed a series of special mouse strains with common genetic backgrounds but differing with respect to these specific H loci. The strains, termed *congenic*, enable individual H loci to be studied for their immunogenic and other properties (Graff et al. 1966a, b). In addition to the autosomal H loci, two sex-linked loci have also been identified (Eichwald and Silmser 1955; Bailey 1965).

Transplantation antigens of the mouse are of unequal immunogenic potency. The most powerful ones, of which more will be said later, belong to the H-2 system. The remainder (non-H-2 system antigens) show a broad spectrum of immunogenicity. The non-H-2 systems cannot be arranged in a simple hierarchy of decreasing immunogenic potency. There is marked variation even within a single system, with some allelic differences provoking rapid graft rejection whilst others do not (Graff et al. 1966a; Hildemann 1970a). Tests for immunogenicity have involved measuring the duration of graft survival, but many other factors, e.g., the vulnerability of a graft to rejection, dose and size of the graft, and immunological status of the host all complicate their interpretation (see Section 15.4.1). Despite this, the tests have been useful for demonstrating that several, individually weak, non-H-2 allelic differences are capable of additive effects (Hildemann 1970) and that multiple non-H-2 differences may provoke graft rejection as rapidly as that induced by an H-2 difference.

The most immunogenic histocompatibility (H) antigen system of the mouse – the H-2 system – is characterised by extreme polymorphism. Each allele of the locus determines a different set of antigenic specificities. To date, eighteen alleles and 27 antigenic specificities have been identified (Gorer and Mikulska 1959; Stimpfling and Snell 1962). It should be emphasized that the great polymorphism of the H-2 system is due not only to the large number of antigenic specificities, but also to the variety of antigenic combinations possible.

The number of specificities determined by each allele varies considerably. According to Graff (1970) the average number is 8, and no allele determines more than 14. However, experience with the HL-A locus, which is believed to be the human analogue of the H-2 system, has shown that definition of any antigenic specificity is a very complicated problem. We will return to this later in some detail but, at this point, merely note the possibility that the definition of many H-2 specificities may require revision in the future. If this occurs, it will also affect the *number* of specificities previously thought to be determined by an allele. In that case, the variation in number of specificities determined by different alleles may turn out to be spurious.

15.2.2. *Human transplantation antigen systems*

Because of the random pattern of mating in human populations, many of the methods successfully applied to mice cannot be used for genetic analysis of human H antigen systems. At present two systems influencing the survival times of human allografts have been definitely identified, and there is some evidence implicating a third. The two well identified systems are ABO and HL-A, and the doubtful third system is P. However, it is generally assumed that there are a large number of further H systems awaiting identification.

The ABO antigens influence the survival of human allografts in accordance with the familiar principles established for red cell transfusions. The data obtained from transplantation of skin and kidneys which can be analysed to test the effect of ABO incompatibility on graft survival are not extensive, but the results conform with those obtained in blood transfusion (Ceppellini et al. 1966, 1969; Gleason and Murray, 1967). In the ABO system, just as in several mouse H systems, particular allelic disparities are more immunogenic than others. For example A_1 skin is more rapidly rejected than A_2 skin by group O recipients (Ceppellini et al. 1966). There are two special considerations applying to the ABO system which should be borne in mind and which may distinguish it from other human H systems, although this is by no means certain yet. Firstly, there is the existence of prior immunity to the A and B antigens, and this makes it difficult to compare the relative immunogenicity of the antigens of this system with those of other systems. Secondly, the distribution of ABO antigens in vascular endothelium (Glynn and Holborow 1959) may have the effect of rendering graft vessels highly susceptible to immunological reactions against ABO antigens, graft rejection occurring as a secondary consequence.

The HL-A system, like the H-2 system, is polymorphic and complex. It is now believed to consist of two closely linked sites on an undetermined autosomal chromosome (Allen et al. 1970; Kissmeyer-Nielsen and Thorsby 1970). Each chromosomal site determines an allelic series of antigens shown as the first (or LA) series and the second (or Four) series. Because normal human cells are diploid, they carry two antigens of each allelic series if heterozygote, or a double dose of one antigen if homozygous. Table 15.1 gives a list of the currently accepted specificities

TABLE 15.1

Calculated on a panel of 84 individuals; gene frequency $= 1 - \sqrt{(1-f)}$ where $f =$ phenotype frequency.

1st Series			*2nd Series*		
Antigen	*Phenotype frequency*	*Gene frequency*	*Antigen*	*Phenotype frequency*	*Gene frequency*
HL-A 1	0.262	0.141	HL-A 5	0.167	0.087
2	0.464	0.268	7	0.298	0.162
3	0.286	0.155	8	0.202	0.107
9	0.262	0.141	12	0.298	0.162
10	0.107	0·055	13	0.071	0.036
11	0.031	0.068	Bt26 (part of LND)	0.060	0.030
Ba*	0.083	0.042	BB*(BB minus HL-A13)	0.107	0.055
Bt 15	0.095	0.049	Maki	0.095	0.049
			Bt 22 (AA)	0.048	0.024
Unidentified alleles		0.081	AJ	0.119	0.061
			(Mapi) Te 17	0.083	0.042
		1.000	R*[a]	0.267	0.146
			Unidentified alleles		0.039
					1.000
8 identified, and at least one unidentified, alleles			12 identified, and at least one unidentified, alleles		

[a] Calculated on basis of panel of 45 for R* specificity.

in each allelic series; it also shows their gene frequency in a panel of individuals from East Grinstead, Sussex, assuming that the HL-A genes are in Hardy-Weinburg equilibrium. It can be seen from the Table that neither allelic series is quite complete, and this is assumed to be so because of as yet unidentified antigens.

Inheritance of HL-A antigens follows Mendelian principles. Each offspring inherits one HL-A bearing chromosomal region (haplotype) from each parent. A haplotype determines two antigens, one of each allelic series. Because crossing over between the chromosomal sites which determine the antigens of the different series is a rare event, antigens of the two series are inherited 'en bloc'. An example of this is shown in Table 15.2.

Identification of HL-A antigens has proved to be an arduous and confusing task. Much of the early confusion was due to the use of different antigen nomenclatures by different laboratories, but this problem has now been resolved by general agreement on terminology (W.H.O. Committee on HL-A Nomenclature, 1968). Precise antigen definition was also impeded by the difficulty in obtaining monospecific sera containing a single HL-A antibody. It was of course recognized that antigen definition would be inaccurate if an antiserum contained more than one antibody, but it was not generally appreciated until very recently that cross-reactive HL-A antibodies exist (Dausset et al. 1969; Svejgaard and Kissmeyer-Nielsen 1968) and that this affects antigen definition. The result of using cross-reactive antibodies is to classify related but different antigens as being identical. Until a non-cross-reacting antibody is found, or one which has a different pattern of cross-reactivity, the true position will not be recognized. A good example of the problem set by cross-reactive antisera is illustrated by antigen Ba (Kissmeyer-Nielsen et al. 1968). This was originally thought to be a single entity because it was defined by a monospecific antiserum. Later, non-cross-reacting sera showed that the Ba antigen was composed of HL-A2 and a second specificity which is termed Ba*. If a panel of individuals is tested, all those who are either Ba*- or HL-A2-positive (or both) will also be positive with the antiserum defining Ba. The distribution of Ba* and HL-A2 is therefore said to be 'included' within that of Ba.

Many of the earlier definitions of HL-A antigens are now recognized as being composite, or serologically cross-reacting groups of antigens. There can be little doubt that this process of antigen dissection will continue, and that some of the currently accepted antigens will be found later to be composite. It is significant that the lymphocytes of unrelated individuals serologically classified as being HL-A identical are nevertheless frequently mutually reactive in mixed lymphocyte cultures (Bach

TABLE 15.2

	Phenotype (HL-A antigens)		Haplotypes			
	1st Series	2nd Series				
Father	1, 2	8, 12	Ⓐ 1, 8		Ⓑ 2, 12	
Mother	3, 9	7, 13	Ⓒ 3, 7		Ⓓ 9, 13	
Sibling 1	1, 9	8, 13	Ⓐ 1, 8		Ⓓ 9, 13	
2	1, 9	8, 13	Ⓐ 1, 8		Ⓓ 9, 13	
3	2, 9	12, 13	Ⓑ 2, 12		Ⓓ 9, 13	
4	2, 3	7, 12	Ⓑ 2, 12		Ⓒ 3, 7	
5	1, 3	7, 8	Ⓐ 1, 8		Ⓒ 3, 7	

The paternal and maternal haplotypes are arbitrarily labelled Ⓐ or Ⓑ and Ⓒ or Ⓓ respectively. Each child inherits one haplotype from each parent. Siblings 1 and 2 are HL-A identical; they share one haplotype D with sibling 3 and have none in common with sibling 4.

et al. 1970; Eijsvoogel et al. 1970). Although other explanations of this observation are possible, a very probable one is that the serological classification of antigenic identity is still an approximation, and that even the more discriminating HL-A antisera show some limited cross-reactivity.

The existence of cross-reactivity has several implications. It might be thought, for example, that the immunogenicity of a given transplantation antigen would depend to some degree on whether the recipient possesses a cross-reacting specificity. This important point has yet to be systematically examined. Because cross-reactivity raises questions about antigen definition, it also affects concepts of the genetic structure of the H antigen system (Batchelor and Sanderson, 1970; Batchelor and Selwood, 1970). Failure to recognize that two antisera are cross-reactive can lead to the false conclusion that the sera are identifying two separate specificities in an individual. Under these circumstances it becomes necessary to postulate a more complex genetic structure in order to accommodate the almost limitless number of antigens determined by the locus. Returning for the moment to the H-2 locus of mice, it is possible that many of what were previously thought to be separate specificities are actually single entities which show varying degrees of cross-reactivity with different H-2 antisera. In that case a simpler genetic interpretation of the H-2 locus might be possible. Great interest has been aroused by the observation that many (but not all) H-2 specificities can be arranged into two allelic series comparable to those of the HL-A system (Thorsby

1970; Snell et al. 1971). Furthermore, the inclusion of some antigens within others is seen in the H-2 system (Shreffler and Klein 1970), just as in the HL-A system, and this implies that much of the complexity, both antigenic and genetic, previously attributed to the H-2 system is artefactual. Although it is possible that the H-2 and HL-A systems may indeed have a different genetic structure, the idea is not an attractive one from an evolutionary point of view, and it is not consistent with the close physico-chemical homology between the two systems (Davies et al. 1968).

15.3. Distribution and chemistry of histocompatibility antigens

Mouse H-2 antigens have been shown to occur on tissue cells from an early embryonic age (Möller, 1962; Edidin, 1964) and they may be found, albeit in varying concentrations, on the cell membranes of all kinds of tissues (Snell and Stimpfling, 1966). Using ferritin-labelled antibody, Aoki et al. (1969) have shown that, whilst spleen and lymph node lymphocytes have relatively high concentrations of H-2 antigens, thymocytes have much lower concentrations and red cells least of all. The distribution of antigens on the cell membrane was found by these workers to be discontinuous but large areas of the membrane were found to be involved. That histocompatibility antigens are poorly expressed on mouse red cells had previously been inferred because red cells are not as good as tissue cells in eliciting antibody formation, they do not absorb antisera very efficiently, and they are virtually ineffective in sensitizing adult mice or rabbits to skin allografts (Medawar 1946, 1959). The reason for the relatively poor immunogenic properties of red cells is likely to be quantitative, for it is known that some H-2 specificities are not at all demonstrable on red cells (Gorer and Mikulska 1959); lack of a suitable carrier molecule could, however, also play a role.

In man the situation appears to be very similar: again, serological tests have shown that HL-A antigens are present on a wide variety of tissues including leucocytes, platelets and even spermatozoa (Fellous and Dausset 1970), but attempts to demonstrate their presence on mature red cells have met with failure (Dausset 1958; Harris and Zervas 1969). It is therefore a matter of some interest that human reticulocytes have been shown to carry several HL-A specificities (Harris and Zervas 1969), an observation that suggests that many HL-A determinants are lost during the course of red cell maturation. Evidently this need not apply to every HL-A antigen, for according to Morton et al. (1969) the rather rare human red cell antigen Bg[a] has almost complete concordance with antigen HL-A7 and may therefore be regarded as an histocompatibility antigen. The relatively feeble expression of histocompatibility antigens on mouse red cells may be presumed to have a similar basis, antigenic loss not having gone to completion here. However, so far as we know, the immunogenicity of mouse reticulocytes has not yet been investigated.

In the mouse there are a number of antigenic systems which have been found on tissue cell membranes, but whose role in transplantation has not yet been determined. They are nevertheless to be regarded as alloantigens because they are not present in all strains and are inherited in Mendelian fashion. The TL (thymus-leukaemia), theta θ and Ly-A/Ly-B antigens belong to this group (see Old and Boyse 1969). The TL system was uncovered by Old et al. (1963) when they demonstrated by serological methods the existence of an antigen specific for radiation-induced leukaemias which was also found to be present on the thymus cells of some, but not all, strains. Recent studies have shown conclusively that, in normal mice, the TL antigens are rigidly restricted to the cells of the thymus and that they are not to be found on spleen or lymph node lymphocytes (Aoki et al. 1969). The TL locus is linked to the H-2 locus, and one of its fascinating features is that its antigens can 'modulate', i.e., disappear from the surface of TL + ve leukaemic cells if a TL + ve leukaemia is grown in TL− ve mice which had been pre-immunized with TL + ve cells. The recognition of θ on thymus cells we owe to the work of Reif and Allen (1964), who showed that it could be present in two allelic forms – θ AKR (in AKR and RF mice) and θ C3H (in most other strains). Unlike TL antigens, θ is present on thymus-derived peripheral lymphocytes as well as on thymocytes, and this makes it possible to distinguish between those peripheral lymphocytes that are thymus and those that are bone marrow-derived (Raff 1970).

It used to be widely held that the antigenicity of tissue cells is wholly dependent on the cells' architectural integrity and viability – a concept destroyed by Billingham et al. (1956), who showed that subcellular preparations obtained from lymphoid tissues sensitize adult mice to skin allografts. This cleared the way for the study of the chemical nature of histocompatibility antigens, and much progress has since been made, largely through the persistent efforts of D. A. L. Davies, B. D. Kahan, A. A. Kandutsch, D. L. Mann, L. Manson, A. R. Sanderson and their colleagues, to name but a few. If progress has at times seemed slow, this merely reflects the great technical difficulties encountered in the study of substances that are both complex and labile. Nathenson (1970) and Reisfeld and Kahan (1970) have recently reviewed this field most admirably, and readers are referred to their articles for detailed references of the more recent work (see also Davies 1968).

Methods used in studying the chemistry of histocompatibility antigens are based on the injection of tissue extracts and their sub-fractions into animals, followed by measurements of immunological reactivity in terms of one of the following criteria: (a) the degree of sensitization or unresponsiveness to skin allografts from the extract donor or donor strain; (b) the ability of the recipient's lymphoid cells to perform immunologically in a graft-*versus*-host assay or to transform *in vitro* to blast cells when cultured in the presence of specific antigens; and (c) antibody formation (chiefly haemagglutinating, cytotoxic or enhancing antibodies). Two other *in vitro* tests have proved useful: (d) the inhibition of haemagglutination or cytotoxicity with tissue extracts, and (e) the macrophage-migration inhibition test, in which macrophages obtained from sensitized donors are prevented from moving out of a capillary tube if the specific antigen(s) is added to the culture medium.* It should be noted that, with the exception of the skin graft test and the graft-*versus*-host assay, these tests do not necessarily *prove* that a given fraction contains antigens that play a role in graft rejection. On the other hand, the *in vitro* tests are generally simpler and more quantitative, and they do give information about the presence or absence of histocompatibility specificity. When used in combination with skin grafting or graft-*versus*-host assays, they have proved to be a most valuable tool, and this is particularly true for the inhibition tests. While most experiments have been done with the H-2 antigens of the mouse, human HL-A antigens have also been intensively studied in recent years.

Nathenson (1970) and Reisfeld and Kahan (1970) have discussed the various methods used in the extraction and solubilization of H antigens. They include exposure of cell suspensions (for reasons of convenience they are nearly always of lymphoid or tumour origin) to ultrasound or low-frequency sound, detergents such as Triton X-100, organic solvents such as butanol, chelating agents (e.g., EDTA), 'autolysis' (i.e., enzymatic degradation by enzymes present within the cells), proteolytic enzymes including trypsin, papain, ficin and pronase, or phospholipase A. Solubilized materials have been purified with the aid of high-speed centrifugation, column chromatography and electrophoresis.

The analytical data of different workers vary somewhat, depending largely on the method used to solubilize, and over the years views regarding the chemical nature of the antigens have changed considerably.

---

* Some soluble fractions obtained by autolysis and papain digestion are strongly and non-specifically toxic to macrophages (personal communication from Dr. N. Staines, Searle Research Laboratories, High Wycombe, England) and some caution is therefore indicated in the application of this test.

It should be pointed out that, in considering the results of chemical investigations, a given extracted fraction may contain the whole native molecule or subunits thereof; knowledge of the substances present in an active fraction need not, therefore, define the chemical nature of the determinant group, which is likely to represent only a small fraction of the whole molecule. Early experiments (Billingham et al. 1956) seemed to implicate deoxyribonucleo-proteins as being involved in graft rejection; but later these authors withdrew this hypothesis (Billingham et al. 1958). Because crude water extracts obtained with the aid of ultrasound were inactivated by periodate oxidation and *Trichomonas foetus* enzymes – treatments that are well-known to destroy the specificity of human blood group substances – and because serological cross-reactions were obtained between H-2 antigens and pneumococcal polysaccharide Type XIV, human blood group substance A, and group A substance extracted from hog gastric mucin, it was suggested that histocompatibility antigens are amino acid-polysaccharide complexes in which the carbohydrate moiety plays an important role in determining specificity (Billingham et al. 1958; Brent et al. 1961). Kandutsch and Reinert-Wenck (1957) arrived at a similar conclusion after studying the antigens that induce immunological enhancement of tumour growth, for their Triton X-100 solubilized antigens were destroyed by periodate as well as by agents causing protein denaturation. Because the preparations from many laboratories contained lipid as well as protein and carbohydrate it was thought for some years that the antigens were lipoproteins, but this view was undermined by the demonstration that lipid is not an essential component (Kandutsch et al. 1965).

Attention was therefore focused on the glycoprotein moiety of the extracts, and the experiments of Shimada et al. (1970) in particular now strongly suggest that antigenic specificity is controlled by their amino acid sequence. Thus it was found that glycoproteins prepared from two mouse strains differing at the H-2 locus ($H-2^b$ and $H-2^k$) could be resolved into peptides of which 90% were identical and 10% different, whereas no detectable difference was found between their carbohydrate moieties (see Nathenson 1970). It is, of course, possible that the apparent absence of carbohydrate differences in these preparations was due to limitations of the techniques used.

H-2 and HL-A preparations have turned out to have very similar physico-chemical properties: although individual analyses differ in detail, depending on the extraction procedure used, they commonly have 70–90% protein, 3–9% carbohydrate and small amounts of sialic acid and glucosamine. Nevertheless, Sanderson et al. (1971) have recently struck a discordant note by describing experiments in which the inhibitory power of low molecular weight (8–10,000) glycopeptides produced by solubilization with papain and further digestion with insoluble pronase was shown to be associated with a high carbohydrate and a low amino acid content. Sanderson et al. propose that both protein and carbohydrate are involved in determining the specificity of histocompatibility antigens, a concept that has also been put forward by Shreffler and Klein (1970) for the mouse H-2 system. Accordingly, the protein would form a molecular backbone and its amino acid sequence would serve as a specific receptor for determinants that are themselves carbohydrate. The situation could therefore be similar to that of the human MN system on red cells, where the specificity of sialo-glycopeptides is thought to reside in the carbohydrate moiety although it has not been possible, so far, to show differences in the composition of the oligopolysaccharides obtained from M and N cells (Lisowska and Morawiecki 1967; Thomas and Winzler 1970). The participation of carbohydrate in determining specificity derives indirect support from the rather remarkable cross-reactivity between histocompatibility and streptococcal antigens (see Rapaport 1968).

There is very great variability in the molecular weight of histocompatibility antigens – weights as small as 10^4 (Sanderson et al. 1971) and as high as 2×10^6 (Hämmerling et al. 1971) have been reported. Most active fractions have a molecular weight of 30–50,000. These apparent discrepancies are likely to be a function of the method of solubilization and therefore of the extent to which the native macromolecules have been split into sub-units. Thus the lowest reported molecular weight substances able to inhibit the cytotoxic action of antibody came from glycopeptides obtained by treatment of higher molecular weight material with insoluble pronase (Sanderson et al. 1971).

There is general agreement that the greatest concentration of histocompatibility antigens is on the cell membrane rather than on intracellular organelles. The evidence for this has come mainly from antibody-binding studies on intact cells (Möller 1961; Davis and Silverman 1968; Aoki et al. 1969), and Haughton (1966) confirmed this by showing that the number of antibody-binding sites does not increase substantially after cell rupture. Whilst many experiments with extracted antigen support this conclusion (see Nathenson 1970), some lines of evidence indicate that histocompatibility antigens may, in addition, be present on microsomal membranes (Dumonde et al. 1963; Ozer and Wallach 1967; Palm and Manson 1968) as well as on plasma membranes (Ozer and Wallach 1967).

The question of whether it is possible to separate fractions carrying the specificity of single determinants is only just beginning to be answered. It appears that at least some of the known H-2 specificities can be separated from one another by gel filtration (Shimada and Nathenson 1967) and ion-exchange chromatography (Summerell and Davies 1969; Davies 1969), but it is too early to say whether this applies to all H-2 specificities or whether, for that matter, the separation is as valid for sensitizing or tolerance-inducing antigens as it is for antibody-binding determinants. This approach may yet turn out to be of great importance in any clinical attempts to induce immunological tolerance, for it could be very advantageous to select as the tolerance-inducing stimulus only the specific antigens that are present in the donor but absent in the recipient; at the same time, such a procedure could free the clinician from his dependence on the organ donor as the source of the tolerogenic stimulus (see Section 15.4.2).

15.4. Immunogenic properties

15.4.1. Transplantation immunity

Examples illustrating the wide range of immunogenicity of tissues and organs are numerous, and this field has been extensively surveyed (Hildemann 1970a, b; Simonsen 1970; Bildsøe et al. 1970; also see the monograph published in honour of G. D. Snell – Billingham and Silvers (eds.) 1970). Before discussing some of these examples it is necessary to summarize briefly current views on the mechanism of allograft rejection; here too the reader is referred to reviews published in the last few years (Russell and Monaco 1965; Brent (ed.) 1965; Wilson and Billingham 1967; Russell and Winn 1970; Brent 1971).

That the rejection of allografts has an immunological basis has been appreciated since it was shown in man (Gibson and Medawar 1943) and in rabbits (Medawar 1944, 1945) that a second graft from the same donor is rejected more rapidly than a first graft, and that this accelerated response is specific for the antigens of the donor. Since then the mechanism of graft rejection has been much studied and it has become clear that two components may be involved, depending on the circumstances in which the allograft is transplanted: (a) a cell-mediated response akin to that of delayed-type hypersensitivity (Brent and Medawar 1967), in which small lymphocytes are strongly implicated (Gowans 1965; Wilson and Billingham 1967; Brent 1971), and (b) a humoral response mediated by antibodies that can frequently be demonstrated in the serum of animals which are rejecting, or have rejected, allografts (Stetson 1963; Winn 1970; Brent 1971). The evidence strongly suggests that

the cell-mediated response is due to receptors on the surface of lymphocytes, and that these resemble 'conventional' free immunoglobulins
(Greaves et al. 1969; Mason and Warner 1970); the humoral antibodies,
on the other hand, can be readily detected by their ability to agglutinate
or lyse red blood cells or tissue cells in suspension, or by their paradoxical
power to promote the induction of immunological enhancement (see
Section 13.4.4).

Which of these two wings of the allograft reaction predominates
depends on a number of factors, mainly on whether the recipient has
been pre-sensitized by prior exposure to the antigens of the graft and
whether the histocompatibility differences between the donor and the
recipient are relatively strong or feeble. Generally, though not always,
the cell-mediated response predominates in solid first-set grafts; in
pre-sensitized recipients circulating antibodies may, however, intervene
decisively as in the hyperacute rejection of kidney grafts (Porter 1965;
Kissmeyer-Nielsen et al. 1966; see Milgrom 1971). Certain kinds of
tissues are undoubtedly more susceptible to the pathogenic effects of
serum antibodies than others; thus skin grafts are relatively refractory,
whilst kidney grafts and grafts of lympho-reticular origin are not (see Winn
1970; Brent 1971). In mice the presence of humoral antibodies is more
difficult to demonstrate when the donor and recipient share the same H-2
('strong') histocompatibility antigens than when they do not, and whilst
this may eventually turn out to be a question of the sensitivity of the
tests used for antibody detection, it is a reasonable presumption that in
many of these relatively 'weak' systems cell-mediated responses pre-
dominate even in second-set responses.

It is now firmly established that the H-2 antigens of the mouse are
positively associated with prompt skin graft rejection and with several
other criteria by which transplantation immunity can be measured, such
as graft-*versus*-host reactions (see Simonsen 1970) and *in vitro* mixed
lymphocyte culture reactions (see Festenstein 1971). Recipients lacking
an H-2 antigen present in the donor can be relied upon to respond
fiercely. (From this it does not follow that 'weak' differences may not,
through an additive effect, provoke strong reactions – see below.)
For the antigens of the human HL-A locus the situation is not nearly
so clear-cut, if only because it is not possible to carry out in man the kind
of experiment that could prove the point decisively; furthermore, it is
most improbable that all antigenic specificities spelled out by this locus
have already been identified. Nevertheless, many attempts to establish
a correlation between the number of HL-A incompatibility differences
and the survival times of skin allografts in normal individuals, or the
survival and function of kidney allografts in immuno-suppressed patients,
indicate that the HL-A system is of great importance.

The evidence is clearest in family studies. The reason for this is that within a family of two parents and their offspring there are only four HL-A haplotypes segregating, if the remote possibility of a cross-over is ignored. Serological recognition of the products of these four alleles is relatively easy even if impure or cross-reacting serological reagents are the only ones available, and therefore the decision as to whether two siblings are HL-A identical or not can be made with accuracy. In contrast, where a large number of different HL-A alleles are segregating, as in any mixed population, classification of two individuals as being HL-A-identical is probably still an approximation. In a mixed population, therefore, one is forced to compare the survival times of obviously HL-A-incompatible grafts with those showing *approximate* HL-A compatibility.

In family studies it has been found that grafts exchanged between HL-A-identical siblings survive on average longer than those made between HL-A-different siblings (or parents). The contrast is very striking when skin grafts are transplanted to otherwise untreated recipients (Amos et al. 1970): HL-A-identical grafts survived for a mean of 24.9 days, those showing one haplotype difference for 14.4 days, and those with 2 haplo-type differences for 11.6 days. Similarly, in immunosuppressed kidney recipients a significantly higher proportion of grafts survive if the donor is HL-A-identical than if he is not (Rapaport et al. 1967; Stickel et al. 1967).

Much of the evidence on the effect of HL-A incompatibility where donor and recipient are unrelated is based on the function and survival of cadaver kidney grafts. Most, but not all laboratories studying this question have reported a positive correlation (Batchelor and Joysey 1969; Batchelor et al. 1971; Morris et al. 1971; Perkins et al. 1971). The steady improvement in both HL-A typing and clinical management of these patients makes it difficult to resolve the controversy over whether HL-A incompatibility has a significant clinical influence on primary kidney transplants; further prospective studies will probably be necessary. But where previous sensitization to HL-A antigens is known to have occurred because of the presence at the time of operation of circulating lymphocytotoxic antibodies reactive with the donor cells, the risk of immediate kidney graft rejection is very high – 80% in the experience of Patel and Terasaki (1969). There seems, therefore, to be little doubt that HL-A compatibility does affect the survival of kidney grafts from unrelated donors, and the argument is only one about the clinical importance of this effect in different circumstances. This conclusion is also supported by the highly significant correlation between HL-A compatibility and the survival of skin from unrelated donors transplanted to severely burned patients (Batchelor and Hackett 1970). Such patients are known to have depressed cell-mediated immune

TABLE

Median survival times (MST) and 95% confidence limits for skin grafts exchanged between

| | | Grafts from C57BL/10ScSn | | | | | |
| | | Female | | | Male | | |
Locus	CR strain	No. reject. Total	MST (days)	95% conf. limits	No. reject. Total	MST (days)	95% conf. limits
H-1	B10·BY	8/8	15	14–16	10/10	15	14–16
H-1	5M	7/7	25	23–27	8/8	26	24–28
H-3	B10·LP-a	9/9	21	20–23	12/14	30	27–33
H-4	21M	5/10	120	46–309	3/4	119	46–311
H-7	47N	22/22	23	21–25	15/15	25	23–26
H-8	57N	4/4	32	26–39	8/9	47	35–63
H-9	45N	8/19	> 400	–	1/11	> 300	–
H-10	9M	14/24	91	67–122	3/14	> 250	–
H-11	10M	10/10	78	63–97	9/9	105	77–144
H-11	55M	4/7	154	52–455	5/8	96	47–201
H-12	12M	7/13	259	132–510	0/12	> 300	–
H-13	14M	10/10	38	33–45	10/10	67	60–75

responses and this presumably exaggerates the difference which was observed in survival times of closely and badly matched skin applied to the same recipient.

Returning to the animal model, mice grafted with H-2-incompatible skin invariably reject their grafts within 12 days of transplantation, whereas differences at other H-loci cause the grafts to be rejected more slowly. This was indicated for the H-3 locus by the work of Counce et al. (1956) and McKhann and Berrian (1961), but it can be illustrated most clearly by comparing numerous congenic pairs (see Section 2). It will be seen from Table 15.3 (taken from Graff et al. 1966a) that many degrees of incompatibility are encountered, and that median survival times (MST – the time at which 50% of grafts are fully rejected) vary from 15 to more than 300 days. (The accuracy of some of these MST's must be regarded as somewhat dubious in view of some of the small groups of mice used, especially as it is not easy to establish end-points for grafts undergoing a long drawn out rejection. However, the data show the general trend clearly enough.) Indeed, such is the feebleness of the antigen(s) involved that recipients differing from their donors at the H-9 locus do not reject skin grafts at all unless great pains are taken to pre-sensitize the recipients. Interestingly, when skin grafts were transplanted reciprocally, MST's often differed substantially.

15.3

congenic resistant (CR) strain pairs. (From Graff et al. 1966a.)

Grafts to C57BL/10ScSn					
Female			*Male*		
No. *reject.* *Total*	*MST* *(days)*	*95%* *conf.* *limits*	*No.* *reject.* *Total*	*MST* *(days)*	*95%* *conf.* *limits*
1/8	> 250	–	1/10	> 250	–
0/5	> 250	–	0/5	> 250	–
5/10	52	24–110	4/6	46	25–84
9/9	25	22–27	9/9	24	21–27
15/15	33	28–40	5/5	47	34–65
5/5	37	21–64	2/5	> 200	–
4/12	> 300	–	0/5	> 300	–
4/5	71	46–110	3/10	> 300	–
7/12	164	101–267	1/6	> 300	–
7/9	71	48–107	5/10	240	80–721
0/15	> 300	–	0/5	> 300	–
3/5	73	22–239	3/5	116	40–330

Another important point emerging from Table 15.3 is that grafts transplanted to females are usually, though not always, rejected faster than grafts transplanted to males. This sex difference can be observed for H-2 incompatibility too, but here rejection occurs so rapidly even in males that the effect may reveal itself by a difference in MST of only a day or two. Nevertheless, such a difference in an H-2-incompatible combination does represent a very significant degree of hyper-reactivity, and this can be shown much more dramatically when graft survival times are artificially lengthened by immunosuppression or the induction of specific unresponsiveness (see Section 15.4.2).

The H-loci listed in Table 15.3 are all autosomal. In order to avoid confusion with the antigens linked with the sex chromosomes (Section 15.2) testing for autosomally controlled histocompatibility differences is always done by selecting donors and recipients of the same sex.

Experiments with congenic mice have established very clearly that it is not so much the histocompatibility loci of the donor that dictate the strength of the response as the interallelic combination of the donor and the recipient. For example, an exchange of skin grafts between the congenic strains C3H/HEDiSn (H-1ᵃ) and C3H.K (H-1ᵇc) revealed that the combination H-1ᵇc → H-1ᵃ represents a considerably stronger incompatibility than the other way about (Hildemann et al. 1970);

such asymmetry of response has been observed in numerous other situations (e.g., Hildemann and Cohen 1967), and on the strength of comparative experiments Hildemann (1970a) has drawn up the following 'pecking order' for the H-1 locus (MST's indicated in brackets): $H\text{-}1^c \rightarrow H\text{-}1^b$ (15) $> H\text{-}1^b \rightarrow H\text{-}1^a$ (25) $> H\text{-}1^a \rightarrow H\text{-}1^b$ (100) $> H\text{-}1^b \rightarrow H\text{-}1^c$ (250). A hierarchical situation of this kind may also apply to human histocompatibility antigens, for Ceppellini et al. (1969) have shown that $A_1 \rightarrow O$ incompatibility is considerably stronger than $A_2 \rightarrow O$.

Apart from interallelic differences and the sex of the host, what other factors enter into the question of immunogenicity of tissue grafts? We will consider, in this order, graft dose, pre-sensitization of the recipients, and the question of whether histocompatibility antigens may have an additive effect; the contribution made by the age of the recipient will be discussed in Section 15.4.4.

Medawar (1944, 1945) first showed that graft dose may influence allograft survival times. Using a genetically heterogeneous collection of rabbits he found that large skin grafts were rejected more rapidly than small grafts. When years later weak histocompatibility barriers were investigated, the question of graft dose assumed even greater importance, though not at all in the same sense as in Medawar's rabbits, for now it was the *small* dose that led to relatively prompt rejection whereas larger skin grafts often showed prolonged survival (Lapp and Bliss, 1967; Hildemann et al. 1970). Indeed, from the earlier studies of McKhann (1964a, b) it is evident that in congenic strains differing at the H-2 locus the balance between immunity and tolerance is greatly dependent on the dose of lymphoid cells injected into the recipients (see Section 15.5). It is impossible, then, to escape the conclusion that graft dose is a vital factor in determining immunogenicity in relatively weak combinations: small doses sensitize, but larger doses may induce immunological tolerance. Conversely, in strong H-2-incompatible situations, in which tolerance cannot be induced in normal animals by a single antigenic stimulus, large doses provide a more effective immunogenic stimulus than small ones, as in Medawar's rabbits.

Evidence concerning the role of pre-sensitization comes from skin grafting (Hildemann et al. 1970), tumour transplantation (Graff et al. 1966a) and graft-*versus*-host assays (see Simonsen 1970). Whilst attempts to presensitize across weak histocompatibility barriers may in fact lead to the induction of partial or complete unresponsiveness (McKhann 1964b; Graff et al. 1966a), accelerated destruction of second-set skin grafts has been observed in many non-H-2 (Hildemann et al. 1970) as well as H-2 (Billingham et al. 1954) incompatible strain combinations. Indeed, Hildemann and his colleagues (see also Klein 1966) find that the weaker the interallelic difference, the greater is the effect of prior sensitization. This is entirely in agreement with Simonsen's observation that the 'factor of immunization' in graft-*versus*-host assays is greater in weak than in strong systems (Simonsen 1962a, b, 1970). (The assay consists essentially of the injection of parental strain spleen cells into young F_1 hybrid recipients: the parental strain cells recognise the antigens inherited by the F_1 hybrid recipient from the other parental strain and, by reacting against them, cause a great deal of proliferation of host cells within the spleen and so, secondarily, splenic enlargement. The 'factor of immunization' is obtained from the ratio of the spleen weight obtained by injecting donor cells pre-sensitized to host antigens and the spleen weight obtained with normal cells.) Simonsen's interpretation of this observation, which has been confirmed in the chicken (Lind and Szenberg 1961; Warner and Szenberg 1964) and in the rat (Elkins 1964; Ford 1967), will be discussed in Section 15.5.

Hildemann et al. (1970) analysed the question of pre-sensitization in congenic mice differing at the H-1 locus. They found that although for first-set grafts the interallelic combination $H\text{-}1^b \rightarrow H\text{-}1^a$ was much stronger than the reciprocal combination $H\text{-}1^a \rightarrow H\text{-}1^b$ (i.e., the MST was shorter), second-set grafts showed a degree of curtailment of survival that was almost equally strong in both combination. These data suggest that pre-sensitization was proportionately more effective in the weaker system, and that pre-sensitization may take precedence over interallelic differences. For the antigens associated with autosomally controlled loci, Hildemann et al. therefore suggest the following 'hierarchy of effects': pre-immunization > interallelic combination > graft dosage > recipient sex. It remains to be seen, however, whether this kind of hierarchy applies to all autosomally directed differences, and clearly other systems need to be studied in similar fashion.

We must now turn our attention to the question: do the weaker histocompatibility antigens reinforce each other when present on the same cell, or is the response they elicit characteristic only for the strongest of them? Unless one postulates antigenic competition between different specificities, or some other negative interaction between them, one might *a priori* expect them to be additive. So it has proved to be. McKhann (1964c), investigating congenic strains differing only at H-1 or H-3 loci, or at both, found that MST's of skin allografts were substantially shorter when donors and recipients differed at both loci than when they differed at only one or the other. He concluded that 'antigenically different receptor sites on or within the cell are highly specific and spatially separated so that immunity against one does not interfere with that against the other'. The more sophisticated studies of

Graff et al. (1966b) are entirely in agreement with McKhann's data, for donor-recipient combinations differing at 2, 3, 4 and more numerous loci were found to give additive effects, i.e., the MST's of skin grafts became shorter as the number of differences increased. However, effects were additive only when the disparity between the strengths of the antigens involved was not too great – a proviso that was found to apply to multiple non-H-2 antigens as well as to combinations of H-2 and non-H-2 antigens. Although they clearly established that there can be a stepwise increase in immunogenicity as the number of histocompatibility differences increases, Graff et al. (1966b) describe an experimental situation in which a ceiling of responsiveness had been reached: multiple non-H-2 antigens having created a strong response (MST = 11.8 days), the addition of a foreign H-2 antigen did not further speed up graft rejection (MST = 11.9 days). Because in the reciprocal combination used in these experiments some further shortening of MST *was* obtained, these workers postulate the existence of a different 'maximum response' for each host.

An interesting complementary study is that of Klein (1966), who analysed congenic mice differing by 1, 2, 3 or more antigens of the H-2 system, non-H-2 differences having been eliminated. Klein reports that in 5 combinations with a single histocompatibility difference the MST's of skin allografts were appreciably greater than in combinations with 2 or more differences, and some of the grafts survived for very long periods without signs of rejection. Not all H-2 antigens are therefore to be regarded as strong, and this highlights the general point that we have, in the past, tended to be too rigid in our views regarding strong and weak antigens. These terms should be used in a purely relative sense. The so-called 'strong' H-2 locus controls a mixed bag of strong, moderately weak and even weak antigens, and likewise the so-called 'weak' loci can present a formidable barrier by virtue of their additive propensities. It is therefore unreasonable to expect the battle of human tissue typing to be fought and won exclusively over the HL-A locus.

Because mixed lymphocyte culture (MLC) tests are being used as an adjunct to tissue typing, we will briefly summarize the most important facts concerning them. Up-to-date reviews of this field by Festenstein (1971) and Bach (1971) are available and further information and references may be obtained from them.

The MLC test depends upon the observation that human lymphocytes 'transform' into pyroninophilic blast cells, many of which divide when cultured in the presence of cells from a genetically different individual (Schrek and Donnelly 1961; Bain et al. 1963; Bain and Lowenstein 1964; Bach and Hirschhorn 1964). Mixtures of cells from identical twins do not show this effect, and a correlation has been found between the degree of genetic disparity and the degree of *in vitro* stimulation; thus, cell mixtures from related individuals do not form as many blast cells as those obtained in cell mixtures from unrelated individuals. The usual method of estimating the degree of stimulation is to measure the amount of radioactive tracer incorporated by the cells after several days of culture. The MLC test has become a useful indicator of histo-incompatibility by the device of blocking the target cells with mitomycin C or some other agent inhibiting cell division, so that the test measures only the reactivity of the responder (recipient) cells to the target (donor) cells.

One of the great attractions of this test is that it can be carried out *in vitro* without sensitizing either the potential donor or the recipient; its principal disadvantage is that it takes several days to complete (this makes it difficult to apply the test to cadaver donors) and that it does not define the antigens responsible for histoincompatibility. The rationale behind the use of peripheral blood leucocytes as target cells, convenience apart, is that both in experimental animals and in man it has been shown that many of the leucocyte antigens are histocompatibility antigens; indeed, from experiments on immunological tolerance one can be reasonably certain that blood leucocytes have all the histocompatibility antigens of that individual (see Section 15.4.2). However, the possible existence of tissue-specific histocompatibility antigens should not be overlooked, a point stressed by Boyse et al. (1970). These workers studied the survival of strain A skin grafts in C57Bl/6 mice that had been lethally irradiated and restored with F_1 hybrid spleen and bone marrow cells. The grafts were destroyed quite rapidly although the lymphocytes as well as the erythrocytes of the recipients were demonstrably of donor origin. Boyse et al. therefore postulate that different skin alloantigens exist in the A and C57Bl/6 strains and that graft rejection was due to the loss of tolerance in the transferred cells to A strain skin alloantigen(s). (They dismiss the possibility that rejection was caused by incomplete destruction of the host's own lymphoid pool.) The strength of these antigens seems surprisingly great and it remains to be seen whether this observation is limited to certain mouse strains and/or to experiments of this particular design; the well known fact that lymphomyeloid cells induce long-lasting tolerance of skin allografts in many strains suggests that this may be so. However, because it is usual to induce tolerance with lymphomyeloid cells or extracts prepared from them, the possible existence of alloantigens specific for different organs clearly needs to be investigated further.

The MLC test has been used in animals as well as in man. In the human situation it appears to correlate quite well with direct skin grafting (Russell et al. 1966; Bach and Kisken 1967) and with serological tests for HL-A antigens (Bach and Amos 1967; Amos and Bach 1968); and genetic analyses with MLC tests mirror the serological findings in that they point to a single genetic locus with a minimum of 20 alleles (Bach and Kisken 1967). As the possible predictive value of present-day serological typing is still a subject for discussion, it is perhaps not too surprising that so far the evidence for a direct correlation between the MLC test and kidney graft survival and function in immuno-suppressed patients is suggestive (Bach 1971) rather than conclusive. In the rat, on the other hand, a negative MLC test has been found to be associated with the prolonged survival of skin, heart and kidney allo-grafts (Bildsøe et al. 1970). Neither in man nor in the rat does the MLC test appear to recognize incompatibility differences controlled by the weaker genetic loci.

In the mouse the picture is somewhat different, for here both H-2 and some non-H-2 incompatibilities may be detected by the MLC test (see Festenstein 1971). In view of what we know about the additive effects of weak loci in skin grafting, it is not unreasonable to assume that positive cultures for mixtures of H-2 compatible cells are likewise caused by the combined effects of weak loci. (Indeed, in the experiments of Rychliková and Ivanyi (1969) the two strains under investigation differed at more than 12 weak loci.) Nevertheless, Festenstein's (1970) finding that in the H-2-compatible strains Balb/c and DBA/2 positive MLC tests appear to be dependent on a single weak locus, casts some doubt on such an interpretation unless it should turn out that the sub-strains used by him are not, after all, H-2-identical.

One of the variables in the presentation of an antigenic stimulus is the route of administration; another, the physical form in which the antigen is administered (Dresser and Mitchison 1968). It is therefore not surprising that some routes of antigen administration are more effective than others in inducing transplantation immunity. For example, in rabbits the intradermal route sensitizes much more strongly than the intravenous route when blood leucocytes (Medawar 1946) or epidermal cell suspensions (Billingham and Sparrow 1955) are injected. By con-trast, in the mouse and the guinea-pig these two routes and others that were investigated sensitized more or less equally well when viable H-2 incompatible lymphoid cells were injected in varying doses (Billingham et al. 1957; but cp. Berrian and McKhann 1960, for H-3 incompatibility). But even in the mouse significant differences between the intraperitoneal and intravenous routes occurred when 'semi-soluble' cell-free tissue extracts were injected into H-2 incompatible recipients – the intraperitoneal but not the intravenous route leading to sensitization (Medawar 1963). In a relatively weak system (C3H and CBA strains) such extracts prolonged rather than curtailed skin allograft survival, and this time the intravenous route was only marginally the more effective in inducing prolongation of survival.

Much of the work discussed above has been done with skin allografts, and it is only in the last few years than an innovation in surgical technique (Lee 1967) has made it possible to study the rejection of organ grafts in genetically defined animals – chiefly in the rat, in which skin graft rejection can be as rapid in the recipients of AgB compatible skin as in an AgB incompatible situation (Stark et al. 1970). The ability to form serum antibodies nevertheless correlates well, as it does in the mouse, with incompatibility at the AgB locus, as the same workers have shown. Leaving aside the observation that, in the rat, kidney allografts are remarkably susceptible to the action of enhancing antibodies (see Section 15.4.3), one of the most interesting points to emerge from this field is that tissues and organs differ in their vulnerability to immunological attack as well as in their immunogenicity. Thus: (a) White and Hildemann (1968), White et al. (1969) and Mahabir et al. (1969) observed that whereas Fischer rat skin grafts transplanted to Lewis recipients showed acute rejection, orthotopically transplanted kidneys survived for more than 200 days, and *vice versa*. The sub-strains used in these experiments are thought to differ at the AgB locus. That differences in both vulnerability and immunogenicity were involved is suggested by the finding that pre-sensitization with skin grafts resulted in the rejection of subsequently transplanted kidneys, whereas the transplantation of skin to animals already carrying well functioning kidneys did not have an adverse effect on the kidneys though the skin grafts themselves were promptly destroyed. (b) Bildsøe et al. (1970) found that in AgB-incompatible rats kidneys were rejected with almost the same speed as skin grafts, but heart grafts survived for variable and often prolonged periods. (c) Freeman and Steinmuller (1969), working with strains carrying the same label as those used by Hildemann and his colleagues, showed that heart as well as skin allografts are rejected acutely (MST's of 13 and 10 days respectively); and (d) L. Lameijer and J. F. Mowbray (personal communication) of St. Mary's Hospital Medical School find that in the August → Wistar combination, which appears to provide an unusually potent histocompatibility difference, there is little to choose between grafts of skin (8–9 days), kidney (6–8 days) and heart (5–8 days) but that liver allografts do very much better (none rejected in an observation period of 3 months). It is difficult to generalize from these data, for surgical procedures as well as strains differed; it may even be unwarranted to assume that strains of the same name are necessarily identical genetically. All that can be inferred at the present time is that some organs fare better than others in certain situations – a point that has also been demonstrated in pigs, which reject skin and kidney allografts very rapidly but tolerate liver transplants for very long periods without any immunosuppressive treatment (Calne et al. 1967).

The question of the differential vulnerability/immunogenicity of organs is bedevilled by the fact that organ grafts usually contain quite large numbers of peripheral blood leucocytes. Our attention has been drawn to the existence of these so-called 'passenger cells' by the work of Hašková et al. (1965) and by the elegant analysis of Steinmuller (1967, 1969), who showed that even skin grafts may contain sufficient numbers of passenger cells to sensitize. This concept has been extended to kidney grafts (Elkins and Guttmann 1968; Guttmann et al. 1969), and the experiments by the latter group suggest that passenger leucocytes provide an important, possibly the most important, source of immunogenic material. The organ transplantation experiments summarized above were all done without prior perfusion, and it seems highly probable that different results will be obtained when this particular variable has been eliminated.

15.4.2. Tolerance

The purpose of this section is not to review the field but to indicate, with the aid of a few selected examples, to what extent histocompatibility differences between donor and recipient may contribute to the induction of tolerance. The subject of immunological tolerance in its widest sense has been well reviewed by Dresser and Mitchison (1968) and by Nossal (1968), and two recent symposia have been devoted to it (see Landy and Braun (eds.) 1969; Nisbet (ed.) 1971).

Tolerance has been defined as a state of specific antigen-induced unresponsiveness. It is true that enhancement too answers this description, but the two phenomena are presumed to differ operationally in that enhancement but not tolerance can be passively transferred with antiserum. Even this dividing line is currently under attack, for the following reasons: (a) low titres of antibodies have been reported in the serum of some mice made tolerant at birth (Voisin et al. 1968), (b) it has been claimed that tolerant mice possess serum substances – presumably antibodies – which block the responses of the animals' lymphocytes to donor antigens (Hellström et al. 1971), and (c) in the rat, the unresponsiveness to kidney allografts that can be induced by pre-treatment with antigenic preparations is frequently accompanied by the formation of humoral antibodies (see the symposium on enhancement, 3rd International Congress of the Transplantation Society, 1971). It has therefore been suggested by Hellström et al. that tolerance and enhancement are fundamentally the same phenomenon – a suggestion that must be taken seriously but which, for the moment, it would be premature to accept as a generalization.*

It is a well-known fact that tolerance of skin allografts as well as organ grafts is most easily induced in foetal or neonatal animals, i.e., when many animals (especially rodents) are still relatively immature from an immunological point of view. But even in neonatal mice injected with donor cells within 24 hours of birth, the ease with which tolerance is induceable is strongly and inversely related to the degree of genetic disparity between donor and recipient, and once again the H-2 locus plays a critical role in this respect. Table 15.4 (Silvers and Billingham 1969) shows that compatibility at the H-2 locus ensures much better results in terms of both the proportion of recipients made tolerant and the number of donor cells required. It will be noted that in some of the H-2-incompatible combinations the proportion of tolerant mice was small or even zero, a result that would be explained in several ways, e.g., (a) a broad front of histocompatibility differences involving both H-2 and numerous non-H-2 loci, (b) greater immunological maturity at birth in certain strains, and (c) fierce graft-*versus*-host reactions resulting in the death of many tolerant animals. As is indicated in Table 15.4, many experiments made use of F_1 hybrid cells, thus circumventing graft-*versus*-host reactions, and in some cases very different results were obtained in experiments involving the same host strain but different donor strains; it follows, therefore, that the degree of antigenic disparity is usually the decisive factor – an observation supported by the work of Zeiss (1966) and Křen et al. (1969) and one that has also been made for tolerance induction of xenogeneic skin grafts (Billingham and Brent 1957).

Another point of interest illustrated by Table 15.4 is that the severity of graft-*versus*-host reactions leading to fatal runt disease (Billingham and Brent 1959) is, as might be expected, *directly* proportional to the degree of genetic disparity between donor and host: in H-2-compatible combinations runt disease does not occur at normal dose levels, and with the weak histoincompatibility difference associated with the X-chromosome even a very large dose of spleen cells failed to cause it.

How important a role the H-2 locus plays in tolerance induction in

---

* *Added in proof.* For full discussion, see L. Brent, 1971, Immunological tolerance 1951–71. *In*: N. W. Nisbet and M. W. Elves, eds.: Immunological tolerance to tissue antigens. Orthopaedic Hospital, Owestry, England. pp. 49–66.

TABLE 15.4

Susceptibility of newborn mice of different strains to the induction of tolerance (skin grafts) and runt disease following inoculation with allogeneic spleen cells. (Data from Silvers and Billingham 1969.)

Donor → recipient strain combinations‡	Compatible at H-2 locus	M.S.T. of skin homografts (days)	Estimated proportion of highly tolerant hosts (%)*	Tolerance susceptibility rating (± to +++)	Proportion of hosts with runt disease (%)*
CBA → A (a, b)	No	10.2 ± 0.3	40 (2×10^6); 90 (10×10^6)	++	40 (10×10^6)
C3H → A (a)	No	~ 10	80 (4–10×10^6)	++	40 (4–10×10^6)
C3H → A (c)	No	11.6 ± 0.7	80 (10×10^6)**	++	
C57 → A (a, d)	No	~ 8	25 (8–10×10^6)**	+	100 (4–10×10^6)
AU → A (a)	No	9.1 ± 0.4	0 (8–10×10^6)**	±	100 (4–10×10^6)
A → CBA (a, e)	No	11.0 ± 0.3	25 (2×10^6); 40 (5×10^6)	+	20 (4–10×10^6)
C57 → CBA (a, f)	No	< 10	60 (20×10^6)**	+	100 (4–10×10^6)
C3H → CBA (g, a)	Yes	~ 15	65 (0.5×10^6); 100 (3–10×10^6)	+++	0 (4–10×10^6)
CBA → C3H (g, a)	Yes	~ 13	100 (4–10×10^6)	+++	0 (4–10×10^6)
A → C3H (a)	No	~ 11	45 (4–10×10^6)	+	70 (4–10×10^6)
AK → C3H (e)	Yes	> 10–11	90 (5–8×10^6)	++	0 (Not known)
C3H → AK (e)	Yes	Not known	70 (5–8×10^6)	++	0 (Not known)
A → C57 (a, f, d)	No	~ 8	0 (20×10^6)**	±	0 (4–10×10^6)†
CBA → C57 (f)	No	< 10	0 (5×10^6)**; 10 (20×10^6)**	±	
A → AU (a)	No	9.0 ± 0.3	50 (4–10×10^6)	+	50 (4–10×10^6)
CBA → AU (a)	No	Not known	5 (4–10×10^6)	±	20 (4–10×10^6)
C57BL/6 ♂ C57BL/6 ♀ (h)	Yes	25 ± 2.5	80 (1×10^5)	+++	0 (50×10^6)

*   Dose of spleen cells given in brackets.

** F_1 hybrid cells used to avoid runt disease.

†   Absence of runt disease ascribed to greater immunological maturity of hosts.

‡   Sources of data as follows:
(a) Billingham and Brent 1959; (b) Billingham and Silvers 1961; (c) White and Hildemann 1968; (d) Jutila and Weiser 1962; (e) Miller 1960; (f) Billingham and Silvers 1962; (g) Argyris 1964); (h) Billingham et al. (1965).

newborn mice is clearly demonstrated by the quantitative analysis of Brent and Gowland (1962). When the dose of donor cells injected into H-2 incompatible and compatible newborn mice was carefully investigated in relation to tolerance induction, there was a 17-fold difference in the number of cells required to induce tolerance in all recipients and a 30-fold difference in the threshold dose at which not a single recipient became tolerant (Figs. 15.1 and 15.2). The shape of the two dose-response curves was different too, the H-2-incompatible experiment showing a much more rapid decline in the proportion of tolerant mice with each halving of antigen dose.

The situation is very similar in the rat, for here too AgB compatibility ensures the successful induction of skin allograft tolerance in newborn animals with quite low doses (c. 1×10^6) of cells of various lymphohaematopoietic origin, including the thymus (Silvers and Billingham 1969), whereas much larger doses are required to surmount an AgB incompatible barrier and thymocytes are virtually ineffective here. The same authors (Billingham and Silvers 1964) had previously shown that, in the mouse, cells of different lymphohaematopoietic origin do not necessarily induce tolerance with the same effectiveness and that thymocytes provide by far the least satisfactory stimulus.

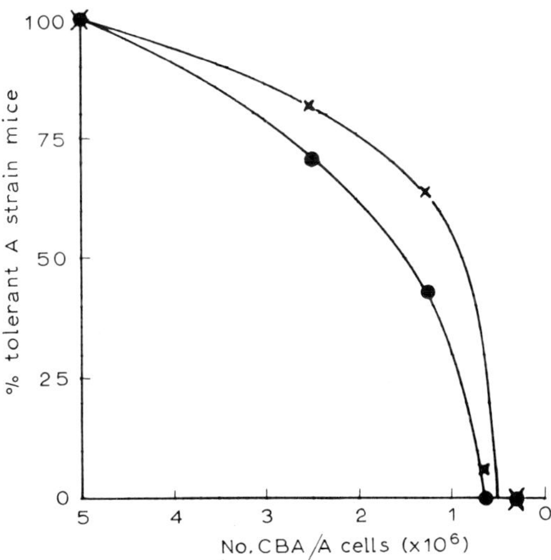

Fig. 15.1. The relationship between antigen dose and the induction of tolerance to skin allografts in newborn mice: H-2 incompatibility. Viable (CBA × A)F₁ spleen cells (H-2^{ak}) were injected intravenously into newborn A strain mice (H-2^a). Survival of test grafts is shown for a minimum of $2 \times$ (×—×) or $5 \times$ (●—●) the MST of the uninjected controls (13 days). (From Brent and Gowland 1962).

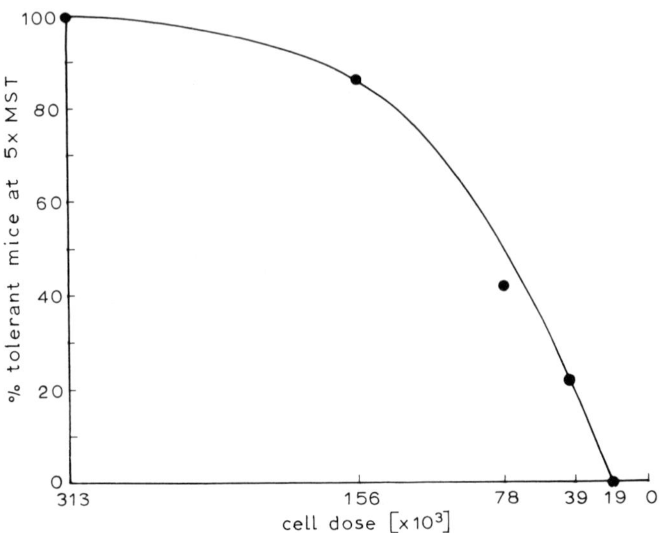

Fig. 15.2. The relationship between antigen dose and induction of tolerance of skin allografts in newborn mice: H-2 compatibility. Viable CBA (H-2^k) spleen cells were injected intravenously into newborn C3H (H-2^k) mice.

The time after birth at which tolerance can be induced with a single inoculum of viable cells is also greatly influenced by the extent of histo-compatibility differences: in the H-2-incompatible strain combination CBA → A there is a rapid fall-off in the percentage of tolerant animals injected intravenously at varying times after birth with a weight-adjusted dose of (CBA × A)F$_1$ hybrid spleen cells, so that not a single mouse injected on the 8th day became highly tolerant (Brent and Gowland 1961). However, a high proportion of congenic mice differing from their donors only at the H-3 locus became tolerant when injected intraperitoneally with 5 × 10^6 cells as late as the 23rd day after birth (McKhann 1964) – a result that is all the more striking compared with the data of Brent and Gowland if it is borne in mind that not only was the dose of cells smaller in McKhann's experiments but the route of injection was less favourable to tolerance induction.

There is now a considerable body of information concerning the induction of unresponsiveness in immunologically mature animals (see Gowland 1965; Nisbet and Elves (eds.) 1971). We have already mentioned the long-term survival of AgB-compatible organ grafts in normal rats (Section 15.4.1); whether these results will turn out to be due to enhancing antibodies or to tolerance as defined above, or to both, remains to be seen. What is certain is that, for skin allografts, too, one can make the

generalization that tolerance in adults can be induced only by the inoculation of very large doses of antigen, usually over a prolonged period,
where H-2 incompatibility is involved, whereas single doses have
overcome H1/H-3 incompatibility (Guttmann and Aust 1961; Martinez
et al. 1962; but see Gowland 1965) and, much more readily, incompatibility at only the H-3 (McKhann 1962; 1964b) and the Y-chromosome-linked
(Mariani et al. 1959) loci.

Although tolerance can be induced more easily across strong H barriers with the aid of immunosuppressive agents (see, for example,
Medawar 1969), even here one finds a marked differential in susceptibility
when comparing strong and weak systems. This is illustrated by the
recent work of Brent and Kilshaw (1970) and Brent et al. (1971) in which
the injection of a single dose of crude tissue extract 16 days before skin
grafting was combined with 3 doses of antilymphocytic serum (ALS) in
the first week after grafting. In a strong system (A → CBA males) this
treatment results in a doubling (sometimes a trebling) of the MST of
the ALS controls, no matter whether the extract is prepared from donor
strain spleen or liver (Fig. 15.3); in a moderately weak system (C3H →
CBA males) as many as 80% of the recipients carried their grafts without
signs of rejection for over a year (Fig. 15.4). These workers believe that
this unresponsiveness is a form of tolerance rather than enhancement.

It remains to be seen to what extent tolerance or enhancement, or

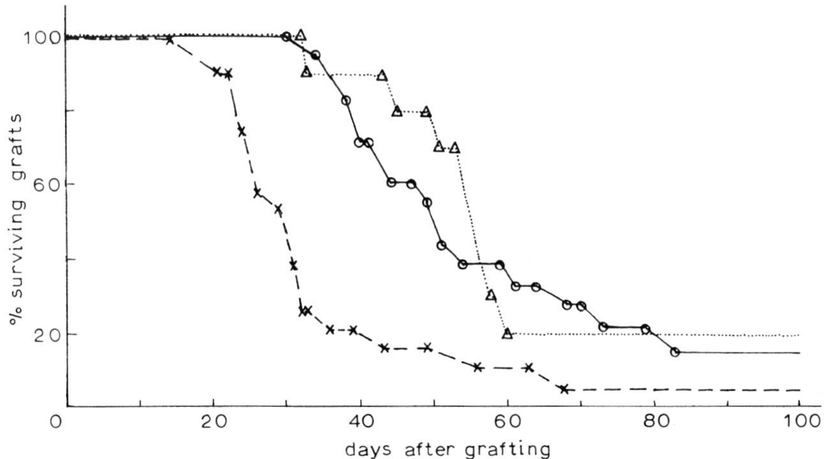

Fig. 15.3. Induction of tolerance to skin allografts in adult mice with tissue extract and
ALS: H-2 incompatibility. Extract from 250 mg wet weight A strain spleen (O—O) or
liver (△—△) was injected intravenously into CBA males 16 days before test-grafting with A
strain skin. 0.5 ml rabbit-anti-mouse ALS was injected on days 2, 4 and 6 after grafting.
×—× mice treated with ALS only.

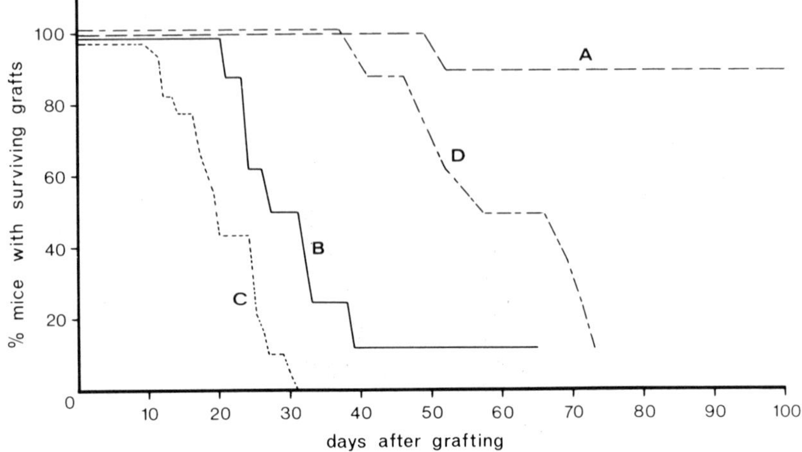

Fig. 15.4. Induction of unresponsiveness to skin allografts in adult mice with tissue extract and ALS: H-2 compatibility. CBA male mice were treated with C3H liver extract and ALS as in the experiment described in Fig. 3, but using a different ALS pool. A. Extract and ALS. B. Extract only. C. No treatment. D. ALS only. (From Brent et al. 1971.)

both, will provide the key to the clinical problem of tissue transplantation. So far as tolerance is concerned, the greatest hope lies in (a) tissue typing, which will in time eliminate *all* HL-A differences and possibly even some of the stronger (and as yet unidentified) of the non-HL-A loci, (b) the production of safe and pure tissue extracts with tolerogenic properties, and (c) the short-term rather than chronic application of immunosuppressive agents. These three approaches used together should, in time, go a long way towards resolving the problem of allograft rejection in man.

We have deliberately refrained from mentioning two other situations in which histocompatibility differences are overridden or evaded: the progressive growth of autochthonous tumours carrying tumour-specific antigens (see, for example, Klein 1966) and the development of the mammalian foetus despite the presence on foetal cells of paternally inherited H antigens (see the review by Simmons 1969). A multiplicity of factors is likely to be involved in both these phenomena, but tolerance is unlikely to be one of them; on the other hand, enhancement (see Section 15.4.3) has recently been invoked as playing a protective role in both (Hellström et al. 1969; Hellström and Hellström 1970).

15.4.3. Enhancement

Since antigenic strength is usually assessed by the survival time of an allograft, any other factors which influence the time of graft survival have to be taken into account. Immunological enhancement is one such factor. There are several reviews describing the phenomenon in detail (Kaliss 1958; Batchelor 1963; Möller and Möller 1966; Batchelor 1968; Hutchin 1968; Snell 1970; Winn 1970) and our intention here is a limited one, namely, to discuss aspects relevant to the concept of antigenic strength, in particular the mechanisms of enhancement.

Enhancement has been defined by Kaliss as the prolongation of graft survival brought about by humoral antibody directed against graft antigens. The antibody causing graft enhancement may be present either because of passive or active immunization. It is now well recognized that enhancement is due to the failure or ineffectual operation of a destructive homograft reaction. Since enhancement is brought about by the action of humoral antibody, a key factor is the vulnerability of grafted tissue to the cytotoxic action of antibody. In general, tissues or cells highly susceptible to this action of antibody either show no enhancement or are enhanced only in specially propitious circumstances (Gorer and Boyse 1959; Gorer and Kaliss 1959; Hellström 1959; Gorer and O'Gorman 1956). Conversely, tissues which are resistant to cytotoxic antibodies are generally, but not always (e.g., skin allografts), more readily enhanced. The chief factor on which the vulnerability of target tissues to antibody appears to depend is the density of antigen sites (Winn 1962; Möller and Möller 1962); lymphoid and myeloid cells which bear a high concentration of antigen sites are highly susceptible whereas other cells, such as certain sarcomas, bear relatively fewer antigen sites per unit surface area and are correspondingly less vulnerable. The importance of antigen site density is that it limits the number of antibody molecules which combine with a target cell and also the rate at which they combine. Since complement fixation, the final step of the processes leading to cytolysis of a target cell, is quantitatively dependent upon the number of antigen-antibody complexes formed, the effect of low antigen site density is to reduce the number of opportunities per cell for the activation of complement (Winn 1962; Möller and Möller 1962).

The type of antibody combining with cellular antigens also influences the amount of complement fixed and the degree of cytolysis produced. Non-complement fixing Fab or $F(ab')_2$ fragments, although capable of combining specifically with antigen, do not cause significant cytolysis (Chard et al. 1967; Chard 1968; Batchelor 1968). In recent studies, using a model system of rabbit antisera and diazotized sheep red cells as the target, Linscott (1970) has analysed the complex interrelationships of antibody class and antigen site density. He showed that, when antigen site density was low, IgM antibody was highly efficient in producing haemolysis, whereas IgG was not. At high site density both classes of antibody were efficient. If target cells were first mixed with IgG antibody and later exposed to IgM, the effect produced again depended upon antigen site density; with low densities, IgG inhibited IgM-induced haemolysis, at high densities it had a potentiating action. Linscott explains the results in terms of the relative abilities of the antibody classes to bind complement. A single molecule of decavalent IgM can fix complement, whereas a doublet of two IgG molecules combining at adjacent sites is required.

It seems highly probable that the same parameters affect the lysis of nucleated cells. 19S antibodies have been shown to be more efficient than 7S antibodies in causing cytolysis of nucleated cells (Andersson et al. 1967), and it is significant that 19S antibodies have not been found to cause enhancement, whereas 7S may do so (Möller 1966). Some mouse allo-antisera have been found on fractionation to contain certain antibodies which combine with target cells as shown by their capacity to induce enhancement, but which have negligible cytotoxic power (Chard 1968; Voisin et al. 1966, 1969; Takasugi and Hildemann 1969).

It has been postulated that enhancement could be due to inhibition of the immunological reflex arc at afferent, central, or efferent levels (Billingham et al. 1956). Passive immunization of a recipient at the same time that antigen is administered may undoubtedly inhibit the development of an immune response (Snell et al. 1960; Uhr and Baumann 1961); i.e., afferent inhibition occurs, and is one probable mechanism of enhancement. In the case of enhancement brought about by active immunization (Snell et al. 1946; Kaliss and Bryant 1958; Chantler and Batchelor 1964) the most plausible explanation is that humoral antibody, synthesized by the host, competes with sensitized lymphocytes for antigen sites. Provided the circumstances are such that humoral antibody has little or no capacity to cause graft damage, its overall effect will be to saturate antigen sites and prevent lymphocyte-mediated graft destruction, i.e., this would be an efferent mechanism. Humoral antibody has been shown to inhibit the graft-destructive effect of lymph node cells both *in vitro* (Brunner et al. 1968; Hellström et al. 1969) and *in vivo* (Batchelor and Silverman 1962; Möller 1963).

Experiments on enhancement of rat kidney grafts also support the interpretation that humoral antibody may compete with sensitized lymphocytes and prevent them from causing graft destruction. AS rats grafted with (AS × August) F_1 kidneys and injected with AS anti-August serum may survive indefinitely despite the removal of their own kidneys (French and Batchelor 1969; see Table 15.5). During the second week after grafting the recipients begin to synthesize detectable titres of anti-August antibodies. At that time graft function deteriorates but later

TABLE 15.5

Median survival time of AS rats receiving renal allografts
after injections of AS anti August enhancing antiserum.

Donor	No. in group	Median survival time (days)
(August × AS)F_1	11	> 120 days*
August	10	23.5

* Indefinitely prolonged survival times.

improves, the blood urea returning to normal limits. If rats bearing enhanced kidneys are subsequently challenged by injection with August spleen cells, a secondary antibody response occurs, but there is no detectable rise in blood urea or clinical sign of graft damage. It seems clear, therefore, that the rats have been immunized but that their grafts continue to survive despite this. It might be argued that immunity had been demonstrated only with respect to humoral antibody, and that tolerance may have been induced in the lymphocyte population, which normally expresses cell-mediated immunity. But this does not seem to be a satisfactory explanation because spleen cells taken from AS rats bearing enhanced kidneys are capable of mounting a graft-*versus*-host reaction when injected into (AS × August) F_1 hybrid rats (French et al. 1971). The strength of the reaction is approximately the same as that produced by spleen cells from normal control AS rats. Reactions fully comparable with those in controls were also observed after injecting spleen cells from recipients which carried enhanced kidneys and which had been further immunized some time after transplantation with August cells. It must be borne in mind that assays for tolerance in these circumstances are complicated by the possibility that what appears to be tolerance may merely be inhibition by antibody of cells competent to react, the antibody having been synthesized by some of the cells in the inoculum. Graft-*versus*-host reactions can be inhibited by suitable passive immunization (Voisin and Kinsky 1962; Batchelor and Howard 1965).

In the preceding discussion on the mechanisms of enhancement, prolonged graft survivals were observed in the various experiments as a consequence of either active or passive immunization. The simplest experiments testing antigenic strength do not involve *prior* immunization of the recipient, and one might therefore question how enhancement could affect the outcome of such a test. Observations by White et al. (1969) and Bildsøe et al. (1970) make it clear that prolonged survival of primary organ allografts can occur despite an incompatibility sufficient to cause rejection of a skin allograft from the same donor (see Section 15.4.1). Hildemann (1970a) reports that allo-antibodies may be detected in the serum in some of these donor-recipient combinations, e.g., Fischer → Lewis rats, and concludes that active immunological enhancement is responsible for the prolonged survivals. It is therefore apparent that prior immunization is not always necessary to cause enhancement, and that the graft itself is capable of providing the type of antigenic stimulus which induces enhancement. It is interesting to note that other examples of 'auto-enhancement' have been observed (Möller 1965).

15.5. Discussion of 'antigenic strength'

It has been customary to explain differences in antigenic strength as being determined either by a property of the antigen or, alternatively, by a property of the recipient's immune response. At present, the evidence indicates that both may affect the results of tests for measuring antigenic strength.

15.5.1. Properties of the antigen

The first possibility to be considered is qualitative. Do strong antigens have physico-chemical features which distinguish them from weak ones? McKhann (1968) has briefly discussed this question and points out that dissociation from the target cell, solubility, rate of production, and inherent immunogenicity of an antigen are all theoretically capable of influencing its strength. Furthermore, immunogenicity need not be necessarily related to the actual determinant so much as the presence of a carrier macromolecule with adjuvant activity. So little is known yet about these factors that we can only speculate at this stage.

The second possibility is that antigenic strength is due to quantitative differences, i.e., strong antigens are those which are present on the cell surface in large numbers whereas those which are sparsely represented are weak. Quantitative differences in antigen site density which affect graft survival times have been most convincingly demonstrated by experiments on allelic dosage. Table 15.5 shows the survival time of August and (August × AS) F_1 hybrid rat kidneys transplanted to AS recipients which have been injected with enhancing antibody (see Section 15.4.3). The mean survival time of grafts involving the double allelic incompatibility is 23.5 days. This contrasts strikingly with the indefinite survival of the F_1 grafts. Similar observations have been made by Lapp and Bliss (1966), who examined the effect of allelic dosage on H-1 incompatible skin grafts in mice. The simplest explanation of these results is that cells with a double allelic incompatibility have more antigen on their surface than do cells with a single allele difference, an interpretation supported by the differential sensitivity of these cells to the lytic action of allo-antibody (Winn 1962). This conclusion is also supported by the results of cadaveric renal transplantation, where a direct correlation has been observed between the number of antigenic incompatibilities of a graft and the risk of rejection (Batchelor and Joysey 1969; Batchelor et al. 1971).

Another problem which is pertinent to the question of whether antigen site density is the basis of antigenic strength, is that of the apparent complexity of strong transplantation antigen systems. However, for reasons discussed in Section 2 this feature of strong H systems may be to some extent artefactual. The concept of a system composed of multiple, pseudo-allelic antigens, as was originally postulated for the H-2 system, envisages a larger number of specificities per cell than the concept of 2 segregant series determining a total of 4 antigenic sites, like the HL-A model. With the former concept in mind, Klein (1967) has shown that the strength of single H-2 specificities may be the same as that of an H-3 difference. This evidence was interpreted as showing that strong antigens are strong because the *total* number of antigenic incompatibilities is greater than in weak differences, but the results could equally well be attributed not to varying numbers of incompatible antigens, but to varying degrees of cross-reactivity of these antigens. Until the question of the genetic and chemical structure of both strong and weak systems has been more clearly resolved, the influence of anti-genic complexity upon the strength of an H system cannot be decided.

Although the evidence cited is strongly suggestive that antigen site density influences antigenic strength, we unfortunately lack the technical means of testing this idea directly. Quantitative detection of the antigens of strong systems with antibody is straightforward enough, but there are no such tests for antigens of the weaker systems. It is unknown whether this is due to a failure of weak antigens to provoke antibody formation even after repeated immunization or whether the level of sensitivity of the test systems used has been too low, but the latter explanation seems more likely.

If antigen site density influences antigenic strength, by what mechan-isms might this occur? Theoretically, both the rate at which immuniza-tion develops (afferent effect) and the rate at which a graft is destroyed (efferent effect) may be involved. The studies of Linscott (1970) cited earlier emphasize the importance of the efferent effect. Discussion of the afferent effect will be deferred until the host response is considered.

One other factor which may have importance in determining antigenic strength is the position which the antigen occupies on the target cell surface. There is some evidence that H-2 specificities are arranged in clusters upon the surface (Cerrotini and Brunner 1967; Boyse et al. 1968; Cresswell and Sanderson 1968) and this may affect both the rate at which immune damage can proceed and immunogenicity. But the evidence indicating clustering of specificities will need to be re-assessed because of the possibility that 'clustering specificities' may not be separate entities, and may merely be a single specificity combining with different but cross-reactive antibodies.

15.5.2. *Properties of the host's immune response*

Simonsen (1962a, b, 1970) has been the originator and chief proponent of the hypothesis that antigenic strength is a direct function of the *number* of antigen-sensitive cells which can recognize an antigen as foreign and react against it. If one accepts that antigen-reactive cells perform on an 'all or none' basis, as was concluded by Brent and Medawar (1966), the violence of an immune response could depend entirely upon the number of cells involved. Simonsen has pointed out that immunization against strong antigens induces only a slight increase in cell-mediated immunity; by contrast, prior immunization against weak antigens induces a proportionately larger increase in the host's responsiveness, i.e., there is a difference in the factor of immunization (see Section 15.4.1). He suggests that the only satisfactory explanation for the differences in the factors of immunization obtained with strong and weak antigens is that a high proportion of immuno-competent cells are genetically capable of reacting against strong, and only a small proportion against weak, antigens. Prior immunization would therefore be expected to cause relatively little change in the *proportion* of cells reacting against strong antigens, but a great change in the proportion of cells reacting against weak antigens.

Although this hypothesis has been persuasively argued, we do not yet have enough facts in our possession to accept it without reserve. Several other factors could be contributory, e.g., the concentration of antigens on the cell surface or the strength of the bond between antigenic sites and lymphocyte receptors. Pursuing for a moment the possibility that the distribution of antigen sites might play a role, it could be argued that strong antigens (as exemplified by H-2 incompatibilities) occur at high, and weak antigens at low, density. In the case of the former, a high proportion of antigen-sensitive cells might be stimulated because of the close proximity of the antigenic sites, even when relatively small numbers of antigen-carrying cells are injected into an animal. In the case of the latter, a low-density distribution might result in the stimulation of only a fraction of the total number of antigen-sensitive cells, but the clone of activated cells would be greatly increased as a result of primary immunization (i.e., the factor of immunization would be high). That high doses of weak antigens may cause tolerance rather than increased sensitivity does not necessarily disqualify this line of reasoning, for the induction of tolerance may well be aided by a low density antigen distribution and a dose-dependent increase in sensitivity would be expected to operate only below the tolerance threshold. A very similar argument could be put forward in terms of a differential binding affinity between antigenic site and lymphocyte receptor. These ideas have been fully discussed by H. Wigzell, G. Möller, J. R. Batchelor and others in the General Discussion of the Symposium on 'Strong and Weak Histocompatibility Antigens' (Transplantation Rev. *3*, 1970), in which W. L. Ford has also made the interesting suggestion that the known facts about the factor of immunization could be explained by the generation of two distinct kinds of cells following stimulation, effector cells and memory cells, and that the proportion in which these cells are generated differs in strong and weak systems.

This discussion has served to emphasize that we do not at present know what causes differences in antigenic strength. Simonsen's hypothesis is certainly attractive in many ways but other candidates cannot be ruled out. That the facts cannot be interpreted wholly in terms of genetic restriction of responsiveness of antigen-sensitive cells emerges from the work of Berrian and McKhann (1960), who showed that immunity against H-3 antigens is more easily elicited if there is concomitant immunization against H-2 antigens.

References

ALLEN, F., B. B. AMOS, J. R. BATCHELOR, W. BODMER, R. CEPPELLINI, J. DAUSSET, C. ENGEL-FRIET, M. JEANNET, F. KISSMEYER-NIELSEN, P. MORRIS, R. PAYNE, P. I. TERASAKI, J. J. VAN ROOD, R. WALFORD, C. ZMIJEWSKI, E. ALBERT, P. MATTIUZ, M. R. MICKEY and A. PIAZZA, 1970, Joint Report of the 4th International Histocompatibility Workshop. *In*: P. I. Terasaki, ed.: Histocompatibility testing 1970. Copenhagen, Munksgaard. pp. 17–44.

AMOS, D. B. and F. H. BACH, 1969, J. Exptl. Med. *128*, 623.

AMOS, D. B., H. F. SEIGLER, J. G. SOUTHWORTH and E. WARD, 1969, Transplant. Proc. *1*, 342.

ANDERSSON, B., H. WIGZELL and G. KLEIN, 1967, Transplantation *5*, 11.

AOKI, T., U. HÄMMERLING, E. DE HARVEN, E. A. BOYSE and L. J. OLD, 1969, J. Exptl. Med. *130*, 979.

ARGYRIS, B. F., 1964, J. Immunol. *92*, 630.

BACH, F. H., 1971, Transplantation in man: pairing of donor and recipient. *In*: J. S. Najarian and R. L. Simmons, eds.: Transplantation. Philadelphia, Lea and Febiger.

BACH, F. H. and D. B. AMOS, 1967, Science *156*, 1506.

BACH, F. H. and W. A. KISKEN, 1967, Transplantation *5*, 1046.

BACH, F. H. and K. HIRSCHHORN, 1964, Science *143*, 813.

BACH, F. H., M. SEGALL, E. DAY and M. L. BACH, 1970, Incompatibility strength of HL-A. *In*: P. I. Terasaki, ed.: Histocompatibility testing 1970. Copenhagen, Munksgaard. pp. 503–513.

BAILEY, D. W., 1965, Transplantation *4*, 531.

BAILEY, D. W. and L. MOBRAATEN, 1964, Genetics *50*, 233.

BAIN, B. and L. LOWENSTEIN, 1964, Science *145*, 1315.

BAIN, B., M. R. VAS and L. LOWENSTEIN, 1963, Federation Proc. *22*, 428.

BARNES, A. D. and P. L. KROHN, 1957, Proc. Roy. Soc. *B146*, 505.

BATCHELOR, J. R., 1963, Guy's Hosp. Rept. *112*, 345.

BATCHELOR, J. R., 1968, Cancer Res. *28*, 1410.

BATCHELOR, J. R. and M. HACKETT, 1970, Lancet 581.

BATCHELOR, J. R. and J. G. HOWARD, 1965, Transplantation *3*, 161.

BATCHELOR, J. R. and V. C. JOYSEY, 1969, Lancet 790.

BATCHELOR, J. R., V. C. JOYSEY and P. E. CROME, 1971, Transplant. Proc. (in press).

BATCHELOR, J. R. and A. R. SANDERSON, 1970, Transplant. Proc. *2*, 133.

BATCHELOR, J. R. and N. H. SELLWOOD, 1970, HL-A sub-loci: are they valid? *In*: P. I. Terasaki, ed.: Histocompatibility testing 1970. Copenhagen, Munksgaard. pp. 243–249.

BATCHELOR, J. R. and M. S. SILVERMAN, 1962, Further studies on interaction between sessile and humoral antibodies in homograft reactions. *In*: G. E. W. Wolstenholme and M. P. Cameron, eds.: CIBA Foundation Symposium on Transplantation. London, Churchill. pp. 216–231.

BERRIAN, J. H. and C. F. MCKHANN, 1960, Ann. N.Y. Acad. Sci. *87*, 106.

BILDSØE, P., S. F. SØRENSEN, Q. PETTIROSSI and M. SIMONSEN, 1970, Transplant. Rev. *3*, 36.

BILLINGHAM, R. E. and L. BRENT, 1957, Proc. Roy. Soc. *B146*, 78.

BILLINGHAM, R. E. and L. BRENT, 1959, Proc. Roy. Soc. *B242*, 439.

BILLINGHAM, R. E., L. BRENT and P. B. MEDAWAR, 1954, Proc. Roy. Soc. *B143*, 58.

BILLINGHAM, R. E., L. BRENT and P. B. MEDAWAR, 1956, Nature *178*, 514.

BILLINGHAM, R. E., L. BRENT and P. B. MEDAWAR, 1956, Transplant. Bull. *3*, 84.

BILLINGHAM, R. E., L. BRENT and P. B. MEDAWAR, 1958, Transplant. Bull. *5*, 377.

BILLINGHAM, R. E., L. BRENT and N. A. MITCHISON, 1957, Brit. J. Exptl. Pathol. *38*, 467.

BILLINGHAM, R. E. and W. K. SILVERS, 1961, J. Exptl. Zool. *146*, 113.

BILLINGHAM, R. E. and W. K. SILVERS, 1962, J. Cell. Comp. Physiol. *60*, 183.

BILLINGHAM, R. E. and W. K. SILVERS, 1964, Some biological differences between thymocytes and lymphoid cells. *In*: V. Defendi and D. Metcalf, eds.: The thymus. Philadelphia, Wistar Institute Press. pp. 41–51.

BILLINGHAM, R. E. and W. K. SILVERS, eds., 1970, Immunogenetics of Transplantation, Transplant. Proc. *2*, pp. 1–178.

BILLINGHAM, R. E., W. K. SILVERS and D. B. WILSON, 1965, Proc. Roy. Soc. *B163*, 61.

BILLINGHAM, R. E. and E. M. SPARROW, 1955, J. Embryol. Exptl. Morphol. *3*, 265.

BITTNER, J. J., 1935, J. Genetics *31*, 471.

BOYSE, E. A., E. M. LANCE, E. A. CARSWELL, S. COOPER and L. J. OLD, 1970, Nature *227*, 901.

BOYSE, E. A., L. J. OLD and E. STOCKERT, 1968, Proc. Natl. Acad. Sci. U.S. *60*, 886.

BRENT, L., ed., 1965, Transplantation of tissues and organs, Brit. Med. Bull. *21*, 97–182.

BRENT, L., 1971, Pathogenic role of delayed hypersensitivity and antibody in allograft reactions. *In*: S. Cohen, G. Cudkowicz and R. T. Cluskey, eds.: Cellular interactions in the immune response. Basel, Karger. pp. 250–263.

BRENT, L. and G. GOWLAND, 1961, Nature *192*, 1265.

BRENT, L. and G. GOWLAND, 1962, Nature *196*, 1298.

BRENT, L., J. A. HANSEN and P. J. KILSHAW, 1971, Transplant. Proc. (in press).

BRENT, L. and P. J. KILSHAW, 1970, Nature *227*, 898.

BRENT, L. and P. B. MEDAWAR, 1966, Proc. Roy. Soc. *B165*, 281.

BRENT, L. and P. B. MEDAWAR, 1967, Brit. Med. Bull. *23*, 55.

BRENT, L., P. B. MEDAWAR and M. RUSZKIEWICZ, 1961, Brit. J. Exptl. Pathol. *42*, 464.

BRUNNER, K. T., J. MAUEL, J. C. CEROTTINI and B. CHAPUIS, 1968, Immunology *14*, 181.

CALNE, R. Y., H. J. O. WHITE, D. E. YOFFA, R. R. MAGINN, R. M. BINNS, J. R. SAMUEL and V. P. MOLINA, 1967, Brit. Med. J. *2*, 478.

CEPPELLINI, R., S. BIGLIANI, E. S. CURTONI and G. LEIGHEB, 1969, Transplant. Proc. *1*, 390.

CEPPELLINI, R., E. S. CURTONI, P. L. MATTIUZ, G. LEIGHEB, M. VISETTI and A. COLOMBI, 1966, Ann. N. Y. Acad. Sci. *129*, 421.

CEROTTINI, J. C. and K. T. BRUNNER, 1967, Immunology *13*, 395.

CHANTLER, S. M. and J. R. BATCHELOR, 1964, Transplantation *2*, 75.

CHARD, T., 1968, Immunology *14*, 583.

CHARD, T., M. E. FRENCH and J. R. BATCHELOR, 1967, Transplantation *5*, 1266.

COUNCE, S., P. SMITH, R. BARTH and G. D. SNELL, 1956, Ann. Surg. *144*, 198.

CRESSWELL, P. and A. R. SANDERSON, 1968, Transplantation *6*, 996.

DAUSSET, J., 1958, Acta Haematol. *20*, 156.

DAUSSET, J., R. L. WALFORD, J. COLOMBANI, L. LEGRAND, N. FEINGOLD, A. BARGE and F. T. RAPAPORT, 1969, Transplant. Proc. *1*, 331.

DAVIES, D. A. L., 1968, Transplantation antigens. *In*: F. T. Rapaport and J. Dausset, eds.: Human transplantation. New York/London, Grune and Stratton. pp. 618–634.

DAVIES, D. A. L., 1969, Transplantation *8*, 51.

DAVIES, D. A. L., A. J. MANSTONE, D. C. VIZA, J. COLOMBANI and J. DAUSSET, 1968, Transplantation *6*, 571.

DAVIES, W. C. and L. SILVERMAN, 1968, Transplantation *6*, 536.

DRESSER, D. W. and N. A. MITCHISON, 1968, Advan. Immunology *8*, 129.

DUMONDE, D. C., S. AL-ASKARI, H. S. LAWRENCE and L. THOMAS, 1963, Nature *198*, 598.

EDIDIN, M., 1964, Transplantation *2*, 627.

EICHWALD, E. J. and C. R. SILMSER, 1955, Transplant. Bull. *2*, 148.

EIJSVOOGEL, V. P., P. TH. A. SCHELLEKENS, B. BREUR-VRIESENDORP, A. VAN LEEUWEN, C. KOCH and J. J. VAN ROOD, 1970, HL-A identity and one-allelic differences in families and unrelated individuals. *In*: P. I. Terasaki, ed.: Histocompatibility testing 1970. Copenhagen, Munksgaard. pp. 523–529.

ELKINS, W. L., 1964, J. Exptl. Med. *120*, 329.

ELKINS, W. L. and R. D. GUTTMANN, 1968, Science *159*, 1250.

FELLOUS, M. and J. DAUSSET, 1970, Nature *225*, 191.

FESTENSTEIN, H., 1970, Transplantation Rev. *3*, 74.

FESTENSTEIN, H., 1971, Lymphocyte transformation in transplantation. *In*: Clinical organ transplantation. Oxford, Blackwell. p. 129.

FORD, W. L., 1967, Brit. J. Exptl. Pathol. *48*, 335.

FREEMAN, J. S. and D. STEINMULLER, 1969, Transplantation *8*, 530.

FRENCH, M. E. and J. R. BATCHELOR, 1969, Lancet 1103.

FRENCH, M. E., J. R. BATCHELOR and H. G. WATTS, 1971, Transplantation *12*, 45.

GIBSON, T., and P. B. MEDAWAR, 1943, J. Anatomy *77*, 299.

GLEASON, R. E. and J. E. MURRAY, 1967, Transplantation *5*, 343.

GLYNN, L. E. and E. J. HOLBOROW, 1959, Brit. Med. Bull. *15*, 150.

GORER, P. A., 1937, Brit. J. Exptl. Pathol. *18*, 31.

GORER, P. A., 1938, J. Pathol. Bacteriol. *47*, 231.

GORER, P. A. and E. A. BOYSE, 1959, Some reactions observed with transplanted reticulo-endothelial cells in mice. *In*: F. Albert and P. B. Medawar, eds.: Biological problems of grafting. Oxford, Blackwell. pp. 193–205.

GORER, P. A. and N. KALISS, 1959, Cancer Res. *19*, 824.

GORER, P. A., J. F. LOUTIT and H. S. MICKLEM, 1961, Nature *189*, 1024.

GORER, P. A. and Z. B. MIKULSKA, 1959, Proc. Roy. Soc. *B151*, 57.

GORER, P. A. and P. O'GORMAN, 1956, Transplant. Bull. *3*, 142.

GOWANS, J. L., 1965, Brit Med. Bull. *21*, 106.

GOWLAND, G., 1965, Brit. Med. Bull. *21*, 123.

GRAFF, R. J., 1970, Transplant. Proc. *2*, 15.

GRAFF, R. J., W. H. HILDEMANN and G. D. SNELL, 1966a, Transplantation *4*, 425.

GRAFF, R. J., W. K. SILVERS, R. E. BILLINGHAM, W. H. HILDEMANN and G. D. SNELL, 1966b, Transplantation *4*, 605.

GREAVES, M. F., G. TORRIGIANI and I. M. ROITT, 1969, Nature *222*, 885.

GUTTMANN, R. D. and J. B. AUST, 1961, Nature *192*, 564.

GUTTMANN, R. D., R. R. LINDQUIST and S. A. OCKER, 1969, Transplantation *9*, 39.

HÄMMERLING, U., D. A. L. DAVIES and A. J. MANSTONE, 1971, Immunochemistry *8*, 7.

HARRIS, R. and J. D. ZERVAS, 1969, Nature *221*, 1062.

HAŠKOVÁ, V., J. CHUTNA and G. BIEGE, 1965, Folia Biol. *11*, 446.

HAUGHTON, G., 1966, Transplantation *4*, 238.

HELLSTRÖM, I., A. C. ALLISON and K. E. HELLSTRÖM, 1971, Nature *230*, 49.

HELLSTRÖM, K. E., 1959, Transplant. Bull. *6*, 411.

HELLSTRÖM, K. E. and I. HELLSTRÖM, 1970, Ann. Rev. Microbiol. *24*, 373.

HELLSTRÖM, K. E., I. HELLSTRÖM and J. BRAWN, 1969, Nature *224*, 914.

HILDEMANN, W. H., 1970a, Transplant. Rev. *3*, 5.

HILDEMANN, W. H., 1970b, Immunogenetics. S. Francisco/Cambridge/London/Amsterdam, Holden-Day. Chpts. 6, 7 and 8.

HILDEMANN, W. H. and N. COHEN, 1967, Weak histo-incompatibilities: emerging immuno-genetic rules and generalizations. *In*: E. S. Curtoni, P. L. Mattiuz and R. M. Tosi, eds.: Histocompatibility testing 1967. Copenhagen, Munksgaard. pp. 13–20.

HILDEMANN, W. H., M. MORGAN and FRAUTNICK, L., 1970, Transplant. Proc. *2*, 24.

HILDEMANN, W. H. and M. TAKASUGI, 1969, Transplant. Proc. *1*, 530.

HUTCHIN, P., 1968, Surg. Gynec. Obstet. *126*, 1331.

JUTILA, J. W. and R. S. WEISER, 1962, J. Immunol. *88*, 621.

KALISS, N. 1958, Cancer Res. *18*, 992.

KALISS, N. and B. F. BRYANT, 1958, J. Natl. Cancer Inst. *20*, 691.

KANDUTSCH, A. A., H. C. JURGELEIT and J. H. STIMPFLING, 1965, Transplantation *3*, 748.

KANDUTSCH, A. A. and U. REINERT-WENCK, 1957, J. Exptl. Med. *105*, 125.

KISSMEYER-NIELSEN, F., S. OLSON, V. PETERSEN and O. FJELDBORG, 1966, Lancet *ii*, 662.

KISSMEYER-NIELSEN, F., A. SVEJGAARD and M. HAUGE, 1968, Nature *219*, 1116.

KISSMEYER-NIELSEN, F. and E. THORSBY, 1970, Transplant. Rev. *4*, 17.

KLEIN, G., 1966, Ann. Rev. Microbiol. *20*, 223.

KLEIN, J., 1966, Folia Biol. *12*, 168.

KLEIN, J., 1967, Strength of histocompatibility genes in mice, *In*: E. S. Curtoni, P. L. Mattiuz and R. M. Tosi, eds.: Histocompatibility testing 1967. Copenhagen, Munks-gaard. pp. 21–28.

KŘEN, V., O. ŠTARK and D. KŘENOVÁ, 1969, Folia Biol. *15*, 188.

LANDY, M. and W. BRAUN, eds., 1969, Immunological tolerance. New York/London, Academic Press. pp. 1–352.

LAPP, W. S. and J. Q. BLISS, 1966, Transplantation *4*, 754.

LAPP, W. S. and J. Q. BLISS, 1967, Immunology *12*, 103.

LEE, S., 1967, Surgery *61*, 771.

LENGEROVÁ, A., 1969, Immunogenetics of tissue transplantation. Amsterdam, North-Holland. pp. 1–270.

LIND, P. E. and A. SZENBERG, 1961, Aust. J. Biol. Med. Sci. *39*, 507.

LINSCOTT, W. D., 1970, Nature *228*, 824.

LISOWSKA, E. and A. MORAWIECKI, 1967, Eur. J. Biochem. *3*, 237.

LITTLE, C. C., 1914, Science *40*, 904.

MAHABIR, R. N., R. D. GUTTMANN and R. R. LINDQUIST, 1969, Transplantation *8*, 369.

MARIANI, T., C. MARTINEZ, J. M. SMITH and R. A. GOOD, 1959, Proc. Soc. Exptl. Biol. Med. *101*, 596.

MARTINEZ, C., F. SHAPIRO and R. A. GOOD, 1962, Induction of immunological tolerance of tissue homografts in adult mice. *In*: M. Hasek, A. Lengerová and M. Vojtisková, eds.: Mechanisms of immunological tolerance. Prague, Czechoslovak Academy of Sciences. pp. 329–335.

MASON, S. and N. L. WARNER, 1970, J. Immunol. *104*, 762.

MCKHANN, C. F., 1962, J. Immunol. *88*, 500.

MCKHANN, C. F., 1964a, Transplantation *2*, 613.

MCKHANN, C. F., 1964b, Transplantation *2*, 620.

MCKHANN, C. F., 1964c, Nature *201*, 937.

MCKHANN, C. F., 1968, Transplantation *6*, 482.

MCKHANN C. F. and J. H. BERRIAN, 1961, J. Immunol. *86*, 170.

MEDAWAR, P. B., 1945, J. Anatomy *78*, 176.

MEDAWAR, P. B., 1945, J. Anatomy *79*, 157.

MEDAWAR, P. B., 1946, Brit. J. Exptl. Pathol. *27*, 15.

MEDAWAR, P. B., 1959, Iso-antigens. *In*: F. Albert, and P. B. Medawar, eds.: Biological problems of grafting. (Blackwell. Oxford, pp. 6–24.

MEDAWAR, P. B., 1963, Transplantation *1*, 21.

MEDAWAR, P. B., 1969, Proc. Roy. Soc. *B174*, 155.

MILGROM, F. and J. KLASSEN, 1971, Immunopathologic studies on allograft reactions. *In*: S. Cohen, G. Cudkowicz and R. T. McCluskey, eds.: Cellular interactions in the immune response. Basel, Karger. pp. 290–296.

MILLER, J. F. A. P., 1960, Brit. J. Cancer *14*, 83.

MÖLLER, E., 1965, J. Natl. Cancer Inst. *35*, 1053.

MÖLLER, E. and G. MÖLLER, 1962, J. Exptl. Med. *115*, 527.

MÖLLER, G., 1961, J. Exptl. Med. *114*, 415.

MÖLLER, G., 1962, J. Immunol. *90*, 271.

MÖLLER, G., 1963, J. Natl. Cancer Inst. *30*, 1153.

MÖLLER, G., 1966, J. Immunol. *96*, 430.

MÖLLER, G. and E. MÖLLER, 1966, *In*: B. Cinader, ed.: Immune cytotoxicity and immunological enhancement in antibodies to biologically active molecules. Oxford, Pergamon. pp. 349–407.

MORRIS, P. J., A. TING and J. FORBES, 1971, Transplant. Proc. *3*, 109.

MORTON, J. A., M. M. PICKLES and L. SUTTON, 1969, Vox. Sang. *17*, 536.

NATHENSON, S. G., 1970, Ann. Rev. Genetics *4*, 69.

NISBET, N. W. and M. W. ELVES, eds., 1971, Immunological tolerance to tissue antigens. Orthopaedic Hospital, Oswestry, England. pp. 1–345.

NOSSAL, G. J. V., 1968, Immunologic tolerance. *In*: F. T. Rapaport, and J. Dausset, eds.: Human Transplantation. New York/London, Grune and Stratton. pp. 643–654.

OLD, L. J. and E. A. BOYSE, 1969, Ann. Rev. Genetics *3*, 269.

OLD, L. J., E. A. BOYSE and E. STOCKERT, 1963, J. Natl. Cancer Inst. *31*, 977.

OZER, J. H. and D. F. H. WALLACH, 1967, Transplantation *5*, 652.

PALM, J. and L. MANSON, 1968, J. Cell Comp. Physiol. *68*, 207.

PATEL, R. and P. I. TERASAKI, 1969, New Engl. J. Med. *280*, 735.

PERKINS, H. A., S. L. KOUNTZ, R. PAYNE and F. O. BELZER, 1971, Transplant. Proc. *3*, 130.

PORTER, K. A. 1965, Brit. Med. Bull. *21*, 171.

PREHN, R. T. and J. M. MAIN, 1958, J. Natl. Cancer Inst. *20*, 207.

RAFF, M. C., 1970, Immunology *19*, 637.

RAPAPORT, F. T., 1968, Heterologous antigens and antibodies in transplantation. *In*: F. T. Rapaport and J. Dausset, eds.: Human transplantation. New York/London, Grune and Stratton. pp. 635–642.

RAPAPORT, F. T., J. DAUSSET, J. HAMBURGER, D. M. HUME, K. KANO, G. M. WILLIAMS, F. MILGROM, 1967, Ann. Surg. *166*, 596.

REIF, A. E. and J. M. V. ALLEN, 1964, J. Exptl. Med. *120*, 413.

REISFELD, R. A. and B. D. KAHAN, Advan. Immunology *12*, 117.

RUSSELL, P. S. and A. P. MONACO, 1965, The biology of tissue transplantation. Boston, Little, Brown and Co.

RUSSELL, P. S., S. D. NELSON and G. J. JOHNSON, 1966, Ann. N.Y. Acad. Sci. *129*, 368.

RUSSELL, P. S. and H. J. WINN, 1970, New Engl. J. Med. *282*, 786, 848 and 896.

RYCHLIKOVÁ, M. and P. IVANYI, 1969, Folia Biol. *15*, 126.

SANDERSON, A. R., P. CRESSWELL and K. I. WELSH, 1971, Nature (in press).

SCHREK, R. and W. J. DONNELLY, 1961, Blood *18*, 561.

SHIMADA, A. and S. G. NATHENSON, 1967, Biochem. Biophys. Res. Comm. *29*, 828.

SHIMADA, A., K. YAMANE and S. G. NATHENSON, 1970, Proc. Natl. Acad. Sci. U.S. *65*, 691.

SHREFFLER, D. C. and J. KLEIN, 1970, Transplant. Proc. *2*, 5.

SILVERS, W. K. and R. E. BILLINGHAM, 1969, Transplantation *8*, 167.

SIMMONS, R. L., 1969, Transplant. Proc. *1*, 47.

SIMONSEN, M., 1962a, The factor of immunization: clonal selection theory investigated by spleen assays of graft-versus-host reaction. *In*: G. E. W. Wolstenholme and M. P. Cameron, eds.: Ciba Foundation Symposium on Transplantation. London, Churchill. pp. 185–209.

SIMONSEN, M., 1962b, Progr. Allergy *6*, 349.

SIMONSEN, M., 1970, Transplant. Rev. *3*, 22.

SNELL, G. D., 1958a, Transplantable tumors. *In*: F. Homburger, ed.: The physiopathology of cancer, 2nd ed. New York, Hoeber-Harper. pp. 293–345.

SNELL, G. D., 1958b, J. Natl. Cancer Inst. *21*, 843.

SNELL, G. D., 1970, Surg. Gynec. Obstet. *130*, 1109.

SNELL, G. D. and H. P. BUNKER, 1965, Transplantation *3*, 235.

SNELL, G. D., M. CHERRY and P. DEMANT, 1971, Transplant. Proc. *3*, 183.

SNELL, G. D., A. M. CLOUDMAN, E. FAILOR and P. DOUGLAS, 1946, J. Natl. Cancer Inst. *6*, 303.

SNELL, G. D. and L. C. STEVENS, 1961, Immunology *4*, 366.

SNELL, G. D. and J. H. STIMPFLING, 1966, Genetics of tissue transplantation. *In*: E. Green, ed.: Biology of the laboratory mouse. New York, McGraw-Hill. pp. 457–491.

SNELL, G. D., H. J. WINN, J. H. STIMPFLING and S. J. PARKER, 1960, J. Exptl. Med. *112*, 293.

STARK, O., D. KŘENOVÁ, V. KŘEN and B. FRENZL, 1970, Folia Biol. *16*, 1.

STEINMULLER, D., 1967, Science *158*, 127.

STEINMULLER, D., 1969, Transplant. Proc. *1*, 593.

STETSON, C. A., 1963, Advan. Immunology *3*, 97.

STICKEL, D. L., D. B. AMOS, C. M. ZMIJEWSKI, J. F. GLENN and R. R. ROBINSON, 1967, Transplantation *5*, 1024.

STIMPFLING, J. H. and G. D. SNELL, 1962, Histocompatibility genes and some immunogenetic problems. *In*: A. P. Cristoffanini, and G. Hoecker, eds.: International Symposium on Tissue Transplantation. University of Chile, Santiago. pp. 37–53.

SUMMERELL, J. M. and D. A. L. DAVIES, 1969, Transplant. Proc. *1*, 479.

SVEJGAARD, A. and F. KISSMEYER-NIELSEN, 1968, Nature *219*, 868.

TAKASUGI, M. and W. H. HILDEMANN, 1969, Transplant. Proc. *1*, 530.

THOMAS, D. B. and R. J. WINZLER, 1970, Biochem. Biophys. Res. Comm. *35*, 811.

THORSBY, E., 1971, Eur. J. Immunol. *1*, 57.

UHR, J. W. and J. B. BAUMANN, 1961, J. Exptl. Med. *113*, 935.

VOISIN, G. A. and R. G. KINSKY, 1962, Protection against runting by specific treatments of newborn mice, followed by increased tolerance. *In*: G. E. W. Wolstenholme and M. P. Cameron, eds.: CIBA Foundation Symposium on Transplantation. London, Churchill. pp. 286–326.

VOISIN, G. A., R. G. KINSKY and F. K. JANSEN, 1966, Nature *210*, 138.

VOISIN, G. A., R. KINSKY, F. JANSEN and C. BERNHARD, 1969, Transplantation *8*, 618.

VOISIN, G. A., R. KINSKY and J. MAILLARD, 1968, Ann. Inst. Pasteur *115*, 855.

WARNER, N. L. and A. SZENBERG, 1964, Aust. J. Biol. Med. Sci. *42*, 100.

WHITE, E. and W. H. HILDEMANN, 1968, Science *162*, 1293.

WHITE, E., W. H. HILDEMANN and Y. MULLEN, 1969, Transplantation *8*, 602.

WILSON, D. B. and R. E. BILLINGHAM, 1967, Advan. Immunology *7*, 189.

WINN, H. J., 1962, Ann. N.Y. Acad. Sci. *101*, 23.

WINN, H. J., 1970, Transplant. Proc. *2*, 83.

World Health Organization Committee on HL-A Nomenclature, 1968, Nomenclature for Factors of the HL-A System. Bull. Wld. Hlth. Org. *39*, 483.

ZEISS, I. M., 1966, Immunology *11*, 597.

CHAPTER 16

Cancer immunity

F. M. BURNET

School of Microbiology, University of Melbourne, Parkville, Victoria

16.1. General aspects of immunogenicity

16.1.1. The established background

In discussing immunogenicity in terms of cancer immunity, one is rather strictly limited by the experimental difficulties of dealing with a type of immune response which is often marginal in activity and which is usually only measurable *in vivo*. Before embarking on such a discussion it is necessary to state certain points which, at least in the author's opinion, can be accepted as established:

(1) 'Cancer immunity' is restricted to phenomena demonstrable either in the autochthonous host or in syngeneic animals by which specific resistance to a clone of malignant cells is shown to have developed as a result of previous exposure to such cells or antigenic material derived from them.

(2) Resistance to transplantation is regarded as strictly analogous to homograft immunity and is basically a form of delayed hypersensitivity mediated by cells which have been spoken of as DH-immunocytes (Burnet 1968).

(3) All types of adaptive immune response are mediated by immunocytes, i.e., lymphoid cells which carry a single type of receptor whose specificity is equivalent to that of antibody which is or could be produced by cells of the same clone. This holds for cells which for morphological or functional reasons are spoken of as antigen-reactive cells, immunocompetent lymphocytes, DH-lymphocytes and plasma cells.

(4) Specific pattern of immune receptor or antibody depends on two genetically-based processes, the first of somatic diversification of pattern – for which either active somatic mutation or some process of intragenomic cross-over between duplicated genes has been suggested – and the second, an apparently rigid phenotypic restriction to one immune pattern and one type of immunoglobulin production. It is convenient

to regard DH-immunocytes as a group of equivalent status to IgG or IgA producers.

(5) The immune response is essentially a selection by antigen of immunocytes with receptors of pattern which will react with sufficient intensity to steric contact with the functioning antigenic determinants, and as a result proliferate to a clone large enough for its effects to become demonstrable.

Justification of these statements can be found in the following reviews: Jerne 1967; Burnet 1969b; Siskind and Benacerraf 1969. Their acceptance will allow a more logical approach to the specific problems of immunogenicity in relation to cancer immunity.

16.1.2. Applications to homograft immunity

From this whole-heartedly selectionist approach there are several aspects of immunogenicity which are equally applicable to homograft immunity and require some consideration:

(1) How do immunocytes (antigen-reactive cells) capable of being stimulated by 'new' antigenic determinants of malignant cells come to be present in the body?

The answer is the same as for any foreign antigen; patterns arise by random diversification of the genetic material provided in the zygote. This may eventually need to be modified in view of Jerne's recent hypothesis (1970) on the direct genetic origin of specificity directed against 'non-self' histocompatibility antigens within the capacity of the species to produce.

(2) Where do the primary immunocytes (antigen-recognition cells – ARC's) wait to be available for selection by antigen?

The only reasonable answer is that until they are 'chosen' by the antigen, they represent a tiny anonymous minority of the small lymphocytes circulating in blood, tissue fluid and lymph, or temporarily held in any of the peripheral accumulations of lymphoid tissue. It is probable that at least in the rabbit, ARC's are also present in the bone marrow (Abdou and Richter 1969a, b). It is still unknown whether such cells represent in part or wholly a less differentiated form than the antigen reactive cells studied in experiments like those of Mitchell and Miller (1968). There may well be a special likelihood that thymus-dependent (TD) cells ancestral to DH-immunocytes concentrate in the 'thymus-dependent areas' of spleen and lymph node as defined by Parrott et al. (1966).

(3) What is the standard process by which antigenic determinants characteristic of new tumour antigens make contact with appropriate immunocyte receptors?

There appear to be two alternative but not necessarily mutually exclusive answers at the present time. The first depends on the hypothesis I have recently developed (Burnet 1969c, 1970a), that it is characteristic of many mobile cells to carry a variety of antigenic determinants (AD) in the lipo-glycoprotein of the cell membrane and to possess a well developed power to transfer such AD's to adjacent cells by contact or propinquity. On this view, lymphocytes or monocytes quite irrespective of any 'antibody-like' receptors they may possess, will when they can make effective contact with the 'foreign' cells, take up the new AD on their surface and in due course lodge in peripheral lymphoid tissue. There they serve as carriers of the AD which, being in essentially the same situation as a genetically appropriate histocompatibility antigen, will react with an appropriate immunocyte by cell to cell contact. The alternative concept of 'peripheral sensitization' favoured by Medawar (1969) and Strober and Gowans (1965) and others, largely from consideration of the problems of kidney transplant rejection, is that amongst the millions of lymphocytes passing through the kidney or other foreign tissue, there will be some with immune receptors capable of picking up the foreign AD from capillary endothelium or elsewhere and thereafter pass to lymphoid tissue where the proliferation stimulated by the contact will take place. It is clear that the first would be more appropriate for a small fragment of tissue, a minimal area skin graft or an initiating tumour while the second would be specially appropriate to an organ connected to the full blood circulation of the host. There is no decisive experimental evidence in favour of either alternative and one should probably remain fully receptive of some other hypothesis yet to be stated.

16.1.3. *Tumour immunity as a manifestation of delayed hypersensitivity*

It is now generally accepted that homograft immunity is a cell-mediated response of the same general quality as delayed hypersensitivity and, as such, mediated by thymus-dependent immunocytes. Cancer immunity would therefore equally be based on delayed hypersensitivity. Before elaborating this contention, however, it may be expedient to present briefly the view which I have been developing in recent years that homograft immunity is the most primitive form of adaptive immunity (Burnet 1968, 1969c, 1970b), and that the standard methods of demonstrating delayed hypersensitivity are rather accidental or artificial developments of the basic quality of an ability to recognize 'new' or 'foreign' antigenic determinants on the surface of mobile cells. By convention, however, delayed hypersensitivity (DH) is what is taken as the characteristic form of cell-based immune responses in contrast to the production of antibody of the various immunoglobulin types. In an attempt to provide in the simplest possible form the essential features of the DH response, I have offered the following scheme (Burnet 1970b):

(1) The immunocytes involved are thymus-dependent. There is no evidence as to whether antigen reactive cells exist with the same relationship to DH-immunocytes as conventional ARC have to plaque-forming cells or plasma cells.

(2) The standard, possibly the only method by which a DH-immunocyte can be specifically stimulated, is by cell to cell contact, the antigenic determinant on a mobile carrier cell (lymphocyte or monocyte) coming into steric contact with the immunocyte receptor which is conceivably located predominantly in the uropod region.

(3) Stimulation results (a) in activation to DNA synthesis and proliferation, (b) in liberation of a variety of pharmacologically active agents which include mitosis-stimulating factors, migration-inhibitory factor, lymph node permeability factor and various proteases and kinins. There is a tendency for any specific immune response to initiate a chain reaction of nonspecific stimulation amongst adjacent cells, (c) in the limit, stimulation results in death of the immunocyte and/or the AD-carrying cell.

A much more speculative addition is to account for the existence and properties of Lawrence's transfer factor which is observed only with DH-provoking immunogens. This was interpreted as essentially a transferable antigenic fragment capable of reversible liberation and attachment to the surface membrane of mobile cells. As we are not directly concerned with transfer factor in cancer immunity, the hypothesis need not be elaborated here.

There has never been any serious doubt since Mitchison's (1955) work that tumour immunity was a cell-mediated function closely analogous to homograft rejection and therefore essentially a delayed hypersensitivity response. It is conventional to study delayed hypersensitivity in guinea-pigs and with the development of the pure line strains 2 and 13, it has recently become possible to study this aspect of cancer immunity directly. Two groups have obtained basically similar results. Oettgen et al. (1968) used Strain 13 guinea-pigs and produced sarcomas by intramuscular injection of methylcholanthrene or dimethylbenzanthracene. Sixteen antigenically distinct tumours were obtained which were lethal by intramuscular injection but which regressed after intradermal injection. Guinea-pigs which had recovered after excision of intramuscular tumour or spontaneously after intradermal implantation showed typical DH-type skin reactions to injection intradermally of tumour cells or extracts. The specificity of the hypersensitivity reactions paralleled that of the capacity to reject an inoculum of living tumour cells. The Bethesda group, Churchill et al. (1968), Zbar et al. (1969a, b) Kronman et al. (1969), used Strain 2 animals given diethylnitrosamine by mouth and induced hepatomas that were transmissible to syngeneic animals and showed similar diversity of antigens and capacity to give typical delayed hypersensitivity reactions.

16.2. The immunogenic qualities of tumours

16.2.1. Histocompatibility antigens

The necessity for limiting serious discussion of the topic to tumours in the autochthonous host or in animals syngeneic with the individual in which it arose has already been stated. It is, however, desirable to mention very briefly one or two points in regard to histocompatibility antigens. In general, a spontaneous tumour is only transmissible to syngeneic animals or to F1 animals of which the original strain is one component. The rules in regard to transplantation in mice which were worked out for tumours (Little 1941) hold equally for skin transplantation. Once a transmissible tumour strain has become well established in a syngeneic strain, it may show less rigid requirements. Much work summarized by Hellström and Möller (1965) has been done with lines of isogenic resistant (IR) mice. These lines, initiated by Snell (1958), are essentially pure line strains differing only in regard to the H2 antigens they carry. Tumours induced in F1 hybrids between 2 IR strains were sometimes transplantable to one or other of the parent strains. A subline from such a tumour grew well in the parental strain and could be shown to have lost the antigen received from the other parental strain (Klein et al. 1960, Bjaring and Klein 1968). This is only the most precisely studied of a wide range of variability in transplantable tumours. Whenever an initially homogeneous tumour clone is maintained where it can proliferate, there are constant opportunities for somatic mutation and for Darwinian selection of any mutant clone which is 'fitter' to survive under the conditions provided by Nature or by the experimenter. 'Progression' may represent some intrinsic change to more vigorous growth but it may equally represent a loss of antigenic groupings by which immune mechanisms of the host could hold it in check.

An important mechanism by which the normal resistance of a mouse or other species to homotransplantation of a tumour strain may be overcome is the enhancement phenomenon (see Kaliss 1958). In many instances if animals of strain B normally resistant to tumour TA which arose in strain A and has subsequently been maintained in A mice, are injected with a relatively large amount of normal A tissue or of tumour inactivated by freezing or some other appropriate method, subsequent inocula of TA tumour will be accepted. The phenomenon is now accepted as resulting from the development of circulating antibody against those histocompatibility antigens of the TA tumour which are not present in the B host. Enhancement is also demonstrable by the passive use of serum from appropriately immunized donors (Kaliss and Molomut 1952). It is well known that if one wishes to produce delayed hypersensitivity in rabbits, the antigen should be given intradermally while intravenous administration, though excellent for antibody production, gives little sensitization. Billingham and Sparrow (1955) (see also Billingham 1957) found, as might be expected, that intravenous administration of dissociated skin epidermal cells from rabbit A into rabbit B allowed subsequent grafts of skin from A to be retained for 16–22 days instead of being rejected within 9 days as is normal. If the epidermal cells were given intraperitoneally there was no significant effect, while intradermal administration induced an accelerated immune rejection of the test graft.

The action of antibody in inducing enhancement is probably complex (Hellström and Möller 1965). On the efferent side, harmless blanketing of antigenic determinants on the target cells by antibody renders them unavailable to stimulate DH-immunocytes to cytotoxic activity. There is also the possibility of an afferent block if antibody prevents the release or transfer to carrier cells of the significant tumour cell antigens.

16.2.2. Tumour-specific antigens

Passing now to cancer immunity proper, *i.e.*, as manifested within a line of animals syngeneic with the primary host in which the tumour arose spontaneously or was experimentally induced, the first point to be discussed quite briefly is the well known difference between the antigenicity of tumours induced by DNA oncogenic viruses and those induced by chemical carcinogens.

Taking polyoma virus as the prototype, any tumour induced in mice or hamsters by inoculation of virus in the new-born animal possesses a new antigenic quality which may involve more than one type of new antigenic determinant but is the same for all tumours irrespective of host or organ involved. Each induced tumour will have, in addition, its own characteristic species and tissue antigens which will become evident in any type of homo- or heterotransplantation (see Habel 1969).

With tumours induced by chemical carcinogens injected intramuscularly or subcutaneously to induce sarcomas in mice or guinea-pigs the result is quite different. As far as it is practicable to replicate experiments, Klein et al. (1960) find that each sarcoma line induced by methylcholanthrene (MCA) in a pure line strain of mice was antigenically distinct from all the other lines. Oettgens et al. (1968) have shown a similar striking diversity in sarcomas induced by MCA in Strain 13 guinea-pigs. The same specificity was evident irrespective of whether the differentiation was demonstrated by transplantation immunity or by tests for delayed hypersensitivity.

Similar findings on sarcomas induced in rats by 3,4-benzpyrene are reported by Alexander et al. (1969) although no direct evidence in regard to delayed hypersensitivity is given. It is of special interest that hepatomas induced in rats by feeding 4-dimethylaminoazobenzene (Baldwin and Barker 1967) or in guinea-pigs with diethylnitrosamine (Zbar et al. 1969b) show the same individuality of antigenic character as the sarcomas.

The accepted interpretation of the unitary nature of the new antigen associated with any oncogenic DNA virus is that portion of the viral genome has been incorporated in the genome of the transformed cell and is able to induce the formation of an appropriate, presumably protein, antigen. It is unlikely that this incorporation is directly related to the malignant character of the transformed cell, but it is associated with a continuing antigenic marker.

According to Habel (1969) there is still considerable uncertainty as to the relationship of the transplantation antigen present on the cell surface and the complement-fixing antigen which is wholly or predominantly in the nucleus.

The diversity of sarcoma antigens is a more interesting and more difficult problem. It is immediately obvious that the new antigen is not directly responsible for the malignant change. A second point which also seems implicit from the findings is that the emergence of one malignant clone in the region where the carcinogen was lodged, inhibits the development of any other malignant clones. It is arguable whether this has yet been fully established but one could not expect to have the consistent experimental results which are reported unless this was the case. There is evidence from the study of tumours that can be induced by the implantation of bland membranes in rat tissue that only one clone of a number of potential candidates is responsible. Klein et al. (1963) have shown that these membrane-induced sarcomas show diverse immunological specificities although they are not as convenient to work with as MCA sarcomas.

There is nothing equivocal about the diversity of tumour antigens to be found in these chemically induced sarcomas. In addition, the specific antigens persist unchanged on passage (Klein and Klein 1962) and must therefore be genetically determined.

16.2.3. The origins of antigenic diversity

Several hypotheses have been offered to account for the diversity. Klein et al. (1957) wondered whether the MCA was directly active in producing inter-cellular variability in antigenic quality as well as in other characteristics. Prehn (1964) adopted a selectionist approach assuming that chemical carcinogens act by selecting cells which had become initially neoplastic by spontaneous random change. A third hypothesis mentioned only to be discarded by Hellström and Möller (1965) is that MCA inactivates latent oncogenic viruses, a sufficient number of different types being present to account for the multiplicity of antigens.

Prehn (1964) entitled his paper, 'A clonal selection theory of chemical carcinogenesis', and the approach I will adopt represents an elaboration of his general hypothesis but with the emphasis almost wholly on antigenic aspects. I would accept the origin of the malignant quality of the initiating cell as by somatic mutation which may or may not have been influenced by the carcinogen. What is specially relevant is that whenever a cell initiates a neoplastic clone, any other individual characteristics it may have will be manifest by all members of the clone. As has been discussed at length elsewhere (Burnet 1970b), this will often allow the manifestation of biochemical or immunological characters which could never have been demonstrated in a single cell.

For some time I have been trying to develop an approach to this problem of antigenic diversity in tumours that would bring it closely into line with other developments implicit in the clonal selection theory of immunity. A theoretical discussion of the background of the present hypothesis is available (Burnet 1970c). The crux of it is that there are sound evolutionary reasons why histocompatibility antigens should have potential variability almost equivalent to that of specific patterns on immunoglobulin molecules.

One assumes that in the process of normal differentiation the stem cells from which in one way or another the initial cell and its descendant sarcoma clone arises, undergo relatively active point mutations at loci coding for plasma-membrane proteins and so giving rise to potential new antigenic determinants (AD) on the cell surface. As long as individual cells carrying a given new AD are in small total numbers, separate from one another and incorporated into normal functional activity, they will not be immunogenic. An elegant demonstration highly relevant to this statement is the finding by Billingham and Silvers (1963) that very small numbers of black melanocytes from Strain 2 guinea-pigs transplanted to white skin areas on histoincompatible Strain 13 animals, would give rise to spreading areas of black pigmentation. When, however, the cell proliferates unduly from neoplastic change and a large uniform clone develops, the condition changes significantly. The new antigenic determinant is carried by, and presumably liberated from many adjacent cells, the changed surface characters of malignant cells may well accentuate this and the new antigenic pattern becomes effectively immunogenic.

16.2.4. Implications for cancer therapy

If immunological surveillance is a reality, there should be at least marginal implications for the application of immunological approaches to cancer therapy. This possibility has been discussed in some detail (Burnet 1971) and only a brief resumé of the approach need be attempted here.

If, as some evidence and all analogy suggests, 'new' antigens in human tumours are widely diverse and that, when a tumour is actively multiplying, there is probably a state of specific immune paralysis involving any relevant immunocytes, attempts to develop tumour-specific immunizing agents seem to be impracticable for the foreseeable future. For the present, laboratory research and cautious clinical experimentation will need to be directed toward means of nonspecific activation of immune responses, particularly of the thymus-dependent system. Perhaps the most important lack is an understanding of the well recognized ineffectiveness of delayed hypersensitivity reactions and other manifestations of the thymus-dependent system in patients with clinical cancer. Any attempt to use what might be called immuno-expressive agents as adjuvants to cancer therapy should be preceded by tests as to whether they could alter this characteristic unresponsiveness. The two visible approaches seem to be the use of bacterial endotoxins and further exploration of the possibility that elderly individuals may be low in hormone levels – oestrogens and thyroxin have been mentioned – and that this may be related to their immunological inadequacy. Another point discussed at some length in the paper referred to is the relatively well established finding that cancer patients show a highly significant difference from equivalent controls in much more rarely giving a history of suffering from allergic conditions. The significance of this has not been explored and offers an interesting field for further research.

16.3. Some evolutionary-genetic speculations

The crux of any discussion of immunogenicity in cancer is to provide some acceptable interpretation of the reasons why a large range of cancers – possibly all malignant tumours – show some antigenic individuality differentiating them from all normal tissues of the host individual. The new antigenic quality is of course usually inadequate to control the malignant clone if this ever escapes beyond early phases of its growth.

In a number of articles (Burnet 1968, 1969a, 1970c), I have developed the theme that the evolutionary basis of adaptive immunity must be sought not as a development of defence against pathogenic or potentially pathogenic micro-organisms but as a means of dealing with either parasitism by organisms closely related to the host, or with potentially pathogenic somatic mutant cells (malignant or hyperplastic). Only in this way does the existence of homograft immunity and of, in Billingham's (1969) words, 'an astounding multiplicity of alleles and pseudo-alleles with corresponding antigenic specificities' become intelligible. The essence of the interpretation was that if it was necessary for good evolutionary reasons to recognize as 'not-self' cyclostome parasitic on larger cyclostomes or neoplastic cells carrying mutant antigenic determinants, two complementary processes were necessary. A diversity of patterns to be recognized needed to be developed as between individuals within the species and a system of cells specialized to recognize foreign configurations entering or appearing in the body. From the first requirement the multiplicity of histocompatibility antigens has developed, from the second the immune system based on immunocytes carrying 'antibody-like' receptors and in part capable of giving rise to antibody-immunoglobulin producing clones.

If the two qualities developed together about the stage when agnathous vertebrates were evolving, it is not unreasonable to suggest that diversification of histocompatibility antigens may have been based on the same principles as are becoming evident for the diversification of immune patterns and their phenotypic restriction. If this is the case it must obviously have important implications in regard to the immunogenicity of neoplastic cells and some elaboration of the hypothesis here seems justified. What will be attempted is to look at HCA diversity from both genetic and somatic genetic angles just as one must look at the diversity of immune pattern from the same points of view.

16.3.1. *Evolution of antigenic diversity*

One's working hypothesis will be that the genes coding for the proteins of cell membranes are subject to a high level of random point mutation and that the result of a significant proportion of mutations is to induce an antigenic change – a new antigenic determinant – without rendering cell or organisms non-viable. It is of the essence of the hypothesis that such mutations occur with similar frequency in germinal and somatic cells.

The frequency of germinal changes in histocompatibility antigen (HCA) qualities is proverbial. It is normally taught that if brother-sister mating in a pure line of mice is replaced by pen-mating for 8 or 10 generations, skin rejection between individuals of the strain can be expected. Lindner (1963), working with CBA sublines, found only a minor degree of rejection but a quantitative study by Bailey and Kohn (1965) using a large F1 population of C57Bl × BALB/c, gave results which indicated that a HCA change of intensity sufficient to cause skin rejection occurred at a rate of slightly over 1% per generation. This is enormously higher than most forms of mutation in mammals. It is implicitly confirmed by general experience and by the extreme complexity of the HCA position in the two mammals which have been most closely studied, man and the house mouse. It is also evident that very similar findings, *viz.*, a multiplicity of loci concerned with HCA's but one locus, corresponding to H2 in mice and HL-A in men, which has both a dominant influence and a very large number of alleles and pseudo-alleles are also characteristic of chickens and rats. Here then, is a basic characteristic of birds and mammals and since homograft rejection is the rule also in lampreys, elasmobranchs and gold-fish, it probably holds for all vertebrates from the cyclostomes upward.

16.3.2. *Somatic diversity of antigens*

Evidence that a similar mutability to a diversity of HCA's is also a feature of somatic cells can be obtained from two sources. The first has already been indicated. We have accepted the origin of antigenic diversity amongst MCA-induced sarcomas and hepatomas induced by oral administration of appropriate agents, as being due to pre-existent diversity amongst the stem cell clones from which the tumour cells derive. This requires that all cell systems in the body from which malignant disease can arise, develop during differentiation clonal differences in potential antigenicity. The differences, insofar as they involve cells from which malignancy can arise, must necessarily be insufficient either to stimulate effective cyto-aggressive action against the clone or, with somewhat less certainty, to induce tolerance. As mentioned previously, it is only when the potential antigen is rendered immunogenic by localized accumulation of a clone and probably a greater ability to liberate the new antigenic determinant, that any immune response can be called into action.

If, however, as we are almost bound to assume, the type and frequency of mutation in somatic cells is parallel to that in germinal cells, we must also assume that major 'H2-type' mutations also occur. Any such changes, however, would probably involve both the elimination of the mutant at an early stage, perhaps even without any necessity for it to show hyperplastic qualities and a *stimulus to proliferation of corresponding immunocytes*. This concept was developed some years ago in discussions with N. L. Warner on some aspects of the Simonsen phenomenon as demonstrated on the chorioallantois (see Warner 1964). The relatively high proportion of competent lymphocytes in adult fowl blood capable of reacting with a given HCA by producing chorioallantoic pocks was ascribed to 'selective pressures favouring these cells'. One of these subsequently discussed (Burnet 1969b) was that somatic mutation would be likely to produce the same range of antigens as are known to have been produced in the species by germinal mutation. This would have provided, on occasion, opportunities for proliferation of reactive immunocytes, so bringing their numbers above what would be expected if the distribution of patterns was wholly random. The same approach was applied (*loc. cit.* p. 635) to the interpretation of the normal lymphocyte transfer reaction of Brent and Medawar (1966) or, in more general terms, to account for the readiness with which rejection of homograft is effected. With the increasing use of the mixed lymphocyte blast transformation reaction it is also evident that there are more than the numbers to be expected of reactive lymphocytes (Wilson et al. 1968; Bach et al. 1969).

Present thoughts on the genetic determinations of the immunoglobulins are still fluid but there seems to be near agreement: (a) that light and heavy chains are synthesized independently at the ribosomal level; (b) that there is evidence of gene duplication, a popular interpretation being that in IgG the light chain involves descendants of 2 modified replicas of a primitive gene and the heavy chain 4 derived from the same gene. (c) At least 2 and probably 3 independent genes are concerned in the production of heavy chains γ and μ in the rabbit (Koshland et al. 1969).

If we picture something similar in relation to cell membrane proteins – with perhaps the dominant H2-type locus broadly equivalent to the region responsible for the 'variable' segments of the immunoglobulin chains – there will be a high possibility that any two cells taken at random will differ in regard to one or more surface antigenic components. As suggested by Mintz's work, the possibility of clonal selection in favour of one or other mutant will always be present but no basis for its discussion yet exists, apart from the varying likelihood of immunological response.

If the hypothesis that somatic mutations will correspond closely to those involving histocompatibility changes at the germinal level is accepted, we must assume that the mutant cells will vary widely in their potential immunogenicity from changes equivalent to a full H2 determinant difference to cells which show no significant 'new' AD. This will provide a continuous spectrum of immunogenicity which may be characterized as follows for the two extremes and an intermediate zone:

(A) 'Strong' difference provoking proliferation of immunocytes of appropriate type and removal of the mutant cells with minimal or no necessity for tumour initiation to render them immunogenic.

(B) Intermediate differences involving a wide diversity of patterns. These will be inadequate to provoke immunocyte proliferation unless a tumour is initiated. In most instances, the initiated tumour will be immunologically eliminated.

(C) No significant antigenic determinant is present which is not found on all standard cells. If such a cell serves to initiate a tumour there is no possibility of its being checked immunologically.

The effect of (A) will be to have available in the body a more than random proportion of immunocytes capable of reacting with major histocompatibility antigens which are within the scope of the genome (germinal or somatic) to produce by point mutation or other mechanism of genetic diversification.

16.3.3. Leads for further work

The suggestion that the multiplicity of histocompatibility antigens may be generated by a process analogous to that responsible for the diversity of immune pattern in antibodies has also been made by Amos (1969) and probably others. The extension to cover somatic diversity which can only become immunologically significant when 'magnified' by clonal proliferation, malignant or otherwise, is a logical but not yet adequately established extension. Its main virtue may be as a guiding theme for fruitful experimentation in the field just opening up of the chemical nature of the histocompatibility (HC) antigens. The cell-membrane is a very complex structure and is probably in life a dynamic structured fabric with lipid polypeptide and carbohydrate aspects, but recent work points strongly toward protein as carrying most of the relevant antigenic determinants. Amino acid analyses have been published and in view of the clinical significance of human HL-A antigens, attempts at amino acid sequence work is bound to follow. If there is, in fact, a hidden multiplicity of HC antigens in human body cells it may be necessary to concentrate on suitable monoclonal tumours or leukaemias to obtain material in quantity and in homogeneous form. The recognition by Putnam (1955) and his successors of the myeloma and Bence-Jones proteins as essentially monoclonal antibodies was of major importance to immunology. If some of the human lymphomas and leukaemias should be as monoclonal as most cases of multiple myelomatosis and carry substantial amounts of plasma-membrane protein, their use might be just as fruitful in the complementary field of histocompatibility.

References

ABDOU, N. I. and M. RICHTER, 1969a, J. Exptl. Med. *130*, 141.

ABDOU, N. I. and M. RICHTER, 1969b, J. Exptl. Med. *130*, 165.

ALEXANDER, P., J. BENSTED, E. J. DELORME, J. G. HALL and J. HODGETT, 1969, Proc. Roy. Soc. *B174*, 237.

AMOS, D. B., 1969, Advan. Immunol. *10*, 251.

BACH, F. H., H. BOCK, K. GRAUPNER, E. DAY and H. KLOSTERMANN, 1969, Proc. Natl. Acad. Sci. U.S. *62*, 377.

BAILEY, D. W. and H. I. KOHN, 1965, Genet. Res. *6*, 330.

BALDWIN, R. W. and C. R. BARKER, 1967, Brit. J. Cancer *21*, 338.

BILLINGHAM, R. E., 1957, Ann. N.Y. Acad. Sci. *64*, 799.

BILLINGHAM, R. E., 1969, Proc. Natl. Acad. Sci. U.S. *63*, 1020.

BILLINGHAM, R. E. and W. K. SILVERS, 1963, Ann. N.Y. Acad. Sci. *100*, 348.

BILLINGHAM, R. E. and E. M. SPARROW, 1955, J. Embryol. Exptl. Morph. *3*, 265.

BJARING, B. and G. KLEIN, 1968, J. Natl. Cancer Inst. *41*, 1411.

BRENT, L. and P. B. MEDAWAR, 1966, Proc. Roy. Soc. *B165*, 281.

BURNET, F. M., 1968, Nature *218*, 426.

BURNET, F. M., 1969a, Acta Path. Microbiol. Scand. *76*, 1.

BURNET, F. M., 1969b, Cellular immunology. Melbourne and Cambridge University Presses.

BURNET, F. M., 1969c, Wissensch. Rundschau *22*(12), 524.

BURNET, F. M., 1970a, The newer immunology: an evolutionary approach. *In*: S. Mudd, ed.: Infectious agents and host resistance. Philadelphia, Saunders. p. 1.

BURNET, F. M., 1970b, Immunological surveillance. Sydney, Pergamon Press.

BURNET, F. M., 1970c, Nature, *226*, 123.

BURNET, F. M., 1971, Israel J. Med. Sci. *7*, 9.

CHURCHILL, W. H., H. J. RAPP, B. S. KRONMAN and T. BORSOS, 1968, J. Natl. Cancer Inst. *41*, 13.

HABEL, K., 1969, Advan. Immunol. *10*, 229.

HELLSTRÖM, K. E. and G. MÖLLER, 1965, Progr. Allergy *9*, 158.

JERNE, N. K., 1967, Cold Spring Harbor Symp. Quant. Biol. *32*, 591.

JERNE, N. K., 1970, personal communication.

KALISS, N., 1958, Cancer Res. *18*, 992.

KALISS, N. and N. MOLOMUT, 1952, Cancer Res. *12*, 110.

KLEIN, G. and E. KLEIN, 1962, Cold Spring Harbor Symp. Quant. Biol. *27*, 463.

KLEIN, G., H. O. SJÖGREN and E. KLEIN, 1963, Cancer Res. *23*, 84.

KLEIN, G., H. O. SJÖGREN, E. KLEIN and K. E. HELLSTRÖM, 1960, Cancer Res. *20*, 1561.

KLEIN, E., G. KLEIN and L. REVESZ, 1957, J. Natl. Cancer Inst. *19*, 95.

KOSHLAND, M. E., J. J. DAVIS and N. J. FUJITA, 1969, Proc. Natl. Acad. Sci. U.S. *63*, 1274.

KRONMAN, B. S., H. J. RAPP and T. BORSOS, 1969, J. Natl. Cancer Inst. *43*, 869.

LINDNER, O. E. A., 1963, Transplantation *1*, 58.

LITTLE, C. C., 1941, The genetics of tumour transplantation. *In*: G. D. Snell, ed.: Biology of the laboratory mouse. Philadelphia, Blakiston. p. 279.

MEDAWAR, P. B., 1969, Proc. Roy. Soc. *B174*, 155.

MITCHELL, G. F. and J. F. A. P. MILLER, 1968, Proc. Natl. Acad. Sci. *59*, 296.

MITCHISON, N. A., 1955, J. Exptl. Med. *102*, 157.

OETTGEN, H. F., L. J. OLD, E. P. MCCLEAN and E. A. CARSWELL, 1968, Nature *220*, 295.

PARROTT, D. M. V., A. B. DE SOUSA and J. EAST, 1966, J. Exptl. Med. *123*, 191.

PREHN, R. T., 1964, J. Natl. Cancer Inst. *32*, 1.

PUTNAM, F. W., 1955, Science *122*, 275.

SISKIND, G. W. and B. BENACERRAF, 1969, Advan. Immunol. *10*, 1.

SNELL, G. D., 1958, J. Natl. Cancer Inst. *21*, 843.

STROBER, S. and J. L. GOWANS, 1965, J. Exptl. Med. *122*, 347.

WARNER, N. L., 1964, Brit. J. Exptl. Path. *45*, 459.

WILSON, D. B., J. L. BLYTH and P. C. NOWELL, 1968, J. Exptl. Med. *128*, 1157.

ZBAR, B., H. T. WEPSIC, H. J. RAPP, J. WHANG-PENG and T. BORSOS, 1969a, J. Natl. Cancer Inst. *43*, 821.

ZBAR, B., H. T. WEPSIC, H. J. RAPP, T. BORSOS, B. S. KRONMAN and W. H. CHURCHILL, 1969b, J. Natl. Cancer Inst. *43*, 833.

CHAPTER 17

Differentiation of immunocytes and the evolution of immunological potential*

NOEL L. WARNER

Laboratory of Immunogenetics, The Walter and Eliza Hall Institute of Medical Research, Melbourne

17.1. Introduction

The injection into a lethally irradiated recipient, of a clone of cells derived from a single immunologically incompetent haemopoietic stem cell, will result in complete repopulation of the immunological and haemopoietic system of the animal. It is thus apparent that the differentiation and development of the many different types of cells which together comprise the immune system is basically controlled by extra-cellular and intercellular factors, which guide a haemopoietic stem cell along different differentiation pathways. It is the intention of this review to discuss the various factors which influence immunocyte differentiation, and to consider in detail, the complete development of the full immune response in an adult animal, from both the phylogenetic and ontogenic aspects.

The clinical and experimental manifestations of immunity can appear in a variety of different forms. These can all be divided into two basic types or a combination of the two types, namely humoral antibody formation and cellular immunity. These two forms of immunity involve different cell types which in some species have been clearly shown to be under the developmental control of different lymphoid organs. Topics to be raised in this discussion include the ontogenic derivation of these different cells, the factors which influence their differentiation, possible cell collaboration in immune responses, and the apparent dissociation of immunity into two types.

In attempting to cover in a general way the developmental origin of the immune system from the earliest recognizable precursor, three

---

* This is publication No. 1418 from The Walter and Eliza Hall Institute.

main areas will be considered. (i) The development of immunocytes through evolution of the invertebrate and vertebrate species; (ii) the development of the adult immune system in an individual member from the earliest stem cell; and (iii) the further differentiation of immunologically competent cells after confrontation with antigen. In all situations, emphasis will be placed on a comparison of the differential behaviour of those cells involved in cellular *versus* humoral immunity.

17.2. The immunocyte complex, definition of categories

The term immunocyte complex was coined by Dameshek (1963) in order to delineate the system of cells involved in immune reactions from other haemopoietic cell series. The active cells involved in mediating the immune responses are antibody-forming plasma cells, and lymphocytes involved in cellular immunity, and these are referred to as immunocytes. In this first use of the term, it was suggested that these arose by differentiation from the immunoblast, which was produced as a result of antigenic contact with either a reticulum cell or another type of small lymphocyte. In view of the current concepts of cell collaboration, which indicate that the original lymphoid cell directly contacted by antigen need not be the direct linear precursor of the active immunocyte, it is important to realize that there is a basic distinction between those cells that respond in some manner, usually proliferation, to contact with antigen, and the actual immunocytes that mediate the immune response.

Accordingly in this review, the term immunocyte is exclusively reserved for those cells which are actively committed in the final productive phase of an immune response, antibody formation or cellular immunity, and this term therefore covers cells of various morphological types. In contrast to the active stage are those cells which are resident in a normal animal and which have the potential to respond in some manner to antigenic contact. This category involves the immunologically competent cell (ICC) defined by Medawar (1963) as referring to the present status or condition of a cell which though capable of an immunological performance is not yet in fact indulging in one. By these criteria, antigen-reactive cells and antigen-sensitive cells are immunologically competent cells, and this again is independent of either the cell morphology, ontogenic derivation, or type of behaviour following the antigenic stimulus. The use of these latter two terms was introduced by Kennedy et al. (1966) in describing the production of antibody-forming cells from a precursor cell challenged with antigen. A recent volume of the Transplantation Reviews (Vol. 1, 1969) deals exclusively with antigen-sensitive cells. Another type of cell which would fall into the ICC category is the antigen binding lymphocyte-like cell described by Byrt and Ada (1969) and Naor and Sulitzeanu (1965).

The haemopoietic stem cell, although having the potential to give rise to ICC, is not itself a member of this category, as it does not directly respond to antigen and does not have antigen-binding surface receptors. Particular emphasis will be placed in this review on the importance of antigen-binding surface receptors as markers for the differentiation level of the particular cell.

A schematic representation of the differing levels of maturity which make up the immunocyte complex is given in Figure 17.1.

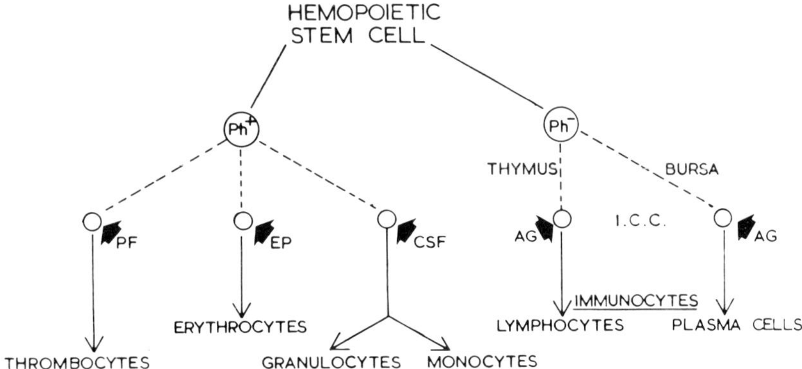

Fig. 17.1. Scheme of haemopoietic stem cell differentiation to mature elements including the immunocyte complex. A speculated lymphoid stem cell differentiates under thymic or bursal influence to immunocompetent cells (ICC). Further differentiation of these cells is then antigen-dependent. Other humoral factors, platelet factors (PF), erythropoietin (EP) and colony-stimulating factor (CSF) are indicated to be involved in other differentiation pathways. Ph indicates the possible presence of a lymphoid stem cell, as based on Philadelphia chromosome studies in chronic granulocytic leukemia.

17.3. The evolution of the immune response

17.3.1. Invertebrate immunity

It has generally been assumed that the development of adaptive immunity is characteristic of only the vertebrate species and that the basic forms of the immune response as recognized in higher vertebrates appeared around the level of the higher cyclostomes such as the lamprey. However, the recent striking demonstration that the hagfish, the earliest living representative of the vertebrates, is fully capable of mediating cellular immunity, clearly indicates that the origins of the immune response may well lie within the invertebrate species, and a more detailed examination of these species for evidence of specific adaptive immunity is fully warranted.

17.3.1.1. Neoplasia and immunity in invertebrates

It is generally considered that cancer, at least malignant cancer, is confined to vertebrates. Burnet (1968) has speculated that the origin of the immune surveillance mechanism may in fact have occurred through a need to counter the onset of malignancy in the vertebrates, with histocompatibility type antigens representing the target antigen for the cellular immune response. It is therefore of relevance to compare the development of cellular immunity and potential to neoplasia in the invertebrates.

Studies on attempts to induce neoplasia in either earthworms (Cooper 1969a) or other insects (Harshbarger 1967) have shown that usually only cellular responses occur which are rather different from those in mammals, and more resemble the reactions of invertebrates to foreign body materials. Clearly malignant cancers were not induced by these treatments which included vertebrate oncogenic virus, chemical carcinogens, and irradiation. It has however been reported that myoblastomas have been regularly observed in Annelids (earthworms) freshly brought in from the wild. Histologically these consisted of acidophilic anaplastic cell clusters in the deeper portions of the inner muscular layer which were not encapsulated. Some of these worms were riddled with tumours and soon succumbed, although of even greater relevance was the observation that occasionally healthy animals had a single tumour which spontaneously regressed. That this regression may have been brought about by a cellular immune response is indicated by transplantation studies with the myoblastomas in which rejection occurred after the initial period of take of the tumour (Cooper 1969a).

These studies although brief, do raise the possibility that the immune surveillance mechanism relevant to suppression of potential neoplasia may also exist in the invertebrates.

17.3.1.2. Cellular immunity

It is fundamental to the wellbeing of the invertebrate just as for vertebrates, that it be able to distinguish between its own body substance and foreign materials of either inert or living types. Much work has been done on the general cellular defense mechanism of invertebrates to such agents as metazooan parasites, foreign bodies, etc. (Salt 1963, 1967; Feng 1967; Huff 1940). The basic process is mediated by blood cells and includes phagocytosis or pinocytosis, nodule formation, encapsulation and storage of particles in fixed cells.

This type of reaction which is the basic non-specific cellular response to foreign material is not however a cell-mediated immune response and the basic evolutionary step we are seeking is the change from a specific contact resulting only in damage and encapsulation to the potential of a specific cell to respond by some degree of proliferation to produce a descendant clone with the same specificity.

Whilst there are many papers which fail to confirm the existence of allotransplantation immunity in invertebrates (reviewed by Favour 1958), several recent papers demonstrating allograft rejection in invertebrates have appeared.

Specific tissue graft rejection in earthworms appears to be well documented (Cooper 1969a, b). Autografts heal in permanently whereas xenografts were eventually rejected, even when the autografts and xenografts were applied together in the same graft bed. Intrafamilial transplants gave a more delayed rejection as compared to interfamilial grafting. When two transplants from the same xenogeneic donor were made five days apart, both were rejected in an accelerated time as compared to the simultaneous application of the two grafts. The rejection of a different third party graft on these animals proceeded at the normal rate. This demonstrates independence and therefore specificity in the immune rejection process as well as the existence of adaptive immunity.

The capacity of earthworms for allograft rejection has also been clearly demonstrated (Dupsat 1964; Cooper and Rubilotta 1969), with the rejection process being of a more delayed and chronic type.

There is accordingly sufficient evidence to indicate that cellular adaptive immune mechanisms capable of discrimination of allo- and xenogeneic antigens has evolved at some stage in the invertebrate species. This mechanism is distinctly different from the pure nonspecific phagocytic encapsulation mechanism mediated by the wandering haemocyte, and further studies are needed to determine (a) whether there are subpopulations of haemocyte-like cells, some involved in specific immunity, others in non-specific reactions, and (b) to define the level in invertebrate evolution, at which a pure amoeba-like phagocytic reaction has evolved into the cellular adaptive immune mechanism.

17.3.1.3. *Humoral immunity*

Two general observations which have been recognized for many years are relevant to the possible existence of antibody-type immunity in invertebrates. (i) There is a widespread occurrence in the fluids of many invertebrates of a variety of agglutinins for vertebrate erythrocytes (reviewed by Cushing et al. 1963) and (ii) insects can acquire resistance to certain pathogenic bacteria. The essential questions to be clarified are whether these agglutinins are mediators of immune responses and whether acquired resistance in invertebrates is mediated by a type of released cell-free product which acts like an antibody. In the context of this review it is of relevance to question whether cellular and humoral immunity show a parallel or separate evolution.

The presence of agglutinins for vertebrate red cells in the haemolymph and other fluids of many invertebrates is by no means indicative of specific antibody synthesis as these substances may rather be akin to the plant phytohaemagglutinins than to natural blood group antibodies. The most significant observation on these substances to date is that they can act as essential opsonins for phagocytosis by invertebrate haemocytes. Tripp (1966) found that *in vitro* phagocytosis of red cells by oyster amoebocytes is markedly enhanced by pretreatment of red cells with oyster haemagglutinins. McKay and Jenkin (1969) showed that phagocytosis of sheep erythrocytes by Yabbie (Australian fresh water crayfish, *Parachoeraps bicarinatus*) haemocytes depended on Yabbie haemagglutinin. In both studies the amount of haemagglutinin in the body fluid could not be increased by preimmunization with erythrocytes, although in McKay and Jenkin's study increased phagocytic activity was observed.

Attempts to induce antibody (or antibody-like) reactivity by preimmunization have almost uniformly failed (Cushing 1967), and this has included attempts with many different types of antigens. In several cases preimmunization has led to an acquired resistance to a particular agent. Specific protective immunity against *P. aeruginosa* was induced in the wax moth larvae (Chadwick 1967) although the period of immunity was relatively brief, being only over 60 hours. Some bactericidal activity was demonstrated in the haemolymph over this same period, although this active factor does not appear to resemble vertebrate antibody as it is dialysable, unaffected by trypsin and of relatively low molecular weight (Stephens and Marshall 1962). The authors have concluded that although this activity may be the closest manifestation to humoral immunity in insects, it is evidently not the chief mechanism responsible for the insects' resistance to most bacterial species.

A somewhat similar lytic substance has been reported (Bang 1967) to appear in infected marine worms after injection with a ciliate Anophrys. This material is absent from normal animals, but again its appearance after injection is very brief and it also does not seem to resemble vertebrate antibody.

In distinction to these previous reports on dialysable materials with antibody-like activities, two recent reports demonstrate the production of a non-dialysable protein-like material with immune activity. The injection of living tetrahymena into male cockroaches produces both protective immunity to subsequent challenge and a ciliate-immobilising activity in the haemolymph (Seamen and Robert 1968). The haemolymph will passively transfer protection and preliminary characterization of the active principle which immobilizes ciliates indicates it is a protein sensitive to heating. Of particular interest is the observation that the active factor moves in acrylamide gel electrophoresis in a region in which a protein band is also present in the normal cockroach haemolymph. This might be interpreted by analogy to vertebrate antibody which, although specifically induced by antigen, may be present in the normal serum. A heat-labile non-dialysable bactericidin has also been produced in spiny lobsters by immunization with bacteria (Evans et al. 1968). In both papers the duration of the immune response was again relatively short and the specificity of the bactericidin is not absolute for the immunizing antigen.

A natural haemagglutinin from the haemolymph of the horseshoe crab has been isolated and partially characterized (Marchalonis and Edelman 1968a). The haemagglutinin is a protein with molecular weight of approximately 400,000 consisting of about eighteen subunits of 22,500 each. These units are held together by non-covalent interactions. This structure differs from that of an immunoglobulin in several respects: (i) only one class of subunit exists, (ii) subunits are not joined covalently, and (iii) subunits do not show the electrophoretic heterogeneity of antibody polypeptide chains. However, these distinguishing marks by no means eliminate the possibility that the haemagglutinin subunit is coded for by a gene resembling that coding for vertebrate immunoglobulins, as some mammalian immunoglobulin molecules contain non-covalent interchain bonds (Abel and Grey 1968), and the haemagglutinin may represent the product of one light chain type gene. It is indeed intriguing that the molecular weight of this subunit is comparable to that of vertebrate light chains and some similarity was observed in amino acid composition.

Endotoxin or a number of vaccines prepared from gram-negative bacteria will confer on Yabbies both a resistance to experimental infections and an increased phagocytic response measured *in vitro* with haemocytes and haemagglutinin-treated vertebrate red cells (McKay and Jenkin 1969). The phagocytic system therefore appears receptive to stimulation for enhanced activity as in vertebrates, although there is a lack of specificity in the response.

At the present time the studies on adaptive immunity in invertebrates might be summarized thus: (i) Phagocytic activity mediated by the wandering haemocyte is present and can be non-specifically stimulated by a variety of agents. The phagocytic activity is greatly enhanced, and possibly even dependent upon a circulating factor such as a haemagglutinin which is behaving like a vertebrate opsonin. (ii) Preimmunization with various antigens does not usually lead to the formation of antibody-like molecules, nor does it increase the amount of the natural haemagglutinins. The physical and chemical properties of most lytic or agglutinating substances studied to date, do not appear to resemble vertebrate antibody, with a few exceptions which may however prove to be the basis of a humoral response. (iii) Specific cellular immunity, showing specificity for different xenografts, and capable of exhibiting specific immunological memory is present at least in the invertebrate Annelids, and further studies on the possible presence of cellular immunity in other invertebrates is clearly warranted.

It therefore appears possible that specific cellular immunity has evolved prior to the development of the capacity to produce a free antibody and that cellular immunity in turn, may have evolved from the wandering haemocyte-mediating phagocytic activity. The step from cellular immunity to humoral immunity may be coincidental with the speculated gene duplication origin of the heavy chain genes from the precursor light chain genes, and this aspect will be discussed in a later section. A summarized scheme of the evolutionary development of immune responses is shown in Figure 17.3 (p. 491).

17.3.2. Development of vertebrate lymphoid tissues

The correlation of morphology with function is inherently a very difficult problem which is further magnified when one examines tissues of many different species. Without functional parameters, which are the essential criteria of the immunocytes, it is extremely problematical that a precise statement as to the presence or absence of, for example, a lymphocyte-like cell, in a given species can be made.

It has been commonly stated that hagfish do not possess a thymus and that their peripheral lymphocyte-like cells may be associated with the thrombocytic or erythroid series (Good et al. 1966). However, as recent studies (Hildeman and Thoenes 1969) have now shown the existence of cellular immunity in the hagfish, there must exist in these animals an immunocyte cell, with a morphology that may or may not resemble higher vertebrate lymphocytes. The blood borne small mononuclear cell would indeed seem to be the most likely candidate.

A summarized listing of the development of lymphoid tissues in evolution is shown in Table 17.1 (see also Figure 17.2).

TABLE 17.1

Phylogenetic development of lymphoid tissues.

Animal class	Thymus	Bursa of Fabricius	Spleen	Lymphatic nodules	Lymph nodes	Lymphatic venules	Tonsils	Appendix	Peyer's patches	Peripheral lymphocytes	Plasma Cells	
											Spleen	Lamina propria
Invertebrates	0	0	0	0	0	–	0	0	0	?	0	0
Agnatha												
Hagfish	0(?)	0	±	–	0	–	0	0	0	+	0	0
Lamprey	±	0	+	–	0	0	0	0	0	+	0	0
Chondrichthyes												
Primitive elasmobranches	++	Rectal	++	–	0	–	0	0	0	+	0	0
Higher elasmobranches	++	Gland?	++	–	0	–	0	0	0	+	+	0
Osteichthyes												
Chondrostei	++	0	+++	–	0	–	0	0	0	+	++	±
Holostei	++	0	+++	–	0	0	0	0	0	+	++	0
Teleostei	++	0	+++	–	0	0	0	0	0	+	+	0
Dipnoi	++	0	+++	–	0	–	0	0	0	+	+	0
Amphibia	++	0	+++	+	0	0	+	0	0	+	++	++
Reptilia	++	±	+++	+	0	±	+	0	±(?)	+	+++	++
Aves	++	++	+++	+	0	±	–	+	Diffuse	+	+++	+++
Mammalia												
Monotremata	++	0	+++	++	0	++	+	++	++	+	+++	+++
Other mammals	++	0	+++	0	++	++	++	++	++	+	+++	+++

0   Sought for but not detected – no published reports of examinations.

+ to +++ Present in differing intensity.

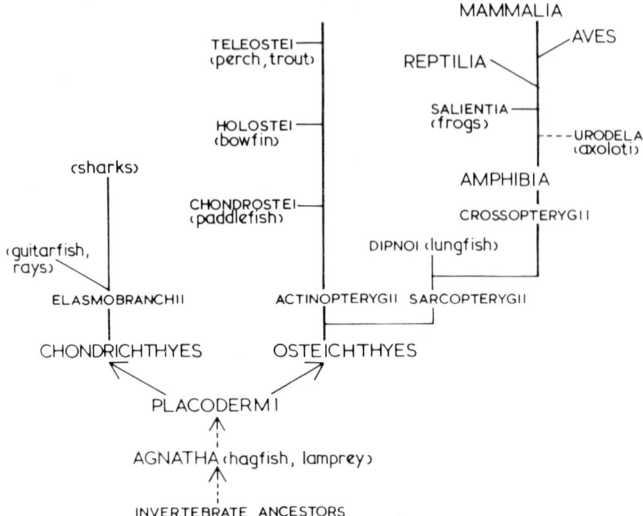

Fig. 17.2. Scheme of evolutionary development of vertebrates studied in regard to immune responses.

17.3.2.1. *Lymphocytes*

As stressed above, the most difficult aspect of morphological development concerns single cell types (as against definable organ structures). According to Fange (1966) it is doubtful whether real lymphocytes are found in invertebrates, although cell types resembling vertebrate lymphocytes have been observed in the coelomic fluid of Annelids (Cameron 1934).

The most primitive chordate, Amphioxus, is reported to have in its gill region tiny excretory ducts covered by ciliated cells called solerocytes which have been suggested to show a relationship to lymphocytes (Willmer 1960).

As mentioned above, the primitive cyclostome hagfish, does indeed possess blood borne small mononuclear cells with a clear resemblance to higher vertebrate lymphocytes. It is not known where these are formed, although it was suggested that free lymphoid-like cells may form by transformation of columnar epithelial cells of the nephrostomes within the Myxine pronephros. However connective tissue and blood vessels are also present within the pronephros.

The blood of the lamprey contains numerous monocytic elements including a family of small, medium and large lymphocytes (Finstad and Good 1964). Focal accumulations of lymphoid cells in all stages of development can also be identified in the primitive spleen. Lymphocytic cells are clearly identifiable in all vertebrate species above these cyclostomes, and in fact it appears that a cell with lymphocyte morphology is present in all vertebrates including hagfish. The lymphocytes of the paddle-fish (a primitive chondrostean) appear to consist of two distinct types, one of which contains primarily a polyribosomal organization while the other has predominantly free individual ribosomes within the cytoplasm (Clauson et al. 1966). This is analogous to the difference noted between avian bursal and thymic lymphocytes (Clauson et al. 1967), and introduces the intriguing possibility of association of this morphological appearance with different immunoglobulin-gene expression.

17.3.2.2. Plasma cells

Although the data on an evolutionary dissociation of cellular and humoral immunity is not fully validated, a separate development of the immunocytes appropriate to these systems is clearly evident.

Whereas lymphocytic cells are evident in both cyclostomes (hagfish and lampreys) and primitive elasmobranchs (for example, horned shark and guitarfish), none of these animals possess true plasma cells, even after antigenic stimulation and despite the production of antibody to some antigens.

The full development of true plasma cells with well developed endoplasmic reticulum composed of ribosome-studded membranes enclosing cisternae is well seen in the higher elasmobranchs such as the leopard shark and particularly in the 'primitive' fishes such as the chondrostean paddlefish (Clauson et al. 1966).

This rather striking appearance of plasma cells at this stage is associated with the development of a far more vigorous humoral antibody response to a wider range of antigens. Plasma cells are regularly observed in all vertebrates higher than the chondrostei with the possible exception that plasma cell incidence and gamma globulin synthesis is relatively poor in some teleost fish (Engle and Woods 1958).

The appearance of plasma cells in the *lamina propria* of the intestine does not parallel the presence of plasma cells in spleen. As indicated in Table 17.1, it is only in Amphibia and higher vertebrates that intestinal plasma cells appear (Good et al. 1966).

In view of the known predominance of IgA producing cells in mammalian intestine (Crabbe et al. 1965) and the speculated later evolutionary development of the α heavy chain locus, it is possible that this gene duplication event may be correlated with the appearance of intestinal plasma cells.

17.3.2.3. *Thymus and bursa of Fabricius*

As previously mentioned the primitive chordate *Amphioxus* does possess small ciliated cells covering the tiny excretory ducts in the gill region and an attempt has been made to homologize the excretory system of *Amphioxus* with the vertebrate thymus (Van Wijhe, reported in Fange 1966). It was suggested that the ciliated cells in the mammalian thymus (Hoshino 1962) might represent the vestige of these cells.

Finstad et al. (1964) have stated that no evidence of thymic tissue or thymic precursor tissue appears in the hagfish. It was suggested by Fange (1966) that the pronephros of Myxine hagfish shows certain resemblance to lympho-epithelial organs such as the thymus and bursa, in that the pronephros may undergo age involution and that there is a suggestive appearance of epithelial to lymphoid transformation. However it is more probable that the pronephros may be the primitive form of a lymph node rather than thymus (see Section 17.3.2.5).

In the ammocete and newly transformed adult lamprey there is a protothymus in the pharyngeal lymphoid tissue. This appears as tiny accumulations of four to twenty lymphoid cells developing in small epithelial follicles within the epithelial tissue lining the pharyngeal gutters.

From the primitive elasmobranch onwards, a clearly demarcated thymus with cortex and medulla is then evident in young animals, and age involution has been observed. In view of the rather small lymphoid accumulation within the pharyngeal epithelial tissue of the lamprey the negative evidence of thymus absence in hagfish should not be too strongly taken. These observations clearly stress the need for careful ontogenic studies on young hagfish with a view to examination of the origin of the peripheral lymphocyte-like cells from a possibly sparse epithelial site. The other possibility to be considered is that a diffusible product of thymic type epithelium may be released and act on immuno-cyte precursors in a site distant from the 'thymic' epithelium. Thus a lympho-epithelial aggregate may not be directly observed.

The bursa of Fabricius which is a lympho-epithelial organ lying distal to the cloaca is thought to be unique to the class Aves. It does appear to be present in all birds studied. The only directly comparable tissue described in the lower fishes is the rectal gland of the elasmobranchs. However this does not contain lymphoid tissue (Good et al. 1966) although it may represent a bursa precursor site. Although Good et al. (1966) have claimed that a clear bursa type tissue does not exist in reptiles or amphibians, Sidky and Auerbach (1968) have demonstrated the existence of bursal-like lymphoid aggregations in both adult snapping turtles and the tortoise *Testudo polyphemus*. These lymphoid aggregations lie directly beneath the mucosa projecting into the cloacal lumen in a fashion somewhat similar to bursa. Functional and ontogenic tests are clearly indicated to confirm or deny the bursal nature of these lymphoid aggregates.

Further considerations on mammalian equivalents of the bursa will be made in a later section.

17.3.2.4. Spleen

The development of the spleen has been quite well characterized for the elasmobranchs and lower bony fishes. However in the hagfish, there is again the morphological problem of the dubious existence of lymphocytes. Finstad et al. (1964) conclude that no clear evidence of lymphopoiesis could be defined, and if present, certainly does not form clear lymphoid foci. Again it must be stressed however that this must remain a tentative conclusion until functional studies can be carried out on cells from the hagfish. The splenic haemopoietic tissue in the hagfish exists as scattered foci through the submucosa of the gut, whereas in the lamprey, a more highly organized tissue mass is located in an infolding of the anterior gut. Lymphoid-like cells are present in both the primitive spleen and protovertebral arch of the lamprey.

A progressively higher order of lymphoid tissue development and organization then proceeds, with clear red and white pulp already present in the primitive sharks.

17.3.2.5. Lymph follicles and lymph nodes

The development of a lymphatic system with well defined lymph nodes appears to be a relatively recent evolutionary event. A system of lymph nodes comparable to mammals does not occur in fish and in seeking for a functional prototype of the lymph node system, two main areas seem likely candidates, either intestine or pronephros. As mentioned previously, hagfish do possess lymphocyte-like aggregations in the pronephros (Fange 1966) and in part of the mesonephros. On purely morphological grounds it is very difficult to determine whether this is thymus-like or lymph node-like. However as the pronephros does appear to drain and filter the coelomic fluid, it was suggested that lymphocyte-like cells may be involved in this process which would be analogous to that of a lymph node function (Willmer 1960). Indeed, specific studies with teleost fish immunized to sheep red blood cells has shown that the pronephros contains even larger members of antibody-forming cells than the spleen, and in view of this observation and the marked morphological similarity to mammalian lymph nodes, it was suggested that the teleost pronephros may represent a primitive prototype of the lymph node (Smith et al. 1967). Some accumulations of lymphoid tissue possibly resembling Peyer's patches, are present in the gut of elasmobranchs, chondrosteans and dipnoans and these appear to resemble primary lymphoid follicles (Good et al. 1968).

One of the earliest forms of lymph node development is the jugular bodies and lymph glands of amphibia. The lymph glands of *Rana catesbiana* have an intricate framework of reticular fibers permeated by a maze of sinusoids containing lymphoid and myeloid cells (Baculi and Cooper 1968). Plasma cells are present in these sites after antigenic stimulation. The juxtajugular bodies are small collections of lymphoid cells lacking in germinal center type organization but definitely involved in immune responses (Evans et al. 1965). These bodies are functionally analogous to lymph nodes in that they selectively trap antigen, although in a nonfollicular localization pattern (Diener and Nossal 1966).

The typical lymph nodule of the echidna (monotreme) appears as a single lymphoid follicle bearing a proliferative area with the characteristics of a germinal center (Diener and Ealey 1965). It floats within the lymph attached only by a small vascular bundle to the wall of the lymphatic. Studies on echidna lymph nodules for localization of labelled antigens (Diener et al. 1967) strongly indicate that each echidna lymph nodule represents a single lymphoid follicle comparable to a cortical follicle in lymph nodes of higher mammals.

The final evolutionary step in lymph node development, namely the multifollicular lymph node, is seen in both marsupials and all higher mammals. A rather nebulous area in lymph node development concerns the different families of birds. Some birds have lymph follicles whereas others do not, and the rationale or evolutionary significance of this is at present quite obscure.

17.3.2.6. *Specialized lymphatic tissue venules*

In higher mammalian vertebrates, the recirculating lymphocyte pool enters the lymph node from the blood through a specialized cuboidal endothelium-lined venule termed the post-capillary venule (Gowans and Knight 1964). The specialized morphology of these venules appears in ontogeny at the time of lymphoid follicle development.

Studies on the phylogeny of these venules (Miller 1969) has shown that they are limited to the lymph nodes and intestinal lymphoid tissue of mammals, including the monotremes which have only the single follicular lymph node. This simultaneous appearance of true lymph nodes and the cuboidal endothelium-lined venules at the same phylogenetic point certainly indicates the functional importance of the venule. Although reptiles and chickens had some cuboidal endothelium of vessels, they were all in splenic arterioles, which is not seen in mammals, and these were not functional sites for lymphocyte transfer from blood to tissue.

It is of interest that although lymphoid tissue is present in the intestine of many lower vertebrates, the specialized venule only appears in intestinal lymphoid tissue concurrent with the lymph node development, suggesting that the recirculation of lymphocytes may not be well developed in lower vertebrates, and this may be a factor in their relatively poorer ability to show immunological memory for circulating antibody formation.

17.3.3. Cellular immunity

If the results of Cooper (1967a, b, c) on skin graft immunity in Annelids are valid in their striking indication of the existence of cellular immunity in invertebrates, then we should expect that all members of the vertebrate species will show cellular immunity. Unfortunately due to the multiple failures of Papermaster et al. (1964) to detect immune responses in hagfish, a concept of the concurrent development of immunity with thymus development in vertebrates higher than the hagfish was proposed (Good and Papermaster 1964). Recent studies have strongly indicated that this is not the case (Hildemann and Thoenes 1969) and are thus more compatible with the concept of evolution of cellular immunity commencing somewhere in the invertebrate phylogeny.

17.3.3.1. Tissue graft rejection

In the studies of Papermaster et al. (1964) the apparent poor ability of the hagfish to heal wounds greatly hampered analysis of skin graft immunity and accordingly their studies were inconclusive. Direct intrahepatic grafts of liver tissue from autologous or homologous sources failed to elicit any differential response in the period of observation.

In a more recent study (Hildemann and Thoenes 1969), different laboratory conditions of housing, temperature and maintenance of the hagfish were employed, and under these more suitable conditions, autografts healed in and wound healing was satisfactorily observed. This accordingly allowed for a more critical evaluation of skin allografts on hagfish. Typical allograft rejection including lymphocytic infiltration, capillary haemorrhage and pigment cell destruction was observed. First set grafts showed a mean survival time of 72 days and thus showed a more chronic type of rejection analogous to that observed with weak histocompatibility antigens in higher vertebrates. When second set grafts were placed shortly after rejection of first set grafts, acute rejection occurred in less than 14 days. Thus immunological memory is clearly present in the hagfish.

As in other studies on antibody production in fish, the elicitation of cellular immunity is temperature dependent, the above observations being recorded at 18.5°C. If grafting is made at lower temperatures (13–15°C), prolonged survival is observed.

Complete allograft rejection was observed in adult lampreys between 21 and 42 days following placement of the grafts (Finstad and Good 1964). A rather chronic allograft rejection was also observed in lamprey ammocetes (Perey et al. 1968) with the onset of rejection occurring usually in the third week. Because of rather intense graft bed inflammation and haemorrhage, it was difficult to assess second set grafts in these animals. The presence of large lymphoblastic-like cells in the graft beds of rejecting allografts was noted and these were similar to those described in mammalian allograft rejection by Scothorne and McGregor (1955).

The existence of immunological memory for skin graft rejection was clearly established (Perey et al. 1968) in both sting-rays and the paddle-fish. In these observations it was noted that first set rejections in these animals, being rather chronic in the time for rejection to be completed, were possibly analogous to observations on graft rejection in mammals where the lymphatic drainage of the graft site is prevented (Barker and Billingham 1967). It was suggested therefore that the slow first set rejection in the lower fishes might be due to lack of lymphatic channels and lymph nodes, although an alternative possibility is that polymorphism of major transplantation antigens is not widespread in these lower forms.

Graft rejection in teleost fishes is well established (Kallman and Gordon 1958) and behaves identically to higher vertebrates in showing requirement for alloantigens and immunological memory. (In two inbred strains of fish parental to F_1 grafts all accepted, F_1 to parental rejected 7–67 days, second set rejected 2–7 days.)

Homograft immunity in both larval and adult amphibians has also been shown to be both temperature dependent, and to show immunological memory (Hildemann and Haas 1959).

17.3.3.2. Delayed hypersensitivity

Reports on classical delayed hypersensitivity in early vertebrates are quite scarce. Papermaster et al. (1964) reported failure to observe any response in hagfish to BCG or old tuberculin. However in view of the temperature at which their hagfish were kept (which does not allow for skin graft rejection to occur) further studies on delayed sensitivity in hagfish are clearly needed.

Delayed skin reactions characterized by induration and inflammation, were observed in lampreys which had previously been given BCG and complete Freund's adjuvant (Finstad and Good 1964). The site of adjuvant injection also showed swelling, discoloration and induration. These Freund's adjuvant injections also stimulated a striking proliferation or accumulation of lymphoid cells in the protovertebral arch.

Delayed skin reactions to Ascaris antigen were induced in holeost fish presensitized with Ascaris in Freund's adjuvant (Papermaster et al. 1964) and reactions to PPD and Freund's adjuvant were observed in teleost fishes (Ridgway et al. 1966). A preliminary report on successful phytohaemagglutinin stimulation *in vitro* of lymphocytes from paddlefish and rays, and of PPD stimulation of lymphocytes from Freund's adjuvant treated lampreys has been made (Olson 1967).

These studies, although brief, support the data on tissue graft immunity in lower vertebrates.

17.3.4. Humoral antibody formation

Although some controversy may still exist concerning the hagfish, it is generally clear that all vertebrate species can produce some circulating humoral antibody on antigenic stimulation. In considering the evolution of the humoral antibody-forming system within vertebrates, we are basically concerned with quantitative changes or degrees of response rather than fundamental qualitative differences. This includes such aspects as temperature dependence, heterogeneity of antibodies, affinity and strength of antibodies and immunological memory. A summary of antibody production in different classes is given in Table 17.2. It is tempting to compare quantitative changes in the antibody response with 'highness or lowness' of the animal in evolution. However in view of the difficulties in clearly defining evolutionary order this may be rather artificial. Thus as stressed by Ching and Wedgwood (1967) it would not be surprising, if advanced forms of animals had a more elaborate immune response than lower forms within a general class, but since the amphibian crossopterygian line branched separately from the main piscine line, caution in comparing different classes is stressed. Several specific aspects of humoral antibody formation will be briefly considered.

In the studies of Papermaster et al. (1964), no detectable antibody was produced to any of six different antigens in hagfish. However Hildemann and Thoenes (1969) have stated that antibody to at least some antigens (such as sheep red cells) can be readily produced in hagfish. This apparent controversy may again involve the question of temperature dependence of antibody production. Ching and Wedgwood (1967) have

TABLE 17.2

Antibody responses in different vertebrate classes.

Class	Group	Ability to respond to different antigens[1]	MW of antibody[2]	Primary titres[3]	Secondary response[4]	Immunoglobulins[5]
Agnatha		Few	14 S, 6.6 S	+	+	L, μ
Chondrichthyes		Few	17 S, 7.0 S	+	+	L, μ
Osteichthyes	Chondrostei	Most	19 S, rare 7 S	++	+	L, μ
	Holeostei	All	?	++	+	?
	Teleostei	All	19 S?	++	+	?
	Dipnoi	All	19 S, 5.9 S[6]	?	?	L, μ, non μ H-chain[7]
Amphibia		All	19 S, rare 7 S	+++	+	L, μ, γ
Reptilia		All	19 S, rare 7 S	+++	+	L, μ, γ
Aves		All	19 S, 7 S, 5.9 S	++++	++	L, μ, γ or IgY[8]
Mammalia		All	19 S, 7 S etc.	++++	++++	L, μ, α, γ, etc.

[1] The ability to respond to several different antigens assuming suitable immunisation schedule.
[2] Approximate molecular weight of commonest occurring antibody.
[3] Approximate level of response in relation to mammals.
[4] Ease of ability to demonstrate immunological memory.
[5] Light and heavy chains detected.
[6] These values from immunoglobulins, not actual antibodies.
[7] Dipnoi have at least two H-chains, a μ and another chain which is not identical to γ.
[8] Leslie and Clem (1969) suggest the avian γ chain is not the true equivalent of mammalian γ.

shown that the Axolotl, (a neotenic urodele) also appears completely unresponsive to antigenic challenge when maintained at 8 to 10°C. Yet at higher temperatures antibody production could be readily detected. Thus the inability of hagfish to produce antibodies (Papermaster et al. 1964) may be due to the low temperatures of maintenance. Studies in the lamprey have involved the use of ten different antigens, and of these only *Brucella* induced an antibody response (Finstad and Good 1966). Restimulation with *Brucella* 30 days after primary injection did elicit an earlier second response and heightened antibody titres. Immunological memory therefore appears to be established at this stage.

Studies by Marchalonis and Edelman (1968b) showed that the sea lamprey was capable of making specific antibody to bacteriophage T2. The neutralization of phage was extremely weak and was similar in this regard to antibody from certain elasmobranchs. Induced antibody formation in lampreys to human erythrocyte antigens has also been observed (Boffa et al. 1967). Antibody activity to bacteriophage was localized in the 6.6S and 14S fractions of lamprey serum. Antigenic analysis of the isolated 6.6S antibody showed similarity, if not identity, to the 14S fraction.

The ability to respond to some, but not all antigens is still evident within the lower elasmobranchs such as the guitarfish. Thus, although bovine serum albumin is cleared from the circulation, no antibody production was detected (Finstad and Good 1966), even after a second challenge. Detectable antibody production occurred in both guitarfish and sharks to haemocyanin, with evidence of immunological memory on second challenge. With both *Brucella* and bacteriophage in these two species, again antigen clearance but no antibody production occurred on primary challenge, whereas antibody developed on second challenge. Marchalonis and Edelman (1965) also observed antibody production to haemocyanin in the smooth dogfish (an elasmobranch), with antibody activity being in the 17S fraction. Sigel and Clem (1966) have shown antibody production in the lemon shark to PR8 virus, chicken erythrocytes and BSA, although it was only under certain conditions and with certain antigens that a secondary response could be demonstrated. Both mercaptoethanol (ME)-sensitive high molecular weight antibody and low molecular weight ME-resistant antibody was produced.

In general it therefore appears that the Chondrichthyes class possesses the ability to produce specific antibody, but it is a relatively weak response in that (i) they respond to some but not all antigens (ii) the levels in a primary antibody response are lower than that in higher vertebrates and (iii) although immunological memory is present, it is somewhat difficult to elicit.

The other main class of fishes, the bonyfish or Osteichthyes follow a separate evolutionary branch to the cartilaginous fish, and in general they show a higher degree of immune responsiveness. In their more primitive members such as the Chondrostean paddlefish, antibody production to all antigens tested occurred, again with noted secondary responses to most antigens. In the holeost fishes such as gars, antibody production to BSA was demonstrated (all ME-sensitive) although no enhanced antibody production occurred on second challenge (Clem and Sigel 1966).

Antibody production in the holeost Amia Calva to many antigens also occurs (Good and Papermaster 1964). Considerably more data is available on antibody production in teleost fishes, and in general it appears that antibody production to all antigens used has been elicited. Immunological memory is more readily demonstrated (Clem and Sigel 1966) at this level. Several studies on antibody-forming cells in teleosts have been reported using the Jerne technique (1963) with isologous fish serum as a source of complement (Chiller et al. 1969). Antibody-producing cells were found in both spleen and the pronephros, the latter organ containing the greater number, and it was suggested that the teleost pronephros may represent a primitive prototype of the mammalian lymph node (Smith et al. 1967). Kinetics of antibody-forming cell development also appears similar to higher vertebrates (Chiller et al. 1969).

Despite a somewhat less complex lymphoid system in amphibians as compared to mammals, excellent antibody production has been reported in these animals. Immunological memory to BSA and t2 coliphage was readily demonstrated, although only primary responses to *S. typhosa* antigen could be elicited (Evans et al. 1966). Similar observations were noted with another bacterial antigen, *Salmonella* flagellin, in that although extremely good primary antibody titres developed, no evidence of a secondary response occurred (Diener and Nossal 1966). In both of these studies the antibody was predominantly high molecular weight and ME sensitive, and although a little ME-resistant antibody was produced, the almost complete conversion to ME-resistant antibody did not occur, as is observed in mammals. In a more detailed study of the cellular events in Anuran antibody formation, a marked similarity to mammals in both numbers and type of antibody-forming cells, was observed. Small and medium lymphocytes played a main role in the early phase, whilst large immature plasma cells were predominant in the later stages (Diener and Marchalonis 1970). Antibody production to heterologous red cells has also been induced *in vitro* with spleen fragments from the toad *Xenopus Laevis* (Auerbach and Ruben).

Antibody production has also been elicited in reptiles to several antigens. However in one study on the turtle (Grey 1966), the response lacked several features of higher mammalian immunity. As in the amphibia, most of the antibody was of high molecular weight and only late in immunization did some ME-resistant antibody appear. By sucrose density-gradient analysis the later antibody was predominantly in the light region. Lack of an anamnestic response was again observed. The continued production of antibody of low avidity persisted without much evidence of a change to higher avidity. As in the amphibian, antibody to *Salmonella* flagellin produced by the primitive reptile the tuatura, was also only 18S immunoglobulin, and no evidence of a secondary response was observed (Marchalonis et al. 1969). *In vitro* culture of spleen fragments from the snapping turtle produced antibody to heterologous red cells with a much shorter latent period than observed *in vivo* (Sidky and Auerbach 1968). Reptiles make only high molecular weight antibodies to *Brucella* (Maung 1963) but are capable of producing 7S antibodies to BSA (Lykakis 1968).

Amphibians and reptiles therefore clearly appear similar to mammals in the intensity of humoral antibody formation and in the cellular component of humoral immunity. However the full complexity of mammalian immunity is not realized in that the antibody population tends to persist in the higher molecular weight form, and with at least some antigens (mainly bacterial), immunological memory cannot be elicited.

17.3.5. *Immunoglobulin synthesis*

The evolutionary origin of the immunoglobulin family of proteins has been studied in various ways. Despite the clear cut distinctions of mammalian immunoglobulins into classes with different properties (Fudenberg and Warner 1970), many chemical and genetic studies have indicated substantial similarities in their structure and genetic control. Studies of the physico-chemical nature of humoral antibodies produced in different species has shown that an IgM type molecule appeared well before an IgG species. A similar pattern occurs ontogenically, in that IgM synthesis precedes IgG synthesis in the developing embryo or foetus (Good and Papermaster 1964; Thorbecke et al. 1968). Sequence studies on mammalian immunoglobulins have provided a scheme of gene duplication of mammalian immunoglobulins which closely parallels the actual phylogenetic data. From the studies of Hill et al. (1966) and Hood et al. (1967) a scheme of gene duplication has been proposed. The light and heavy chains of immunoglobulins were derived from an ancestral gene that determines the sequence of a protein containing about 110 residues. This ancestral gene first showed contiguous duplication giving rise to a primitive light chain gene. A further contiguous duplication led to the heavy chain, and complete duplication led to the κ and λ subtypes. The heavy gene in turn, yielded by a series of complete duplications, each of the major types of heavy chain genes, this process being continued extensively right up to the highest primate species man, in which at least ten heavy chain types are present (Warner 1969).

The present data is also compatible with the evolution of the different H-chain genes by separate contiguous duplications from the L-chain genes, or alternatively, should the variable gene represent a separate genetic entity, complete duplications may be limited only to the constant part of the heavy chains. However in view of the close linkage of the different heavy chain genes (Natvig et al. 1967; Herzenberg 1964), and the absence of linkage of H to L-chain genes, it is more probable that only one contiguous L-chain duplication occurred.

Detailed data on the isolated immunoglobulins of different vertebrate species closely parallels the interpretation of sequence data in showing an increasing complexity of immunoglobulin polypeptide chain types with the more recent vertebrate species. Several of the key specific aspects in the phylogenetic development include the following studies.

The sea lamprey is the lowest vertebrate in which data has been obtained on the chain structures of the immunoglobulin molecules (Marchalonis and Edelman 1968b). Antibody activity is present in both 14S and 6.6S fractions of serum. Antigenic analysis of the purified 6.6S immunoglobulin showed apparent identity to the heavier fraction. The 6.6S unit consisted of two types of chain, L-chains of mol. wt. 25,000 and a heavy chain of mol. wt. 70,000. This latter chain was analogous to mammalian μ chains and to the heavy chains of elasmobranchs in starch gel electrophoresis. A point of distinction from most IgM types is that the L and H polypeptides were linked *via* weak interactions without interchain disulphide bonds. This suggests that the firmer interchain bond of immunoglobulins appeared at some time after the emergence of the L and μ chains.

Analysis of the immunoglobulins in several different species of elasmobranchs has again shown the existence of molecules with the same L and H polypeptide components, but of differing molecular size. The smooth dogfish (Marchalonis and Edelman 1965) and the lemon shark (Clem and Small 1967) both have antibody activity in the 17S and 7S fractions, the immunoglobulins of these two fractions having identical light chains and heavy chains (mol. wt. 70,000), the latter resembling mammalian μ chains.

The existence of this 7S IgM molecule therefore appears to date back to the earliest vertebrate forms, and it is of interest that it has persisted to the present time, in that 7S IgM responses have been detected in a variety of human pathological conditions (Rothfield et al. 1965; Stobo and Tomasi 1967; Solomon 1969).

In distinction to the existence of these two forms of IgM molecules in elasmobranchs in which the heavier form is fully susceptible to 2 ME treatment, the chondrostean paddlefish, poly-don spathula, contains all its antibody activity in a macroglobulin fraction which was not reduced by 2 ME under ordinary conditions (Fish et al. 1966). The presence of $2M$ urea together with 2-mercaptoethanol was required for a loss of antibody activity to occur.

Relatively little direct data is available on the higher members of the Osteichthyes, although Marchalonis and Edelman (1968b) mention that only μ type H-chains were observed in both holostean and teleost fishes.

The Australian lungfish is a member of the Dipnoi group, which branched just prior to the crossopterygions which in turn are ancestral to the higher vertebrates. This is accordingly at a rather key level in immunoglobulin phylogeny. Analysis of the immunoglobulins of the lungfish (Marchalonis 1969) has shown that it does indeed possess more than one H-chain type. A serum 19.4S immunoglobulin closely resembled other vertebrate IgM globulins in both chain structure, size and electrophoretic analysis of the heavy chain. The other immunoglobulin was of 5.9S with heavy chain of mol. wt. 40,000. The light chains of the two types were identical. This rather unique heavy chain of the 5.9S molecule did not correspond to mammalian γ chains in either electrophoretic behaviour or size, instead it may resemble an immunoglobulin of comparable size (5.7S) in the duck (Grey, 1967).

Immunoglobulin heavy chain heterogeneity into several classes is then clearly apparent with all species above and including the amphibians. The anuran amphibian *Rana catesbiana* possesses two classes corresponding in all parameters to IgM and IgG (Marchalonis and Edelman 1966). In this instance the G type heavy chain has a mol. wt. of 53,600. Studies of a primitive reptile the tuatura, also show the presence of two distinct H-chain types, one μ type and a second which cannot be definitively classified, but resembles γ chain (Marchalonis et al. 1969).

Avian immunoglobulins are heterogeneous with a γM and γG like globulin being clearly evident. A recent study has however questioned the validity of terming the 7S immunoglobulin in chickens as IgG (Leslie and Clem 1969). The 7.1S immunoglobulin isolated from serum was shown to contain H-chains of mol. wt. 67,500, whereas the 19S molecule has H-chains of 70,000 mol. wt. This 7S molecule is therefore not strictly analogous to mammalian IgG, in which the γ chain has a mol. wt. of 50,000 or to the α chain of mol. wt. 60,000. It was proposed by these authors that this major 7S component of chicken serum be termed IgY. Other studies have demonstrated the existence of anaphylactic antibodies in chickens and ducks, thus indicating the existence of more H-chain types in birds (Kubo and Benedict 1968; Grey 1967b).

The continuing complexity of immunoglobulin polypeptide chain evolution in higher vertebrates is quite evident with the increasing list of human L and H-chain types (Warner 1969). Since this is rather away from the scope of this review, these will not be further discussed save to stress that immunoglobulin evolution had not reached its finite end with the emergence of the mammals, and studies such as those of Shuster et al. (1969) clearly indicate the development of H-chain subclasses occurring within the higher primate species.

17.3.6. *Phylogenetic dissociation of cellular and humoral immunity*

One of the clear impressions from a study of the phylogeny of immunity is the emergence of a more complex system of immune responses with the developing vertebrate species. This is apparent in both morphology and structure of the lymphoid tissues, such as the relatively late appearance of lymph nodes, in the case of development of immunological memory, which may indeed correlate with efficient use of lymph nodes, and at the molecular level in terms of greater numbers of types of immunoglobulin molecules. In general the degree of intensity of antibody responses increases also, with only very low activity being evident in the lamprey and marked temperature dependence being apparent. However despite this increasing complexity with vertebrate evolution, it must be stressed that in the most primitive vertebrate species studied, both cellular immunity involving lymphocyte mediated graft rejection, and the production into serum of a circulating antibody, are present. At the morphological level these are represented by mononuclear cells with noted structural differences correlating with their function as a protein-secreting or non-secreting cell, and are already apparent in the paddlefish and possibly earlier species.

In considering the relationship of the development of cellular to humoral immunity we must therefore concentrate at either the invertebrate or earliest vertebrate level. In the absence of structural data on the various factors associated with immunity in invertebrates, it is impossible at present to make firm conclusions on this development. However a provisional hypothesis is presented in Fig. 17.3, which is mainly intended to suggest several points.

(i) The cellular origin of both series probably lies in the wandering haemocyte.

(ii) At some stage an immunoglobulin like gene developed perhaps coding for a protein of length 110 amino acids, which was synthesized at a relatively low level.

(iii) A dissociation occurred, in that one cell line emerged which was capable of active secretion of this product and possibly occurred concomitantly with gene duplication to the complete L-chain size.

(iv) A non-secreting series persisted which still synthesized enough of the recognition unit to allow for surface recognition of foreign materials. Whether this material is indeed an intact L-chain or a variable half fragment, remains to be determined. In view of the apparent demonstration of immunological memory in Annelids, this surface unit would seem to be specific, and on interaction with antigen to stimulate cell division.

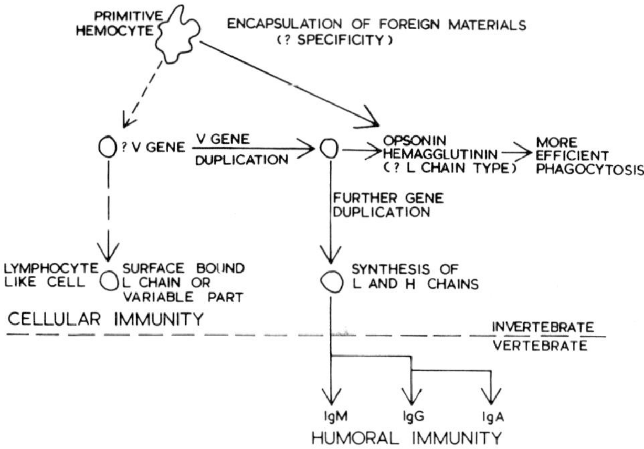

Fig. 17.3. Proposed scheme of evolutionary development of the immune responses from invertebrate to vertebrate animals.

(v) Further L-chain contiguous duplication gave rise to the μ chain gene possibly at the level of vertebrate evolution, and further gene duplication is clearly confined to later vertebrates.

A detailed scheme is clearly beyond the scope of present data and further studies on the chemical nature of invertebrate 'antibodies' or recognition structures are needed. It will also be important to identify the nature of the cells synthesizing invertebrate opsonins or haemagglutinins, in order to ascertain whether they represent a separate cell series from the phagocytic cells, and if so, whether their differentiation is already controlled by a separate inducer.

17.4. The differentiation of immunologically competent cells

The complete ontogenic development of the immunocyte system within a single individual can be conveniently separated into two main components. It is apparent that when an antigen is given to a young adult animal, some type of cell reacts in some way with this antigen and by a process of differentiation produces the actual effector cell, the immunocyte. However it is also clear that this initial cell type which reacts with antigen is itself showing evidence of immune differentiation, since this response to antigen is not a property of all cells in the body. Accordingly immunocyte differentiation can be conveniently divided into (i) antigen-independent events leading up to the development of the immunologically competent cells which have never previously encountered antigen, and (ii) the differentiation that is induced by the antigen.

17.4.1. Cell types involved prior to antigen induced differentiation

Whilst the fertilized egg is obviously the ultimate progenitor cell of an immunologically competent cell (ICC) just as it is of any other differentiated cell, there are identifiable stages in differentiation between these two extremes. The haemopoietic stem cell could more reasonably be considered to be the starting point for consideration of differentiation toward the ICC. This cell is committed along haemopoietic pathways, but in a monophyletic approach, can still be influenced into different mature haemopoietic elements. As indicated in Figure 17.1, there is at least one other major stage between the haemopoietic stem cell and the ICC. This concerns a separation between immune differentiation (lymphocytes and plasma cells), versus erythroid, granulocytic and megakaryocytic pathways. The philadelphia chromosome (Ph[1]) is an abnormal small chromosome which has been found in malignant cells of nearly all cases of chronic granulocytic leukaemia (Nowell and Hungerford 1961; Tough et al. 1961; Sandberg et al. 1962). It is not present in skin cells (Tough et al. 1961), nor is it present in lymphocytes stimulated to divide by phytohaemagglutinin (Nowell and Hungerford 1961). However, although it was originally thought to be unique to the myeloid series, other studies have shown that the Ph[1] chromosome is present in both nucleated erythroid cells and probably in megakaryocytic cells (Frei et al. 1964). Thus it appears that there may be an initial commitment of a stem cell into either immune or non-immune haemopoietic pathways. Further studies on stem cell relationships to immunity will be discussed in the following section.

In our original division of differentiation of immunocytes, into pre-

and post-antigen induced stages, it was inferred that there is a cell type which responds to antigen in some manner. Whilst the eventual outcome of antigen-induced differentiation will be considered later, it is relevant at this stage to indicate our means of directly assessing the presence of these cells and of quantitating their number in a given population. The term antigen sensitive cell has been applied to those cells which react to antigen by producing antibody-forming cells, rather than producing antibodies directly. Thus the term antigen-sensitive cells originally implied a precursor cell which directly gave rise by cell divisions to the antibody-forming cell. In view of the more recent work by several groups on cell collaborations in immunity (see Section 17.5), it is apparent that some cells can respond to antigen by division without directly giving rise to antibody-forming cells. Such cells have been termed antigen-reactive cells (Miller and Mitchell 1969) in distinction from 'antibody-forming cell precursors' which are the true direct precursors of antibody-producing cells.

The assay system of Kennedy et al. (1965) and Playfair et al. (1965) is a measure of antigen-sensitive cells and is based on the clonal expansion of an antigen-stimulated cell in the environment of an irradiated recipient spleen. This assay was originally used with heterologous red cells as antigens but has also been modified to work with bacterial antigens (Armstrong and Diener 1968). By these tests, a normal mouse spleen contains approximately 1 in 10^5 cells which can respond to sheep erythrocytes by proliferation and differentiation to antibody-forming cells (Kennedy et al. 1966) and 1 in 10^6 cells responsive to *Salmonella* flagellin (Armstrong and Diener 1968).

As outlined previously the ICC (immunocompetent cell) is a broader term which simply implies a response in a cell following antigenic stimulation. This term therefore also includes cells involved in cellular immune reactions which would obviously not be scored in a Kennedy type of assay. These cells mediate transplantation immune reactions and whilst there are many quantitative measures for degrees of reactivity in this type of response, there are very few assays for directly scoring numbers of competent cells in a population. One of the most direct assays in this regard is the development of lesions on the chorioallantoic membrane (CAM) of fertile chick eggs which have been inoculated with adult fowl leucocytes (Boyer 1960; Szenberg et al. 1962). In this system approximately 1 in 10^3 to 1 in 10^4 lymphocytes are ICC, although a higher figure of 1–2% is proposed by Nisbet et al. (1969).

Finally, considerable emphasis will be given in this review (see 17.4.7) to those cells which can directly be shown to interact with antigen, in systems which do not require any subsequent activity on behalf of the test cells. These are direct assay systems which either visualize antigen binding to cells in a normal animal by the use of radioactively labelled antigen and autoradiography (Naor and Sulitzeanu 1967; Byrt and Ada 1969; Humphrey and Keller 1970), or demonstrate their elimination by binding to an antigen-coupled particle (Singhai and Wigzell 1970).

17.4.2. Haemopoietic stem cells

Lethal doses of irradiation will almost completely deplete all elements of the haemopoietic system. Recovery of this system can be attained by the injection of cell suspensions of bone marrow, fetal liver or yolk sac. Precursor cells (termed haemopoietic stem cells) present in these populations are capable of both self-renewal and differentiation into all haemopoietic elements. This includes the repopulation of both myeloid and lymphoid tissues (Ford et al. 1966; Micklem et al. 1966) from the same bone marrow cell suspension. At this stage it was not clear whether the same precursor cell could give rise to both lymphoid and myeloid elements, or whether there were separate precursor cells.

Haemopoietic stem cells can be directly assayed by their ability to rapidly proliferate in the environment of an irradiated spleen and form macroscopically visible colonies (Till and McCulloch 1961). This involves both proliferation with differentiation into mature elements of erythroid, granulocytic and megakaryocytic elements and self-renewal proliferation (Lewis and Trobaugh 1964). In this system, it was shown with cytological markers, that each colony represented the clonal expansion of a single stem cell and that colony-forming cells can indeed differentiate into either erythroid or granulocytic elements (Wu et al. 1967). Using a chromosome marker technique it has also been shown that a high proportion of cells in the thymus and lymph nodes of either irradiated (Ford et al. 1966) or unirradiated mice (Wu et al. 1968) injected with bone marrow are derived from the marrow inoculum. The studies of Wu et al. (1968) indicate that haemopoietic colony-forming cells, erythroblasts, granulocytes, thymic cells and cells of lymph nodes, may all belong to the same clone. However it is still not certain whether the haemopoietic colony-forming cells actually give rise to the lymphoid descendants, or whether colony-forming cells and lymphoid cells have an as yet unidentified precursor.

Specific evidence of restoration of immunological competence to a lethally irradiated animal by the progeny of a single haemopoietic clone has been presented by Trentin et al. (1967). Lethally irradiated mice were given small numbers of bone marrow from normal adult (CBA × T_6)F_1 mice. Cell suspensions were prepared from the resulting haemopoietic colonies (4–13 per spleen) and used to repopulate another group of lethally irradiated mice. Mice surviving more than 30 days were then challenged with three different antigens. As indicated by the T_6 marker chromosome, the haemopoietic and lymphoid systems of these re-populated mice were all of donor origin. Antibody production occurred to all antigens used in these mice. These experiments therefore indicate that haemopoietic cells derived from spleen colonies which do not contain lymphoid cells, effectively repopulate the lymphoid system. The active donor cells involved, probably being stem cells produced in large numbers within the colonies by self renewal proliferation.

Cell marker experiments in normal embryonic or foetal animals have also strongly implied that there is a seeding of stem cells *via* the blood stream into the embryonic myeloid organs and into the primary lymphoid organs, where their differentiation is directed accordingly into the different myeloid and lymphoid types (Moore and Owen 1967). These experiments will be covered in more detail in 17.4.5.

Haemopoietic stem cells are first formed in the early yolk sac probably from cells that migrate out of particular regions of the primitive streak. Many of these differentiate within the blood islands of the yolk sac into first generation erythrocytes, although others divide to produce more stem cells. The mouse yolk sac has been shown to contain *in vivo* colony-forming cells which are capable of producing granulocytic, megakaryocytic and erythroid spleen colonies, and cells which are capable of repopulating the lymphoid and myeloid tissue of lethally irradiated hosts (Moore and Metcalf 1970). These experiments also showed that the development of intraembryonic haemopoiesis, par-ticularly in foetal liver, is dependent on colonization by yolk sac haemo-poietic cells. It therefore appears firmly established that there is a *de novo* formation of haemopoietic stem cells in the yolk sac, which then seed out *via* the blood stream into other sites, both myeloid and lym-phoid, and that both stem cell self renewal and myeloid differentiation occur within foetal liver, bone marrow and to a certain extent spleen, whereas it is predominantly differentiation to lymphoid elements that occurs in the primary lymphoid organs. This pathways is schematically presented in Figure 17.4.

The possible existence of a specific lymphoid stem cell has been indicated by Ford et al. (1968). They studied the repopulation of lymphoid tissues of lethally irradiated mice injected with a mixture of syngeneic bone marrow and lymph node cells. Each of these donor cell types were chromosomally marked. Initially lymph node derived cells predominated in the recipients' lymphoid tissues as expected from previous studies (Ford and Micklem 1963). However instead of an eventual complete replacement of bone marrow-derived cells, which

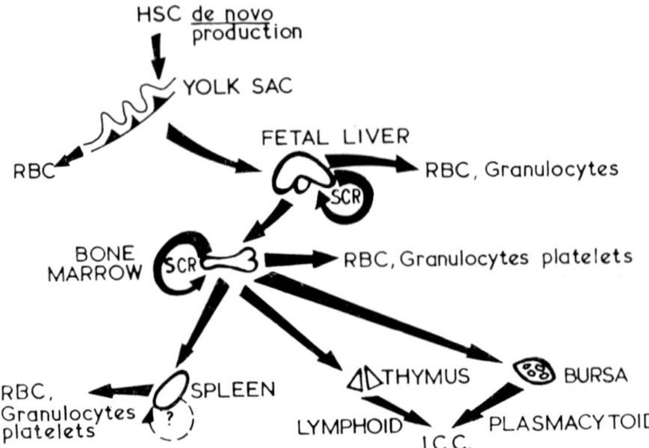

Fig. 17.4. Pathway of haemopoietic stem cell (HSC) differentiation. *De novo* formation occurs in the yolk sac and stem cells then seed to foetal liver, bone marrow and spleen where differentiation to blood elements occurs. Immunocompetent cell differentiation (ICC) occurs via stem cell seeding to thymus or bursa.

would be expected if lymphoid tissue renewal were dependent on haemopoietic stem cell differentiation, approximately 19% of lymph node derived mitoses persisted between 56 and 77 weeks after cell transfer. This strongly raises the possibility that there exists in lymphoid tissue a cell which can undergo self-renewal and limited differentiation to only lymphoid elements. Such a cell might fall in the position depicted in Figure 17.1 as the Ph[1]-negative precursor cell.

Further evidence consistent with a direct lineage between the haemopoietic stem cell and the lymphocyte is the finding that a specific anti-rat thymocyte serum, will completely inactivate both ICC (measured by a graft-*versus*-host assay) and haemopoietic stem cells (Field and Gibbs 1968). This may well indicate a common membrane surface antigen of the two cell types, thus suggesting a direct relationship between them, although a non-specific 'mouse' antigen may well be involved. Pretreatment of bone marrow cell suspensions with specific anti-light chain immunoglobulin sera does not appear to alter the number of colonies produced on injection into irradiated mice (Warner, 1971a), and hence immunoglobulin gene expression is not activated in the haemopoietic stem cell.

17.4.3. *Primary and secondary lymphoid organs*

Haemopoietic stem cells are capable of undergoing specific differentiation towards elements of the haemopoietic system, providing that they encounter the appropriate inducers of differentiation. It is at this level that the definitive commitment of the stem cell towards the ICC occurs.

This occurs through an interaction of the stem cell with an appropriate environment which either through cell contact or the effect of a diffusible product (inducer) initiates the expression of certain genes which identify that cell as belonging to the ICC category. This event appears to occur only in certain parts of the lymphoid system. Thus our distinction between primary and secondary level lymphoid organs relates to the level of differentiation occurring in the immune development. Differentiation to the ICC level occurs in primary lymphoid organs, and this is still an antigen-independent step. The further differentiation of the ICC into an immunocyte is antigen-induced and occurs in secondary level lymphoid organs. As will be stressed later (17.4.7), differentiation to ICC is proposed to involve the derepression and activation of at least one immunoglobulin-structural gene in the cell. It is also proposed that this occurs in primary level lymphoid organs. This scheme is diagrammatically represented in Figure 17.5. Whether induction of stem cell differentiation occurs through interaction with a diffusible factor or involves more intimate cell-cell interaction is not at present clear, however in several other inductive systems direct cell interaction does appear to be required (Lilien and Moscona 1967) and it is probable that epithelial mesenchymal tissue interaction is also involved in ICC differentiation (Auerbach 1969).

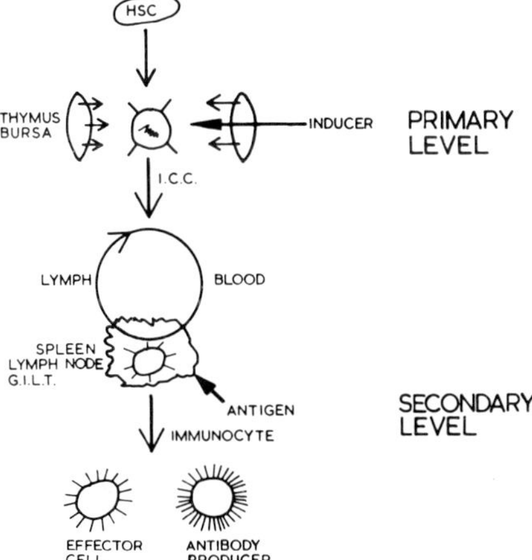

Fig. 17.5. Primary and secondary level lymphoid organs. Haemopoietic stem cells (HSC) pass through the primary level organs for induction to the immunocompetent cell stage (ICC) and then join the recirculating lymphocyte pool and thence fixed lymphoid tissues such as spleen, lymph node and gastro – intestinal tract lymphoid tissue (GILT). It is in this secondary level, that antigenic stimulation leads to immunocyte development of both effector cells for cellular immunity and antibody-producing plasma cells.

Primary lymphoid organs include the thymus, the bursa of Fabricius in birds, and possibly a mammalian equivalent of the bursa. Several features of thymus and bursa are uniquely those of primary lymphoid organs and are clearly distinct from secondary level lymphoid organs. These are summarized in Table 17.3.

TABLE 17.3

Distinguishing features of primary and secondary level lymphoid organs.

Property	Primary lymphoid tissue	Secondary lymphoid tissue
Embryonic origin of stromal cells	Epithelial (Ectoendodermal junctions)	Mesenchymal
Timing of lymphopoiesis	First (Mouse, fetal)	Second (Mouse, neonatal)
Lymphopoietic activity	High, approx. 1%	Low, approx. 0.1%
Lymphopoiesis dependence on antigen	No	Yes
Lymphopoiesis in germ-free animals	Normal	Considerably reduced
Repopulation after irradiation	Haemopoietic stem cells	Lymphoid cells
Persistence in life	Involution at maturity	Throughout life
Effects of embryonic, or neonatal removal	Profound immunological deficiency	Only slight local effects
Content of lymphoid cells	ICC	Immunocytes and ICC

Primary lymphoid organs are derived from ecto-endodermal junctions in association with gut epithelium, and accordingly are frequently referred to as lympho-epithelial organs. They are the first organs to become lymphoid, the timing of this being related to the gestation period of the animal. In small animals such as chickens, mice and rats the primary lymphoid organs show lymphoid development well before birth, whereas peripheral secondary lymphoid tissue is evident only after birth. Lymphopoiesis is about ten times higher in thymus than lymph nodes (Metcalf 1964) and is independent of antigenic stimulation. In germ-free animals which are under far less antigenic challenge during fetal life, lymphopoiesis in secondary organs is greatly reduced but is unaffected in thymus and bursa (Gordon 1959; Thorbecke et al. 1957). Primary lymphoid organs can only be repopulated after irradiation by haemopoietic stem cells whereas lymphoid cells will repopulate secondary lymphoid tissues (Ford and Micklem 1963). Consistent with their function, removal of primary lymphoid organs at a time prior to or early in immune ontogeny, will lead to immunological deficiencies, whereas removal of a secondary lymphoid organ only deletes a small proportion of ICC and immunocytes. Primary lymphoid organs contain primarily ICC, although later in life some entry and settling of plasma cells occurs. Accordingly the primary lymphoid organs are not the sites of local immune reactions, which occur mainly in secondary level lymphoid organs.

17.4.4. Role of the thymus in immunity

Despite many bursts of research activity on the thymus gland relatively few well documented facts on its function existed prior to 1960. In the mid 1940's Furth (1946) and later Law (1952) and Kaplan (1950) established that thymectomy prevents the development of lymphoid leukaemia in mice. In 1956 Metcalf then demonstrated that saline extracts of thymus tissue would produce a lymphocytosis when injected into baby mice, and this was a specific property of thymic extracts. The active principle in these extracts was termed lymphocytosis-stimulating factor. The current era of intense thymic research which has firmly established the role of the thymus in immunity then commenced in 1961 with the demonstrations of immunological deficiency created by neonatal thymectomy (Miller 1961; Good et al. 1962).

As many complete books and reviews have since appeared which specifically deal with the role of the thymus in immunity, this topic will not be extensively covered here, and the reader is referred to several of these review articles (Metcalf 1966; Miller and Osoba 1967; Goldstein and Mackay 1969). Specific attention will be given only to those aspects which relate to the differentiation of the ICC .

17.4.4.1. Stem cell-thymus interactions

The twelve day old mouse foetal thymus rudiment is composed of a single epithelio-mesenchymal rudiment. This can be removed from the animal and cultured *in vitro* or *in vivo* for seven days, during which time complete lymphoid development occurs (Auerbach 1965). Thus the 12 day foetal thymic rudiment contains the cells that are required for lymphoid differentiation. When the rudiments were separated into epithelial and mesenchymal components and cultured separately or in combination, it was clearly demonstrated that the mesenchyme is essential for lymphoid differentiation to occur, although this differentiation occurs within the epithelial component (Auerbach 1961). These studies clearly demonstrate the importance of embryonic interaction in differentiation. However, it was concluded in these studies that the precursor cell of the lymphocyte was indeed of epithelial origin. The alternative possibility, however, is that the 12-day old foetal thymic epithelial rudiment, already has received an immigrant haemopoietic stem cell from the blood, and this is the true precursor of the lymphocyte. This latter alternative has now been decisively proven by the work of Moore and Owen (1967a, b). In experiments utilizing the sex chromosome markers with parabiosed chick embryos of opposite sexes, an inflow of blood borne stem cells into the chick embryo thymic rudiment was clearly demonstrated. It was proposed that embryonic lymphopoiesis is therefore dependent upon an initial dynamic cellular interflow, similar to the continued cellular migration streams in adult haemopoiesis. The studies of Auerbach indicated that mesenchyme is also essential for thymic lymphopoiesis, but the mesenchyme can be derived from any source including non-thymic. Accordingly, since lymphopoiesis occurs in the epithelial rudiments, it must be concluded that under a non-specific mesenchymal direction, thymic epithelium directs or induces lymphoid differentiation in the haemopoietic stem cell.

That this differentiation is indeed toward an ICC was demonstrated by Umiel et al. (1968). Mouse foetal liver cells which include many haemopoietic stem cells, cannot themselves induce graft-*versus*-host reactions. However if they are cultivated for several days in combination with thymic tissue, they do acquire immunological competence.

Foetal liver cells can also be shown to contain the precursors of ICC in *in vivo* models, in which their passage through a thymus of a host animal is essential for them to become actual ICC capable of inducing a graft-*versus*-host reaction (Tyan and Cole 1966; Tyan, Cole and Nowell 1966).

Precursors of some antibody-forming cells have also been shown to be present in foetal liver which also required passage through a thymic environment for their maturation to ICC (Tyan et al. 1969). This was demonstrated for a synthetic polypeptide antigen (T, G,)-A-L, in which virtually no antibody production occurred in thymectomized, irradiated mice given foetal liver cells. However the resulting antibody response to sheep red cells was surprisingly, only minimally reduced, although the number of anti-sheep cell forming plaques in the spleen was reduced to 10% of that observed in control irradiated non-thymectomized mice.

These results therefore stress that precursors of ICC exist in embryonic haemopoietic tissues, and under a thymic influence will become ICC, predominantly committed to cellular immunity.

The content of ICC within thymic cell suspensions is generally considered to be rather low, and in some studies thymic cells from neonatal mice were as competent as adult thymic cells (Thorbecke and Cohen 1964). Studies in chickens (Warner 1964) with the Simonsen chorioallantoic membrane assay for ICC has indicated that the avian thymus does contain ICC capable of initiating graft-*versus*-host reactions, and that the number of these cells within the thymus remains at a fairly constant level throughout life. The ratio of cortex to medulla was altered in various ways, and it was concluded from these studies that the thymic cortical lymphocytes are not ICC, but that a competent population of cells exists throughout life in the medulla.

The recent introduction of a technique for directly demonstrating the presence in normal lymphoid populations, of cells which specifically can react with antigen (Naor and Sulitzeanu 1967; Byrt and Ada 1969; Humphrey and Keller 1970), has recently been applied to thymic cell suspensions. In a preliminary study with young adult mouse thymus cells, only a small proportion of cells, 1 per 10^5, were found to react with ^{131}I-labelled *Salmonella* flagellin or haemocyanin, whereas about 1 in 10^4 spleen cells reacted with flagellin and 1 in 10^3 with haemocyanin. In a more recent study (Dwyer and Mackay 1970b), human foetal thymus has been examined for reactivity with ^{125}I-labelled flagellin. Approximately 1 cell in 50 showed some degree of labelling with thymi from 20–22 week foetuses. This number fell with increasing age of the donor thymus, and a 39 year old thymus contained about 1 in 2×10^3. At the foetal stage, the number in thymus was about 20 fold higher than in blood, whereas by adult life the situation is reversed (Dwyer and Mackay 1970a). Studies of grain counts over labelled foetal thymic cells showed an exponential decline in relation to cell frequency. The existence of antigen-binding lymphocyte in the foetal thymus suggests that antibody patterns arise independently of antigenic stimulation and that the thymus may be the main site for the origin of these patterns (Burnet 1967). The extremely high number of these cells in foetal thymus appears however contrary to the view that specific patterns against all antigenic determinants arise in thymus and are carried by separate cells. Aspects of this problem will be discussed later (Section 17.4.7).

17.4.4.2. Thymus seeding to other organs
If it is proposed that ICC arise within the thymus by differentiation from stem cells, then it is equally necessary that they then leave the thymus and become available for reaction with antigen, since not all antigens penetrate into the thymic environment (Weiss 1963; Clark 1963, 1964). In an animal like the mouse it was calculated that approximately 40 to 65% of all new lymphocytes are produced in the thymus (Metcalf and Nakamura 1962). However since the weight of the thymus remains relatively constant over a long period, this high level of lymphopoiesis must either be balanced by an equivalent amount of cell death or of cell migration from the organ.

Attempts to demonstrate cell migration from the thymus have involved two main approaches. Studies with chromosomally marked thymus grafts have definitely shown that cells derived from these thymic grafts settle in host lymph nodes (Harris and Ford 1964; Leuchars et al. 1964). However in these experiments it is possible that the seeding is the result of the mechanical disruption involved in thymus grafting and occurs only in the first few days.

Studies with multiple thymus grafts in which mice carried 5–20 times the normal weight of thymus, failed to reveal any evidence of extensive cell seeding to secondary lymphoid organs (Matsuyama et al. 1966). It was concluded that relatively few cells ($<$ 1%) produced in the thymus leave the organ, and instead are destroyed within three or four days. A more direct approach to the study of thymic cell migration is by *in situ* labelling of thymic cells with tritiated nucleosides followed by subsequent examination of peripheral lymphoid tissue for labelled cells.

This approach has been followed by Nossal and Gorrie (1964), Murray and Woods (1964), Weissman (1967) and Linna and Stillstrom (1966). Nossal (1964) utilizing direct intrathymic arterial infusion of tritiated thymidine in young adult guinea-pigs showed that over 0.2% of mesenteric lymph nodes were labelled and presumed derived from thymus. It was estimated that approximately 1 in 100 newly formed small lymphocytes came from the thymus. Studies in newborn guinea-pigs showed a higher migration of around 1–2% immigrant cells. Similar studies by Linna and Stillstrom (1966) and Linna (1967) used specific activity of tritiated DNA measurements and also concluded that there was a significant transport of DNA from the thymus to spleen, presumably in the form of migrating cells.

The added precaution of simultaneous whole body infusion of cold nucleoside with the intra-thymic arterial hot nucleoside infusion was included by Weissman (1967) in a study of thymic cell seeding in the rat. This study strongly indicates that in the newborn animal up to 20% of the cells in splenic white pulp or in the lymph nodes are thymus-derived cells, and for adult rats the values are lower, approximately 3%.

These various studies seem to indicate that although the bulk of thymic cells are probably destroyed within the organ after a life span of a few days, some cells do leave, and particularly in newborn animals, may play a major role in lymphoid development in secondary lymphoid organs. The true significance of intra-thymic death of many cells is still unanswered, although it has been implied to be of great relevance to certain selective theories of immunity (Burnet 1967; Jerne 1969).

The eventual fate of the migrating thymocytes is more clearly defined. The studies of Schooley and Kelly (1964), Miller et al. (1967) and

Goldschneider and McGregor (1968) show a marked reduction in the number of thoracic duct lymphocytes in thymectomized animals, which in turn represent the recirculating lymphocyte pool passing through lymph nodes, spleen and intestinal lymphoid tissue (Gowans 1964; Gowans and McGregor 1965). Migrating thymocytes therefore appear to leave the thymus *via* the blood stream (Sainte-Marie and Leblond 1964), enter the recirculating lymphocyte pool, where they may settle in the thymus-dependent areas (Parrott et al. 1966) of lymph nodes and spleen.

Thymus-derived lymphocytes carry a specific isoantigen (θ) present on thymus cells. The theta (θ) isoantigen is present in brain and thymus (Reif and Allen 1966) and is detected by specific isoantisera made against C3H or CBA thymocytes. Approximately 60–80% of lymph node lymphocytes and 20–40% of splenic lymphocytes carry the θ antigen on their surface. This population is strikingly reduced in mice which have been depleted of thymus-derived lymphocytes by chronic anti-lymphocyte serum treatment, or thymectomy (Raff 1969; Schlesinger and Yron 1969). This antigen accordingly serves as a very useful thymus-derived cell marker.

17.4.4.3. Thymus and immunity

The essential role of the thymus for the full ontogenic development of immunity is now well established and has been reviewed in detail elsewhere (Miller and Osoba 1967). A brief summary of the main points follow and can best be considered in two sections, (a) transplantation immunity and delayed hypersensitivity, and (b) immunoglobulin synthesis and antibody production.

(a) In general it is quite evident that in all species studied, where thymectomy has been performed at an early stage of development, cell-mediated immune responses are strikingly depressed. Thus skin homografts from allogeneic animals of different major histocompatibility types will be accepted or show prolonged rejection by neonatally thymectomized mice (Miller 1962; Good et al. 1962), rats (Arnason et al. 1964; Fisher and Fisher 1965), chickens (Warner and Szenberg 1962; Aspinall et al. 1963), and hamsters (Sherman et al. 1964). In several other species however, lymphoid maturation occurs well before birth, and accordingly neonatal thymectomy has little effect in depressing immunity, for example, in the dog (Fisher et al. 1965). Neonatal thymectomy of germ-free mice does not cause as extensive a depression of skin graft immunity as in conventional thymectomized mice (Miller et al. 1967b) suggesting that in some manner, other factors, perhaps involving bacterial contamination, endotoxins and cross-reacting antigens, act to further reduce the number of ICC available in the already limited population of these cells.

Delayed hypersensitivity reactions to various antigens are clearly depressed in neonatally thymectomized mice (Kantor and Miller unpublished observations; Moir et al. 1964), rats (Arnason et al. 1962; Messini et al. 1964), and chickens (Janković and Isvaneski 1963; Cooper et al. 1966). This depression also parallels a depression in the incidence and severity of experimental autoimmune diseases in thymectomized animals, in which it is suspected that cell-mediated immunity plays the major pathogenic role (Arnason et al. 1965; Janković and Isvaneski 1963; Janković et al. 1965).

It should be stressed that the measurement of these three parameters of immunity, skin graft rejection, delayed hypersensitivity and experimental autoimmunity, is made in terms which cannot at present be directly related to numbers of ICC in the lymphocyte pool. Studies which assess the ability of peripheral lymphoid populations to induce graft-*versus*-host reactions are a little more direct, and certainly indicate that there is a depression in the responsiveness of the population (Good et al. 1962; Dalmasso et al. 1962; Miller et al. 1967a; Rieke 1966).

(b) Neonatal thymectomy does not appear to have a very profound effect on circulating immunoglobulin levels. In one study of thymectomized mice (Humphrey et al. 1964) the only major change detected was a spasmodic elevation of IgA levels in some mice, which approached in a few cases a myeloma-like appearance in restriction of electrophoretic heterogeneity. Although another report appears to present a contrary result in that IgA levels are reported to be subnormal (Arnason et al. 1964b), this is not the case as there is a difference in terminology, and the IgA of Arnason is not in the accepted IgA class of Fahey et al. (1964) and is probably IgG_1. Indeed, in a study by Fahey et al. (1965) IgG_1 and IgG_2 levels tended to be lower than normal and this was due to an increased catabolism of these proteins; IgA levels were again found to be occasionally high. Moderately elevated immunoglobulin levels were also observed in another study (Bazin and Duplan 1966). Congenital absence of the thymus in man is also associated with normal immunoglobulin production (Lischner and di George 1969).

Immunoglobulin synthesis, although not quantitated, also appears normal in thymectomized chickens (Cooper et al. 1967).

It is thus clear that in all species studied, the presence or absence of the thymus in the embryonic or neonatal period is of no consequence to the development of immunoglobulin synthesis. Although neonatal thymectomy does not cause any striking changes in immunoglobulin synthesis, the ability to produce certain antibodies is severely depressed.

An association of the thymus with antibody formation had been periodic-ally contemplated for many years (Fichtelius 1957) and has now been definitely shown for many different antigens in various animal species (see Miller and Osoba 1967). The essential point is that some but not all antigens, will provoke a normal antibody response in neonatally thymec-tomized animals. The specific rationale for the division of antigens into thymus-dependent and thymus-independent is not clear, and further-more an antigen which will not elicit antibody responses in thymecto-mized animals of one species, may do so in another species (Lind 1970).

There are two alternative possibilities in this regard: (i) the apparent separation of thymus-dependent and independent antigens is a real phenomenon, or (ii) the development of all potential antibody responses is under thymic control but with some antigens sufficient maturation of the thymus-controlled stage in antibody formation has occurred prior to birth, that is, before the time of neonatal thymectomy. This is consis-tent with studies demonstrating a distinct time difference in the ability of normal foetal animals to respond to different antigens (Šterzl and Silverstein 1967). However this explanation is not compatible with the studies performed in adult thymectomized, lethally irradiated mice which have been given syngeneic bone marrow. In these animals the same antigens which fail to elicit antibody responses in neonatally thymectomized animals, also fail in these mice. Furthermore, adult thymectomized mice which have not been irradiated will also eventually become relatively incapable of responding to these same thymus-dependent antigens (Taylor 1964; Miller 1965; Metcalf 1965).

In general, antigens which are foreign erythrocytes, serum globulins or albumins will not produce antibody responses in thymectomized mice, whereas bacterial antigens will do so. A clear-cut distinction of this type is not possible however, as antibody responses to synthetic antigens such as a copolymer of four amino acids (Tyr, Glu, Ala, Lys) are also totally thymus-dependent. The depression by thymectomy of the res-ponse to sheep red cells is also only quantitative rather than absolute (Tyan et al. 1969; Sinclair and Millican 1967).

Although it first appeared that the absence of thymic development in man (thymic agenesis) was associated with depression of cellular immunity but not of humoral immunity, Lischner and di George (1969) have recently stressed that most of these observations were made in individuals with only incomplete thymic development, rather than a true agenesis. In one child with total absence of the thymus, immunoglobulin levels were quite normal (at least prior to the more terminal stages), but no antibody production could be detected to triple antigen, Salk vaccine or measles. A low level of isohaemagglutinin was present but did not show the usual increase in titre. They accordingly suggested that total absence of the thymus would be associated with total absence of antibody-producing potential.

Studies in chickens, although not extensive, have not revealed any depression in the ability of neonatally thymectomized chickens to produce circulating antibodies, despite a marked depression in cellular immunity (Warner and Szenberg 1962; Graetzer et al. 1963; Cooper et al. 1964). In one of these studies human γ-globulin was used as antigen, which is an antigen which fails to elicit antibody production in thymectomized mice. Unfortunately, sheep red blood cells have not been tried as an antigen in thymectomized chickens.

In more recent studies aimed at elucidating the mechanism of involvement of thymic cells in antibody production, a distinct response to antigenic challenge can be invoked in thymic cells (Davies et al. 1966). It is important to stress that these studies which involve cell collaboration are events occurring under antigenic direction, and are thus a separate problem from that of the thymic control of the development of immunocompetent cells with potentiality for antibody production. These studies will be considered in a later section.

It therefore appears that, although the thymus of chickens does not play any essential role in the development of humoral immunity, the mammalian thymus does so for some but perhaps not all antibody responses. This comparison between avian and mammalian thymic involvement will be further taken up in considering the mammalian equivalent of the avian bursa of Fabricius (see Section 17.4.6).*

17.4.4.4. Thymic humoral factors

In discussing the haemopoietic stem cell origin of thymus-derived immunocompetent cells it was speculated that the thymus induces the differentiation of these stem cells through an agent produced by some cell type resident in the pre-lymphoid thymus.

This conclusion is supported by studies on the ability of thymic tissues to induce the restoration of immunological competence in a neonatally thymectomized animal. Direct evidence that the thymus produces a humoral factor which can act in the development of immunological competence comes from the demonstration that thymus grafts contained in cell impermeable millipore chambers will restore immune

---

* Recent observations (Rouse and Warner, unpublished) have shown that neonatally thymectomised chickens which are also injected with a specific duck antichicken thymus serum, are still capable of making normal levels of antibody to brucella antigen, but not to horse erythrocytes or heterologous proteins. Thus the chicken thymus may function in certain antibody responses in similar fashion to the mouse thymus.

competence to neonatally thymectomized mice. These animals do not suffer from wasting disease (Levey et al. 1963) and can reject skin grafts (Osoba and Miller 1964) and make antibodies to sheep red cells. Allogeneic thymic tissue enclosed within diffusion chambers will restore the capacity to reject skin grafts derived from the same strain as the thymus graft donor (Osoba 1965). Accordingly this inductive action toward immune competence is not strain-specific and does not involve the imprinting of specific recognition patterns. The initial implantation of intact thymus grafts in chambers results in massive destruction of cortical cells. This might indicate the possibility that immune restoration is mediated by a nucleic acid adjuvanticity effect on the few remaining competent cells present in thymectomized animals, since nucleic acids can act as powerful adjuvants (Braun and Nakano 1967). This is unlikely to be the sole explanation however as the introduction of lethally irradiated thymus cell suspensions do not restore immunocompetence in neonatally thymectomized mice (Miller and Mitchell 1968).

Restoration of immunocompetence may be associated with a product from the epithelial component of the thymus graft. Grafts of thymic epithelial reticulum will result in lymphoid and immunological reconstitution of neonatally thymectomized mice (Metcalf 1966; Hays 1967). Carcinogen-induced thymic non-lymphoid tumours can also restore immuno-deficient animals (Stuttman et al. 1968), as measured by prevention of early mortality and restoration of allograft immunity and graft-*versus*-host reactivity. Immunological recuperation could occur in the absence of complete morphological recovery of the lymphoid tissues. This biological function of the tumour was lost after repeated transplantation, which coincided with a change in morphology of the tumour from a pleomorphic type comprising spindle cells, reticuloendothelial cells and multinucleated cells to a population of large irregular anaplastic cells.

Several electron microscopic studies of the thymus have described a characteristic cell type found in the thymic medulla of a variety of animal species (Clark 1963; Hoshino 1963; Mandel 1968). These are termed cystic epithelial cells and were shown by Clark (1966) to secrete a sulphated mucopolysaccharide, and the activity of these cells correlated with the degree of lymphopoiesis in the thymus. This was considered (Clark 1968) to be circumstantial evidence for the hypothesis that the product of these cells is a lymphopoietic hormone. However, studies of the development of these cells (Mandel 1970) show that in ontogeny they appear after lymphopoiesis is well established. Further studies on their function are clearly warranted.

In vitro studies on thymus-induced restoration of immune competence to sublethally irradiated spleen fragments have also shown that a diffusible material from the thymus may be involved (Auerbach and Globerson 1967), in that separation of the thymus fragment from the irradiated spleen by a millipore membrane still permitted restoration of competence. That this effect may be on stem cells was indicated by the additional need of bone marrow, if lethal irradiation were used.

These various approaches all appear to indicate the existence of a hormonal type of material synthesized and perhaps secreted by a thymic (? epithelial) cell which is responsible for the induction of stem cell differentiation into immunocompetence. The direct approach of using soluble thymic extracts to induce immune restoration has however led to a rather confusing pattern of results. The existence of a humoral factor(s) from the thymus capable of stimulating lymphopoiesis in peripheral populations has been clearly and unquestionably demonstrated (Metcalf 1966). Metcalf (1956) recorded increased numbers of circulating lymphocytes in newborn mice and thymectomized adults injected with a heat-labile extract of mouse thymus. Gregoire and Duchateau (1956) described hyperplasia of rat lymphoid tissues with extracts of rabbit and pig thymus. In both of these early studies the authors indicated that the source of the active principle was medullary in origin. Enhanced lymphopoiesis induced by allogeneic thymus extracts has been demonstrated by thymidine incorporation in several recent series of studies (Klein et al. 1965; Trainin et al. 1967). This effect is not always specific for thymic extracts and it was shown that the use of thymectomized recipients increased the sensitivity and specificity for thymic extract-induced proliferation (Trainin et al. 1967). The factor described by Metcalf and Trainin is heat-labile and non-dialysable (Metcalf 1964). Some partial purification of this material has been achieved (Trainin et al. 1967; Hand et al. 1967) and the latter group indicated a basic protein of molecular weight around 17,000. Several other reports of glycoproteins with 'thymic factor activity' have also been made (Bernardi 1965; Comsa 1965). The factor of Klein et al. (1965), termed thymosin, appears to be a heat-stable, dialysable and carbohydrate-containing protein (Goldstein et al. 1966).

This array of lymphopoietic (mitogenic) factors from the thymus is reminiscent of the mitogenic factors described in extracts or supernatant fluids from sensitized lymphocytes involved in delayed hypersensitivity reactions (Lawrence and Landy 1969). This type of activity may therefore not be thymus-specific (but perhaps still be thymus-derived lymphocyte dependent) and is therefore not the type of inducing factor involved in haemopoietic stem cell differentiation. To firmly establish the presence of a true factor for inducing immune differentiation, the assay system must involve a demonstration of immunological reconstitution to neo-natally thymectomized animals. Although thymosin has been shown to induce some measure of skin graft rejection by neonatally thymecto-mized mice (Goldstein et al. 1970), it does not lead to any immune re-constitution of the antisheep red cell response in thymectomized mice (Sprent and Miller 1970; Goldstein et al. 1970). Prevention of the neonatal thymectomy wasting syndrome by thymic extracts has been shown by De Somer et al. (1963) and Trainin et al. (1966). Repeated injections of extracts of calf thymus or of mouse thymus have partially restored immunological competence to neonatally thymectomized mice as measured by either transplantation immune competence or antibody formation (Trainin and Linker-Israel 1967; Trainin et al. 1967; Law and Agnew 1968; Small and Trainin 1967). In analysing this restorative effect with an *in vitro* assay of graft-*versus*-host reactivity, Trainin et al. (1969) have shown that spleen cells from neonatally thymectomized mice will gain immune competence when incubated in syngeneic thymus extract for one hour prior to testing. Extracts from spleen or lymph node did not confer this activity. In view of this rapid activation, it becomes difficult to regard this action as a true induction of differentiation unless it be considered that stem cell proliferation toward a 'lymphoblastic' type of cell occurs in a thymectomized animal, and thymic factor acts in a rapid manner involving de-repression of genes involved in the anti-gen recognition site of lymphocytes. Alternatively, these experiments might indicate that thymus-derived cell division is an essential pre-requisite of certain immune responses and that a 'mitogenic factor' present in thymus, might initiate cell division in the small proportion of thymus-derived cells still present in spleens of neonatally thymecto-mized mice. Such an effect could possibly be induced by either an adjuvant-like action of nucleotides in the thymus extracts or by some other unknown mitogenic agent.

It seems clear at present that none of these thymic factors are behaving in analogous fashion to erythropoietin (Fisher 1968), bone marrow colony-stimulating factor (Metcalf 1969) or other regulators of haemo-poiesis (Metcalf and Moore 1971). Further study on this line would be greatly aided by the development of a method for *in vitro* cultivation of lymphoid cells from bone marrow precursors.

17.4.5. *Role of the bursa of Fabricius in immunity*

The *bursa of Fabricius* is a lymphoid organ unique to the class Aves. It is situated on the distal side of the *cloaca* and is connected to it by a short bursal duct. Its relevance to the development of immunity was first recognized by Glick (Glick et al. 1956) in showing that surgically bursectomized chickens were extremely poor at antibody synthesis. In its general growth behaviour the bursa resembles the thymus rather than peripheral lymphoid organs such as spleen or lymph node (Warner 1967; Warner and Szenberg 1964). In this article, discussion of the bursal function will be mainly restricted to aspects of differentiation.

17.4.5.1. Stem cell-bursa interactions

The embryonic bursa becomes fully lymphoidal several days prior to hatching. The earliest recognizable lymphoid cells appear around day fifteen of incubation, and develop in the nodules which form from epithelial budding of the surface epithelium. On the basis of light and electron microscopic observations it was proposed that medullary (and probably cortical) lymphocytes were directly derived from undifferentiated epithelial cells (Ackerman and Knouff 1959, 1964; Ackerman 1962). It was also suggested that the relatively strong alkaline phosphatase activity in the sub-epithelial mesenchyme of the bursa might be involved in lympho-epithelial nodule formation, and that this activity might be the direct target of testosterone suppression of nodule formation (Ackerman and Knouff 1963).

Direct morphological examination however cannot ascertain whether or not earlier immigrant cells have entered the developing bursa and then differentiated into lymphocytes. Moore and Owen (1965) using parabiotic chick embryos of opposite sex clearly demonstrated with chromosome markers that such an inflow of immigrant cells does occur into the bursa at the time of earliest lymphopoiesis. Up to 50% of dividing cells in the 15–20 day embryonic bursa were of partner origin. Analysis of other lymphoid organs confirmed the general concept of a migration stream of blood-borne haemopoietic precursor cells moving through chick tissues, and within the bursa, being differentiated into lymphoid cells.

In view of the relative unavailability of inbred lines of chickens, there have only been a few studies on attempts at restoration of immune competence with bursal grafts or cells. Bursal grafts in allogeneic recipients, although rejected have given some restoration of immune competence (Isaković et al. 1963). Several reports on restoration by bursal extracts or bursal grafts in millipore chambers have been made (Janković and Leskowitz 1965; St. Pierre and Ackerman 1965; Glick 1960; Janković et al. 1967) although in many cases the effects were marginal and most recipients used were not totally agammaglobulinaemic and could form minimal amounts of antibody. Restoration by bursal extracts might therefore again only involve an adjuvant-mediated type of stimulation of the already existing immune potential. Further studies on the mechanism of bursal induction of stem cell differentiation to antibody-forming precursors are clearly needed.

Recent studies have indicated that differentiation of stem cells within the bursa proceeds as far as an actual immunoglobulin-synthesizing cell. It is to be stressed however, that this does not imply differentiation to an actual antibody-secreting cell but rather, that in the absence of antigen, bursa-induced differentiation does lead to activation (de-repression) of the immunoglobulin structural genes. At the morphological level it is apparent that bursal lymphocytes are distinctly different from thymic lymphocytes and from most of the peripheral small lymphocyte population. Bursal lymphopoiesis shows clear evidence of maturation changes in the embryonic period (Sherman and Auerbach 1966), and the typical bursal lymphocyte shows considerable evidence of cytoplasmic ribosomal activity (Clauson et al. 1967) consistent with the data on its ability to synthesize some immunoglobulin.

Immunoglobulin synthesis in chickens has been shown to first occur in the bursa of Fabricius (Thorbecke et al. 1968). When fragments of embryonic bursa, thymus, or spleen are cultured *in vitro* with ^{14}C-labelled amino acids, only bursal fragments show synthesis of immunoglobulins, which are exclusively IgM with 18d embryos and only one week later IgG synthesis appears. This sequence was also observed with germ-free chick embryos, perhaps indicating a lack of involvement of antigenic stimulation in this synthesis. Using an even more sensitive system involving detection of immunoglobulin-containing cells by fluorochrome-labelled goat antibodies to chicken μ, γ and light chains, Cooper et al. (1970) and Kincade and Cooper (1970) have shown the presence of IgM-containing cells in the embryonic bursal follicles as early as day fourteen. IgG-containing cells were also first detected in the bursa, appearing around embryonic day nineteen to twenty-one. Very few immunoglobulin-containing cells appeared in other sites until hatching and the few observed all contained IgM. After hatching, a rapid increase in IgM-containing cells, and then IgG-containing cells occurred in spleen and other peripheral sites. Grossi et al. (1968) has also observed immunoglobulin-containing cells in the bursal follicles of the newly hatched chicken.

These studies are therefore consistent in clearly demonstrating that activation of immunoglobulin gene synthesis first occurs in bursal lymphoid cells and must involve a fairly rapid activation. Moore and Owen (1965) demonstrated stem cells in the bursa on day thirteen, only one day before the presence of IgM can be found. Following induction of immunoglobulin synthesis, bursal lymphocytes then appear to move out from the bursa and colonize the peripheral lymphoid tissues. Cells with identical morphological features to bursal lymphocytes have been found in the splenic germinal centres (Clawson et al. 1967) of normal chickens but not in bursectomized irradiated chickens. The sequence of appearances of immunoglobulin-containing cells described above (bursa then peripheral tissues) is also compatible with the concept of direct seeding. By a technique of local labelling of bursal cells with tritiated thymidine, it has also been shown that a transport of cells from the bursa to the spleen and thymus occurs (Woods and Linna 1965). The significance of this latter observation is not clear, although it is compatible with earlier observations (Thorbecke et al. 1957) demonstrating the presence of germinal centres in the young adult avian thymus.

One of the more fundamental questions still to be completely elucidated, concerns the possible antigen recognition-specificity of bursal lymphocytes. The preceding consideration of immunoglobulin synthesis has concerned immunoglobulin classes as defined by antisera to the constant regions of the heavy chains. It is also relevant to question whether molecules synthesized in the bursa are intact in also possessing a variable region of defined antibody specificity.

Antibody-forming cells do not usually appear in the bursa following -conventional routes of immunization (Dent and Good 1965; Glick 1967). This however may only imply that the bursa does not directly receive antigen, rather than indicating an inability for generating antibody-specific patterns.

A direct approach to this problem involves cell transfer studies with bursal cell suspensions. Using B-histocompatibility locus-isogenic chickens Gilmour et al. (1970) have shown that bursal cell suspensions will transfer the capacity to produce antibodies to *Brucella abortus* to neonatally x-irradiated recipients. With 4 week-old donors, bursal cell suspensions were more efficient than spleen cells in this regard, but with older donors (10–11 weeks) spleen cells were more efficient, and in both cases thymus cells were much less efficient than either of the other two cell types. As this reversion sequence parallels the relative immunoglobulin synthetic capacity of bursa and spleen, it suggests that bursal cells are the direct precursors of the potential antibody-forming cells. This is further corroborated by the observation that spleens of bursectomized donors were incapable of cell transfer of antibody production (Gilmour et al. 1970; Cain et al. 1967).

However, in view of the evidence of cell collaboration in mammalian systems (see later section), the possibility exists that a bursal cell behaves in the manner of collaborating with thymic cells in certain antibody responses in mice (Miller and Mitchell 1969) and aids in the induction of antibody synthesis by another cell type. The data on immunoglobulin synthesis in bursa is somewhat contrary to this notion and specific studies on cell collaboration in avian systems are urgently required. It was observed by Gilmour et al. (1970) that with sheep erythrocytes as antigen, bursal cells were inefficient at transfer of antibody formation, whereas spleen cells were quite competent. This again indicates the possibility that with this antigen, another cell type, possibly of thymic origin, might be needed for collaboration with the bursal cells in order to induce the antibody response. If the antibody response to *Brucella* is purely of bursal type (that is, thymus independent), we must also consider the possibility that collaboration might have occurred between two different bursal cell types, one destined to produce the antibody and the other involved in inducing activity of the former. In the absence of any direct evidence we can only speculate, and possibly consider the simpler interpretation, namely that antigen directly contacting the bursal cell can stimulate its clonal expansion into an immunoglobulin-synthesizing cell. The fact that most bursal medullary cells fluoresce with antiglobulin (H-chain) reagents is in support of this concept.

An even more direct approach is to ascertain whether bursal cells can specifically bind labelled antigens. Several authors (Naor and Sulitzeanu 1967; Byrt and Ada 1969; Humphrey and Keller 1970) have shown that mouse lymphoid spleen cells will specifically bind radio-labelled antigens. This is not a property of adult thymus cells (Byrt and Ada 1969), nor of peripheral lymphocytes (Dwyer and Mackay 1970) in agamma-globulinaemic humans (Naor et al. 1969). In preliminary studies Dwyer and Warner (1971) have found that embryonic bursal cells will bind ^{125}I-labelled flagellin as early as 14 days of incubation, and very little activity is detected in embryonic thymus or spleen. This binding is mediated by a surface immunoglobulin molecule of as yet undefined class, but most likely IgM (cf. Warner et al. 1970). If further studies confirm the present view that this technique in mammals does not detect thymus-derived cells, it will reinforce the idea that bursal cells are therefore direct precursors of antibody-forming cells (at least for some antigens) and are expressing both the v and c regions of the immunoglobulin polypeptide chains.

17.4.5.2. Bursa-controlled development of the immune response

The essential role of the bursa of Fabricius for the development of the humoral antibody response was first shown by Glick et al. (1956). It was subsequently shown (Meyer et al. 1959; Mueller et al. 1960) that a more complete prevention of antibody-forming capacity could be achieved by the injection of 19-nortestosterone into 5 day chick embryos, this procedure resulting in a failure of bursal development. Further studies with bursectomized chickens by various groups (Warner et al. 1962; Warner et al. 1969; Cooper et al. 1965; Isaković et al. 1963; Pierce et al. 1966) have fully confirmed that the bursa is required in embryonic and neonatal life for the development of the potential for antibody formation. As these studies have been considered in some detail elsewhere (Warner 1967; Warner and Szenberg 1964), we will only consider here several of the more controversial aspects.

The various studies by different groups with bursectomized chickens have involved the use of a wide range of antigens, including heterologous red cells and proteins, bacterial, viral and protozoal antigens and more defined chemical haptens. In all cases depression or abolition of the antibody response was observed in bursectomized chickens. This clearly indicates that the bursa is involved in development of potential for the synthesis of *all* types of antibody molecules, and does not parallel the apparent thymic dependence or independence of certain antibody responses in mammals. A block in antibody-forming potential following bursectomy- could therefore involve a specific interference with the mechanism of de-repression of the immunoglobulin structural genes, with or without the necessity of infering that the bursa also controls the generation of antibody diversity. Several reports have in fact argued that the immunoglobulin levels of bursectomized chickens do not necessarily bear a relationship to the antibody-forming potential of the animal (Van Meter et al. 1969; Carey and Warner 1964; Pierce et al. 1966). These and other results (Claflin et al. 1966; Rose and Orlans 1968; Janković and Isaković 1966) tend to show that bursectomized chickens can make some immunoglobulins, and primary, and particularly secondary antibody responses. This has led to some controversy as it is interpreted by some groups to indicate that other non-bursal factors might play a role in development of antibody-forming potential, or that only certain stages in plasma cell development may be blocked in bursectomized animals. A simpler explanation consistent with all the observations, is that bursectomy is frequently incomplete, in the sense that some peripheralization of bursal cells has occurred before the bursectomy. As the recent studies of Cooper et al. (1970) and Dwyer and Warner (1971) have indicated that bursa-induced differentiation to immunoglobulin synthesis occurs as early as embryo day fourteen, only a complete prevention of all bursal lymphoid development might be expected to totally suppress antibody and immunoglobulin formation. All available experimental data is totally consistent with this concept. Thus, surgical bursectomy alone several weeks after hatching has very little effect on potential antibody synthesis (Chang et al. 1957; Mueller et al. 1960). If irradiation is combined with adult bursectomy, some depression in antibody response is however observed (Sato and Suzuki 1969). Bursectomy at hatching has a marked though not complete suppressive action on primary but not secondary antibody synthesis and on IgG but not IgM synthesis. Bursectomy at hatching combined with irradiation has a more marked effect in reducing subsequent IgM and IgG immunoglobulin synthesis (Van Meter et al. 1969; Cooper et al. 1966) but the reduction is still not complete (Rose and Orlans 1968). Surgical bursectomy in the late embryonic period (day 18–19, however, has a much more profound depressive effect on both subsequent antibody and immunoglobulin synthesis (Cooper et al. 1969; Van Alten et al. 1968). Hormonal bursectomy given before any bursal lymphoid development can cause total agammaglobulinaemia (Warner et al. 1969). That this complete depression does not occur in all birds is not unexpected, since administration of the hormone several days after lymphoid follicle development has commenced, does not totally suppress lymphoid differentiation (Warner and Burnet 1961). Differential rates of testosterone uptake by the outbred embryos might therefore explain the absence of 100 percent uniform total agammaglobulinaemia. That it does occur at all, and lead to persistence of complete agammaglobulinaemia and lack of antibody formation well into adult life, strongly infers that the bursa is the sole site of control (induction) of differentiation of the antibody-secreting cell line.

That this effect is not due to other non-specific actions of the hormonal treatment, is indicated by recent studies (Cooper at al. 1970) in which marked suppression of IgM synthesis was induced by the repeated embryonic injection of heterologous anti-μ chain antibodies.

17.4.5.3. *Dissociation of immunity*

The preceding considerations on the effects of neonatal removal of primary lymphoid organs clearly indicate that in both mammals (Miller and Osoba 1967) and in chickens (Warner 1967), the thymus controls the development of the lymphocyte-mediated system of cellular immunity, and has no effect at all on immunoglobulin ontogeny nor on many antibody responses. Studies in chickens show that the bursa controls the ontogeny of all types of immunoglobulin synthesis and therefore the ability to synthesize and secrete circulating antibodies of all specificities.

These results led to the concept of a complete dichotomy of immunity into two cell series, plasmacytic and lymphocytic, which respectively control the development of humoral and cellular immunity (Warner et al. 1962; Warner 1967).

Evidence of this dissociation of immunity is also to be seen in studies on the immunocompetence of primary lymphoid organs themselves.

Thus, whereas the thymus contains many cells competent for inducing graft-*versus*-host reactions (Warner 1964), the bursa is relatively incompetent in this regard (Warner 1965; Cain et al. 1967). Bursal cell suspensions contain more plasma cells and higher natural antibody levels than do thymic cell suspensions (Warner 1965) and, as previously discussed, contain antigen-reactive cells to at least some antigens (Gilmour et al. 1970).

The concept of a dichotomy of immune responses has been fully confirmed by various groups and is also clearly evident in many clinical syndromes involving depression of the immune response (see review, Cooper et al. 1967). Lischner and di George (1969), however, have recently questioned the validity of a complete dissociation between cellular and humoral immunity in thymic agenesis in man. It was claimed that in *complete* agenesis of the thymus all antibody-producing capacity was depressed as well as the cellular immune response.

Various recent studies have stressed that dissociation of immunity is an absolute qualitative phenomenon at least as regards immunoglobulin synthesis *versus* cell mediated immunity (Warner et al. 1969). The essential questions still to be answered concern the interaction of cell types in immune responses (see Section V). In the current terminology of 'T' and 'B' cells (Roitt et al. 1969) for the thymus-dependent and independent components of the immune response, it is often considered that 'B' represents the bone marrow-derived cells involved in the direct lineage of the antibody-forming cells (Mitchell and Miller 1968). However, as 'T' cells may also be originally bone marrow-derived (from haemopoietic stem cells), 'B' should be thought of as representing the bursal equivalent component in mammals which involves induction of stem cells to potential immunoglobulin synthesis. The basic questions concerning the nature of cells in collaboration for immune responses include:

(i) What is the source of 'B' cells in mammals?

(ii) Do 'B' cells carry antibody specificity (v gene expression)?

(iii) In cellular immunity do 'T' cells collaborate with 'T' cells, and if so, are they both of the same or different type?

(iv) Are there true thymus-independent antibody responses which do not involve 'T' cells?

(v) If so, does antigen directly stimulate a 'B' cell or can 'B' cells interact with each other?

(vi) In chickens, the precise relation of Thymic and Bursal cells to 'T' and 'B' interactions must still be demonstrated.

17.4.6. *Mammalian equivalents of the bursa of Fabricius*

Before the question of possible cell interactions in thymus-independent systems can be evaluated, the source of induction of immunoglobulin gene activation in mammals (bursal equivalent) must first be determined. There are two basic alternatives, in that either the mammalian thymus has incorporated both the avian thymus and bursal functions (cf. Lischner and di George 1969), or, that a separate bursal equivalent site does exist in mammals.

Neonatally thymectomized, and adult thymectomized, irradiated, bone marrow-protected mice, show no evidence of depression of immunoglobulin synthesis. Furthermore, recent studies with immunoglobulin allotypic markers have shown that the 'B' line of cells is the direct progenitor of the antibody-producing cells in cell collaboration experiments (Jacobson et al. 1970). These results strongly indicate that the mammalian thymus has not assumed the bursal function of induction of immunoglobulin synthesis. In searching for a mammalian bursal equivalent there are two essential components or functions of the avian bursa to be considered, (i) the production of an inducer (bursal hormone?) for differentiation to immunoglobulin synthesis, and (ii) the actual site of action of this inducer on the haemopoietic stem cell. In chickens both these events appear to occur within the bursa, but in mammals they may be separated. There is no direct evidence at present to support the view that the bone marrow fulfils both these criteria. It has been claimed that the bone marrow contains antigen-reactive cells (Singhal and Richter 1968; Armstrong et al. 1969; Singhal and Wigzell 1970), although other studies with rabbits (Abdou and Richter 1970) introduce the possibility that these cells, like those in the *sacculus rotundus*, may be more advanced and be actual antibody-forming cells derived from some cross-antigenic stimulation. Immunoglobulin synthesis by foetal bone marrow cells has been directly demonstrated in one study (Matsen et al. 1967).

The other main view of bursal equivalents was first proposed by Cooper et al. (1966) and holds that haemopoietic stem cells migrate to lympho-epithelial tissues in the gastro-intestinal tract for differentiation to immunoglobulin synthesis. It was first thought that appendix fulfilled this role (Archer et al. 1964) and although some suppression of antibody formation occurred after appendectomy, the results were not very striking (Sutherland et al. 1964, 1965; Konda and Harris 1966). The tonsils were also briefly considered for this role on the basis of clinical studies with certain immunoglobulin deficiency syndromes (Peterson et al. 1965).

Most of the recent experimental data in rabbits points towards a central role of the Peyer's patch lymphoid tissue (Cooper et al. 1966, 1968; Perey et al. 1968). In reviewing this data Cooper et al. (1970) have listed a series of similarities between bursa and Peyer's patch tissues, which include thymus independent development (Matsaniotis et al. 1966) and high mitotic activity (Meuwissen et al. 1968). Several of the other proposed similarities, such as antigen-independent development, source of plasma cell precursors and being a relatively aloof site from execution of antibody responses *in vivo,* are by no means certain and various studies indicate that the Peyer's patches do not fulfil these criteria. The key evidence that the Peyer's patches are both sites for the receipt of haemopoietic stem cells and of first immunoglobulin synthesis *in utero,* are totally lacking. In fact, in studies with chromosome-marked transfused bone marrow cells, the pattern of cellular repopulation of the Peyer's patches resembled lymph nodes and not thymus (Evans et al. 1967). Furthermore, when fragments of Peyer's patch tissue from newborn mice were cultured *in vitro* with ^{14}C-labelled amino acids, no immunoglobulin synthesis was detected unless the donor was at least 2 weeks of age (Warner and Moore 1969). Mesenteric lymph nodes however showed some synthetic activity around 3–5 days of age. Fichtelius (1967) has suggested that the entire epithelium in chondrosteans and the epithelium covering the Peyer's patches in mammals may act as bursal epithelium. In considering the immunoglobulin synthesis data in newborn mice Warner and Moore (1969) have proposed that although the epithelium may act in this fashion, the actual act of induction of differentiation in stem cells does not occur in this site, but occurs in other sites of stem cell location which the factor may reach *via* blood or lymphatic drainage, for example, the mesenteric lymph nodes.

Further precise definition of the mammalian bursal equivalent must be made, and should involve studies on the potential of 'bursal candidates' to synthesize immunoglobulin and to collaborate with thymic cells in inducing antibody formation. Various mammalian species must also be carefully examined, as it may turn out that Peyer's patch, *sacculus rotundus* and appendix all function in a bursal manner in rabbits, but perhaps not in mice or other species.

17.4.7.   *Immunoglobulin-gene expression in differentiation*

Synthesis of immunoglobulin molecules by a cell is an absolute proof of the immunocompetent or immunocyte differentiation state of the cell. Classical antibody-secreting cells are unquestionably well differentiated members of the plasmacytic series. At the electron microscopic level they are clearly primarily concerned with protein synthesis and secretion (de Petris et al. 1963; Bosman et al. 1969).

This stage has been reached in a gradual process, and by tracing back the lineage to a cell with the earliest detectable expression of immunoglobulin synthesis, one would identify the first site of induction of immunocompetent cell differentiation. This is based on the concept that the antigen-recognition cell or immunocompetent cell which has not yet been stimulated by antigen, nevertheless carries a specific antibody-like surface receptor which will permit its specific union with antigen (Mitchison 1968).

Considerable interest has recently developed in identifying the nature of the receptor site on immunocompetent cells which interact with antigen. Direct visualization of the interaction between normal lymphoid cells and antigen has been made possible by two techniques, the rosette-forming cell method and the antigen-binding cell method. Naor and Sulitzeanu (1967), Byrt and Ada (1969), and Humphrey and Keller (1970) have demonstrated that lymphoid cell suspensions from mice contain a small proportion of cells which avidly react with ^{125}I-labelled protein antigens. Although cell types such as macrophages and polymorphs show labelling, electron microscopic studies have confirmed that a proportion of small lymphocyte-like cells also directly bind labelled antigen (Mandel et al. 1969). The antigen appears to bind preferentially to certain localized areas of the cell membrane, rather than uniformly over the entire surface (Mandel et al. 1969), in similar fashion to the patchy distribution of H-2 antigen (Aoki et al. 1969) on lymphocytes. Antigen-binding lymphocytes are also present in the blood of normal adults (Dwyer and Mackay 1969) but not of agammaglobulinaemic patients (Naor et al. 1969). As these cells are also found in embryonic bursa (Dwyer and Warner 1971), it appears at present that only the 'B' cells are capable of giving this reaction. Further studies with appropriate cell surface markers of 'T' and 'B' cells such as theta (Reif and Allen 1964; Raff 1969; Schlesinger and Yron 1969) and PC-1 (Old et al. 1970) respectively, are clearly needed to confirm this view.

Pretreatment of normal lymphoid cell suspensions with specific rabbit anti-mouse immunoglobulin sera prior to application of the labelled antigen, has shown that antibodies to either L chains or μ chains will completely prevent uptake of labelled antigen (Warner et al. 1970; Ada et al. 1970). Antibodies to γ_2, γ_1 and α chains were without effect in this regard.

It therefore appears that a surface-bound IgM molecule acts as the receptor site for antigen on unprimed normal lymphoid cells. This is clearly consistent with the observation that bursal cells first synthesize IgM immunoglobulin. Studies with malignant populations of lymphoid cells have also shown the presence of surface IgM on Burkitt lymphoma cells (Klein et al. 1967), chronic lymphatic leukaemic cells (Johansson and Klein 1970) and certain lymphoid leukaemia cells in mice (Warner 1970). These latter cases may therefore represent the malignant counterparts of the normal lymphoid population of cells which are not active antibody-secreting cells, but have sufficient immunoglobulin gene synthesis to produce some surface-bound immunoglobulin. Whether this surface-bound IgM protein is in the normal 19S polymeric form, or exists as the 7S subunit remains to be determined.

Antigen-binding lymphoid cells specific for antigens on sheep erythrocytes have been identified by the rosette technique (Zaalberg 1964; Nota et al. 1964). Although this technique measures antibody-secreting cells, a certain proportion of minimally or non-secreting lymphoid cells also give rosette formation. With lymphoid cells from non-immunized mice, it is not at present clear whether only 'B' cells, or both 'T' and 'B' cells are measured by this technique. Anti-θ serum has been claimed to suppress rosettes in one study with non-immune cells (Greaves and Hogg 1970), but to be without effect in another study (Schlesinger 1970). Inhibition of rosettes with anti-lymphocyte sera and cells from normal mice, does however validate their classification as lymphocytes (Bach and Antoine 1968).

Further clarification of this point is badly needed. The nature of the immunoglobulin receptor on rosette-forming cells from unimmunized animals is also still to be fully clarified. Anti-Fab sera do cause complete inhibition, but the nature of the heavy chain type (if present) is still uncertain (Greaves and Hogg 1970).

A variety of techniques have demonstrated the presence of immunoglobulins on the surface of mouse lymphoid cells (see reviews Sell and Asofsky 1968; Greaves 1970). These include immunofluorescence (Raff et al. 1970), mixed antiglobulin reactions (Coombs et al. 1970), cell electrophoresis (Bert et al. 1969), immuno-electron microscopy (Hammond and Kline 1970), enzymatic methods (Sercarz and Modabber 1968) and immunoautoradiography (Raff et al. 1970; Bankhurst et al. 1971).

These, and other techniques such as antiglobulin-induced stimulation of lymphocytes (Sell and Asofsky 1968; Sell et al. 1970), are all liable to the problem of detecting cytophilic immunoglobulin binding on the surface of normal lymphoid cells. Indeed several unusual findings which are currently interpreted as indicating the presence of multiple H-chain classes or allotypes on cells (Sell et al. 1970; Greaves 1970) might conceivably be caused by such a phenomenon. Although it is generally considered that lymphocytes do not carry immunoglobulin cytophilic receptors, some recent studies throw considerable caution in accepting this conclusion (Uhr 1965; Nussenzweig et al. 1971; Coulson et al. 1967; Basten et al. 1970). In a recent study with purified mouse thoracic duct cells, Basten et al. (1970) have shown the 'production' of antigen-binding cells by passive treatment of normal cells with an IgG fraction of a mouse antiserum. Further work on all methods of identifying antigen-binding cells must rigorously examine for the detection of cytophilic binding.

That the antigen binding technique of Ada and Byrt does not involve passive antibody binding, is indicated by the inactivation of immune responsiveness to a specific antigen, when normal lymphoid cells are incubated with heavily radiolabelled flagella antigen (Ada and Byrt 1969). Immune responsiveness to other unlabelled antigens was not abolished. This has also been confirmed by Humphrey and Keller (1970) using haemocyanin and a synthetic amino acid copolymer antigen.

The fundamental question of the possible presence of immunoglobulin receptors on 'T' cells has still to be fully answered.* Greaves et al. (1970) have shown that specific anti-light chain or anti-Fab sera will inhibit the lymphocyte proliferative response induced by tuberculin and HL-A antigens. Mason and Warner (1970) have shown that pretreatment of normal mouse spleen cells with specific rabbit anti-mouse light chain sera will abolish the capacity of these cells to induce graft-*versus*-host reactions. This inhibitory activity of the antiserum is specific, in that it can be removed by absorption with purified light chains, and no inhibition of the haemopoietic stem cell activity of the spleen cell suspension is observed with the serum treatment. The inhibitory effect was not found with pretreatment of spleen cells by any of the known anti-heavy chain sera. These results therefore indicate the possibility that the graft-*versus*-host reactive immunocompetent cells do carry surface light chains, possibly without expressing a heavy chain gene. An alternative possibility, that a known heavy chain is combined with the light chain, but is held deeper in the cell membrane (Greaves 1970), is rendered somewhat unlikely in view of the complete inability to detect heavy chain synthesis in cultures of spleens from agammaglobulinaemic bursaless chickens (Warner et al. 1969) which can nevertheless initiate normal cellular immune responses (Szenberg and Warner 1967). The third possibility, that a new immunoglobulin, 'IgX', is involved in the 'T' cell receptor site must also be considered a major possibility.

The mechanism of immune suppression by anti-L chain pretreatment probably involves clearance in the liver, of the opsonized spleen cells, as preliminary studies with chromium-labelled cells have shown a marked liver uptake of injected cells which were pretreated with anti-light chain sera (Sprent et al. 1970). In parallel fashion to the studies

---

* Recent studies have now directly demonstrated immunoglobulin components on the surface of 'T' cells. This subject is extensively discussed in another review (Warner 1971b).

with malignant lymphomas carrying surface IgM receptors, it may also be possible to approach the question of surface immunoglobulin on 'T' cells, by examining thymomas or thymus-derived lymphomas for immunoglobulin synthesis. In preliminary studies (Warner 1971c), free light chain synthesis without heavy chain synthesis, was detected *in vitro* with several mouse lymphomas. This may indicate the true state of the appropriate non-malignant cell, or be a further example of change in immunoglobulin synthesis, with serial tumour transplantation, leading to free light chain synthesis as is frequently observed with plasma cell tumours (Coffino et al. 1970; Warner 1970b).

Further work in this area must involve a clear delineation of the nature of the immunoglobulin synthesized by lymphoid cells from non-immunized animals, and must be correlated with cell surface markers to identify the type of lymphoid cell concerned (for example, θ, LyA, LyB for 'T' cells, PC-1 for 'B' cells).

17.5. *Antigen-induced differentiation of immunocytes*

The continued proliferation and differentiation of the immunocompetent cell is dependent upon antigenic stimulation. Many factors enter into this process, each of which is in itself a major topic well beyond the scope of this chapter, and many are covered in other chapters of this book. These factors include the role of macrophage processing, the form and type of antigenic presentation (dose, adjuvant, size, route etc.), the presence or absence of pre-existing specific antibody and various other factors.

Recent studies have indicated that one of the main events involved after antigenic stimulation, is the phenomenon of cell collaboration, which for many antibody responses (if not all) is an obligatory step, if the antibody response is to develop.

This section will therefore be restricted to a brief summary of the effects of antigen on both the 'T' and 'B' cell lines, as regards their essential collaboration to initiate the final stage of antibody secretion.

17.5.1. *Cell collaboration in antibody formation*

It is now well established that the primary immune response to various antigens requires the interaction of two lymphoid cell types, one derived from the thymus and one from the bone marrow. The first reports of collaboration involved the direct use of thymus cell suspensions with bone marrow cells. Claman et al. (1966) showed that combinations of thymus and bone marrow, but neither alone, would transfer the ability to irradiated recipients, to make anti-sheep erythrocyte antibody. Miller and Mitchell (1968) then showed that thymus cell suspensions would restore antisheep red cell antibody-forming capacity to neonatally thymectomized mice. Thymus cells were as effective as thoracic duct cells in this system. Previous studies with irradiated recipients given thymus cells or grafts had shown that thymus cells responded to antigenic stimulation with a burst of mitotic activity (Davies et al. 1966). but did not appear to be capable of producing antibody (Davies et al. 1967). By means of a chromosome marker method, it was then directly shown that all the antibody-forming cells produced in thymus-bone marrow collaboration, were indeed direct progeny of the bone marrow and not the thymus cell population (Nossal et al. 1968). Restoration of antibody-forming capacity could be achieved in adult thymectomized, lethally irradiated mice which were protected with bone marrow and given thoracic duct lymphocytes. When the lymphocytes were obtained from a semi-allogeneic donor, it was again shown by the use of anti-H2 sera, that the antibody-forming cells were mainly of bone marrow origin and not of thoracic duct derivation (Mitchell and Miller 1968a).

A modified system of cell collaboration involved the use of thymus-derived cells collaborating with bone marrow cells. When thymic cells and antigen are injected into lethally irradiated recipients, proliferation of thymic cells occurs (Davies et al. 1966; Miller and Mitchell 1969). When spleens of these animals are then taken 5–7 days later and combined with normal bone marrow cells and the antigen, excellent collaboration for antibody production occurs (Mitchell and Miller 1968b; Miller 1971). This is an antigen-specific phenomenon and the same antigen must be given on both occasions. Shearer and Cudkowicz (1969) using this two-step design, have shown that thymus, but not bone marrow, contains antigen-reactive cells (ARC) capable of initiating the immune response to sheep red cells. The thymic ARC proliferate in response to the antigen and these thymus derived cells, which were termed specific inducer cells (Shearer and Cudkowicz 1969) then interact with the marrow precursors of plaque-forming cells to initiate the antibody-forming clone. It was estimated that each ARC generated 80–800 inducer cells in four days by way of a minimum of 6–10 divisions.

In the two step experiments of Miller (1971) it is clear that 'antigen-educated' thymus-derived cells are far more competent to collaborate with bone marrow cells than are thymocytes themselves. It is not clear at present whether this represents a quantitative or a qualitative difference between 'T' cells from the thymus *versus* the antigen-educated thymus-derived cells. The population of spleen cells containing the antigen-educated thymus-derived cells would contain a far higher proportion of antigen-specific cells and accordingly the same *absolute* number of thymic antigen-specific cells may be found, for example, in 50 million thymocytes and in only 5 million educated thymic cell suspensions. An alternative possibility is that the thymus-derived cell may now be qualitatively more efficient, in perhaps possessing an antigen-specific receptor of high affinity, analogous to the development of higher affinity antibody populations in *in vivo* immunizations (Steiner and Eisen 1967). Further studies on this aspect are in progress.

These experiments clearly demonstrate that the thymus-derived cell which proliferates in response to antigen, does carry a receptor site specific for antigen. Further evidence for the antigen specificity of the thymus-derived cell comes from experiments with tolerant mice. If adult mice are rendered tolerant to sheep red blood cells, their thoracic duct lymphocytes are no longer capable of collaborating with normal bone marrow-derived cells to produce a specific antibody response (Miller and Mitchell 1970). In this experiment, thymus cells from tolerant donors were still as effective at collaborating with bone marrow cells as were normal thymic cells. This may only indicate that the state of tolerance to the sheep red cell antigen did not exist at the thymic lymphocyte level, perhaps because of insufficient penetration in the thymus of the antigen concerned. Using a soluble protein antigen of the type known to be capable of inducing tolerance at the thymic cell level (Isaković et al. 1965; Taylor 1968), Chiller et al. (1970) were able to demonstrate that thymus cells from mice tolerant to human γ-globulin were incapable of collaborating with normal bone marrow cells.

These results on tolerance, and the experiments on antigen specificity of the thymus derived cell collaboration, indicate that the thymic 'T' cell lineage, carries a surface receptor site which is antigen-specific, and is accordingly most likely to at least involve the variable region of an immunoglobulin polypeptide chain. At the present time no direct data on the immunoglobulin nature of the receptor site on these collaborating 'T' cells is available. Experiments are now in progress to elucidate this point (see Warner 1971b).

The possible nature and antigenic specificity of the receptor site in the 'B' cell compartment is at present still unclear. Using the same approaches as described above for the 'T' cells, bone marrow derived cells on transfer to irradiated recipients with antigen did not show any evidence of containing antigen-reactive cells capable of initiating a response to sheep erythrocytes (Shearer and Cudkowicz 1969). Quantitative changes in the 'B' cell compartment may however have occurred.

Taylor (1968, 1969) was unable to demonstrate tolerance in the bone marrow compartment with bovine serum albumin as the antigen. Similarly Miller and Mitchell (1970) could find no evidence for 'B' line tolerance to sheep erythrocytes, when bone marrow cells from tolerant donors were interacted with normal thymus cells and transferred to irradiated recipients. In preliminary studies with sheep erythrocyte tolerant mice, Playfair (1969) has claimed to show tolerance at the bone marrow cell level. Unfortunately a series of essential controls are lacking from these experiments (see Miller and Mitchell 1970) and it is accordingly difficult to conclude that the data do show tolerance at the bone marrow level. Bone marrow cells from mice tolerant to human γ-globulin were found to be incapable of collaborating with normal thymus cells for the initiation of an antibody response (Chiller et al. 1970).

At the present time it is somewhat difficult to be dogmatic about a statement on the antibody specificity of the bone marrow cell. The experiments of Chiller et al. do seem to clearly indicate that tolerance can be induced at the 'B' cell level. This work involves a high zone tolerance with a diffusible antigen, whereas the study of Miller and Mitchell (1970) involves a cyclophosphamide-induced tolerance to red cells. It may well be that the mechanism of tolerance induction in this latter system specifically involves deletion of the thymus-derived cells without affecting the bone marrow cell population.

A direct interaction of bone marrow cells with antigen has been demonstrated in several other assay systems. Laskov (1968) has shown that marrow cells of unprimed mice form rosettes *in vitro* with sheep erythrocytes. Normal bone marrow cells from rabbits have been shown to proliferate on direct challenge with antigen (Singhal and Richter 1968; Singhal et al. 1968). Specific removal of these cells on antigen-coated bead columns indicates the presence of preformed antibody molecules on the outer surface of this cell population (Singhal and Wigzell 1970). Induction of a specific state of unresponsiveness to antigen has also been produced *in vitro* with normal rabbit bone marrow cells (Singhal and Wigzell 1970). In contrast to these studies, Byrt and Ada (1969) found in mouse bone marrow a very high proportion of cells capable of binding ^{125}I-labelled antigen. However, unlike the antigen-binding cells in spleen, the uptake of antigen by bone marrow cells could not be blocked by anti-immunoglobulin pretreatment. Some doubt on the inherent specificity of 'B' line cells still exists, and again it must be emphasized that different species may well behave differently in this regard.

Cell collaboration, although only recently recognized, has been shown to be involved in the well-studied phenomenon of carrier specificity in anti-hapten antibody responses (Ovary and Benacerraf 1963). Mitchison (1968a), using a cell transfer system, has described an antigen-focusing effect of carrier-specific cells in inducing anti-hapten cells to antibody formation. Mice were immunized with the conjugate nitro-iodophenacetyl-ovalbumin (NIP-OA) and their spleen cells were transferred to irradiated recipients. These failed to produce anti-NIP antibody in response to NIP-BSA, but did so, if they were simultaneously given spleen cells from mice immune to BSA. Mitchison (1968b) has also dissociated this co-operative function of the anti-BSA cells from their ability to produce anti-BSA antibody, in that the co-operative function reached a peak much earlier after primary immunization than did actual antibody formation.

A direct link between the observations on hapten-carrier recognition, and thymus-bone marrow interaction has recently been made by Miller (1971). Spleen cells from mice primed with dinitro-phenacetyl-ovalbumin (NNP-OA), failed to react on transfer to irradiated recipients when challenged with NNP on chicken γ-globulin (NNP-CG). However if the spleen cells were combined *in vitro* with thymus-derived cells from spleens of irradiated mice given thymic cells and chicken γ-globulin, a marked anti-hapten response occurred.

That the hapten-carrier effect has its basis in cell collaboration, has led to the proposal that the 'T' cell, by virtue of a cell surface bound antibody-like receptor, traps antigen at a critical site where it can more readily stimulate the hapten-specific antibody precursor 'B' cell (Mitchison 1968a, 1969). This implies that the tolerant 'T' cell is incapable of collaborating, by virtue of its inability to bind antigen on its surface. In a recent study (Miller et al. 1971a), this concept has been seriously questioned, and a more active role of the 'T' cell implied. The experiments involved attaching a specific antigen to the surface of the tolerant cell. Normal thoracic duct cells treated *in vitro* with a chicken anti-mouse lymphocyte globulin, collaborated with normal bone marrow cells to produce an anti-chicken γ-globulin response. Thoracic duct cells from mice previously rendered tolerant to chicken γ-globulin were incapable of this collaboration, even when directly coated with chicken γ-globulin, by the chicken anti-mouse lymphocyte globulin. In this system, tolerant 'T' cells are therefore shown to be incapable of 'antigen focusing', even though they do carry the antigen on their surface. An active participation of the 'T' cell is indicated. The fact that tolerant 'T' cells do not collaborate, with 'B' cells, seems to indicate that 'T' cell action does not occur through either non-specific provision of nucleosides, or by providing non-specific antigen precursors of macrophages. The experiment on antigen-coated tolerant cells indicates that the 'T' cell also does not act merely as an antigen-coated particle which 'focuses' hapten determinants on the 'B' cell. The possibility of information transfer for antibody specificity has not been strictly eliminated, and must still be considered as a possible mechanism. It is clear from allotype (Jacobson et al. 1970) and immunoglobulin class studies (Cudkowicz et al. 1969), that the constant region of the immunoglobulin molecule that is produced in the antibody response is determined by the 'B' cell line. If information transfer is involved, it can therefore only involve the variable specificity region of the antibody molecule.

17.5.2. *Cell collaboration in cellular immunity*

Attempts to demonstrate collaboration between thymic and bone marrow cells for the induction of graft-*versus*-host reactivity have uniformly failed to demonstrate any collaboration (Cole and Davis 1968; Stuttman and Good 1969). No evidence of collaboration was found between foetal liver and either adult or foetal thymus (Tyan 1969; Tyan and Cole 1966). In recent studies with the killer cell assay against tumour cells bearing foreign H-2 antigens, Miller et al. (1971) could find no evidence for collaboration between thymus- and non-thymus-derived cells. Such a collaboration is inherently unlikely, as thymus cell suspensions themselves are very competent for inducing graft-*versus*-host reactivity (Cohen et al. 1963; Warner 1964). The possibility however exists, that collaboration between two cell types within the thymus may occur. This possibility receives considerable support from recent studies of Cantor et al. (1970) and Cantor and Asofsky (1970). Using graft-*versus*-host reactions in mice, with spleen cells from young and old NZB mice it was found that mixtures of the two cell populations, neither of which alone produced a reaction, were competent in inducing a response. Synergistic responses were also observed with mixtures of thymus and spleen from young BALB/c mice. Changes in the ratio between the two cell populations greatly affected the degree of response, and the results clearly seem to indicate that both populations were interacting to result in an increased level of competence, much greater than could be accounted for merely by an additive response. The data also show that both populations must have the genetic disposition to mount the graft-*versus*-host reaction.

Further studies in the area of possible collaboration in cellular immunity, as it applies to transplantation immunity and delayed hypersensitivity are clearly warranted. The striking carrier specificity of all delayed hypersensitivity responses, clearly argues for the possibility of an essential cell collaboration in mediating the response. Cell collaboration may also be of considerable importance in developing an immune response to weak tumour antigens, and some preliminary studies (Colnaghi et al. 1970) have indicated that the additional presence of another antigen, such as H-2, may more readily lead to a tumour-specific immune response, perhaps through a hapten-carrier type of cell collaboration.

References

ABDOU, N. I. and M. RICHTER, 1970, J. Immunol. *104*, 1087.

ABEL, C. A. and H. M. GREY, 1968, Biochemistry 7, 2682.

ACKERMAN, G. A., 1962, J. Cell Biol. *13*, 127.

ACKERMAN, G. A. and R. A. KNOUFF, 1959, Am. J. Anat. *104*, 163.

ACKERMAN, G. A. and R. A. KNOUFF, 1963, Anat. Record *146*, 23.

ACKERMAN, G. A. and R. A. KNOUFF, 1964, Lymphocytopoietic activity in the bursa of Fabricius. *In*: R. A. Good and A. E. Gabrielsen, eds.: The thymus in immunobiology. New York, Hoeber-Harper. pp. 123–146.

ADA, G. L. and P. BYRT, 1969, Nature *222*, 1291.

ADA, G. L., P. BYRT, T. MANDEL and N. L. WARNER, *in*: J. Sterzl, ed.: Developmental aspects of antibody formation and structure. Prague, in press.

AOKI, T., V. HAMMERLING, E. DE HARVEN, E. A. BOYSE and L. J. OLD, 1969, J. Exptl. Med. *130*, 979.

ARCHER, O. K., D. E. R. SUTHERLAND and R. A. GOOD, 1964, Lab. Invest. *13*, 259.

ARMSTRONG, W. D. and E. DIENER, 1968, J. Exptl. Med. *129*, 371.

ARMSTRONG, W. D., E. DIENER and G. SHELLAM, 1969, J. Exptl. Med. *129*, 393.

ARNASON, B. G., B. D. JANKOVIC, B. H. WAKSMAN and C. WENNERSTEIN, 1962, J. Exptl. Med. *116*, 177.

ARNASON, B. G., B. D. JANKOVIC and B. H. WAKSMAN, 1964a, The role of the thymus in immune reactions in rats. *In*: R. A. Good and A. E. Gabrielsen, eds.: The thymus in immunobiology. New York, Hoeber-Harper. pp. 492–501.

ARNASON, B. G., S. T. DE VAUX, C. CYR and J. B. SHAFFNER, 1964b, J. Immunol. *93*, 915.

ASPINALL, R. L., R. K. MEYER, M. A. GRAETZER and H. E. WOLFE, 1963, J. Immunol. *90*, 872.

AUERBACH, R., 1961, Develop. Biol. *3*, 336.

AUERBACH, R., 1965, Experimental analysis of lymphoid differentiation in the mammalian thymus and spleen. *In*: R. L. de Haan and H. Ursprung, eds.: Organogenesis. New York, Holt, Rinehart and Winston. p. 539.

AUERBACH, R., 1970, *in*: J. Sterzl, ed.: Developmental aspects of antibody formation and structure. Prague, in press.

AUERBACH, R. and L. N. RUBEN, 1969, personal communication.

BACH, J. F. and B. ANTOINE, 1968, Nature *217*, 658.

BACULI, B. S. and E. L. COOPER, 1968, J. Morphol. *126*, 463.

BANG, F. B., 1967, Federation Proc. *26*, 1680.

BANKHURST, A. and N. L. WARNER, 1971, J. Immunol., in press.

BARKER, C. F. and R. E. BILLINGHAM, 1967, Transplantation *5*, 962.

BASTEN, T., N. L. WARNER and J. F. A. P. MILLER, 1970, unpublished observations.

BAZIN, H. and J. F. DUPLAN, 1966, Rev. Franc. d'Etudes Clin. et Biol. *11*, 987.

BERNARDI, G. and J. COMSA, 1965, Experientia *21*, 416.

BERT, G., A. L. MASSARO, D. L. DI COSSANO and M. MAJA, 1969, Immunology *17*, 1.

BOFFA, G. A., J. M. FINE, A. DULHON and P. AMOUCH, 1967, Nature *214*, 700.

BOSMAN, C., J. D. FELDMAN and E. PICK, 1969, J. Exptl. Med. *129*, 1029.

BOYER, G. S., 1960, Nature *185*, 327.

BRAUN, W. and M. NAKANO, 1967, Science *157*, 819.

BURNET, F. M., 1967, Cold Spring Harbor Symp. Quant. Biol. *32*, 1.

BURNET, F. M., 1968, Nature *218*, 426.

BYRT, P. and G. L. ADA, 1969, Immunology *17*, 503.

CAIN, W. A., W. P. WEIDANZ and M. D. COOPER, 1967, Federation Proc. *26*, 571.

CAMERON, G. R., 1934, J. Pathol. Bacteriol. *38*, 44.

CANTOR, H. and R. ASOFSKY, 1970, J. Exptl. Med. *131*, 235.

CANTOR, H., R. ASOFSKY and N. TALAL, 1970, J. Exptl. Med. *131*, 223.

CHADWICK, J. S., 1967, Federation Proc. *26*, 1675.

CHANG, T. S., M. S. RHEINS and A. R. WINTER, 1957, Poultry Sci., *36*, 735.

CHILLER, J. M., G. S. HABICHT and W. O. WEIGLE, 1970, Proc. Natl. Acad. Sci. U.S. *65*, 551.

CHILLER, J. M., H. O. HODGINS and R. S. WEISER, 1969, J. Immunol. *102*, 1202.

CHING, Y. C. and R. J. WEDGWOOD, 1967, J. Immunol. *99*, 191.

CLAFLIN, A. J., O. SMITHIES and R. K. MEYER, 1966, J. Immunol. *97*, 693.

CLAMAN, H. N., E. A. CHAPERON and R. F. TRIPLETT, 1966, J. Immunol. *97*, 828.

CLARK, S. L., JR., 1963, Am. J. Anat. *112*, 1.

CLARK, S. L., JR., 1964, The penetration of protein and colloidal materials into the thymus from the blood stream. *In*: V. Defendi and D. Metcalf, eds.: The thymus, Wistar Inst. Symp. Monog. No. 2. Philadelphia, Wistar Inst. Press. pp. 9–31.

CLARK, S. L., JR., 1966, Cytological evidences of secretion in the thymus. *In*: G. E. W. Wolstenholme and R. Porter, eds.: Ciba Found. Symp, The thymus. London, Churchill. pp. 3–30.

CLARK, S. L., JR., 1968, J. Exptl. Med. *128*, 927.

CLAUSON, C. C., M. D. COOPER and R. A. GOOD, 1967, Lab. Invest. *16*, 407.

CLAUSON, C. C., J. FINSTAD and R. A. GOOD, 1966, Lab. Invest. *15*, 1830.

CLEM, L. W. and M. M. SIGEL, 1966, Immunological and immunochemical studies on holostean and marine teleost fishes immunized with bovine serum albumin. *In*: R. T. Smith, P. A. Miescher and R. A. Good, eds.: Phylogeny of immunity. Gainesville, Univ. of Florida Press. pp. 209–217.

CLEM, L. W. and P. A. SMALL, 1967, J. Exptl. Med. *125*, 893.

COFFINO, P., R. LASKOV and M. D. SCHARFF, 1970, Science *167*, 186.

COHEN, M. W., G. J. THORBECKE, G. M. HOCHWALD and E. B. JACOBSON, 1963, Proc. Soc. Exptl. Biol. Med. *114*, 242.

COLE, L. J. and W. E. DAVIS, 1968, Exptl. Hematol. *16*, 21.

COLNAGHI, M. J., G. DELLA-PORTA, M. BOROCCHI, G. CARBONE and S. MENARD, 1970, Abstr. 10th Int. Canc. Congr. Houston. p. 209.

COMSA, J., 1965, Am. J. Med. Sci. *250*, 113.

COOMBS, R. R. A., B. W. GURNER, C. A. JANEWAY, A. B. WILSON, P. G. H. GELL and A. S. KELUS, 1970, Immunology *18*, 417.

COOPER, E. L., 1969a, Natl. Cancer Inst. Monogr. *31*, 655.

COOPER, E. L., 1969b, Science *166*, 1414.

COOPER, E. L. and L. M. RUBLIOTTA, 1969, Transplantation *8*, 220.

COOPER, M. D., W. A. CAIN, P. VAN ALTEN and R. A. GOOD, 1969, Int. Arch. Allergy *35*, 242.

COOPER, M. D., A. E. GABRIELSEN and R. A. GOOD, 1967, Ann. Rev. Med. *18*, 113.

COOPER, M. D., P. W. KINCADE and A. R. LAWTON, 1970, *In*: B. M. Kagan and E. R. Stiehm, eds.: Immunologic incompetence. Chicago, Year Book Med. Publ., in press.

COOPER, M. D., D. Y. PEREY, M. F. MCKNEALLY, A. E. GABRIELSEN, D. E. R. SUTHERLAND and R. A. GOOD, 1966b, Lancet *i*, 1388.

COOPER, M. D., D. Y. PEREY, M. F. MCKNEALLY, A. E. GABRIELSEN, D. E. R. SUTHERLAND and R. A. GOOD, 1968, Int. Arch. Allergy, *33*, 6.

COOPER, M. D., R. D. A. PETERSON and R. A. GOOD, 1965, Nature *205*, 143.

COOPER, M. D., R. D. A. PETERSON, M. A. SOUTH and R. A. GOOD, 1966, J. Exptl. Med. *123*, 75.

COULSON, A. S., B. W. GURNER and R. R. A. COOMBS, 1967, Int. Arch. Allergy *32*, 264.

CRABBE, P. A., A. CARBONARA and J. F. HEREMANS, 1965, Lab. Invest. *14*, 235.

CUDKOWICZ, G., G. M. SHEARER and R. L. PRIORE, 1969, J. Exptl. Med. *130*, 481.

CUSHING, J. E., 1967, Federation Proc. *26*, 1666.

CUSHING, J. E., N. L. CALAPRICE and G. TRUMP, 1963, Biol. Bull. *125*, 69.

DALMASSO, A. P., C. MARTINEZ and R. A. GOOD, 1962, Proc. Soc. Exptl. Biol. Med. *110*, 205.

DAMESHEK, W., 1963, Blood *21*, 243.

DAVIES, A. J. S., E. LEUCHARS, V. WALLIS and P. C. KOLLER, 1966, Transplantation *4*, 438.

DAVIES, A. J. S., E. LEUCHARS, V. WALLIS, R. MARCHANT and E. V. ELLIOTT, 1967, Transplantation *5*, 222.

DENT, P. B. and R. A. GOOD, 1965, Nature *207*, 491.

DE PETRIS, S., G. KARLSBAD and B. PERNIS, 1963, J. Exptl. Med. *117*, 849.

DE SOMER, P., P. DENYS, JR. and R. LEYTEN, 1963, Life Sci. *11*, 810.

DIENER, E. and E. H. M. EALEY, 1965, Nature *208*, 950.

DIENER, E., E. H. M. EALEY and J. S. LEGGE, 1967, Immunology *13*, 339.

DIENER, E. and J. MARCHALONIS, 1970, Immunology, in press.

DIENER, E. and G. J. V. NOSSAL, 1966, Immunology *10*, 35.

DUBSAT, P., 1964, Compt. Rend. Acad. Sci. *259*, 4177.

DWYER, J. and I. R. MACKAY, 1970a, Lancet *i*, 164.

DWYER, J. and I. R. MACKAY, 1970b, Lancet *i*, 1199.

DWYER. J. and N. L. WARNER, 1971, Nature, New Biology *229*, 210.

ENGLE, R. L., JR., K. R. WOODS and J. H. PERT, 1958, J. Clin. Invest. *37*, 892.

EVANS, E. E., S. P. KENT, M. H. ATTLEBERGER, C. SEIBERT, R. E. BRYANT and B. BOOTH, 1965, Ann. N.Y. Acad. Sci. *126*, 629.

EVANS, E. E., S. P. KENT, R. E. BRYANT and M. MOYER, 1966, Antibody formation and immunological memory in the marine toad. *In*: R. T. Smith, P. A. Miescher and R. A. Good, eds.: Phylogeny of immunity. Gainesville, Univ. of Florida Press. pp. 218–226.

EVANS, E. P., D. A. OGDEN, C. E. FORD and H. S. MICKLEM, 1967, Nature *216*, 36.

EVANS, E. E., B. PAINTER, M. L. EVANS, P. WEINHEIMER and R. T. ACTON, 1968, Proc. Soc. Exptl. Biol. Med. *128*, 394.

FAHEY, J. L., W. F. BARTH and L. W. LAW, 1965, J. Natl. Cancer Inst. *35*, 663.

FAHEY, J. L., J. WUNDERLICK and R. MISHELL, 1964, J. Exptl. Med. *120*, 243.

FANGE, R., 1966, Comparative aspects of excretory and lymphoid tissue. *In*: R. T. Smith, P. A. Miescher and R. A. Good, eds.: Phylogeny of immunity. Gainesville, Univ. of Florida Press. pp. 141–145.

FAVOUR, C. B., 1958, Ann. N.Y. Acad. Sci. *73*, 590.

FENG, S. Y., 1967, Federation Proc. *26*, 1685.

FICHTELIUS, K. E., 1957, Trans. 6th Congr. Europ. Soc. Hematology. Basel, S. Karger. p. 10.

FICHTELIUS, K. E., 1967, Exptl. Cell Res. *46*, 231.

FIELD, E. O. and J. E. GIBBS, 1968, Nature *217*, 561.

FINSTAD, J. and R. A. GOOD, 1964, J. Exptl. Med. *120*, 1151.

FINSTAD, J. and R. A. GOOD, 1966, Phylogenetic studies of adaptive immune responses in the lower vertebrates. *In*: R. T. Smith, P. A. Miescher and R. A. Good, eds.: Phylogeny of immunity. Gainesville, Univ. of Florida Press. pp. 173–188.

FINSTAD, J., B. W. PAPERMASTER and R. A. GOOD, 1964, Lab. Invest. *13*, 490.

FISH, L. A., B. POLLARA and R. A. GOOD, 1966, Characterization of an immunoglobulin from the paddlefish (Polyodon spathula). *In*: R. T. Smith, P. A. Miescher and R. A. Good, eds.: Phylogeny of immunity. Gainesville, Univ. of Florida Press. pp. 99–104.

FISHER, B., E. R. FISHER, S. LEE and A. SAKAY, 1965, Transplantation *3*, 49.

FISHER, E. R. and B. FISHER, 1965, Transplantation *14*, 546.

FISHER, J. W., 1968, Ann. N.Y. Acad. Sci. *149*, 1.

FORD, C. E. and H. S. MICKLEM, 1963, Lancet *i*, 359.

FORD, C. E., H. S. MICKLEM, E. P. EVANS, J. G. GRAY and D. A. OGDEN, 1966, Ann. N.Y. Acad. Sci. *129*, 283.

FORD, C. E., H. S. MICKLEM and D. A. OGDEN, 1968, Lancet *i*, 621.

FREI, E., J. H. TIJO, J. WANG and P. P. CARBONE, 1964, Ann. N.Y. Acad. Sci. *113*, 1073.

FUDENBERG, H. H. and N. L. WARNER, 1970, Advan. Human Genetics *1*, 131.

FURTH, J., 1946, J. Gerontol. *11*, 46.

GILMOUR, D. G., G. A. THEIS and G. J. THORBECKE, 1970, J. Exptl. Med. *132*, 134.

GLICK, B., 1960, Poultry Sci. *39*, 1097.

GLICK, B., T. S. CHANG and R. G. JAAP, 1956, Poultry Sci. *35*, 224.

GLICK, B. and S. WHATLEY, 1967, Poultry Sci. *46*, 1587.

GLOBERSON, A. and R. AUERBACH, 1967, J. Exptl. Med. *126*, 223.

GOLDSCHNEIDER, I. and D. D. MCGREGOR, 1968, J. Exptl. Med. *127*, 155.

GOLDSTEIN, A. L., F. D. SLATER and A. WHITE, 1966, Proc. Natl. Acad. Sci. U.S. *56*, 1010.

GOLDSTEIN, A. L., Y. ASANUMA, J. R. BATTISTO, M. A. HARDY, J. QUINT and A. WHITE, 1970, J. Immunol. *104*, 359.

GOLDSTEIN, G. and I. R. MACKAY, 1969, The human thymus. London, Heinemann.

GOOD, R. A., A. P. DALMASSO, C. MARTINEZ, O. K. ARCHER, J. C. PIERCE and B. W. PAPER-MASTER, 1962, J. Exptl. Med. *116*, 773.

GOOD, R. A., J. FINSTAD, B. POLLARA and A. E. GABRIELSEN, 1966, Morphologic studies on the evolution of the lymphoid tissues among the lower vertebrates. *In*: R. T. Smith, P. A. Miescher and R. A. Good, eds.: Phylogeny of immunity. Gainesville, Univ. of Florida Press. pp. 149–168.

GOOD, R. A., A. E. GABRIELSEN, B. POLLARA, H. GEWARZ and J. FINSTAD, 1968, Phylogenetic development of the lymphoid tissue and immunologic capacity among the lower verte-brates. *In*: B. Cinader, ed.: Regulation of the antibody response. Springfield, Thomas. pp. 212–231.

GOOD, R. A. and B. W. PAPERMASTER, 1964, Advan. Immunol. *4*, 1.

GORDON, H. A., 1959, Ann. N.Y. Acad. Sci. *78*, 208.

GOWANS, J. L., 1964, The migration of lymphocytes into lymphoid tissue. *In*: R. A. Good and A. E. Gabrielsen, eds.: The thymus in immunobiology. New York, Hoeber-Harper. pp. 255–272.

GOWANS, J. L. and E. J. KNIGHT, 1964, Proc. Roy. Soc. *B. 195*, 275.

GOWANS, J. L. and D. D. MCGREGOR, 1965, Progr. Allergy *9*, 1.

GRAETZER, M. A., H. R. WOLFE, R. L. ASPINALL and R. I. C. MEYER, 1963, J. Immunol. *90*, 878.

GREAVES, M. F., 1970, Transplantation Rev. *5*, in press.

GREAVES, M. F. and N. M. HOGG, 1970, *in*: A. Cross, T. Kosunen and O. Mäkelä, eds.: Proceedings of the Third Sigrid Julius Symposium on Cell Co-operation in the Immune Response. New York, Academic Press, in press.

GREGOIRE, C. and C. DUCHATEAU, 1956, Arch. Biol. (Liège) *67*, 269.

GREY, H. M., 1966, *in*: R. T. Smith, P. A. Miescher and R. A. Good, eds.: Phylogeny of immunity. Gainesville, Univ. of Florida Press. p. 227.

GREY, H. M., 1967a, J. Immunol. *98*, 811.

GREY, H. M., 1967b, J. Immunol. *98*, 820.

GROSSI, C. E., V. GENTA, M. FERRARINI and D. ZACCHEO, 1968, Rev. Franc. d'Etudes. Clin. Biol. *5*, 497.

HAMMOND, E. and E. KLINE, 1970, Exptl. Cell Res., in press.

HAND, T., P. CASTER and T. D. LUCKEY, 1967, Biochem. Biophys. Res. Commun. *26*, 18.

HARRIS, J. E. and C. E. FORD, 1964, Nature *201*, 884.

HARSHBARGER, J. C., 1967, Federation Proc. *26*, 1693.

HAYS, E. F., 1967, Blood *29*, 29.

HERZENBERG, L. A., 1964, Cold Spring Harbor Symp. Quant. Biol. *29*, 455.

HILDEMANN, W. H. and R. HAAS, 1959, J. Immunol. *83*, 478.

HILDEMANN, W. H. and G. H. THOENES, 1969, Transplantation 7, 506.

HILL, R. L., R. DELANEY, R. E. FELLOWS, JR. and H. E. LEBOVITZ, 1966, Proc. Natl. Acad. Sci. U.S. 56, 1762.

HOOD, L. E., W. R. GRAY, B. G. SANDERS and W. J. DREYER, 1967, Cold Spring Harbor Symp. Quant. Biol. 32, 133.

HOSHINO, T., 1962, Exptl. Cell Res. 27, 615.

HOSHINO, T., 1963, Z. Zellforsch. 59, 513.

HUFF, C. G., 1940, Physiol. Rev. 20, 68.

HUMPHREY, J. H. and H. KELLER, 1970, *in*: J. Šterzl, ed.: Developmental aspects of antibody formation and structure. Prague, in press.

HUMPHREY, J. H., D. M. V. PARROTT and J. EAST, 1964, Immunology 7, 419.

ISAKOVIĆ, K., B. D. JANKOVIĆ, L. POPESKOVIĆ and D. MILOSEVIĆ, 1963, Nature 200, 273.

ISAKOVIĆ, K., S. B. SMITH and B. H. WAKSMAN, 1965, J. Exptl. Med. 122, 1103.

JACOBSON, E. B., J. L'AGE-STEHR and L. A. HERZENBERG, 1970, J. Exptl. Med. 131, 1109.

JANKOVIĆ, B. D., K. ISAKOVIĆ and J. HOWAT, 1967, Experientia 23, 1062.

JANKOVIĆ, B. D. and M. ISVANESKI, 1963, Int. Arch. Allergy 23, 188.

JANKOVIĆ, B. D., M. ISVANESKI L. POPESOVIĆ and K. MITROVIĆ, 1965, Int. Arch. Allergy 26, 18.

JANKOVIĆ, B. D. and S. LESKOWITZ, 1965, Proc. Soc. Exptl. Biol. Med. 118, 1164.

JERNE, N. K., 1970, Europ. J. Immunol. 1.

JERNE, N. K. and A. A. NORDIN, 1963, Science 140, 405.

JOHANSSON, B. and E. KLEIN, 1970, Clin. Exptl. Immunol. 6, 421.

KELLMAN, K. O. and M. GORDON, 1958, Ann. N.Y. Acad. Sci. 73, 599.

KANTOR, F. S. and J. F. A. P. MILLER, 1969, Unpublished observations.

KAPLAN, H. S., 1950, J. Natl. Cancer Inst. 11, 83.

KENNEDY, J. C., L. SIMINOVITCH, J. E. TILL and E. A. MCCOULLOCH, 1965, Proc. Soc. Exptl. Biol. Med. 120, 868.

KENNEDY, J. C., J. E. TILL, L. SIMINOVITCH and E. A. MCCULLOCH, 1966, J. Immunol. 96, 973.

KINCADE, P. W. and M. D. COOPER, 1970, Federation Proc. 29 (2), 1449.

KLEIN, E., G. KLEIN, J. S. NADKARNI, J. J. NADKARNI, H. WIGZELL and P. CLIFFORD, 1967, Lancet *ii*, 1068.

KLEIN, J. J., A. L. GOLDSTEIN and A. WHITE, 1965, Proc. Natl. Acad. Sci. U.S. 53, 812.

KONDA, S. and T. N. HARRIS, 1966, J. Immunol. 97, 805.

KUBO, R. T. and A. A. BENEDICT, 1968, Proc. Soc. Exptl. Biol. Med. Sci. 129, 256.

LASKOV, R., 1968, Nature 219, 973.

LAW, L. W., 1952, J. Natl. Cancer Inst. 12, 789.

LAW, L. W. and M. D. AGNEW, 1968, Proc. Soc. Exptl. Biol. Med. 127, 953.

LAWRENCE, H. S. and M. LANDY, eds., 1969, Mediators of cellular immunity. New York, Academic Press.

LESLIE, G. A. and L. W. CLEM, 1969, J. Exptl. Med. 130, 1337.

LEUCHARS, E., A. M. CROSS and A. DAVIES, 1964, Nature 203, 1189.

LEVEY, R. H., N. TRAININ and L. W. LAW, 1963, J. Natl. Cancer Inst. 31, 199.

LEWIS, J. P. and F. E. TROUBAUGH, 1964, Nature 204, 589.

LILIEN, J. E. and A. A. MOSCONA, 1967, Science 157, 70.

LIND, P. E., 1970, Int. Arch. Allergy 37, 258.

LINNA, J., 1967, Int. Arch. Allergy 31, 313.

LINNA, J. and J. STILLSTROM, 1966, Acta Pathol. Microbiol. Scand. 68, 465.

LISCHNER, H. W. and A. M. DI GEORGE, 1969, Lancet *ii*, 1044.

LYKAKIS, J. J., 1968, Immunology 14, 799.

MCKAY, D. and C. JENKIN, 1969, Immunology *17*, 127.

MANDEL, T., 1968, Aust. J. Exptl. Biol. *46*, 755.

MANDEL, T., 1970, Z. Zellforsch., in press.

MANDEL, T., P. BYRT and G. L. ADA, 1969, Exptl. Cell Res. *58*, 179.

MARCHALONIS, J. J., 1969, Aust. J. Exptl. Biol. Med. Sci. *47*, 405.

MARCHALONIS, J. J., E. H. M. EALEY and E. DIENER, 1969, Aust. J. Exptl. Biol. Med. Sci. *47*, 367.

MARCHALONIS, J. J. and G. M. EDELMAN, 1965, J. Exptl. Med. *122*, 601.

MARCHALONIS, J. J. and G. M. EDELMAN, 1966, J. Exptl. Med. *124*, 901.

MARCHALONIS, J. J. and G. M. EDELMAN, 1968a, J. Mol. Biol. *32*, 453.

MARCHALONIS, J. J. and G. M. EDELMAN, 1968b, J. Exptl. Med. *127*, 891.

MASON, S. and N. L. WARNER, 1970, J. Immunol. *104*, 762.

MATSANIOTIS, N., E. APOSTOLOPOULOU and J. VLACHOS, 1966, J. Ped. *69*, 576.

MATSEN, J. M., E. M. HEIMLICH and R. J. BUSSER, 1967, Ann. Allergy *25*, 607.

MATSUYAMA, M., M. WIADROWSKI and D. METCALF, 1966, J. Exptl. Med. *123*, 559.

MAUNG, R. T. 1963, J. Pathol. Bacteriol. *85*, 51.

MEDAWAR, P. B., 1963, Introduction: Definition of the immunologially competent cell. *In*: G. E. W. Wolstenholme and J. Knight, eds.: Ciba Foundation Study Group No. 16. Boston, Little Brown and Co. pp. 1–3.

MESSINI, M., G. P. CENCI and G. CUCCHI, 1964, Lancet *ii*, 180.

METCALF, D., 1956, Brit. J. Cancer *10*, 442.

METCALF, D., 1964, The thymus and lymphopoiesis. *In*: R. A. Good and A. E. Gabrielsen, eds.: The thymus in immunobiology. New York, Hoeber-Harper. pp. 150–179.

METCALF, D., 1965, Nature *208*, 1336.

METCALF, C., 1966, The thymus. *In*: Recent results in cancer res., Vol. 5. New York, Springer-Verlag.

METCALF, D. and T. BRADLEY, 1970, *in*: A. S. Gordon, ed.: Regulation of haematopoiesis. New York, Appleton-Century Crofts. in press.

METCALF, D. and M. A. S. MOORE, 1971, Haemopoietic cells. Frontiers in Biology, Vol. 24. Amsterdam, North-Holland.

METCALF, D. and K. NAKAMURA, 1962, Lymphocyte production and differentiation in the preleukaemic mouse thymus. *In*: L. Severi, ed.: The morphological precursors of cancer. Perugia, Perugia Univ. Press. pp. 269–278.

MEUWISSEN, H. J., G. KAPLAN and D. Y. PEREY, 1968, Federation Proc. *27*, 718.

MEYER, R. K., M. A. RAO and R. L. ASPINALL, 1959, Endocrinology *64*, 890.

MICKLEM, H. S., C. E. FORD, E. P. EVANS and J. GRAY, 1966, Proc. Roy. Soc. Ser. *B165*, 78.

MILLER, J. F. A. P., 1961, Lancet *ii*, 748.

MILLER, J. F. A. P., 1962, Ann. N.Y. Acad. Sci. *99*, 340.

MILLER, J. F. A. P., 1965, Nature *208*, 1337.

MILLER, J. F. A. P., 1971, *in*: A. Cross, T. Kosunen and O. Mäkelä, eds.: Proceedings of the Third Sigrid Julius Symposium on Cell Co-operation in the Immune Response. New York, Academic Press, in press.

MILLER, J. F. A. P., K. BRUNNER, J. SPRENT and P. RUSSELL, 1971b, Transplantation Proc., in press.

MILLER, J. F. A. P., P. DUKOR, G. A. GRANT, N. R. SINCLAIR and E. SACQUET, 1967b, Clin. Exptl. Immunol. *2*, 513.

MILLER, J. F. A. P. and G. F. MITCHELL, 1968, J. Exptl. Med. *128*, 801.

MILLER, J. F. A. P. and G. F. MITCHELL, 1969, Transplantation Rev. *1*, 3.

MILLER, J. F. A. P. and G. F. MITCHELL, 1970, J. Exptl. Med. *131*, 675.

MILLER, J. F. A. P., G. F. MITCHELL and N. S. WEISS, 1967a, Nature *214*, 992.

MILLER, J. F. A. P. and D. OSOBA, 1967, Physiol. Rev. *47*, 437.

MILLER, J. F. A. P., J. SPRENT, T. BASTEN, N. L. WARNER, J. BREITNER, G. ROWLAND, J. HAMILTON, H. SILVER and J. MARTIN, 1971a, J. Exptl. Med., in press.

MILLER, J. J., 1969, Lab. Invest. *21*, 484.

MITCHELL, G. F. and J. F. A. P. MILLER, 1968a, J. Exptl. Med. *128*, 821.

MITCHELL, G. F. and J. F. A. P. MILLER, 1968b, Proc. Natl. Acad. Sci. U.S. *59*, 296.

MITCHISON, N. A., 1968, Symp. Int. Cell Biol. *7*, 29.

MITCHISON, N. A., 1968a, Transplantation immunology. *In*: N. A. Mitchison, J. M. Greep and J. C. M. Hattinga Verschure, eds.: Organ transplantation today. Amsterdam, Excerpta Medica Found. pp. 13–23.

MITCHISON, N. A. 1968b, Recognition of antigen. *In*: K. B. Warren, ed.: Differentiation and immunology. New York, Academic Press. pp. 29–42.

MITCHISON, N. A., 1969, *in*: M. Landy and W. Braun, eds.: Immunological tolerance. New York, Academic Press.

MORI, R., K. NOMOTO and K. TAKAYA, 1964, Proc. Japan Acad. *40*, 772.

MOORE, M. A. S. and D. METCALF, 1970, Brit. J. Haematol. *18*, 279.

MOORE, M. A. S. and J. J. T. OWEN, 1965, Nature *208*, 956.

MOORE, M. A. S. and J. J. OWEN, 1967, Lancet *ii*, 658.

MOORE, M. A. S. and J. J. T. OWEN, 1967a, J. Exptl. Med. *126*, 715.

MUELLER, A. P., H. R. WOLFE and R. K. MEYER, 1960, J. Immunol. *85*, 172.

MURRAY, R. G. and P. A. WOODS, 1964, Anat. Record *150*, 113.

NAOR, D., Z. BENWICH and G. CIVIDALLI, 1969, Aust. J. Exptl. Biol. Med. Sci., *47*, 759.

NAOR, D. and D. SULITZEANU, 1967, Nature *214*, 687.

NATVIG, J. B., H. G. KUNKEL and T. GEDDE-DAHL, JR., 1967, Genetic studies of the heavy chain subgroups of γG globulin. *In*: J. Killander, ed.: Nobel Symposium III. Gamma globulins. Stockholm, Almquist and Wiksell. pp. 313–328.

NISBET, N. W., M. SIMONSEN and M. ZALESKI, 1969, J. Exptl. Med. *129*, 459.

NOSSAL, G. J. V., 1964, Ann. N.Y. Acad. Sci. *120*, 171.

NOSSAL, G. J. V., A. CUNNINGHAM, G. F. MITCHELL and J. F. A. P. MILLER, 1968, J. Exptl. Med. *128*, 839.

NOSSAL, G. J. V. and J. GORRIE, 1964, Studies of the emigration of the thymic cells in young guinea pigs. *In*: R. A. Good and A. E. Gabrielsen, eds.: The thymus in immunobiology. New York, Hoeber-Harper. pp. 288–290.

NOTA, N. R., M. LIACOPOULOS-BRIOT, C. STIFFEL and G. BIOZZI, 1964, Compt. Rend. Acad. Sci. *259*, 1277.

NOWELL, P. C. and D. A. HUNGERFORD, 1961, J. Natl. Cancer Inst. *27*, 1013.

NUSSENZWEIG, V., 1971, *in*: A. Cross, T. A. Kosunen and O. Mäkelä, eds.: Proceedings of the Third Sigrid Julius Symposium on Cell Co-operation in the Immune Response. New York, Academic Press, in press.

OLSON, G. B., 1967, Federation Proc. *26*, 357.

OSOBA, D., 1965, J. Exptl. Med. *122*, 633.

OSOBA, D. and J. F. A. P. MILLER, 1964, J. Exptl. Med. *119*, 177.

OVARY, Z. and B. BENACERRAF, 1963, Proc. Soc. Exptl. Biol. Med. *114*, 72.

PAPERMASTER, B. W., R. M. CONDIE, J. FINSTAD and R. A. GOOD, 1964, J. Exptl. Med. *119*, 105.

PARROTT, D. M. V., M. A. B. DE SOUSA and J. EAST, 1966, J. Exptl. Med. *123*, 191.

PEREY, D. Y. E., J. FINSTAD, B. POLLARA and R. A. GOOD, 1968, Lab. Invest. *19*, 591.

PETERSON, R. D. A., M. D. COOPER and R. A. GOOD, 1965, Am. J. Med. *38*, 579.

PIERCE, A. E., R. C. CHUBB and P. L. LONG, 1966, Immunology *10*, 321.

PLAYFAIR, J. H. L., 1969, Nature *222*, 882.

PLAYFAIR, J. H. L., B. W. PAPERMASTER AND L. J. COLE, 1965, Science *149*, 998.

RAFF, M. C., 1969, Nature *224*, 378.

RAFF, M. C., M. STEINBERG and R. TAYLOR, 1970, Nature *225*, 553.

REIF, A. E. and J. M. U. ALLEN, 1964, J. Exptl. Med. *120*, 413.

REIF, A. E. and J. M. U. ALLEN, 1966, Nature *209*, 521.

RIDGWAY, G. J., H. O. HODGINS and G. W. KLONTZ, 1966, The immune response in teleosts. *In*: R. T. Smith, P. A. Miescher and R. A. Good, eds.: Phylogeny of immunity. Gainesville, Univ. of Florida Press. pp. 199–207.

RIEKE, W. O., 1966, Science *152*, 535.

ROITT, I. M., M. F. GREAVES, G. TORRIGIANI, J. BROSTOFF and J. H. L. PLAYFAIR, 1969, Lancet *ii*, 367.

ROSE, M. E. and E. ORLANS, 1968, Nature *217*, 231.

ROTHFIELD, N. F., B. FRANGIONE and E. C. FRANKLIN, 1965, J. Clin. Invest. *44*, 62.

SAINTE-MARIE, G. and G. P. LEBLOND, 1964, Thymus-cell population dynamics. *In*: R. A. Good and A. E. Gabrielsen, eds.: The thymus in immunobiology. New York, Hoeber-Harper. pp. 207–226.

ST PIERRE, R. L. and G. A. ACKERMAN, 1965, Science *147*, 1307.

SALT, G., 1963, Parasitology *53*, 527.

SALT, G., 1967, Federation Proc. *26*, 1671.

SANDBERG, A. A., T. ISHIHARA, L. H. CROSSWHITE and T. S. HAUSCHKA, 1962, Blood *20*, 393.

SATO, K. and K. SUZUKI, 1969, Poultry Sci. *48*, 1195.

SCHLESINGER, M., 1970, Nature *226*, 1254.

SCHLESINGER, M. and I. YRON, 1969, Science *164*, 1412.

SCHOOLEY, J. C. and L. S. KELLY, 1964, Influence of the thymus on the output of thoracic-duct lymphocytes. *In*: R. A. Good and A. E. Gabrielsen, eds.: The thymus in immunobiology. New York, Hoeber-Harper. pp. 236–253.

SCOTHORNE, R. J. and I. A. MCGREGOR, 1955, J. Anat. *89*, 283.

SEAMEN, G. R. and N. L. ROBERT, 1968, Science *161*, 1359.

SELL, S. and R. ASOFSKY, 1968, Progr. Allergy *12*, 86.

SELL, S., J. A. LOWE, and P. G. H. GELL, 1970, J. Immunol. *104*, 103.

SERCARZ, E. E. and F. MODAKKER, 1968, Science *159*, 884.

SHEARER, G. M. and G. CUDKOWICZ, 1969, J. Exptl. Med. *130*, 1243.

SHERMAN, J. D., M. M. ADNER, and W. DAMESHEK, 1964, Blood *23*, 375.

SHERMAN, J. D. and R. AUERBACH, 1966, Blood *27*, 371.

SHUSTER, J., N. L. WARNER and H. H. FUDENBERG, 1969, Ann. N.Y. Acad. Sci. *162*, 195.

SIDKY, Y. A. and R. AUERBACH, 1968, J. Exptl. Zool. *167*, 187.

SIGEL, M. M. and L. W. CLEM, 1966, Immunologic anamnesis in elasmobranchs. *In*: R. T. Smith, P. A. Miescher and R. A. Good, eds.: Phylogeny of immunity. Gainesville, Univ. of Florida Press. pp. 190–197.

SINCLAIR, N. R. S. C. and D. MILLICAN, 1967, Clin, Exptl. Immunol. *2*, 269.

SINGHAL, S. K. and M. RICHTER, 1968, Int. Arch. Allergy *33*, 493.

SINGHAL, S. K., M. RICHTER and D. G. OSMOND, 1968, Int. Arch. Allergy *34*, 224.

SINGHAL, S. K. and H. WIGZELL, 1970, J. Exptl. Med. *131*, 149.

SMALL, M. and N. TRAININ, 1967, Nature *216*, 377.

SMITH, A. M., M. POTTER and E. B. MERCHANT, 1967, J. Immunol. *99*, 876.

SOLOMON, A., 1969, J. Immunol. *102*, 496.

SPRENT, J., T. BASTEN, N. L. WARNER and J. F. A. P. MILLER, 1970, Unpublished observations.

SPRENT, J. and J. F. A. P. MILLER, 1970, Unpublished observations.

STEINER, L. A. and H. N. EISEN, 1967, J. Exptl. Med. *126*, 1161.

STEPHENS, J. M. and J. H. MARSHALL, 1962, Canad. J. Microbiol. 8, 719.
ŠTERZL, J. and A. M. SILVERSTEIN, 1967, Advan. Immunol. 5, 337.
STOBO, J. D. and T. B. TOMASI 1967, J. Clin. Invest. 46, 1329.
STUTTMAN, O. and R. A. GOOD, 1969, Proc. Soc. Exptl. Biol. Med. 130, 848.
STUTTMAN, O., E. J. YUNIS and R. A. GOOD 1968, J. Natl. Cancer Inst. 41, 1431.
SUTHERLAND, D. E. R., O. K. ARCHER and R. A. GOOD, 1964, Proc. Soc. Exptl. Biol. Med. 115, 673.
SUTHERLAND, D. E. R., O. K. ARCHER, R. D. A. PETERSON, E. ECKERT and R. A. GOOD, 1965, Lancet i, 130.
SZENBERG, A. and N. L. WARNER, 1967, Brit. Med. Bull. 23, 30.
SZENBERG, A., N. L. WARNER, F. M. BURNET and P. E. LIND, 1962, Brit. J. Exptl. Pathol 43, 129.
TAKAHASHI, T., L. J. OLD and E. A. BOYSE, 1970, J. Exptl. Med., 131, 1325.
TAYLOR, R. B., 1964, Immunology 7, 595.
TAYLOR, R. B., 1968, Nature 220, 611.
TAYLOR, R. B., 1969, Transplantation Rev. 1, 114.
THORBECKE, G. J. and M. W. COHEN, 1964, In: V. Defendi and D. Metcalf, eds.: The thymus. Wistar Inst. Symp. Monogr. No. 2. Philadelphia, Wistar Inst. Press. pp. 33–39.
THORBECKE, G. J., H. A. GORDON, B. WOSTMAN, M. WAGNER and J. A. REYNIERS, 1957, J. Infect. Dis. 101, 237.
THORBECKE, G. J., N. L. WARNER, G. M. HOCHWALD and S. H. OHANIAN, 1968, Immunology 15, 123.
TILL, J. E. and E. A. MCCULLOCH, 1961, Radiation Res. 14, 213.
TOUGH, I. M., W. M. COURT-BROWN, A. G. BAIKIE, K. E. BUCKTON, D. G. HARNDEN, P. A. JACOBS, M. J. KING and J. A. MCBRIDE, 1961, Lancet i, 411.
TRAININ, N., A. BEJERANO, M. STRAHILEVITCH, D. GOLDRING and M. SMALL, 1966, Israel J. Med. Sci. 2, 549.
TRAININ, N., M. BURGER and A. M. KAYE, 1967, Biochem. Pharmacol. 16, 711.
TRAININ, N. and M. LINKER-ISRAEL, 1967, Cancer Res. 27, 309.
TRAININ, N., M. SMALL and A. GLOBERSON, 1969, J. Exptl. Med. 130, 765.
TRENTIN, J., N. WOLF, V. CHENG, W. FAHLBERG, D. WEISS and R. BONHAG, 1967, J. Immunol. 98, 1326.
TRIPP, M. R., 1966, J. Invertebrate Pathol. 8, 478.
TYAN, M. L., 1970, Proc. Soc. Exptl. Biol. Med. 132, 1183.
TYAN, M. L. and L. J. COLE, 1966, Transplantation 4, 557.
TYAN, M. L., L. J. COLE and P. C. NOWELL, 1966, Transplantation 4, 79.
TYAN, M. L., L. A. HERZENBERG and P. R. GIBBS, 1969, J. Immunol. 103, 1283.
UHR, J. W., 1965, Proc. Natl. Acad. Sci. U.S. 54, 1599.
UMIEL, T., A. GLOBERSON and R. AUERBACH, 1968, Proc. Soc. Exptl. Biol. Med. 129, 598.
VAN ALTEN, P. J., W. A. CAIN, R. A. GOOD and M. D. COOPER, 1968, Nature 217, 358.
VAN METER, R., R. A. GOOD and M. D. COOPER, 1969, J. Immunol. 102, 370.
WARNER, N. L., 1964, Aust. J. Exptl. Biol. Med. Sci. 42, 401.
WARNER, N. L., 1965, Aust. J. Exptl. Biol. Med. Sci. 43, 439.
WARNER, N. L., 1967, Folia Biol. 13, 1.
WARNER, N. L., 1969, Med. J. Aust. ii, 506.
WARNER, N. L., 1971a, Transplantation Proc. 3, 848.
WARNER, N. L., 1971b, in: Contemporary topics in immunobiology. New York, Plenum Press. In press.
WARNER, N. L., 1971c, in: Lindahl-Kiesling, Alm and Hanna, eds.: Morphological and fundamental aspects of immunity. New York, Plenum Press.

WARNER, N. L., 1971d, Abstr. 10th International Cancer Congress, Houston. p. 237.

WARNER, N. L. and F. M. BURNET, 1961, Aust. J. Biol. Sci. *14*, 580.

WARNER, N. L., P. BYRT and G. L. ADA, 1970, Nature *226*, 942.

WARNER, N. L., J. UHR, G. J. THORBECKE and Z. OVARY, 1969, J. Immunol. *103*, 1317.

WARNER, N. L. and M. A. S. MOORE, 1969, Unpublished observations.

WARNER, N. L. and A. SZENBERG, 1962, Nature *196*, 784.

WARNER, N. L. and A. SZENBERG, 1964, Ann. Rev. Microbiol. *18*, 253.

WARNER, N. L., A. SZENBERG and F. M. BURNET, 1962, Aust. J. Exptl. Biol. Med. Sci, *40*, 373.

WEISS, L., 1963, Anat. Record *145*, 413.

WEISSMAN, I. L., 1967, J. Exptl. Med., *126*, 291.

WILLMER, E. N., 1960, *In*: Cytology and Evolution. New York, Academic Press.

WOODS, R. and J. LINNA, 1965, Acta Pathol. Microbiol. Scand. *64*, 470.

WU, A. M., J. E. TILL, L. SIMINOVITCH and E. A. MCCULLOCH, 1967, J. Cell Physiol. *69*, 177.

WU, A. M., J. E. TILL, L. SIMINOVITCH and E. A. MCCULLOCH, 1968, J. Exptl. Med. *127*, 455.

ZAALBERG, O. B., 1964, Nature *202*, 123.

Dragons teeth: or immunology in the future

P. G. H. GELL

Department of Experimental Pathology, The Medical School, University of Birmingham

> *'Tis mute, the word they went to hear on high Dodona mountain*
> *When winds were in the oakenshaws and all the cauldrons rolled . . . .*

> A. E. Housman.

As I look back at the varied chapters of this book, there is no role left except to play the oracle; and I remember the fate of past prophets whose shrines I have once visited.

If one sees Dodona now, ruinous, lonely and inaccessible in its bowl of low treeless hills, it becomes clear that the oracles of the Gods are no longer available to us: we have to take a cold look at the cold future on our own. But Futurology is in fashion: now more than ever one has to end up on a rising note of query. It is fairly evident where as scientists we think we are going: less so whom we are dragging along unwillingly with us.

One thing is clear enough, that immunologists in common with other scientists will accelerate the process of pumping power into a social structure which is hardly competent to contain it, and forcing the possibilities of choice upon our fellows to whom this enlarged freedom is an embarrassment. Scientific activity generates power: the megaton explosion and the ability to cure cancer are powers of exactly the same kind. For our own science of immunology we are well advised to forecast not only the exciting technical advances which are likely in the next few decades, but also, so as to be aware in time, the social and political tensions which they may engender. Forty years ago, such a look forward would have shown a bold prospect of the progressive control of disease – diphtheria, poliomyelitis, malaria: a humane and gentlemanly programme, with only the tangential problem of over-population to worry us a little. We need to be more wary now.

Not that malaria, still less say schistosomiasis and other tropical diseases, are indeed controlled: but the problems are mainly techno-logical, political, not scientific. Immunology has clearly much to contribute yet in these fields, but our chief interests are elsewhere. These, stated in terms of power, are, the control of the immune response (which is directly relevant to the subject of this book) and the control of the genome. I say 'stated in terms of power' because I believe that the basic nature of the scientist, as opposed to the technologist, is the fascination of finding out how nature, and the rest of the universe, actually works; disinterested curiosity, in fact. But this knowledge gives the power to intervene in natural phenomena; wherever power is involved, one has to consider the implications of its possible use. Hence in this short term forecast, much of which will be sufficiently obvious to anyone aware of the trends of modern work, I intend to spend time in discussing the possible social impact of advances in biological knowledge, as well as in speculating on the technical advances themselves.

The control of the immunological response

Control of the immunological response first became manifest as an aim because of the work on homografting. From this, such thinking has found an application to the control of the allergic and auto-allergic (auto-immune) diseases – much commoner cases in a hospital at present than are grafted patients; and possibly to the treatment of established cancers, commoner still. Its most important application may be to the universal phenomenon, old age.

Nearly everyone will agree that immunosuppression as used at present is a crude form of therapy, a pre-Listerian kind of surgery. More sophisticated use of antigens is aimed at adjusting the overall specific immune response up or down, at deviating the kind of immune mechanism activated (antibodies or cellular sensitivity) and at altering the balance of the kinds of antibody produced. These general methods comprise tolerance induction, feedback suppression of antibody, adjuvant immunization, immune deviation and precise analysis of the geography and cytotoxic properties of antibodies and allergized cells. In grafting and in cancer therapy we are aiming at strictly opposed results, in the one retention and in the other rejection. So the aim is specific tolerance towards a graft, and the breaking of tolerance towards a cancer: at the suppression of cytotoxic antibodies and the stimulation of enhancing antibodies towards a graft: at precisely the reverse towards a cancer. Likewise at the suppression or the stimulation of cellular sensitivity? This is more problematic, until the biological role of cellular sensitivity and its relationship to non-antibody dependent cytotoxicity on the one hand, and to antibody production on the other, gets a little clearer. But it is obvious that manipulation rather than blunderbuss suppression of the immune response will become more and more understood in the future both by the proper use of antigens, and by the preparation of anti-cell sera of specificity for particular cell populations.

This manipulation of immunity by use of antigens has been practised for years, though blindly, in the treatment of that commonest of hypersensitivity diseases, hay-fever – sufferers from this tend to produce IgE antibodies, (which are presumably meant to clear our guts of parasites), against all sorts of irrelevant particulate antigens: hyposensitization by subcutaneous injection may or may not affect the sensitivity of end organs but certainly induces the production of antibodies in other classes, mainly IgG. One would suppose that we ought to stimulate them to produce antibodies of IgA class, which should be more effective in protecting the mucous membranes, in spite the lack of correlation so far of the success of conventional hyposensitization with the level of specific IgA antibodies: or at best to find some way of deviating their responses away from the IgE class, possibly even in the direction of delayed sensitivity. One can envisage this kind of approach being applied to other Type I hypersensitivities.

In other extrinsic allergies, and in many of the 'auto-immune' diseases, antibody production seems to be a sign that the immunity system is involved, rather than a cause of the disease per se; but they are always an indication of an abnormal immune system at a deeper level, anomalies of the response to antigens, with an ill-defined genetic basis. Apart from total immunosuppression, with its accompanying dangers, our ability to bring them under control will depend in part on a better understanding of the genetic basis of the response to particular antigens, and in part on a more sophisticated approach to immunological control as discussed above.

But there is one correlation which must be of some significance, that of the increase of cancer with age and the increase of auto-allergic antibodies with age. By the age of 60 about 50% of subjects tested have detectable auto-allergic antibodies (Whittingham et al. 1969). At this age, something begins to go wrong with the immune system; it loses discrimination. Apart from the possibly relevant specific diseases of the elderly (heart disease in particular), and apart from the failure of 'surveillance' which may allow cancers to grow, one cannot, as an immunologist, doubt that this immunological collapse plays a part in the ageing process as such. Once recognised, we are bound to try and do something about it.

An alternative or additional theory about ageing is that put forward informally by E. J. Field, that much of the characteristic picture of senility is the result of a slow virus infection. If this theory, admittedly rather 'far out' at present, has a germ of truth in it, immunologists cannot fail to be interested, as we all are with regard to the other slow virus diseases such as scrapie, and for that matter herpes simplex, in the state of tolerance which is implied. Breaking of tolerance is another aspect of control of the immune system, about which we are learning at a great rate: perhaps we can use it to cure senility. Perhaps by proper immunological techniques we can raise the normal age of healthy survival to 90 years or more.

Social impact of control of the immune system

Control of the deterioration of individual organs by grafting, control of deterioration of the whole organism in ageing: what problems do they raise? As far as grafting goes, we can quite reasonably envisage a time fairly soon when organ grafting will be as safe as any other internal operation – say a 5% mortality or less. Its use will then only be limited by the time and expense of the operation, and the availability of suitable organs. With the immunological problems solved, and possibly with improvements in regenerating nerve connections, it should be technically feasable to graft practically any organ.

There are two social (as opposed to moral) problems raised by grafting. One is the supply of organs, which has been sufficiently discussed elsewhere: the other is the probably inescapable fact that the operation will always be relatively elaborate and expensive, even if not dangerous. Thus the health services of the world will be faced with a difficult problem of priorities. Suppose that every patient with a seriously diseased lung, heart, liver, kidney or intestine could be saved – if one took enough trouble. Who will get the treatment? It is not cynical, in view of the intolerable pressures which are exercised by a dying parent, child or friend, to expect that the operations will be confined to those, individuals or nations, who can pay for them. If the kind, as opposed to the availability, of treatment given to the rich is different from that given to the poor, the whole tendency of modern medicine will be negated.

The postponement of old age, unless it involves grafting, and there is no reason why it should, might well be comparatively cheap and simple. It poses other problems, which have been raised before in imaginative literature: chiefly the continuing domination of the old over the young. Our social system, which puts a premium on the wisdom and experience of the elders, is geared to a time when the average age of death was 45 or less: if a man is not wise and experienced by 45, he is not likely ever to be. Supposing he sits at the head of the table for 45 years more? So we may be adding fuel to the fires of the two grumbling revolutions of our time, that of the poor against the rich, and the young against the old. Surely it is time that we discussed these problems now, rather than postponing them until they are taken out of our hands, for good or ill, by the ruling forces of society.

The control of the genome

In control of the genome, we do not face but side-step the immunological problem, either by making use of an extreme form of tolerance by the production of 'mosaics' or by getting inside the recognition organ of the cell, the cell membrane, by cell hybridization techniques, or ultimately by 'DNA grafting'. The final goal of this kind of work is the creation of an organism according to a predetermined genetic formula. This is no doubt a long way off, but the cell-biologists have certainly made a good start. Mosaics of a kind with which any immunologist is familiar have been little exploited as yet, perhaps because, using immuno-competent cells, we have been too discouraged by the G.v.H. reaction; but anyway the greater possibilities lie in intervention at a much earlier stage, with the gametes and blastocysts. Any 20-year old postgraduate with neat fingers can produce from blastocyst fusion (McLaren and Bowman 1969) a mosaic of two distinct genomes, which is perfectly stable and viable. True, this is in mice; but the application of such results to man is not a matter of whether we can, but of whether we dare to: anything which we can do to our small murine brothers we can do to each other. Before me now is the photograph by Shettles of a 100-cell human blastocyst, fertilized and cultivated *in vitro*, for which 'there was no discernable contraindication for a successful transfer' into the maternal uterus (Shettles 1971). The possibilities of monkeying with this plastic bit of human slime are considerable.

If there is no experimental block to the cultivation of gametocytes- and one cannot really see why they should be more resistant to *in vitro* conditions than any other sort of cell – one can envisage the long-term culture, or preservation of male gametocytes instead of the preservation of the much more differentiated and tender spermatozoon: and their maturation and use when required for *in vitro* fertilization, or indeed their use as such by some cell-fusion trickery avoiding the spermatozoal stage altogether. When in the future some patrician, a young Olympic runner with a first in History at Oxbridge-Harvard, is killed in a polo accident, can we look forward to the time when his cultured testes will be regarded as a National Heritage?

It is easy to be frivolous; yet it really is the case that genetic engineering is not a sort of journalist's turnip-ghost which any professional scientist can treat with scepticism and a curling lip, but is with us now, in some forms at least, in the sober columns of the scientific press. Many intelligent and sensitive scientists discount such fears as fantasies, because they cannot envisage doing such things as working on human gametocytes themselves. But what has upset the non-scientists is that genetic interference can be shown to be *possible.* If it is possible in principle it is high time, they say, that the moral attitude of the scientist towards it were defined: and there is little evidence that scientists have much use, or aptitude, for the taking of moral attitudes.

As immunologists, working to neutralize immunity, we tread indeed in a delicate area, like cows blundering in a minefield. The immune function preserves not just the boundaries between species, but the boundaries between individuals: it keeps Joe different from Jimmy, and Mary from Kate. We trespass here on another contemporary tension which the creative artists have discovered for us to worry about, the problem of identity. Who am I? when I have Arthur's kidney, and Bill's liver, and Jones' adrenals and Mr. Smith's heart? or when I am a mosaic of what was meant to be Paul and Virginia? Who am I, when I can be created by someone no better than myself?

Dragon's teeth

Cadmus, the African, killed the primitive dragon – the forces of ignorance and nature. He then took and sowed the dragon's teeth; it seemed the natural thing to do. No doubt they would sprout and bear a crop of benefit to humanity. Sprout they did indeed, a decorative crop of armed men: those bird-headed regiments who move in frozen procession around archaic Greek vases. One dropped a gauntlet, his neighbour picked it up and slapped his face with it: true to their nature, the rest took up sides and fought; using fast cars, complex chemical gases and defoliants, drugs which paralyse the will, virus aerosols to which their own side were immune, sophisticated verbal and visual propaganda. As each gained power by knowledge and experiment he used it to oppress and destroy his neighbour. A large part of the primaeval forest in which the old dragon had lived for aeons quickly became a shambles, a heap of rubbish. This is where we come in. Eventually, the story goes on, now in terms of prophecy, only a few exhausted men were left. In the barren wilderness they had created, they helped Cadmus to build the pretty but intellectually undistinguished city of Thebes. I find myself quite incapable of interpreting this particular oracle.

References

WHITTINGHAM, S., J. IRVINE, I. R., MACKEY, S. MARSH and D. G. COWLING, 1969, Australasian J. Med. *18*, 130.
MCLAREN, A. and P. BOWMAN, 1969, Nature *224*, 238.
SHETTLES, L. B., 1971, Nature *229*, 343.

Author index

Numbers in italics refer to listing in the references

Aalseth, B. L., 137, *150*
Abbott, A., 60, *80*, 90, *109*
Abdou, N. I., 290, *298*, 453, *465*, 517, *528*
Abel, C. A., 473, *528*
Abelson, N. M., 55, *85*
Aboulafia, R., 229, *234*
Abrahams, I., 235, 236, *237*, *238*
Abramoff, P., 274, *298*, 386, *388*
Abuelo, J. G., 13, *38*, 75, *80*
Ackerman, G. A., 510, *528*, *535*
Ackroyd, J. F., 74, *80*
Acton, R. T., 473, *530*
Ada, G. L., 36, *39*, *42*, 54, 60, 61, 64, *80*, *83*,
    84, *85*, 90, 91, 94, *109*, *111*, 113, *130*, 207,
    210, 213, 217, *223*, 469, 494, 501, 513,
    519, 521, 525, *528*, *533*, *537*
Adams, C., 178, 179, *202*
Adams, E., 347, *363*
Adams, H., 378, *388*
Adams K. M., 307, *332*
Adant, M., 8, *38*
Adelsberger, L., 263, *270*
Adkinson, N. K., 207, *223*
Adler, F. L., 26, 27, 28, *38*, 55, *80*, 114, *129*,
    133, *149*, 274, 282, 296, *298*, *299*, *333*,
    378, *388*
Adner, M. M., 503, *535*
Adriano, S. M., 249, *249*
Agarossi, G., 291, *299*
Agbayani, B. F., 228, *228*
Agnello, V., 24, *41*
Agnew, H. D., 356, *362*
Agnew, M. D., 509, *532*
Ahmed, K., 387, *388*
Ainsworth, G. C., 227, *228*
Aisenberg, A. C., 382, *388*
Aizawa, Y., 383, *389*
Ajello, L., 242, *249*
Akiba, T., 385, *393*
Al-Askari, S., 220, *223*, 420, *447*

Albert, E., 413, *445*
Albertazzi, C., 404, *408*
Albright, J. F., 28, *38*
Alexander, H. L., 73, *80*
Alexander, M., 374, 375, *390*
Alexander, P., 458, *465*
Alford, R. H., 172, 191, *197*, *201*
Alford, Jr., C. A., 168, 185, *197*
Alkins, B. J., 26, *39*
Allen, F., 413, *445*
Allen, J. M. U., 503, 519, *535*
Allen, J. M. V., 268, *270*, 417, *450*
Allen, P. Z., 128, 146, 148, *149*
Allende, M. F., 180, *200*
Allerhand, J., 233, *234*
Allison, A. C., 94, *111*, 114, 118, 121, 122,
    128, *130*, 157, 163, 168, 178, 179, 180,
    182, 185, 186, 187, 188, 190, *197*, *199*,
    200, *202*, 207, *224*, 395, 397, 406, *408*,
    432, *448*
Allison, J. L., 376, *388*
Almeida, J., 168, *199*
Almeida, J. D., 176, *197*
Altemeier, W. A., 216, *223*
Altman, P. L., 242, *249*
Alvord, E. C., 401, *407*
Alvord, Jr., E. C., *130*
Amano, T., 33, *39*
Amberson, J. M., 234, *238*
Ambrose, C. T., 348, 349, *360*, 387, *388*
Amiel, L., 381, *388*
Amies, C. R., 112, *128*
Amkraut, A. A., 27, *38*, 65, *80*, 128, 139,
    146, 148, *149*, *151*
Ammann, A. J., 168, 172, *197*, *202*
Amos, D. B., 26, *38*, 231, *233*, 413, 423,
    430, *445*, *450*, 464, *465*
Amouch, P., 485, *528*
Anderer, F. A., 28, *38*, 56, *80*
Anderson, H. W., 383, *388*

544

Subject index